Dendritic Cells in Clinical Immunology

Dendritic Cells in Clinical Immunology

Editor: Jeremy Collins

AMERICAN
MEDICAL PUBLISHERS
www.americanmedicalpublishers.com

AMERICAN
MEDICAL PUBLISHERS
www.americanmedicalpublishers.com

Cataloging-in-Publication Data

Dendritic cells in clinical immunology / edited by Jeremy Collins.
p. cm.
Includes bibliographical references and index.
ISBN 979-8-88740-041-9
1. Dendritic cells. 2. Dendritic cells--Therapeutic use. 3. Clinical immunology.
4. Immunopathology. I. Collins, Jeremy.
QR185.8.D45 D46 2023
616.079--dc23

American Medical Publishers,
41 Flatbush Avenue,
1st Floor, New York,
NY 11217, USA

ISBN 979-8-88740-041-9 (Hardback)

Contents

Preface

Dendritic cells are powerful antigen presenting cells which are significant for initiating the primary immune response. They travel to the lymph nodes when activated, where they interact with B and T cells to instigate and develop the adaptive immune response. They are the principal regulators of the immune system response and perform this function by linking the specificity of the adaptive response with the microbial sensing features of the innate immune system. Furthermore, these cells are effective in antigen presentation and are capable of acclimatizing to produce right amount of T cells as a response to a particular pathogen. Dendritic cells are also helpful in directing the immune system to react to foreign substances, simultaneously avoiding autoimmune responses. Altered function of dendritic cells is recognized to have a crucial role in autoimmune diseases and allergies, such as inflammatory bowel disease and lupus erythematosus. This book provides comprehensive insights into the role of dendritic cells in immunology. It is a valuable compilation of topics, ranging from the basic to the most complex advancements in this area of study. Those in search of information to further their knowledge will be greatly assisted by this book.

The information contained in this book is the result of intensive hard work done by researchers in this field. All due efforts have been made to make this book serve as a complete guiding source for students and researchers. The topics in this book have been comprehensively explained to help readers understand the growing trends in the field.

I would like to thank the entire group of writers who made sincere efforts in this book and my family who supported me in my efforts of working on this book. I take this opportunity to thank all those who have been a guiding force throughout my life.

Editor

1

Understanding the Functional Properties of Neonatal Dendritic Cells: A Doorway to Enhance Vaccine Effectiveness?

*Nikos E. Papaioannou [1], Maria Pasztoi [1] and Barbara U. Schraml [1,2]**

[1] Biomedical Center, Institute for Cardiovascular Physiology and Pathophysiology, Ludwig-Maximilians-University Munich, Munich, Germany, [2] Walter-Brendel-Centre of Experimental Medicine, University Hospital, Ludwig-Maximilians-University Munich, Munich, Germany

***Correspondence:**
Barbara U. Schraml
barbara.schraml@med.uni-muenchen.de

Increased susceptibility to infectious diseases is a hallmark of the neonatal period of life that is generally attributed to a relative immaturity of the immune system. Dendritic cells (DCs) are innate immune sentinels with vital roles in the initiation and orchestration of immune responses, thus, constituting a promising target for promoting neonatal immunity. However, as is the case for other immune cells, neonatal DCs have been suggested to be functionally immature compared to their adult counterparts. Here we review some of the unique aspects of neonatal DCs that shape immune responses in early life and speculate whether the functional properties of neonatal DCs could be exploited or manipulated to promote more effective vaccination in early life.

Keywords: dendritic cell (DC), DC subsets, early life immunity, vaccination, immune system development, T cell activation, innate immunity, DC targeting

INTRODUCTION

Early life immune balance is essential for survival and establishment of healthy immunity in later life. The neonatal period in mammals represents a critical window, in which the immune system has to keep a fine balance between efficient pathogen defense and maintenance of tolerance against a continuous flood of commensal microbes and environmental antigens (1–4). Reduced inflammatory capacity is an inherent feature of early life immunity that has been attributed to an altered repertoire of immune cells, as well as a relative functional immaturity of immune cells in early compared to later life (2–5). For example, the T and B cell pools are not fully expanded at birth and are biased to generate T helper (Th) 2 type responses compared to a more Th1 type response in adults (1). Neonatal, but not adult, monocytes and neutrophils potently suppress T cell activation *in vitro* and therefore strongly resemble myeloid derived suppressor cells (6). Although neutrophil-like myeloid derived suppressor cells show microbicidal activity (6), the inflammation-induced trafficking of neutrophils, as well as their ability to form extracellular traps, are reduced in fetal and early life compared to adult (7–9). Fetal monocytes are transcriptionally distinct from their adult counterparts and fetal, as well as, neonatal monocytes show distinct responsiveness to inflammatory stimuli than adult monocytes (10–14). Macrophages first develop before birth and are thought to aid in tissue remodeling during development, whereas they acquire their full-blown immune functions with increasing age (11, 14). Microglia of the brain for instance gain an immune-related gene signature over time and in response to microbial signals (15). Additionally, the existence of specific immune regulatory cells of erythroid origin in early life has been suggested to dampen inflammatory responses (4, 16).

As a result of these immune alterations, neonates exhibit an increased susceptibility to infections (2, 5). In humans, pathogens that are often asymptomatic in adults, such as *Haemophilus influenzae* type B, *Bordetella pertussis* and *Streptococcus pneumoniae*, account for the death of more than two million infants per year world-wide (17). Dendritic cells (DCs) have been implicated to promote immune responses to these pathogens in adults (18–21). It is possible to immunize infants under one year against these pathogens, but a single immunization does not necessarily provide immediate protection, or as in the case of *H. influenzae* type B, antibody titers may not persist (17). For other pathogens, such as rotavirus, immunization is first possible few weeks after birth leaving infants at risk of infection, when the disease is most severe (17, 22). The efficacy, success and challenges of vaccines in early life, as well as existing efforts to improve their effectiveness have recently been reviewed elsewhere (17). Here we focus on the functional differences between DCs in early and adult life. DCs sense the presence of pathogens or damage via so called pattern recognition receptors (PRRs) and initiate innate, as well as adaptive immune responses through cytokine production and antigen presentation (23–25). In their function as immune sentinels DCs have been extensively targeted to increase vaccine effectiveness and DC based vaccines hold promise in adults (26). However, as other immune cells, DCs in early life differ from their adult counterparts in phenotype and function, raising the question, whether targeting DCs could be used to elicit protective immunity in infants and increase vaccine effectiveness. Although most of the data discussed here derive from mouse studies, parallels likely exist in humans, as DC subsets and functions appear highly conserved across species (23, 25).

DENDRITIC CELLS DEVELOP AS FUNCTIONALLY DISTINCT SUBSETS

Among DCs, we distinguish two main functionally and developmentally distinct cell lineages. Conventional or classical DCs (cDCs) are remarkable activators of adaptive immune responses with a remarkable capacity to capture, process, and present antigens to T cells (23–25, 27). Plasmacytoid DCs (pDCs) on the other hand are critical for defense against viruses, because of their capacity to respond to viral antigens and secrete type I interferons (IFN) (28, 29). Most of our knowledge about the development of these cells is based on studies in adult mice. In adults, DCs have a short lifespan and rely on constant replenishment from bone marrow-derived hematopoietic stem cells (30, 31). cDCs and pDCs were long thought to derive from a common myeloid precursor, the so-called common dendritic cell progenitor (CDP) (32, 33). Within this progenitor fraction, expression of the C type lectin receptor CLEC9A/DNGR-1 distinguishes cells with cDC-restricted developmental potential (34). These cDC restricted CDPs further differentiate into pre-cDCs, which leave the bone marrow and seed lymphoid and non-lymphoid tissues (31, 35) where they differentiate into the two main cDC1 and cDC2 subsets in response to environmental cues (23–25, 27). Of note, the signals that regulate cDC differentiation in tissues remain poorly defined and recent studies indicate that the commitment of pre-cDCs toward cDC1 or cDC2 may already be imprinted in the bone marrow (36, 37). In contrast to cDCs, pDCs exit the bone marrow as fully differentiated cells (38) and only a fraction of pDCs appears to belong to the myeloid lineage, whereas the majority of pDCs arises from lymphoid progenitors (39).

In adults cDC1 and cDC2 are developmentally and functionally distinct cell subsets that can be distinguished based on their differential dependence on transcription factors (23–25, 27). While cDC1 rely on BATF3, ID2 and IRF8 for their development, cDC2 require the transcription factors IRF4, ZEB2, and RELB and are additionally influenced by Notch2 signaling and retinoic acid (23–25, 27). Although not yet investigated in detail, at least some of these developmental pathways are conserved with age, as cDC1-like cells are missing in spleen, mesenteric lymph node and intestinal lamina propria of neonatal BATF3-deficient mice (40, 41). Additionally, DCs in early and late life require FMS-like tyrosine kinase 3 ligand (FLT3L) for their development (42, 43). In adults cDC1 can be reliably identified across tissues by expression of XCR-1, DNGR-1, and CD205 (23 25, 27). In addition, CD8α and CD24 mark cDC1 in lymphoid tissues (23–25, 27). The integrin CD103 marks cDC1 in non-lymphoid tissues, although it is also expressed on a subset of intestinal cDC2 (23–25, 27). cDC2 on the other hand are marked by expression of CD11b, CD172a, and CLEC4A4 (23–25, 27). Functionally, cDC1 are exceptional activators of $CD8^{+}$ T cells, in part for their superior activity to cross-present cell associated antigens (23–25, 27). cDC1 are additionally dominant inducers of Th1 polarized immune responses due to their strong capacity to produce IL-12 (23–25, 27). In contrast, cDC2 are generally thought to be more efficient at activating $CD4^{+}$ T cell and inducing Th2- or Th17-biased effector responses (23, 24, 44, 45). Since cDC1 and cDC2 have unique functions in immunity and can be distinguished by expression of select surface markers, they are attractive targets for the manipulation of immune responses in adults (26).

ALTERED SUBSET DISTRIBUTION OF DENDRITIC CELLS IN EARLY LIFE

Although DCs reportedly can be found in mice as early as embryonic day 17, the DC compartment of newborn mice is not fully developed and subject to dynamic age-dependent changes during development (46, 47). In mice the neonatal period includes the first 10 days after birth, which correlates to the first 28 days of life in humans (1, 17). However, it is important to note that in terms of immune development there is substantial temporal variation between mice and humans in early life (48). In murine neonates the DC compartment in lymphoid and non-lymphoid organs is much smaller than that of adults and hallmarked by distinct DC subset distribution (46, 47). The frequency of splenic cDCs at birth is about ten-fold lower than that of adult spleen and, similarly, neonatal splenic pDCs are seven-fold lower in terms of frequency compared to their adult counterparts (46, 47). This is also reflected in lower numbers of DCs in neonatal spleen, which is not fully developed at birth in terms of organ architecture and size (46, 47). By about 5 weeks of age, when the total splenic cellularity reaches adult levels, both cDC and pDC numbers also reach adult levels (46, 47). A relative scarcity of DCs in newborn mice is also evident in other organs, such as thymus, lymph nodes, lung and intestine (47, 49–53). Altered immune responses and infection susceptibility in early life could therefore simply be a by-product of low DC numbers. Administration of the DC growth factor FLT3L leads to a strong increase in DC numbers in neonatal mice and results in increased resistance to *Listeria monocytogenes* (*L. monocytogenes)* and herpes simplex virus 1 (HSV-1) (43). Similarly, administration of FLT3L significantly enhances resistance of neonates to the intestinal parasite *Cryptosporidium parvum* by increasing the number of intestinal $CD103^+$ cDCs, which include both cDC1 and a fraction of cDC2 (54).

In adults, the cDC compartment is dominated by cDC2, while in early life cDC1 appear to be the dominant cDC subtype in spleen and lymph nodes (46, 47, 51). In thymus, cDC1 remain the dominant cDC population also in adults, possibly owing to a unique requirement of this cell type in ensuring central T cell tolerance (55). A systematic analysis of DC subset distribution with age across non-lymphoid organs has not been performed, with one exception being the lung, where cDC1 outnumber cDC2 in neonates, but this relationship is inversed in adults (50). It is important to note that most of these studies relied on the use of surface markers to identify cDC subsets. Notably, within the first 6 days of life, cDC1 from spleen and mesenteric lymph node lack CD8α, although they do express CD24, CLEC9A/DNGR-1, and CD205 (40, 46, 47). Expression of XCR-1 on neonatal cDC1 has not been investigated. These data have led to the suggestion that $CD8\alpha^-$ cDC1 may represent a progenitor of bona fide cDC1 (40) and indicate that the use of surface markers to define cDC subsets in early life needs to be approached with caution. A summary of surface markers expressed on neonatal and adult DCs can be found in **Figure 1**.

Why DC subset distribution differs between neonates and adults is unclear. It is possible that DC differentiation may be intrinsically programmed to generate a functionally adapted DC repertoire that meets the needs of immune responses in early life. However, age-specific changes in specific organ environments could alter DC subset development. cDC1 in neonatal mediastinal lymph nodes express lower levels of CD103 than cDC1 from adult mediastinal lymph nodes (49). This difference in CD103 expression has been attributed to the unique cytokine environment of the lung in early life, such as low expression of GM-CSF (49). Thus, the DC compartment of neonates differs from that of adults in terms of cell number, subset distribution and marker expression.

DENDRITIC CELL FUNCTION IN NEONATES VS. ADULTS

It is well established that neonatal DCs in both mice and men are functionally distinct from DCs in adults, which has been suggested to represent a level of functional immaturity. In mice, early life cDCs produce lower levels of pro-inflammatory cytokines than their adult counterparts. In the first week of life, splenic cDC1 produce lower amounts of IL-12 in response to CpG or after *in vivo* poly I:C treatment (40, 47). Similarly, splenic cDC2 produce less IFN-γ after stimulation with IL-12 and IL-18 compared to their adult counterparts and pDCs produce less IFN-α after combined treatment with CpG, GM-CSF, IL-4 and IFN-γ than pDCs from 6-week old mice (47). Interestingly, when cDC1 from Balb/C rather than C57BL/6 mice were analyzed, CpG-induced IL-12 production did not differ between cDC1 from 7-day old and adult mice (46). In cDC1 from C57BL/6 mice CpG-induced IL-12 production in early life can be augmented by addition of GM-CSF, IFN-γ, and IL-4 to culture conditions, however, the level of IL-12 produced still does not reach that of adult cDC1 (40, 47). These data indicate that some pathogen sensing pathways are fully functional in early life cDCs and that cytokine production of neonatal cDCs may at least in part be augmented through the use of additional costimulatory signals, which in turn could be used to boost immune responses in early life.

A key property of DCs is their ability to activate naïve T cells. Early life cDCs express lower basal levels of major histocompatibility complex class II (MHCII) and costimulatory molecules compared to adult cDCs (43, 47, 49) but expression of these molecules can be induced, for instance upon CpG stimulation *in vivo* (46). Despite these differences, splenic cDC1 and cDC2 from 1-week-old mice are able to induce allogeneic $CD4^+$ T cell proliferation *in vitro* to a similar extent as the same subsets from 6-week old mice (47). In the first week of life, $CD8\alpha^-$ cDC1 phagocytose *L. monocytogenes* and cross-present *L. monocytogenes*-derived antigens to $CD8^+$ T cells as efficiently as adult cDC1 (40). However, while cDC1 from adults respond to this pathogen in a predominantly pro-inflammatory manner, neonatal cDC1 additionally produce the anti-inflammatory cytokine IL-10, which suppresses $CD8^+$ T cell activation (40). Accordingly, IL-10 blockade augments the antigen-specific $CD8^+$ T cell proliferation induced by neonatal $CD8\alpha^-$ cDC1 *in vitro* (40). Whether this IL-10 production has an impact on pathogen burden *in vivo* has not been examined, but these results indicate that the response to *L. monocytogenes* is intrinsically different between cDC1 from neonatal and adult mice. Following infection with respiratory syncytial virus (RSV) 7-day-old mice show an altered $CD8^+$ T cell response to that is hallmarked by an epitope shift toward $D^bM_{187-195}$, rather than the K^dM2_{82-90} epitope that is immunodominant in adults (49). This epitope shift can be partially rescued by administration of costimulatory signals *in vivo* (51), suggesting that lower levels of costimulatory molecules on cDCs contribute to the observed epitope bias. However, it is noteworthy, that cDC1 from 7-day-old RSV infected mice preferentially present $D^bM_{187-195}$

cDC1		
Mouse	Adult	Neonate
CD11c	+	+
MHCII	+	+↓
CD8α	+	-
CD24	+	+
CLEC9A	+	+
CD205	+	+
CD103	+	+↓
XCR-1	+	n.d.
CD86	+	+↓
CD80	+	+↓

cDC2		
Mouse	Adult	Neonate
CD11c	+	+
MHCII	+	+↓
CD11b	+	+
CD172a	+	+
CLEC4A4	+	+
CD4	+/-	-
CD86	+	+↓
CD80	+	+↓

Human	Adult	Fetus/Neonate
CD11c	+	+ (CB)
HLA-DR	+	+↓(CB)
CD141	+	+ (FT)
CLEC9A	+	+ (FT)
XCR-1	+	n.d.
CD86	+	+↓(CB)
CD80	+	+↓(CB)
CD40	+	+↓(CB)

Human	Adult	Fetus/Neonate
CD11c	+	+ (CB)
HLA-DR	+	+↓(CB)
CD1c	+	+ (FT)
CD11b	+	+ (FT)
CD172a	+	+ (FT)
CD86	+	+↓(CB)
CD80	+	+↓(CB)
CD40	+	+↓(CB)

CB: Cord Blood FT: Fetal Tissues

FIGURE 1 | Overview of typical surface markers expressed on cDC subsets from mice and humans in early and adult life. (+) marker is expressed, (–) marker is not expressed or is expressed by a small fraction of cells, n.d., not determined; (↓) lower expression; CB, cord blood; FT, fetal tissues; cDC, conventional dendritic cell; MHCII, major histocompatibility complex class II; CLEC, C-type lectin domain family; HLA, human leukocyte antigen.

epitopes (49, 51), indicating that early life cDCs may exhibit intrinsic differences in antigen processing. Notably, epitope bias may also be found in humans, as infants infected with RSV show age-dependent differences in antibody specificities (56). cDC1 are also required for generating antigen-specific $CD8^+$ T cell responses to rotavirus, a major cause of childhood gastroenteritis (41). Interestingly, neonatal Batf3-deficient mice have a stronger impairment in the antigen-specific $CD8^+$ T cell response to rotavirus than adults, yet, Batf3 deficiency delays viral clearance only minimally in neonates (41). These data suggest, that *in vivo* other immune mechanisms are put in place that compensate for a lack of cDC1 in this case.

Antigen exposure in early life can elicit both Th1 and Th2 responses (1, 57, 58), however generates a strong bias for Th2 recall responses later in life. This has been partially attributed to a T cell intrinsic Th2 bias in early life but also to the altered cytokine production of cDCs in the first weeks of life, such as low-level IL-12 production (59, 60). Immunization with OVA before postnatal day 6 leads to an upregulation of IL-13 receptor α (IL-13Rα) in antigen specific Th1 cells (59). During secondary exposure to OVA, IL-13Rα expression renders antigen-specific Th1 cells sensitive to IL-4-induced apoptosis, thus leading to Th2-biased recall responses (58, 59). Exogenous administration of IL-12 or adoptive transfer of IL-12 competent cDCs from adult mice reverses the Th2-biased recall response (59), indicating that the low level IL-12 production by cDCs in early life exerts lasting effects on immunity. Why functional differences between neonatal and adult DCs exist, is unclear but several studies suggest that the neonatal environment functionally imprints DCs. As an example, in the developing lung IL-33 produced by epithelial cells during alveolarization on postnatal day 14 suppresses the ability of pulmonary cDC2 to produce the Th1 cytokine IL-12 (50). IL-33 instead promotes OX40L expression, which in turn leads to a stronger ability of cDC2 to promote Th2-biased responses and allergy (50). Th17 responses can be mounted in neonatal mice, for instance after infection with

Yersinia enterolytica (61), but early life Th17 responses are damped by T cell derived IL-4 (62). The role of neonatal DCs in this process has not been investigated in detail.

Functional differences between early life and adult DCs have also been observed in humans. cDC2 from fetal spleen respond differently to various PAMPs than adult splenic cDC2 and as in mice, the response in the fetus is marked by higher production of anti-inflammatory cytokines (63). Although human fetal splenic cDC2s can induce allogeneic T cell proliferation, they limit T-cell-derived TNF-α production in an arginase 2-dependent manner and promote differentiation of Foxp3$^+$ regulatory T cells (63). pDCs from cord blood exhibit a severe defect in IFN-I secretion upon TLR9 stimulation with CpG when compared to pDCs from peripheral blood in adults, whereas the cytokine response to influenza A or human immunodeficiency virus is similar (64, 65). Collectively, these data show that the response of neonatal DCs to pathogens differs from that of adults in many ways, however, some signaling pathways induce immune responses that are comparable to those in adults.

NEONATAL DENDRITIC CELLS AS TARGETS FOR VACCINATION?

The unique properties of neonatal cDCs discussed above likely contribute to the relative ineffectiveness of vaccines in early life (**Figure 2A**) and it will be important to determine to what extent tailoring vaccines to the properties of early life DCs can be used to boost immunity. Similarities in surface receptor expression exist between neonatal and adult cDC subsets in both mice and humans (**Figure 1**) and specific targeting of cDC subsets holds promise for immunization in adults (26). Subset specific targeting using selectively expressed surface receptors can induce protective immunity in murine neonates. Targeting OVA to cDC1 via antibodies directed against CLEC9A with poly I:C as adjuvant on postnatal day 3 efficiently protects murine neonates against lethal challenge with OVA-expressing *L. monocytogenes* in adulthood (40). Whether targeting cDC2 in early life can induce protective immunity remains to be investigated. The prominent capacity of cDC2 to migrate to draining lymph nodes from the lung (50) indicates that they may be potent targets for initiating T cell responses. But several functions of neonatal cDC2 have not been studied in detail and it is unclear whether they induce effector T cell responses and promote T follicular helper cell differentiation and concomitant antibody production as efficiently as their adult counterparts.

Synergistic use of TLR agonists greatly increases the Th1 polarizing capacity of human adult DCs (66) and thus the use of defined PRR agonists may be used to promote immunity in early life. A recent study showed that stimulation with multiple TLR agonists elicits stronger secretion of Th1 polarizing cytokines from total human cord blood mononuclear cells than stimulation with a single TLR agonist, however, in cord blood cDCs a single TLR agonist induced stronger pro-inflammatory cytokine production than a combinatorial treatment (67). Agonists of the stimulator of interferon genes (STING) induce expression of costimulatory molecules on neonatal bone marrow derived DCs *in vitro* and promote secretion of IFN-β (68). *In vivo*

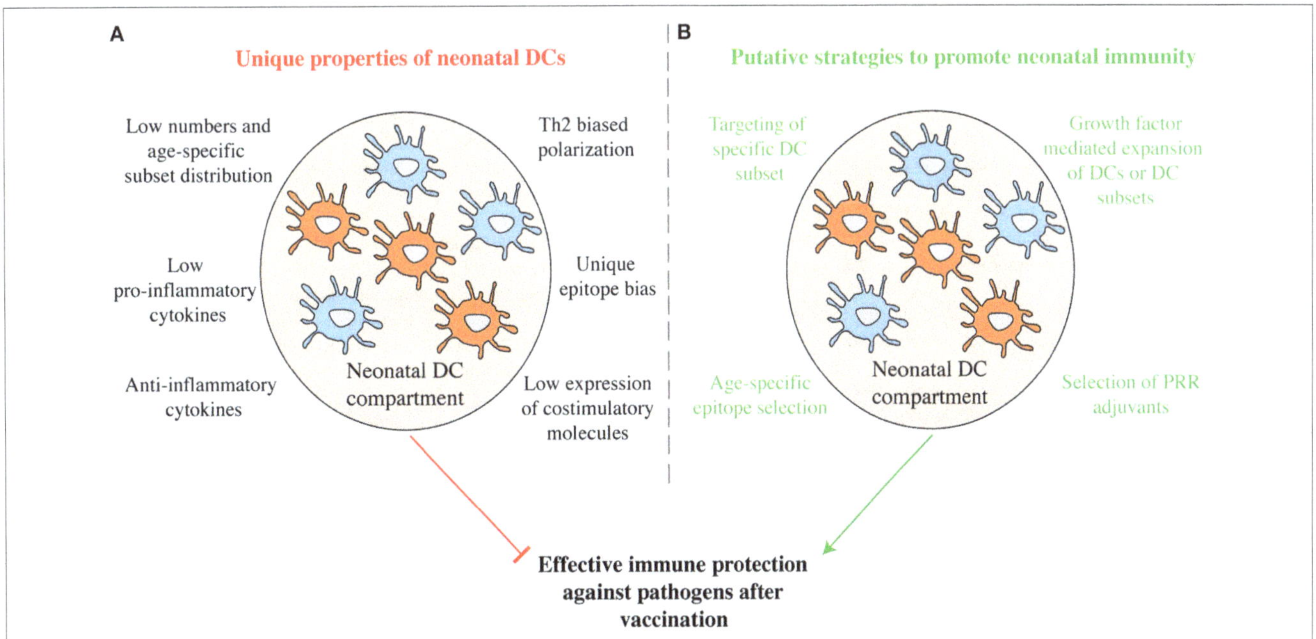

FIGURE 2 | Manipulation of the neonatal DC compartment as putative strategy to promote immunity. **(A)** Some of the functional properties that characterize neonatal DCs are shown. Taken together they may inhibit efficient immunity in currently used vaccination protocols. **(B)** Exploiting the unique functions of neonatal DCs may prove promising in developing more efficient vaccination protocols tailored to early life. Through age-specific epitope selection, DC subset specific epitope delivery, the combinatorial use of select PRR agonists as adjuvants, as well as via the manipulation of the DC compartment using growth factors, increased protective humoral and cellular immunity may be promoted.

administration of STING agonists in alum in neonatal mice promotes germinal center formation, IFN-γ production by antigen specific T cells, as well as increased antibody titers (68). Taken together these data highlight that the correct choice of adjuvant, either alone or in combination, is important for the design of effective vaccine strategies (17).

Immunization critically depends on the pathogen epitope selected to be vaccinated against. In neonatal mice, T cell responses are directed against a distinct set of antigenic epitopes compared to adults (49, 51). Similarly, in human infants neutralizing antibodies against RSV are preferentially generated against a distinct array of viral epitopes than in adults (56). Thus, selection of age-specific epitopes may also serve as a strategy to foster early life immunity and may help to circumvent deprivation of antigen by pre-existing maternal antibodies (17). At the same time, expanding the DC compartment or specific DC subsets using growth factors may ultimately shift epitope bias and cytokine production. Understanding the functional and developmental properties of neonatal cDCs and how to manipulate them may potentially be used to increase the effectiveness of neonatal immunization beyond what is possible today (**Figure 2B**). However, immune responses in early life are complex and vaccine effectiveness is influenced by a wide array of factors, including preexisting maternal antibodies (17). Therefore, further studies, especially in humans, are required to better understand the unique aspects of DC development and function in neonates and in early life, as well as the interplay of DCs with other components of the immune system, in order to fully capture whether DCs could be exploited to alter early life vaccination.

AUTHOR CONTRIBUTIONS

NP and BS wrote the manuscript with assistance from MP. NP designed the figures. All authors provided critical feedback throughout the writing process.

REFERENCES

1. Adkins B, Leclerc C, Marshall-Clarke S. Neonatal adaptive immunity comes of age. *Nat Rev Immunol.* (2004) 4:553–64. doi: 10.1038/nri1394
2. Kollmann TR, Kampmann B, Mazmanian SK, Marchant A, Levy O. Protecting the newborn and Young infant from infectious diseases: lessons from immune ontogeny. *Immunity* (2017) 46:350–63. doi: 10.1016/j.immuni.2017.03.009
3. Zhang X, Zhivaki D, Lo-Man R. Unique aspects of the perinatal immune system. *Nat Rev Immunol.* (2017) 17:495–507. doi: 10.1038/nri.2017.54
4. Dowling DJ, Levy O. Ontogeny of early life immunity. *Trends Immunol.* (2014) 35:299–310. doi: 10.1016/j.it.2014.04.007
5. PrabhuDas M, Adkins B, Gans H, King C, Levy O, Ramilo O, et al. Challenges in infant immunity: implications for responses to infection and vaccines. *Nat Immunol.* (2011) 12:189–94. doi: 10.1038/ni0311-189
6. He YM, Li X, Perego M, Nefedova Y, Kossenkov AV, Jensen EA, et al. Transitory presence of myeloid-derived suppressor cells in neonates is critical for control of inflammation. *Nat Med.* (2018) 24:224–31. doi: 10.1038/nm.4467
7. Nussbaum C, Gloning A, Pruenster M, Frommhold D, Bierschenk S, Genzel-Boroviczeny O, et al. Neutrophil and endothelial adhesive function during human fetal ontogeny. *J Leukoc Biol.* (2013) 93:175–84. doi: 10.1189/jlb.0912468.
8. Sperandio M, Quackenbush EJ, Sushkova N, Altstätter J, Nussbaum C, Schmid S, et al. Ontogenetic regulation of leukocyte recruitment in mouse yolk sac vessels. *Blood* (2013) 121:e118–28. doi: 10.1182/blood-2012-07-447144
9. Yost CC, Cody MJ, Harris ES, Thornton NL, McInturff AM, Martinez ML, et al. Impaired neutrophil extracellular trap (NET) formation: a novel innate immune deficiency of human neonates. *Blood* (2009) 113:6419–27. doi: 10.1182/blood-2008-07-171629
10. Ulas T, Pirr S, Fehlhaber B, Bickes MS, Loof TG, Vogl T, et al. S100-alarmin-induced innate immune programming protects newborn infants from sepsis. *Nat Immunol.* (2017) 18:622-632. doi: 10.1038/ni.3745
11. De Kleer, Stanislas Goriely I. Ontogeny of myeloid cells. *Front Immunol.* (2014) 9:432. doi: 10.3389/fimmu.2014.00423
12. Krow-Lucal ER, Kim CC, Burt TD, McCune JM. Distinct functional programming of human fetal and adult monocytes. *Blood* (2014) 123:1897–904. doi: 10.1182/blood-2013-11-536094
13. Hoeffel G, Chen J, Lavin Y, Low D, Almeida FF, See P, et al. C-Myb+ erythro-myeloid progenitor-derived fetal monocytes give rise to adult tissue-resident macrophages. *Immunity* (2015) 42:665–78. doi: 10.1016/j.immuni.2015.03.011
14. Ginhoux F, Guilliams M. Tissue-resident macrophage ontogeny and homeostasis. *Immunity* (2016) 44:439–49. doi: 10.1016/j.immuni.2016.02.024
15. Thion MS, Low D, Silvin A, Chen J, Grisel P, Schulte-Schrepping J, et al. Microbiome influences prenatal and adult microglia in a sex-specific manner. *Cell* (2018) 172:500–16.e16. doi: 10.1016/j.cell.2017.11.042
16. Elahi S, Ertelt JM, Kinder JM, Jiang TT, Zhang X, Xin L, et al. Immunosuppressive CD71+ erythroid cells compromise neonatal host defence against infection. *Nature* (2013) 504:158–62. doi: 10.1038/nature12675
17. Whittaker E, Goldblatt D, McIntyre P, Levy O. Neonatal immunization: rationale, current state, and future prospects. *Front Immunol.* (2018) 9:532. doi: 10.3389/fimmu.2018.00532
18. Dunne PJ, Moran B, Cummins RC, Mills KHG. CD11c+CD8alpha+ dendritic cells promote protective immunity to respiratory infection with *Bordetella pertussis*. *J Immunol.* (2009) 183:400–10. doi: 10.4049/jimmunol.0900169
19. Latz E, Franko J, Golenbock DT, Schreiber JR. Haemophilus influenzae type b-outer membrane protein complex glycoconjugate vaccine induces cytokine production by engaging human toll-like receptor 2 (TLR2) and requires the presence of TLR2 for optimal immunogenicity. *J Immunol.* (2004) 172:2431–38. doi: 10.4049/jimmunol.172.4.2431
20. Heesters BA, Carroll MC. The role of dendritic cells in *S. pneumoniae* transport to follicular dendritic cells. *Cell Rep.* (2016) 16:3130–37. doi: 10.1016/j.celrep.2016.08.049
21. Colino J, Shen Y, Snapper CM. Dendritic cells pulsed with intact *Streptococcus pneumoniae* elicit both protein- and polysaccharide-specific immunoglobulin isotype responses *in vivo* through distinct mechanisms. *J Exp Med.* (2002) 195:1–13. doi: 10.1084/jem.20011432
22. Levy O, Goriely S, Kollmann TR. Immune response to vaccine adjuvants during the first year of life. *Vaccine* (2013) 31:2500–05. doi: 10.1016/j.vaccine.2012.10.016
23. Merad M, Sathe P, Helft J, Miller J, Mortha A. The dendritic cell lineage: ontogeny and function of dendritic cells and their subsets in the steady

state and the inflamed setting. *Annu Rev Immunol.* (2013) 31:563–604. doi: 10.1146/annurev-immunol-020711-074950

24. Durai V, Murphy KM. Functions of murine dendritic cells. *Immunity* (2016) 45:719–36. doi: 10.1016/j.immuni.2016.10.010
25. Guilliams M, Ginhoux F, Jakubzick C, Naik SH, Onai N, Schraml BU, et al. Dendritic cells, monocytes and macrophages: a unified nomenclature based on ontogeny. *Nat Rev Immunol.* (2014) 14:571–8. doi: 10.1038/nri3712
26. Kastenmuller W, Kastenmüller K, Kurts C, Seder RA. Dendritic cell-targeted vaccines — hope or hype? *Nat Rev Immunol.* (2014) 14:705–11. doi: 10.1038/nri3727
27. Pakalniškyte D, Schraml BU. Tissue-specific diversity and functions of conventional dendritic cells. *Adv Immunol.* (2017) 134:89–135. doi: 10.1016/bs.ai.2017.01.003
28. Swiecki M, Colonna M. The multifaceted biology of plasmacytoid dendritic cells. *Nat Rev Immunol.* (2015) 15:471–85. doi: 10.1038/nri3865
29. Reizis B. Regulation of plasmacytoid dendritic cell development. *Curr Opin Immunol.* (2010) 22:206–11. doi: 10.1016/j.coi.2010.01.005
30. Liu K, Waskow C, Liu X, Yao K, Hoh J, Nussenzweig M. Origin of dendritic cells in peripheral lymphoid organs of mice. *Nat Immunol.* (2007) 8:578–83. doi: 10.1038/ni1462
31. Liu K, Victora GD, Schwickert TA, Guermonprez P, Meredith MM, Yao K, et al. *In vivo* analysis of dendritic cell development and homeostasis. *Science* (2009) 324:392–7. doi: 10.1126/science.1170540
32. Naik SH, Sathe P, Park H-Y, Metcalf D, Proietto AI, Dakic A, et al. Development of plasmacytoid and conventional dendritic cell subtypes from single precursor cells derived *in vitro* and *in vivo*. *Nat Immunol.* (2007) 8:1217–26. doi: 10.1038/ni1522
33. Onai N, Obata-Onai A, Schmid MA, Ohteki T, Jarrossay D, Manz MG. Identification of clonogenic common Flt3+M-CSFR+ plasmacytoid and conventional dendritic cell progenitors in mouse bone marrow. *Nat Immunol.* (2007) 8:1207–16. doi: 10.1038/ni1518
34. Schraml BU, van Blijswijk J, Zelenay S, Whitney PG, Filby A, Acton SE, et al. Genetic tracing via DNGR-1 expression history defines dendritic cells as a hematopoietic lineage. *Cell* (2013) 154:843–58. doi: 10.1016/j.cell.2013.07.014
35. Ginhoux F, Liu K, Helft J, Bogunovic M, Greter M, Hashimoto D, et al. The origin and development of nonlymphoid tissue CD103 +DCs. *J Exp Med.* (2009) 206:3115–30. doi: 10.1084/jem.20091756
36. Grajales-Reyes GE, Iwata A, Albring J, Wu X, Tussiwand R, KC W, et al. Batf3 maintains autoactivation of Irf8 for commitment of a CD8α+ conventional DC clonogenic progenitor. *Nat Immunol.* (2015) 16:708–17. doi: 10.1038/ni.3197
37. Schlitzer A, Sivakamasundari V, Chen J, Bin Sumatoh HR, Schreuder J, Lum J, et al. Identification of cDC1- and cDC2-committed DC progenitors reveals early lineage priming at the common DC progenitor stage in the bone marrow. *Nat Immunol.* (2015) 16:718–28. doi: 10.1038/ni.3200
38. Cisse B, Caton ML, Lehner M, Maeda T, Scheu S, Locksley R, et al. Transcription factor E2-2 is an essential and specific regulator of plasmacytoid dendritic cell development. *Cell* (2008) 135:37–48. doi: 10.1016/j.cell.2008.09.016
39. Rodrigues PF, Alberti-Servera L, Eremin A, Grajales-Reyes GE, Ivanek R, Tussiwand R. Distinct progenitor lineages contribute to the heterogeneity of plasmacytoid dendritic cells. *Nat Immunol.* (2018) 19:711–22. doi: 10.1038/s41590-018-0136-9
40. Torres D, Köhler A, Delbauve S, Caminschi I, Lahoud MH, Shortman K, et al. IL-12p40/IL-10 producing preCD8α/Clec9A+ dendritic cells are induced in neonates upon listeria monocytogenes infection. *PLoS Pathogen.* (2016) 12:e1005561. doi: 10.1371/journal.ppat.1005561
41. Sun T, Rojas OL, Li C, Ward LA, Philpott DJ, Gommerman JL. Intestinal Batf3-dependent dendritic cells are required for optimal antiviral T-cell responses in adult and neonatal mice. *Mucosal Immunol.* (2016) 10:775–88. doi: 10.1038/mi.2016.79
42. Durai V, Bagadia P, Briseño CG, Theisen DJ, Iwata A, Davidson JT IV, et al. Altered compensatory cytokine signaling underlies the discrepancy between Flt3 -/-and Flt3l -/-mice. *J Exp Med.* (2018) 215:1417–35. doi: 10.1084/jem.20171784
43. Vollstedt S, Franchini M, Hefti HP, Odermatt B, O'Keeffe M, Alber G, et al. Flt3 ligand-treated neonatal mice have increased innate immunity against intracellular pathogens and efficiently control virus infections. *J Exp Med.* (2003) 197:575–84. doi: 10.1084/jem.20021900
44. Satpathy AT, Briseño CG, Lee JS, Ng D, Manieri NA, KC W, et al. Notch2-dependent classical dendritic cells orchestrate intestinal immunity to attaching-and-effacing bacterial pathogens. *Nat Immunol.* (2013) 14:937–48. doi: 10.1038/ni.2679
45. Persson EK, Uronen-Hansson H, Semmrich M, Rivollier A, Hägerbrand K, Marsal J, et al. IRF4 transcription-factor-dependent CD103+CD11b+ dendritic cells drive mucosal T helper 17 cell differentiation. *Immunity* (2013) 38:958–69. doi: 10.1016/j.immuni.2013.03.009
46. Sun CM. Ontogeny and innate properties of neonatal dendritic cells. *Blood* (2003) 102:585–91. doi: 10.1182/blood-2002-09-2966
47. Dakic A, Shao QX, D'Amico A, O'Keeffe M, Chen WF, Shortman K, et al. Development of the dendritic cell system during mouse ontogeny. *J Immunol.* (2004) 172:1018–27. doi: 10.4049/jimmunol.172.2.1018
48. Mold JE, McCune JM. Immunological tolerance during fetal development: from mouse to man. *Adv Immunol.* (2012) 115:73–111. doi: 10.1016/B978-0-12-394299-9.00003-5
49. Ruckwardt TJ, Morabito KM, Bar-Haim E, Nair D, Graham BS. Neonatal mice possess two phenotypically and functionally distinct lung-migratory CD103+ dendritic cell populations following respiratory infection. *Mucosal Immunol.* (2018) 11:186–98. doi: 10.1038/mi.2017.28
50. de Kleer IM, Kool M, de Bruijn MJW, Willart M, van Moorleghem J, Schuijs MJ, et al. Perinatal activation of the interleukin-33 pathway promotes type 2 immunity in the developing lung. *Immunity* (2016) 45:1285–98. doi: 10.1016/j.immuni.2016.10.031
51. Ruckwardt TJ, Malloy AMW, Morabito KM, Graham BS. Quantitative and qualitative deficits in neonatal lung-migratory dendritic cells impact the generation of the CD8+ T cell response. *PLOS Pathog.* (2014) 10:e1003934. doi: 10.1371/journal.ppat.1003934
52. Torow N, Yu K, Hassani K, Freitag J, Schulz O, Basic M, et al. Active suppression of intestinal CD4+TCRαβ+ T-lymphocyte maturation during the postnatal period. *Nat Commun.* (2015) 6:7725. doi: 10.1038/ncomms8725
53. Bain CC, Bravo-Blas A, Scott CL, Gomez-Perdiguero E, Geissmann F, Henri S, et al. Constant replenishment from circulating monocytes maintains the macrophage pool in the intestine of adult mice. *Nat Immunol.* (2014) 15:929–37. doi: 10.1038/ni.2967
54. Lantier L, Lacroix-Lamandé S, Potiron L, Metton C, Drouet F, Guesdon W, et al. Intestinal CD103+ dendritic cells are key players in the innate immune control of *Cryptosporidium parvum* infection in neonatal mice. *PLOS Pathog.* (2013) 9:e1003801. doi: 10.1371/journal.ppat.1003801
55. Ardouin L, Luche H, Chelbi R, Carpentier S, Shawket A, Montanana Sanchis F, et al. Broad and largely concordant molecular changes characterize tolerogenic and immunogenic dendritic cell maturation in thymus and periphery. *Immunity* (2016) 45:305–18. doi: 10.1016/j.immuni.2016.07.019
56. Goodwin E, Gilman MSA, Wrapp D, Chen M, Ngwuta JO, Moin SM, et al. Infants infected with respiratory syncytial virus generate potent neutralizing antibodies that lack somatic hypermutation. *Immunity* (2018) 48:339–49.e5. doi: 10.1016/j.immuni.2018.01.005
57. Adkins B, Du R-Q. Newborn mice develop balanced Th1/Th2 primary effector responses *in vivo* but are biased to Th2 secondary responses. *J Immunol.* (1998) 160:4217–24.
58. Li L, Lee H-H, Bell JJ, Gregg RK, Ellis JS, Gessner A, et al. IL-4 utilizes an alternative receptor to drive apoptosis of Th1 cells and skews neonatal immunity toward Th2. *Immunity* (2004) 20:429–40. doi: 10.1016/S1074-7613(04)00072-X
59. Lee H-H, Hoeman CM, Hardaway JC, Guloglu FB, Ellis JS, Jain R, et al. Delayed maturation of an IL-12-producing dendritic cell subset explains the early Th2 bias in neonatal immunity. *J Exp Med.* (2008) 205:2269–80. doi: 10.1084/jem.20071371
60. Ridge JP, Fuchs EJ, Matzinger P. Neonatal tolerance revisited: turning on newborn T cells with dendritic cells. *Science* (1996) 271:1723–6. doi: 10.1126/science.271.5256.1723
61. Echeverry A, Saijo S, Schesser K, Adkins B. Yersinia enterocolitica promotes robust mucosal inflammatory T-cell immunity in murine neonates. *Infect Immun.* (2010) 78:3595–608. doi: 10.1128/IAI.01272-09
62. Debock I, Delbauve S, Dubois A, Pétein M, Leo O, Goldman M, et al. Th17 alloimmunity prevents neonatal establishment of lymphoid

chimerism in IL-4-deprived mice. *Am J Transplant.* (2012) 12:81–9. doi: 10.1111/j.1600-6143.2011.03778.x

63. McGovern N, Shin A, Low G, Low D, Duan K, Yao LJ, et al. Human fetal dendritic cells promote prenatal T-cell immune suppression through arginase-2. *Nature* (2017) 546:662–6. doi: 10.1038/nature 22795
64. Danis B, George TC, Goriely S, Dutta B, Renneson J, Gatto L, et al. Interferon regulatory factor 7-mediated responses are defective in cord blood plasmacytoid dendritic cells. *Eur J Immunol.* (2008) 38:507–17. doi: 10.1002/eji.200737760
65. Zhang X, Lepelley A, Azria E, Lebon P, Roguet G, Schwartz O, et al. Neonatal Plasmacytoid Dendritic Cells (pDCs) display subset variation but can elicit potent anti-viral innate responses. *PLoS ONE* (2013) 8:e52003. doi: 10.1371/journal.pone.00 52003
66. Napolitani G, Rinaldi A, Bertoni F, Sallusto F, Lanzavecchia A. Selected Toll-like receptor agonist combinations synergistically trigger a T helper type 1–polarizing program in dendritic cells. *Nat Immunol.* (2005) 6:769–76. doi: 10.1038/ni1223
67. Surendran N, Simmons A, Pichichero ME. TLR agonist combinations that stimulate Th type I polarizing responses from human neonates. *Innate Immun.* (2018) 24:240–51. doi: 10.1177/1753425918771178
68. Borriello F, Pietrasanta C, Lai JCY, Walsh LM, Sharma P, O'Driscoll DN, et al. Identification and characterization of stimulator of interferon genes as a robust adjuvant target for early life immunization. *Front Immunol.* (2017) 8:1772. doi: 10.3389/fimmu.2017.01772

2

Poly(I:C) Potentiates T Cell Immunity to a Dendritic Cell Targeted HIV-Multiepitope Vaccine

*Juliana de Souza Apostólico [1,2], Victória Alves Santos Lunardelli [1,2], Marcio Massao Yamamoto [3], Edecio Cunha-Neto [2,4], Silvia Beatriz Boscardin [2,3] and Daniela Santoro Rosa [1,2]**

[1] Laboratory of Experimental Vaccines, Department of Microbiology, Immunology and Parasitology, Federal University of São Paulo, São Paulo, Brazil, [2] Institute for Investigation in Immunology (iii)—INCT, São Paulo, Brazil, [3] Department of Parasitology, Institute of Biomedical Sciences, University of São Paulo, São Paulo, Brazil, [4] Laboratory of Clinical Immunology and Allergy (LIM60), School of Medicine–University of São Paulo, São Paulo, Brazil

***Correspondence:**
Daniela Santoro Rosa
dsantororosa@gmail.com

Cellular immune responses are implicated in resistance to HIV and have been considered for the development of an effective vaccine. Despite their safety profile, subunit vaccines need to be delivered combined with an adjuvant. In the last years, *in vivo* antigen targeting to dendritic cells (DCs) using chimeric monoclonal antibodies (mAb) against the DC endocytic receptor DEC205/CD205 was shown to support long-term T cell immunity. Here, we evaluated the ability of different adjuvants to modulate specific cellular immune response when eight $CD4^+$ HIV-derived epitopes (HIVBr8) were targeted to $DEC205^+$ DCs *in vivo*. Immunization with two doses of αDECHIVBr8 mAb along with poly(I:C) induced Th1 cytokine production and higher frequency of HIV-specific polyfunctional and long-lived T cells than MPL or CpG ODN-assisted immunization. Although each adjuvant elicited responses against the 8 epitopes present in the vaccine, the magnitude of the T cell response was higher in the presence of poly(I:C). Moreover, poly(I:C) up regulated the expression of costimulatory molecules in both cDC1 and cDC2 DCs subsets. In summary, the use of poly(I:C) in a vaccine formulation that targets multiple epitopes to the DEC205 receptor improved the potency and the quality of HIV-specific responses when compared to other vaccine-adjuvant formulations. This study highlights the importance of the rational selection of antigen/adjuvant combination to potentiate the desired immune responses.

Keywords: HIV, multiepitope vaccine, dendritic cell targeting, DEC205, adjuvants

INTRODUCTION

Vaccine induced T cell immunity is required for effective protection against intracellular pathogens responsible for diseases classified as global threats like AIDS, tuberculosis, malaria, and also against cancer. The ability of dendritic cells (DCs) to uptake, process and present antigens is crucial to induce and regulate T cell immunity (1). Thus, activation of DCs has been considered key in vaccines designed to induce cellular immunity (2). DCs express a wide range of receptors including pattern recognition receptors (PRRs), like toll-like receptors (TLRs), cytosolic receptors, and C-type lectin receptors, that are able to recognize pathogen- or damage- associated molecular patterns (PAMPs or DAMPs, respectively) (3). The nature of the signal delivered to the DC does not only affect the magnitude of T cell responses, but also influences the generation of memory precursors and the overall quality of immune response (4, 5).

Human and mouse DCs can be divided in two major subsets: plasmacytoid DCs and conventional/myeloid DCs with specific functions in the steady state (6–8). Recently, DCs were classified based on their ontogeny in conventional type 1 DCs (cDC1) and conventional type 2 DCs (cDC2) (9, 10). Conventional type 1 DCs encompass lymphoid CD8α^+ and non-lymphoid CD103$^+$, both of which express DEC205. DEC205 also known as CD205 is a C-type lectin endocytic receptor and was the first identified DC-specific receptor (11). DEC205 is highly expressed on cDC1, but can also be found on thymic epithelial cells, Langerhans cells and, at relatively low levels, on B cells (12, 13). Recently, synthetic CpG oligonucleotides (ODNs), a potent immunostimulator, were identified as ligands that bind to the surface DEC205 (14, 15).

A promising strategy to improve vaccine efficacy is to selectively target the desired antigen to a DC subset by linking it to a monoclonal antibody (mAb) against the specific DC receptor. During the last decade, several reports revealed the feasibility of *in vivo* antigen targeting to cDC1 using a mAb against DEC205 (αDEC205) to improve both humoral and cellular responses (2, 16–20). Vaccination with DEC205 targeted antigens also induced protection in different infection and tumor models (21–23). However, for this particular receptor, inflammatory signals such as adjuvants must be co-administered with the targeted antigen to induce DC maturation, cellular immunity and avoid tolerance (24–26).

Different microbial products such as TLR ligands have been characterized and used as adjuvants to trigger intracellular signaling cascades that result in cytokine production, up regulation of costimulatory molecules and DCs maturation (27–30). Mouse conventional DC subsets differentially express a broad repertoire of TLRs that result in different activating phenotypes and adaptive immunity (31). The co-delivery of TLR ligands and DEC205 targeted antigens has been shown to significantly improve vaccine immunogenicity in mice and in non-human primates (16).

Polyinosinic:polycytidylic acid [poly(I:C)] is a synthetic analog of viral double-stranded RNAs (dsRNAs) that activates TLR3 and RIG-I-like receptors (retinoic acid-inducible gene -I- like receptors, or RLRs) (32). Poly(I:C) is the most commonly administered adjuvant in mice in the context of DC-targeted vaccines using αDEC205 mAbs fused with proteins of interest (18). This strategy has already been tested with chimeric mAbs containing proteins derived from dengue virus (33), *Trypanosoma cruzi* (34), *Plasmodium* sp (26, 35, 36), *Mycobacterium tuberculosis* (37), *Yersinia pestis* (22), *Toxoplasma gondii* (23), HIV (21, 38, 39) and also from tumors (40). The excellent results obtained with this adjuvant, justified its use in clinical trials. To improve poly I:C stability (32) in humans, a modified version (poly-ICLC) was developed and used in different trials (41, 42).

Monophosphoryl lipid A (MPL), a chemically derivative of bacterial lipopolysaccharide (LPS), is a TLR4 agonist that preferentially activates the TIR-domain-containing adapter-inducing interferon-β (TRIF) signaling pathway to drive the production of Th1 cytokines and activate CD4$^+$ T cells (43) (44, 45). MPL is the first and only TLR ligand licensed in a human vaccine (Melacine™, approved as a melanoma vaccine). More recently, other MPL-containing vaccines became available (Fendrix™ and Cervarix™, both from GSK) (46). CpG oligodeoxynucleotides (ODN) are unmethylated CpG motifs that interact with endosomal TLR9 and lead to proinflammatory cytokine production by DCs (47). B type ODN has a protective phosphorothioate backbone that protects it from nuclease digestion and enhances its half-life *in vivo* (48). Several clinical trials were conducted and CpG ODN emerged as a potent adjuvant to induce high antibody titers more quickly and after fewer doses (49, 50). Moreover, CpG ODN has been used along with αDEC205 mAb to target HIV and *Plasmodium* proteins (51, 52).

Here, we used eight promiscuous HIV-derived CD4$^+$ T cell epitopes (HIVBr8) fused with αDEC205 to target CD11c$^+$ CD8α^+ DCs in the presence of different TLR ligands. The hierarchy of adjuvant potency shows that poly(I:C) is a superior adjuvant for the multiepitope DC-targeted vaccine in magnitude, breadth, and longevity.

MATERIALS AND METHODS

Generation of the Fusion Monoclonal Antibody (mAb)

Plasmids encoding the light and heavy chain of the mouse αDEC205 antibody were kindly provided by Dr. Michel C. Nussenzweig (The Rockefeller University, New York, USA). The plasmid encoding the heavy chain of the mouse DEC205 fused to eight HIV-1 epitopes was previously described and contains the following epitopes: p6 (32-46), p17 (73-89), pol (785-799), gp160 (188-201), rev (11-27), vpr (65-82), vif (144-158), and nef (180-194) (39).

Expression and Purification of αDECHIVBr8 mAb

The production of αDECHIVBr8 mAb [original clone NLDC145 (24)] was performed after transient transfection of human embryonic kidney (HEK) 293T cells (ATCC, CRL-11268) exactly as described elsewhere (33). Briefly, 293T cells were cultured in 150 mm plates (Sarstedt) under standard conditions in Dulbecco's modified Eagle's medium (Invitrogen) supplemented with 1% (v/v) antibiotic-antimycotic (Invitrogen), 1% (v/v) l-glutamine (Invitrogen), and 5% (v/v) Ultra low IgG Fetal Bovine Serum (Invitrogen). When cell confluence reached 70%, 293T cells were transfected using 10 μg of the plasmids encoding the light and the heavy chains in the presence of 150 mM NaCl and 0.45 mg/mL polyethyleneimine (PEI) (Sigma Aldrich). After 7 days in culture at 37°C with 5% CO_2, the culture supernatants containing secreted antibodies were collected by centrifugation at 1,000 x g for 30 min at 4°C and filtered through 0.22 μM membrane. The chimeric αDECHIVBr8 mAb was precipitated by addition of ammonium sulfate (Sigma Aldrich) to 60% of the total culture volume, and resuspended/dialyzed overnight against PBS at 4°C. After purification by affinity chromatography with protein G beads column (GE Healthcare), fusion mAb was dialyzed against PBS, resolved on a SDS-12% polyacrylamide gel, quantified, and stored at −20°C until use.

Mice

Female BALB/c (H-2^d) mice with 6-to 8-week old were purchased from Centro de Desenvolvimento de Modelos Experimentais para Medicina e Biologia (CEDEME)- Brazil. Mice were housed and manipulated under specific-pathogen-free (SPF) conditions at the animal care facility of the Division of Immunology, Federal University of São Paulo (UNIFESP).

Immunization

Groups of six mice were immunized twice, 2 weeks apart, with 4 μg of αDECHIVBr8 mAb by intraperitoneal (I.P) route in the presence of the following adjuvants: 50 μg of poly(I:C) (Invivogen), 20 μg of Monophosphoryl Lipid A (MPL) (Invivogen), or 10 μg of CpG ODN 1826 (Invivogen). The amount of adjuvants used was previously determined (53). Control groups were immunized with 4 μg of αDECHIVBr8 in the absence of adjuvant or with PBS only.

Spleen and Mesenteric Lymph Node Cell Isolation

Fifteen and sixty days after the administration of the second dose (boost), mice were deeply anesthetized by ketamine/xylazine solution (300 and 30 mg/kg, respectively) and mesenteric lymph nodes and the spleen were aseptically removed. After obtaining single cell suspensions, cells were washed in 10 mL of RPMI 1640 (Gibco). Splenic red blood cells were lysed with 1 mL of ACK solution (150 mM NH_3Cl, 10 mM $KHCO_3$, 0.1 mM EDTA) for 2 min at room temperature. After two additional washes with RPMI 1640, splenocytes and lymph node cells were then resuspended in R10 (RPMI supplemented with 10% of fetal bovine serum, 2 mM L-glutamine, 1% v/v vitamin solution, 1mM sodium pyruvate, 1% v/v non-essential amino acids solution, 40 μg/mL of Gentamicin, 5 x 10^{-5} M 2-mercaptoetanol (all from Gibco) and 20 μg/mL of Cyprofloxacin (Ciprobacter, Isofarma). The viability of cells was evaluated using 0.2% Trypan Blue exclusion dye to discriminate between live and dead cells. Cell concentration was estimated with the aid of a cell counter (Countess, Invitrogen) and adjusted in cell culture medium.

Cytokine Determination

One million splenocytes were incubated for 48 h in the presence of pooled HIV-1 peptides (5 μM) or medium alone as negative control. Culture supernatants were harvested and stored at −20°C until analysis. IL-2, IL-4, IL-6, IL-10, IL-17, IFNγ, and TNFα were detected simultaneously using mouse Th1/Th2/Th17 cytokine bead array (CBA) kit (BD Pharmingen), according to the manufacturer's instructions. The range of detection was 20–5,000 pg/mL for each cytokine.

T Cell ELISpot Assay

The ELISpot assay was performed using mouse IFNγ ELISpot Ready-SET-Go! (eBiosciences) according to manufacturer's instructions. Splenocytes from immunized mice were obtained as described and assayed for their ability to secrete IFNγ after *in vitro* stimulation with individual or pooled HIV-1 peptides (5 μM) or medium alone as negative control. Spots were counted using an AID ELISPOT Reader System (Autoimmun Diagnostika GmbH, Germany). The number of IFN-γ producing cells/10^6 splenocytes was calculated after subtracting the negative control values and the cutoff was 15 SFU per million splenocytes.

Analysis of HIV-Specific Proliferation and Intracellular Cytokine Production by Flow Cytometry

To analyze HIV-specific T cell expansion, proliferation, and cytokine production, splenocytes from immunized mice were labeled with carboxyfluorescein succinimidyl ester (CFSE) (54). In summary, freshly isolated splenocytes were resuspended (50 × 10^6/mL) in PBS and labeled with 1.25 μM of CFSE (Molecular Probes) at 37°C for 10 min. The reaction was quenched with RPMI 1640 supplemented with 10% FBS (R10) and cells were washed/resuspended with R10. Cells were cultured in 96-well round-bottomed plates (5 × 10^5/well in triplicate) for 5 days at 37°C and 5% CO_2 with medium alone or with pooled HIV-1 peptides (5 μM). After 4 days, cells were restimulated with pooled HIV-1 peptides (5 μM) in the presence of 2 μg/mL anti-CD28 (BD Pharmingen) and Brefeldin A- GolgiPlugTM (BD Pharmingen) for further 12 h. After the incubation period, cells were washed with FACS buffer (PBS with 0.5% BSA and 2 mM EDTA) and surface stained with anti-mouse CD3 APCCy7 (clone 145-2C11), CD4 PerCP (clone RM4-5), and CD8 Pacific Blue (clone 53-6.7) monoclonal antibodies for 30 min at 4°C. Cells were fixed and permeabilized using Cytofix/Cytoperm™ kit (BD Pharmingen), according to manufacturer's instructions. After permeabilization, cells were washed with Perm/Wash buffer (BD Biosciences) and stained with anti-mouse IL2 PE (clone JES6-5H4), TNFα PECy7 (clone MP6-XT22), and IFNγ APC (clone XMG1.2) monoclonal antibodies for 30 min at 4°C. Following staining, cells were washed twice and resuspended in FACS buffer. All antibodies were from BD Pharmingen. Samples were acquired on a FACSCanto II flow cytometer (BD Biosciences) and then analyzed using FlowJo software (version 9.9, Tree Star, San Carlo, CA). To analyze cellular polyfunctionality, we used the Boolean gate platform (FlowJo software) to create combinations of the three cytokines (IL-2, TNFα, and IFNγ) within the $CFSE^{low}$ population (cells that have undergone at least one cycle of division) resulting in seven distinct patterns. Polyfunctionality was defined as the ability of cells to exert at least two functions. The gating strategy, illustrated using data from one representative experiment, is shown in **Figure S1**. The frequencies of cytokine producing cells were calculated by subtracting the frequency of cells that were stimulated *in vitro* with HIV peptides by the frequency of the cells that were cultured in the presence of medium alone (background). For each experiment performed, unstained and all single-color controls were processed to allow proper compensation.

Expression of Costimulatory Molecules on DC Surface

Mice were immunized once with 4 μg of αDECHIVBr8 mAb combined with the different adjuvants (poly(I:C), MPL or

CpG ODN 1826). After 12 h, splenocytes were stained with biotinylated anti-mouse CD3 (clone 145-2C11), CD19 (clone 1D3), and CD49b (clone DX5). After 30 min, cells were washed with FACS buffer and stained with streptavidin APCCy7, anti-mouse CD11c APC (clone HL3), IAIE PE (clone 2G9), CD8 Pacific Blue (clone 53-6.7), CD40 FITC (clone 3.23), CD80 PerCP (clone 16-10A1), and CD86 PECy7 (clone GL1). Samples were acquired on a FACSCanto II flow cytometer (BD Biosciences) and then analyzed using FlowJo software (version 9.9, Tree Star, San Carlo, CA). For each experiment performed, unstained and all single-color controls were processed to allow proper compensation. Three million events were acquired in a live lymphocyte gate.

Data Analysis

Statistical significance (p-value) was calculated by Two-way ANOVA followed by Bonferroni *post hoc* test or unpaired t-test (different time points comparison). Statistical analysis and graphical representation of data was performed using GraphPad Prism version 7.0 software.

RESULTS

Multiepitope Targeting to DEC205$^+$ DCs With Different Adjuvants Induces Type 1 Cytokine Production

To examine the effect of different adjuvants on HIV-specific cellular immune response, mice were immunized with two doses of αDECHIVBr8 mAb in the presence of the TLR agonists poly(I:C), MPL or CpG ODN 1826. Fifteen or Sixty days after the boost, splenocytes from immunized mice were incubated with pooled HIV-1 peptides to analyze specific cytokine production. First, we evaluated IFNγ production by ELISpot assay (**Figure 1A**). We observed that 15 days after the boost splenocytes from mice immunized with αDECHIVBr8 mAb combined with poly(I:C) presented higher number of specific IFNγ producing cells (716 SFU/10^6 cells) when compared to the groups immunized in the presence of MPL or CpG ODN 1826 (404 and 286 SFU/10^6 cells, respectively). Moreover, a significant difference was observed between MPL and CpG ODN 1826 groups (**Figure 1A**, left). Sixty days after the boost, we detected the same profile albeit with lower magnitude. Mice immunized with αDECHIVBr8 combined with poly(I:C) displayed 514 SFU/10^6 cells while MPL and CpG ODN 1826 presented 284 and 142 SFU/10^6 cells, respectively (**Figure 1A**, right). A comparison between 15 and 60 days revealed a significant decrease in the magnitude for poly(I:C) ($p < 0.001$), CpG ODN 1826 ($p < 0.001$), and MPL ($p < 0.01$) immunized groups. Splenocytes from mice immunized with αDECHIVBr8 in the absence of adjuvant or PBS (control groups) presented negligible numbers of IFNγ producing cells.

We also analyzed the cytokine profile by CBA assay using supernatant culture of splenocytes stimulated with pooled HIV peptides. Splenocytes from mice that received αDECHIVBr8 combined with poly(I:C) produced higher levels of IFNγ when compared to MPL or CpG ODN 1826, corroborating the ELISpot findings (**Figure 1B**). Interestingly, in the poly(I:C) adjuvanted group IFNγ production was even higher 60 days after the boost when compared to the 15 days time point ($p < 0.001$). Poly(I:C) also induced superior IL-2 production 15 days after the boost (**Figure 1C**, left). However, 60 days after the boost, IL-2 production significantly decreased in the group immunized with αDECHIVBr8 plus poly(I:C) and increased in the group that received the mAb in the presence of MPL ($p < 0.001$) (**Figure 1C**, right). IL-2 production by the group that received the mAb with CpG ODN 1826 slightly increased 60 days after the boost when compared to 15 days time point ($p < 0.001$). Regarding TNFα production 15 days after the boost, we observed that αDECHIVBr8 mixed with MPL produced the highest levels (**Figure 1D**). TNFα levels increased 60 days after the boost for the poly(I:C) group ($p < 0.001$) and decreased for the CpG ODN 1826 group ($p < 0.05$). No difference was observed for the MPL immunized group. Inflammatory IL-6 (**Figure 1E**) was higher in the group immunized with αDECHIVBr8 plus MPL 15 days after boost, but at the later time point the levels of this cytokine significantly decreased ($p < 0.01$). In contrast, 60 days after the boost with mAb and poly(I:C), IL-6 ($p < 0.01$) production increased considerably. IL-10 (**Figure 1F**) was superior in the poly(I:C) immunized group in both time points followed by MPL immunized group. However, after 60 days, IL-10 production decreased in the MPL ($p < 0.001$) and in the CpG ODN 1826 ($p < 0.05$) groups. Of note, IL-4 and IL-17 production was below the assay detection limit (data not shown). Taken together, these results indicate that different adjuvants induce a type 1 immune response when multiple HIV-antigens are delivered to CD8α$^+$ DCs by the endocytic receptor DEC205.

Poly(I:C) Promotes Robust and Long-Lived Polyfunctional T Cell Responses

In an attempt to evaluate HIV-specific CD4$^+$ and CD8$^+$ T cell responses, splenocytes from immunized mice were labeled with CFSE and pulsed *in vitro* with HIV-1 peptides. After culture, the frequency of CD3$^+$CD4$^+$CFSE^{low} (**Figure 2A**) and CD3$^+$CD8$^+$CFSE^{low} (**Figure 2B**) were evaluated by flow cytometry. Fifteen days after boost, splenocytes from mice that received αDECHIVBr8 along with poly(I:C) presented higher frequency of proliferating CD4$^+$ (9.96%) and CD8$^+$ (5.90%) T cells when compared to MPL immunized groups (6.83 and 4.86%, respectively). In contrast, CpG ODN 1826 displayed the lowest frequency of proliferating T cells. The same profile was observed 60 days after the boost, with the group that received αDECHIVBr8 plus poly(I:C) displaying higher CD4$^+$ (11.30%) and CD8$^+$ (6.17%) specific proliferation when compared to MPL (CD4$^+$CFSE^{low} 4.86% and CD8$^+$CFSE^{low} 2.47%) or CpG ODN 1826 (CD4$^+$CFSE^{low} 3.60% and CD8$^+$CFSE^{low} 1.31%) (**Figures 2A,B** right, respectively). Comparative analyses showed significant difference on the frequency of CD4$^+$CFSE^{low} cells between 15 and 60 days only for the group that received αDECHIVBr8 plus MPL ($p < 0.05$). Regarding the CD8$^+$ T cell compartment (CD8$^+$CFSE^{low} cells), a significant difference was observed for MPL ($p < 0.05$) or CpG ODN 1826 ($p < 0.01$) groups. In contrast, mice immunized with αDECHIVBr8

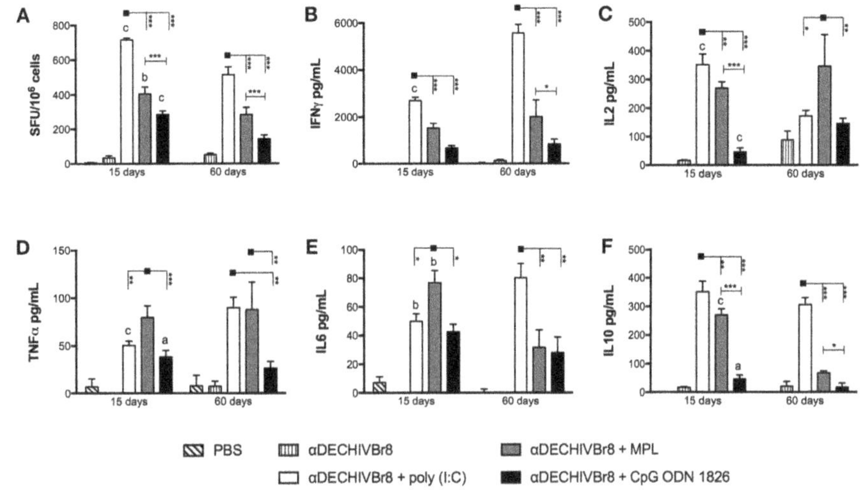

FIGURE 1 | Properties of HIV-specific cellular imune response after immunization with multiepitope αDECHIVBr8 mAb in the presence of adjuvants. BALB/c mice ($n = 6$) were immunized with two doses of 4 μg of αDECHIVBr8 along with poly(I:C), MPL or CpG ODN 1826. Control groups received αDECHIVBr8 only or PBS. Fifteen and sixty days after the boost the splenocytes were **(A)** cultured in the presence of pooled HIV-1 peptides (5 μM) for 18 h to evaluate the number of IFN-γ producing cells by ELISpot assay. SFU, spot forming units. Cutoff = 15 SFU/10^6 cells and is represented by the dotted line. **(B–F)** cultured in the presence of pooled HIV-1 peptides for 48 h to measure IFNγ **(B)**, IL2 **(C)**, TNFα **(D)**, IL6 **(E)**, and IL10 **(F)** in culture supernatants by flow cytometry. Data were analyzed by two-way ANOVA followed by Bonferroni *post hoc* test or unpaired *t-test* (different time points comparison) $^*p < 0.05$, $^{**}p < 0.01$; $^{***}p < 0.001$; a $p < 0.05$; b $p < 0.01$; c $p < 0.001$ when 15 days was compared to 60 days time point. Data represent mean ± SD and are representative of 3 independent experiments.

in the presence of poly(I:C) displayed similar frequency of proliferating $CD4^+$ and $CD8^+$ T cells in all time points. To further characterize the functional profile of antigen-specific T cells, we assessed the ability of single cells to proliferate and produce the cytokines IFNγ, TNFα, and IL2 individually or simultaneously. The flow cytometry profile demonstrated that immunization with αDECHIVBr8 mAb along with poly(I:C) induced higher frequency of $CD4^+$ T cells that proliferated and produced $IFN\gamma^+IL2^+TNF\alpha^+$ or $IFN\gamma^+TNF\alpha^+$ simultaneously or only one cytokine (IFNγ or TNFα) 15 or 60 days after the boost (**Figures 3A,B**, respectively). Interestingly, for the poly(I:C) and MPL groups 60 days after the boost, the frequency of polyfunctional $CD4^+$ T cells that proliferated and produced IFNγ, TNFα, and IL-2 simultaneously decreased, leading to an increase in the double or single cytokine producers (**Figure 3**–pie charts). Moreover, αDECHIVBr8 mixed with poly(I:C) also displayed higher frequency of proliferating $CD8^+$ T cells that produce IFNγ or TNFα 15 or 60 days after the boost when compared with other groups (**Figures 3C,D**, respectively). Similarly to what was observed with the CD4 compartment at the later time point (60 days), there was also a shift in the $CD8^+$ T cell polyfunctional profile in all groups when compared to 15 days after the boost; the frequency of three cytokine producing cells diminished while the single cytokine producers augmented (**Figure 3** pie charts). Altogether, these results demonstrated that immunization with two doses of αDECHIVBr8 along with poly(I:C) induced higher and long-lasting specific polyfunctional $CD4^+$ and $CD8^+$ T cells responses.

Poly(I:C) Increases Epitope Coverage

To assess the breadth of T cell responses, splenocytes from immunized mice were incubated with single HIV-1 peptides present in the fusion vaccine and the number of IFNγ producing cells was determined by ELISpot. Fifteen days after last dose (**Figure 4A**), all adjuvants tested were able to induce positive responses against all peptides, albeit at different magnitudes (poly(I:C) > MPL > CpG ODN). At a later time point (**Figure 4B**), poly(I:C), and CpG ODN adjuvanted groups sustained IFNγ production against all peptides (head-to-head comparison in **Figures S2A,C**). On the contrary, in the MPL group, the magnitude of the response was more significantly reduced when we compared the 15 and 60 days time points (**Figure S2B**). Thus, multiepitope *in vivo* targeting to $DEC205^+$ DCs when combined with poly(I:C) induced broad, potent and long-lasting T cell responses.

Differential Expression of Costimulatory Molecules in Splenic DCs Subsets

To further characterize phenotypic differences among the adjuvants, we compared the maturation status of splenic DCs after *in vivo* administration of the mAb combined with poly(I:C), MPL or CpG ODN 1826. The gating strategy, illustrated using data from one representative experiment, is shown in **Figure S3**. Twelve hours after injection, $CD11c^+CD8\alpha^+$ DCs from poly(I:C) group considerably up-regulated the expression of CD80 compared to other groups (**Figures 5A,B**). CpG ODN 1826 slightly increased CD80 expression only when compared to MPL. However, none of the adjuvants up regulated CD80 expression on $CD11c^+CD8\alpha^-$ DCs. Furthermore, poly(I:C) was the only adjuvant to significantly up regulate CD86 expression in both DCs subsets (**Figures 5C,D**). Similarly, we observed a significant increase in the MFI of CD40 molecule by poly(I:C) in both DCs subsets when compared to other adjuvants (**Figures 5E,F**). In addition, to assess whether DC activation could occur

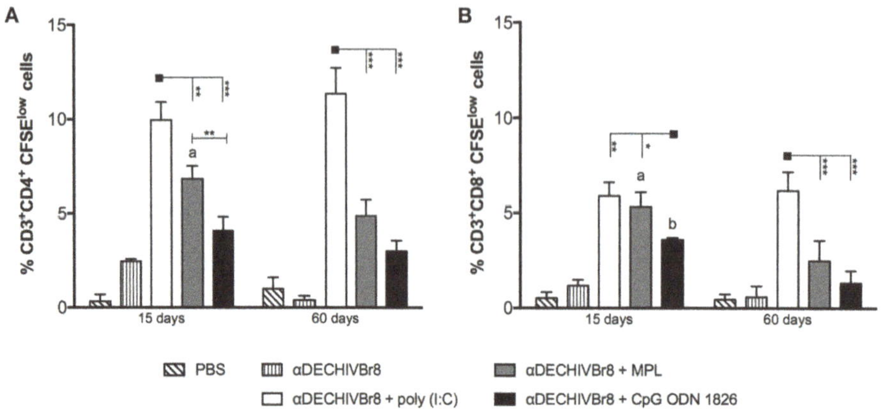

FIGURE 2 | Immunization with αDECHIVBr8 mAb in the presence of poly(I:C) induces robust HIV-specific T cell proliferation. BALB/c mice ($n = 6$) were immunized as in **Figure 1**. Fifteen and 60 days after the boost the splenocytes were labeled with CFSE and cultured in the presence of pooled HIV-1 peptides (5 μM) for 5 days to evaluate specific proliferation. CFSE dilution on gated **(A)** $CD3^+CD4^+$ or **(B)** $CD3^+CD8^+$ cells was used as readout for antigen-specific proliferation. One million events were acquired in a live lymphocyte gate. Data were analyzed by two-way ANOVA followed by Bonferroni *post hoc* test or unpaired *t-test* (time points comparison). $^*p < 0.05$, $^{**}p < 0.01$; $^{***}p < 0.001$. a $p < 0.05$; b $p < 0.01$; c $p < 0.001$ when 15 days was compared to 60 days time points. Data represent mean ± SD and are representative of 3 independent experiments.

earlier than 12 h, we analyzed the expression of costimulatory molecules 6 h after injection, and observed the same pattern of CD80, CD86, and CD40 expression in both DCs subsets (**Figures S4A–C**, respectively). We also analyzed the activation profile on mesenteric lymph nodes and the same pattern of expression was observed (data not shown). Taken together, these results strength the idea that poly(I:C) is a superior adjuvant than MPL or CpG ODN 1826 since it up regulates costimulatory molecules in both splenic DCs subsets ($CD8\alpha^+$ and $CD8\alpha^-$).

DISCUSSION

Antigen targeting to DCs through DEC205 endocytic receptor is an effective way to enhance antigen uptake. However, the induction of cell immunity is only accomplished when αDEC205 chimeric mAbs are delivered together with an adjuvant (55–57). Adjuvants enhance immunity to vaccine antigens by influencing the magnitude, breadth/immunodominance, and persistence of immune responses (27). Hence, the choice of the adjuvant formulation is of utmost importance to induce the desired immune response (58). Although a limited number of vaccine adjuvants are currently licensed for human use (aluminum salts, MF59, AS03, and AS04), several compounds have entered clinical trials with demonstrated efficacy (27).

Antigen targeting to DCs through DEC205 receptor is used as a vaccination strategy to induce strong antigen-specific immune responses against several pathogens (26, 34, 55) and tumors In the HIV vaccine scenario, antigen targeting to cDC1 through DEC205 was performed using the full-length gag (p24) protein (21, 51, 59–62). The success in different pre-clinical studies using mice and non-human primates (16) quickly pushed forward the translation of this strategy to humans. Recently, two phase I clinical trials (NCT01889719 and NCT01127464) delivered HIV p24 using a human αDEC205 mAb plus poly-ICLC as adjuvant. Promising results were obtained when a human αDEC205 mAb fused to the full-length tumor antigen NY-ESO-1 was administered together with poly-ICLC (41, 42). In fact, three phase I/IIb clinical trials are currently under way (NCT02166905, NCT03206047, NCT03358719) and two others are already completed (NCT01522820, NCT00948961, NCT01834248).

Previously, we generated an αDEC205 multiepitope fusion mAb (αDECHIVBr8) to target eight promiscuous $CD4^+$ T cell epitopes from several HIV proteins to cDC1s. The αDECHIVBr8 mAb was administered to mice in the presence of poly(I:C) as adjuvant and compared to DNA plasmid immunization in homologous and heterologous prime-boost regimens. We found that αDECHIVBr8 homologous prime-boost regimen induced stronger T cell immune responses against all epitopes when compared to homologous DNA vaccination (39). Here, we compared the adjuvant properties of poly(I:C), MPL, and CpG ODN 1826 to induce HIV-specific cellular immune response when formulated with the fusion αDECHIVBr8 mAb. To our knowledge, this is the first time that multiple epitopes derived from different proteins of the same pathogen are targeted *in vivo* to DCs and tested in the context of different adjuvants. This is an important issue since adjuvants can influence immunodominance by altering the immune repertoire of CD4 T cell responses (63). Overall, our data reveal the potential of poly(I:C) as a superior adjuvant for the development of a multiepitope-based vaccine that targets $CD8\alpha^+$ DCs through the DEC205 endocytic receptor.

Initially, we found that poly(I:C) induced higher magnitude of specific IFNγ producing cells and also Th1 cytokine production when compared to MPL or CpG ODN 1826. Likewise, Longhi et al. showed that poly(I:C) is a more potent adjuvant to induce specific immune responses against a DC-targeted HIV gag protein (51). Indeed, poly(I:C) has been the most commonly administered adjuvant with DC-targeted vaccines using αDEC205 mAbs fused with full length proteins from

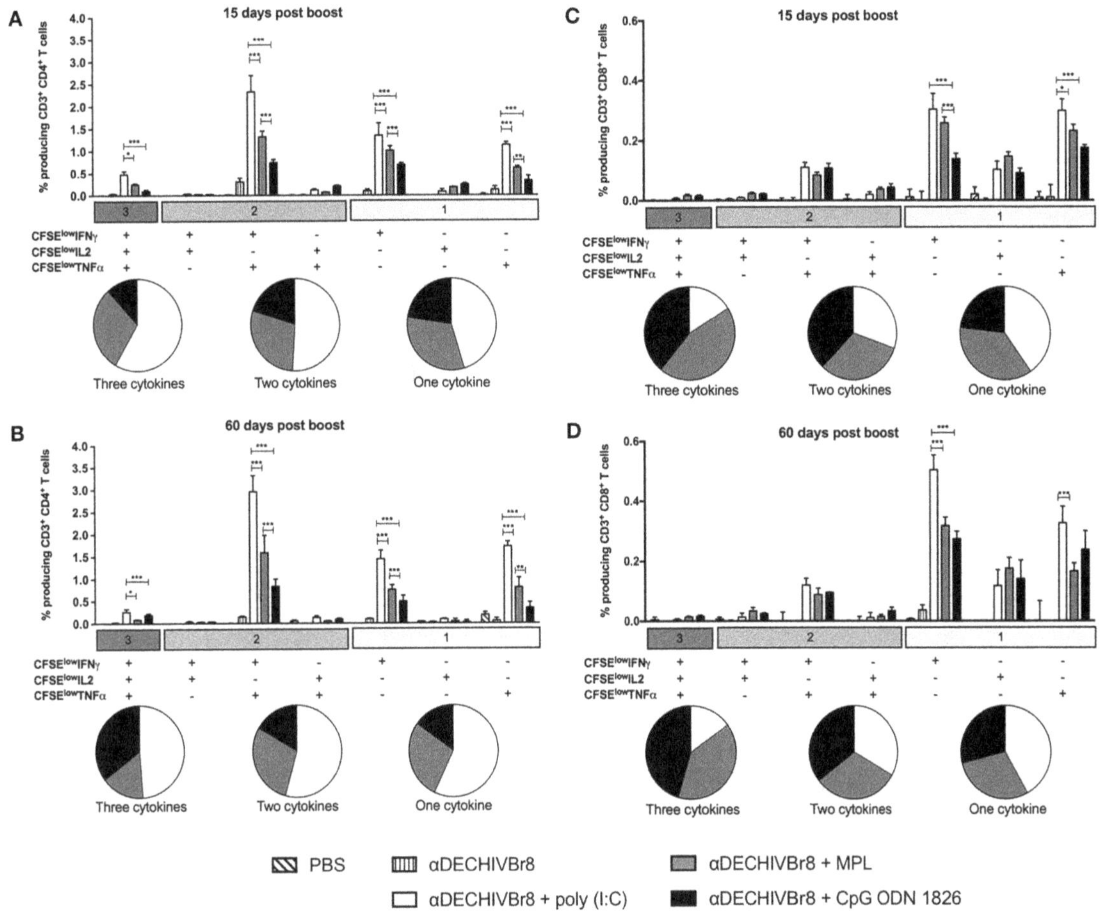

FIGURE 3 | Poly(I:C) induces superior polyfunctional and long-lived HIV- specific T cell responses. BALB/c mice ($n = 6$) were immunized as in **Figure 1**. The splenocytes were labeled with CFSE and cultured in the presence of pooled HIV-1 peptides (5 μM) to evaluate specific proliferation and cytokine production by multiparameter flow cytometry. After gating on proliferating ($CFSE^{low}$) and cytokine-producing cells, boolean combinations were created using FlowJo software to determine the frequency of each response based on all possible combinations of cytokine-producing $CD4^+$ T cells **(A,B)** and $CD8^+$ T cells **(C,D)** 15 and 60 days after the boost. Pie charts represent the proportion of T cells producing 1, 2, or all 3 cytokines. One million events were acquired in a live lymphocyte gate. Data were analyzed by two-way ANOVA followed by Bonferroni *post hoc* test.$^*p < 0.05$, $^{**}p < 0.01$; $^{***}p < 0.001$. Data represent mean ± SD and are representative of 3 independent experiments.

different pathogens in both mice and non-human primates (21–23, 33–39, 60).

Poly(I:C) is sensed by TLR3 and RLR receptors, and triggers up regulation of costimulatory molecules, strong type I IFN production by DCs and Th1 responses (32). Type I IFNs mediate the adjuvant effect of poly(I:C) acting as a third signal by promoting and sustaining clonal expansion of T cells (64–68). Indeed, our results demonstrate that immunization with αDECHIVBr8 along with poly(I:C) also induced higher frequency of proliferating $CD4^+$ and $CD8^+$ T cells. Moreover, we found that administration of the αDECHIVBr8 mAb concomitant with poly(I:C) induced higher frequency of specific polyfunctional T cells, i.e., cells that proliferated and simultaneously produced Th1 cytokines (IFNγ, IL2, and TNFα). Ours results corroborate with previous reports showing the development of polyfunctional T cells after HIV gag protein targeting to DCs along with poly(I:C) (21, 38, 62). Additionally, the presence of polyfunctional T cells is also a hallmark after vaccinia and yellow fever virus vaccinations (69, 70), and correlates with non-progressive HIV infection (71, 72). Recent HIV vaccine trials suggest that a broad (multiple specificities) and potent (high magnitude) response against conserved epitopes would be a desirable attribute of a T-cell based vaccine (73, 74). Indeed, vaccine induced broad T cell responses conferred protection after simian immunodeficiency virus challenge (75). We showed that poly(I:C) and MPL induced T cell responses against all epitopes (broad responses) present in the αDECHIVBr8 fusion mAb, although poly(I:C) was more potent. Likewise, Teixeira et al. demonstrated the ability of a bacterial adjuvant (*Propionibacterium acnes*) to expand the breath of a multiepitope DNA-based HIV vaccine (76).

A central feature of successful vaccines is their ability to induce immunological memory. Cross-sectional studies of smallpox and yellow fever vaccines showed that specific humoral and

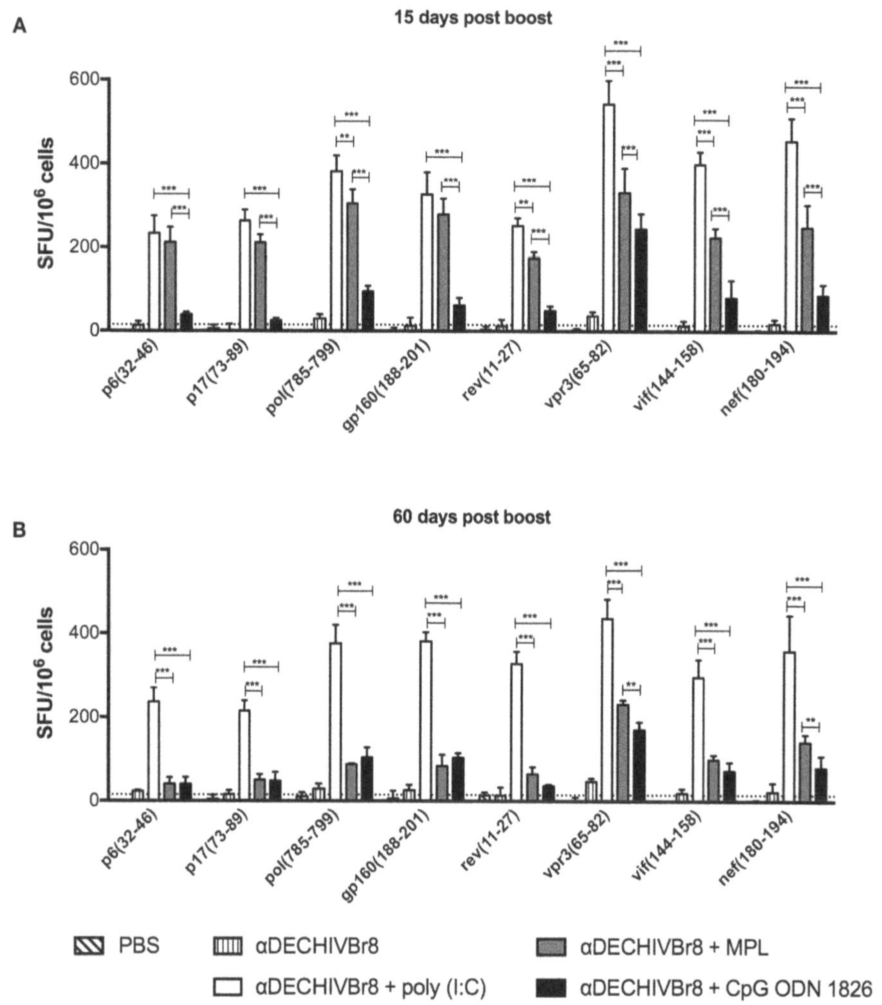

FIGURE 4 | Multiepitope DC targeting in the presence poly(I:C) induces broad T cell responses. BALB/c mice ($n = 6$) were immunized as described in **Figure 1**. **(A)** Fifteen and **(B)** 60 days after the boost the splenocytes were cultured with single HIV-1 peptides (5 μM) for 18 h to evaluate the number of IFN-γ producing cells by ELISpot assay. SFU, spot forming units. Cutoff = 15 SFU/10^6 cells and is represented by the dotted line. Data were analyzed by two-way ANOVA followed by Bonferroni *post hoc* test. $^{**}p < 0.01$; $^{***}p < 0.001$. Data represent mean ± SD and are representative of 4 independent experiments.

T cell responses can be detected for many years (77, 78). When we analyzed the longevity of the immune response, only poly(I:C) vaccine group had sustained T cell proliferation and IFNγ responses against all peptides ~2 months after the second immunization. It is important to note that MPL was the second most potent adjuvant tested and better to induce pro-inflammatory cytokines such as TNFα and IL-6. Previous reports provided evidence that MPL, a TLR2, and TLR4 agonist, is effective to induce TNFα, IL-10, and IL-12 production (44, 79). MPL induced a broad T cell response after the boost but narrowed after 2 months. Previous reports using αDEC205 mAb fused with HIV gag protein showed that MPL or LPS were as effective as poly(I:C) to induce specific humoral responses but less potent to induce Th1 $CD4^+$ T cell immunity (38, 51).

Interestingly, immunization with αDECHIVBr8 in the presence of CpG ODN induced weak T cell responses and narrowed epitope positivity. B class CpG ODN is a fully phosphorothioate TLR9 agonist that binds to surface DEC205 receptor (14, 15) and could therefore compete with the fusion αDEC205 mAb for cellular uptake. Our data are in line with a previous study demonstrating that immunization with αDEC-Gag plus CpG ODN 1826 induces lower frequency of responding $CD4^+$ T cells compared with poly(I:C) (51).

Anti-DECHIVBr8 combined with poly(I:C) was the most effective strategy to modulate DC activation by up regulating costimulatory molecules in a more pronounced way in the $CD11c^+$ $CD8\alpha^+$ subset but also in $CD11c^+$ $CD8\alpha^-$ DCs. This may be due to the fact that $CD8\alpha^+$ $DEC205^+$ DCs express higher levels of TLR3 when compared to $CD8\alpha^-$ DCs (2, 18, 80). As a consequence of DC maturation, poly(I:C) enhanced T cell immunity. As stated before, it was shown that poly(I:C) was most effective to induce Th1 $CD4^+$ T cell immunity compared to LPS or CpG ODN 1826 using the HIV gag targeted protein (51).

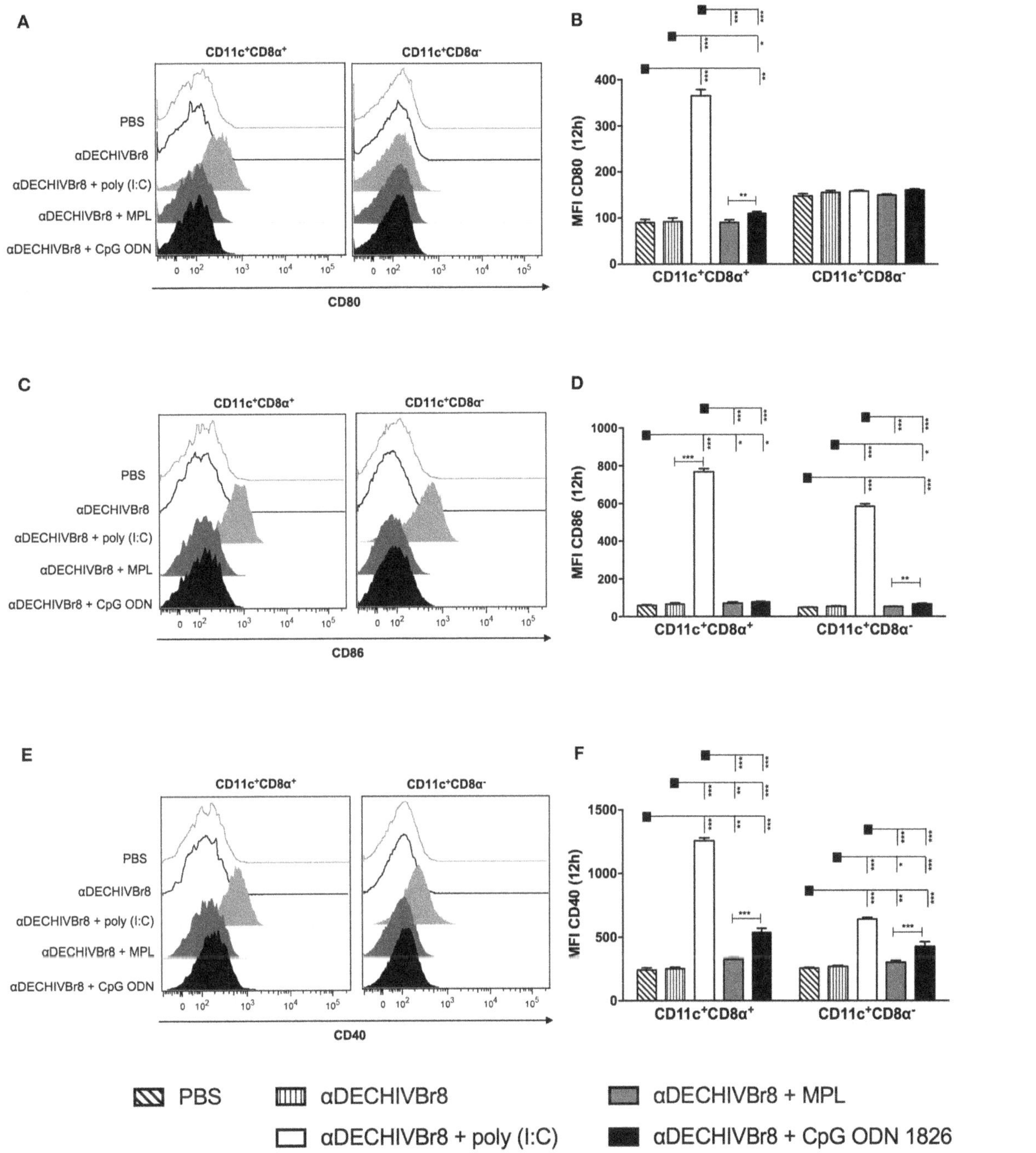

FIGURE 5 | DC targeting in the presence of different adjuvants modulates the expression of costimulatory molecules in splenic DC subsets. BALB/c mice ($n = 5$) were injected with 4 μg of αDECHIVBr8 plus poly(I:C), MPL or CpG ODN 1826. Control groups received αDECHIVBr8 only or PBS. After 12 h the splenocytes were labeled with fluorescent antibodies and 3 million events were acquired. Initial gating included a single cell gate followed by selection of $CD3^-CD19^-CD49b^-$ population. DCs were identified as $CD11c^+$ $IAIE^+$, subsequently gated on $CD8\alpha^+$ and $CD8\alpha^-$ and the median fluorescence intensity (MFI) of CD80 **(A,B)**, CD86 **(C,D)**, and CD40 **(E,F)** was determined in each DC subset. Data were analyzed by two-way ANOVA followed by Bonferroni *post hoc* test. $^*p < 0.05$, $^{**}p < 0.01$; $^{***}p < 0.001$. Data represent mean ± SD and are representative of 3 independent experiments.

The use of mouse model to select an adjuvant may be a caveat since the pattern of expression of TLR in the target DEC205$^+$ DC subset can differ between human and mouse (18). However, the adjuvant effect after antigen targeting does not necessarily rely on the direct activation of its respective TLR. For example, the effect of poly(I:C) on cDC1 is mediated by type I IFN receptor (51) suggesting that it is possible to have immune activation even if the targeted DC does not express a certain TLR.

Collectively, the observations demonstrate that combination of poly(I:C) with multiepitope targeting to DEC205$^+$ DCs modulates DC activation and elicits strong, broad, polyfunctional, and long-lived Th1 responses superior to other adjuvants both in quantity and quality. Therefore, the pursuit of a safe and effective T cell-based vaccine may benefit from the proper association of multiple epitope targeting to DC populations using a potent adjuvant formulation.

AUTHOR CONTRIBUTIONS

JA, SB, and DR conceived and designed the experiments. JA, VL, MY, and DR performed the experiments. JA, VL, and DR analyzed the data and prepared the figures. DR, SB, and EC-N contributed with reagents and materials. JA, VL, SB, and DR wrote the manuscript. SB, EC-N, and DR performed the final review of the article. All authors read and approved the final article.

ACKNOWLEDGMENTS

We thank Mr. Geová Santos for assistance in the animal facility.

REFERENCES

1. Lopez-Bravo M, Ardavin C. *In vivo* induction of immune responses to pathogens by conventional dendritic cells. *Immunity.* (2008) 29:343–51. doi: 10.1016/j.immuni.2008.08.008
2. Cohn L, Delamarre L. Dendritic cell-targeted vaccines. *Front Immunol.* (2014) 5:255. doi: 10.3389/fimmu.2014.00255
3. Iwasaki A, Medzhitov R. Control of adaptive immunity by the innate immune system. *Nat Immunol.* (2015) 16:343–53. doi: 10.1038/ni.3123
4. Joshi NS, Cui W, Chandele A, Lee HK, Urso DR, Hagman J, et al. Inflammation directs memory precursor and short-lived effector CD8(+) T cell fates via the graded expression of T-bet transcription factor. *Immunity.* (2007) 27:281–95. doi: 10.1016/j.immuni.2007.07.010
5. Sarkar S, Teichgraber V, Kalia V, Polley A, Masopust D, Harrington LE, et al. Strength of stimulus and clonal competition impact the rate of memory CD8 T cell differentiation. *J Immunol.* (2007) 179:6704–14. doi: 10.4049/jimmunol.179.10.6704
6. Shortman K, Naik SH. Steady-state and inflammatory dendritic-cell development. *Nat Rev Immunol.* (2007) 7:19–30. doi: 10.1038/nri1996
7. Villadangos JA, Schnorrer P. Intrinsic and cooperative antigen-presenting functions of dendritic-cell subsets *in vivo*. *Nat Rev Immunol.* (2007) 7:543–55. doi: 10.1038/nri2103
8. Steinman RM, Idoyaga J. Features of the dendritic cell lineage. *Immunol Rev.* (2010) 234:5–17. doi: 10.1111/j.0105-2896.2009.00888.x
9. Guilliams M, Ginhoux F, Jakubzick C, Naik SH, Onai N, Schraml BU, et al. Dendritic cells, monocytes and macrophages: a unified nomenclature based on ontogeny. *Nat Rev Immunol.* (2014) 14:571–8. doi: 10.1038/nri3712
10. Guilliams M, Dutertre CA, Scott CL, McGovern N, Sichien D, Chakarov S, et al. Unsupervised high-dimensional analysis aligns dendritic cells across tissues and species. *Immunity.* (2016) 45:669–84. doi: 10.1016/j.immuni.2016.08.015
11. Kraal G, Breel M, Janse M, Bruin G. Langerhans' cells, veiled cells, and interdigitating cells in the mouse recognized by a monoclonal antibody. *J Exp Med.* (1986) 163:981–97.
12. Inaba K, Swiggard WJ, Inaba M, Meltzer J, Mirza A, Sasagawa T, et al. Tissue distribution of the DEC-205 protein that is detected by the monoclonal antibody NLDC-145. I Expression on dendritic cells and other subsets of mouse leukocytes. *Cell Immunol.* (1995) 163:148–56.
13. Merad M, Sathe P, Helft J, Miller J, Mortha A. The dendritic cell lineage: ontogeny and function of dendritic cells and their subsets in the steady state and the inflamed setting. *Annu Rev Immunol.* (2013) 31:563–604. doi: 10.1146/annurev-immunol-020711-074950
14. Lahoud MH, Ahmet F, Zhang JG, Meuter S, Policheni AN, Kitsoulis S, et al. DEC-205 is a cell surface receptor for CpG oligonucleotides. *Proc Natl Acad Sci USA.* (2012) 109:16270–5. doi: 10.1073/pnas.1208796109
15. Caminschi I, Meuter S, Heath WR. DEC-205 is a cell surface receptor for CpG oligonucleotides. *Oncoimmunology.* (2013) 2:e23128. doi: 10.4161/onci.23128
16. Trumpfheller C, Longhi MP, Caskey M, Idoyaga J, Bozzacco L, Keler T, et al. Dendritic cell-targeted protein vaccines: a novel approach to induce T-cell immunity. *J Intern Med.* (2012) 271:183–92. doi: 10.1111/j.1365-2796.2011.02496.x
17. Apostolopoulos V, Thalhammer T, Tzakos AG, Stojanovska L. Targeting antigens to dendritic cell receptors for vaccine development. *J Drug Deliv.* (2013) 2013:869718. doi: 10.1155/2013/869718
18. Kastenmuller W, Kastenmuller K, Kurts C, Seder RA. Dendritic cell-targeted vaccines–hope or hype? *Nat Rev Immunol.* (2014) 14:705–11. doi: 10.1038/nri3727
19. Park CG. Vaccine strategies utilizing C-type lectin receptors on dendritic cells *in vivo*. *Clin Exp Vaccine Res.* (2014) 3:149–54. doi: 10.7774/cevr.2014.3.2.149
20. Macri C, Dumont C, Johnston AP, Mintern JD. Targeting dendritic cells: a promising strategy to improve vaccine effectiveness. *Clin Transl Immunol.* (2016) 5:e66. doi: 10.1038/cti.2016.6
21. Trumpfheller C, Finke JS, Lopez CB, Moran TM, Moltedo B, Soares H, et al. Intensified and protective CD4+ T cell immunity in mice with anti-dendritic cell HIV gag fusion antibody vaccine. *J Exp Med.* (2006) 203:607–17. doi: 10.1084/jem.20052005
22. Do Y, Koh H, Park CG, Dudziak D, Seo P, Mehandru S, et al. Targeting of LcrV virulence protein from Yersinia pestis to dendritic cells protects mice against pneumonic plague. *Eur J Immunol.* (2010) 40:2791–6. doi: 10.1002/eji.201040511
23. Lakhrif Z, Moreau A, Herault B, Di-Tommaso A, Juste M, Moire N, et al. Targeted delivery of *Toxoplasma gondii* antigens to dendritic cells promote immunogenicity and protective efficiency against toxoplasmosis. *Front Immunol.* (2018) 9:317. doi: 10.3389/fimmu.2018.00317
24. Hawiger D, Inaba K, Dorsett Y, Guo M, Mahnke K, Rivera M, et al. Dendritic cells induce peripheral T cell unresponsiveness under steady state conditions *in vivo*. *J Exp Med.* (2001) 194:769–79. doi: 10.1084/jem.194.6.769
25. Bonifaz L, Bonnyay D, Mahnke K, Rivera M, Nussenzweig MC, Steinman RM. Efficient targeting of protein antigen to the dendritic cell receptor DEC-205 in the steady state leads to antigen presentation on major histocompatibility complex class I products and peripheral CD8+ T cell tolerance. *J Exp Med.* (2002) 196:1627–38. doi: 10.1084/jem.20021598
26. Boscardin SB, Hafalla JC, Masilamani RF, Kamphorst AO, Zebroski HA, Rai U, et al. Antigen targeting to dendritic cells elicits long-lived T cell help for antibody responses. *J Exp Med.* (2006) 203:599–606. doi: 10.1084/jem.20051639
27. Coffman RL, Sher A, Seder RA. Vaccine adjuvants: putting innate immunity to work. *Immunity.* (2010) 33:492–503. doi: 10.1016/j.immuni.2010.10.002
28. Kwissa M, Nakaya HI, Oluoch H, Pulendran B. Distinct TLR adjuvants differentially stimulate systemic and local innate immune responses in nonhuman primates. *Blood.* (2012) 119:2044–55. doi: 10.1182/blood-2011-10-388579
29. Gutjahr A, Tiraby G, Perouzel E, Verrier B, Paul S. Triggering intracellular receptors for vaccine adjuvantation. *Trends Immunol.* (2016) 37:P716. doi: 10.1016/j.it.2016.08.005
30. McElrath MJ. Adjuvants: tailoring humoral immune responses. *Curr Opin HIV AIDS.* (2017) 12:278–84. doi: 10.1097/COH.0000000000000365
31. Hemmi H, Akira S. TLR signalling and the function of dendritic cells. *Chem Immunol Allergy.* (2005) 86:120–35. doi: 10.1159/000086657

32. Martins KA, Bavari S, Salazar AM. Vaccine adjuvant uses of poly-IC and derivatives. *Exp Rev Vaccines.* (2015) 14:447–59. doi: 10.1586/14760584.2015.966085
33. Henriques HR, Rampazo EV, Goncalves AJ, Vicentin EC, Amorim JH, Panatieri RH, et al. Targeting the non-structural protein 1 from dengue virus to a dendritic cell population confers protective immunity to lethal virus challenge. *PLoS Negl Trop Dis.* (2013) 7:e2330. doi: 10.1371/journal.pntd.0002330
34. Rampazo EV, Amorim KN, Yamamoto MM, Panatieri RH, Rodrigues MM, Boscardin SB. Antigen targeting to dendritic cells allows the identification of a CD4 T-cell epitope within an immunodominant *Trypanosoma cruzi* antigen. *PLoS ONE.* (2015) 10:e0117778. doi: 10.1371/journal.pone.0117778
35. Tewari K, Flynn BJ, Boscardin SB, Kastenmueller K, Salazar AM, Anderson CA, et al. Poly(I:C) is an effective adjuvant for antibody and multi-functional CD4+ T cell responses to Plasmodium falciparum circumsporozoite protein (CSP) and alphaDEC-CSP in non human primates. *Vaccine.* (2010) 28:7256–66. doi: 10.1016/j.vaccine.2010.08.098
36. Amorim KN, Rampazo EV, Antonialli R, Yamamoto MM, Rodrigues MM, Soares IS, et al. The presence of T cell epitopes is important for induction of antibody responses against antigens directed to DEC205(+) dendritic cells. *Sci Rep.* (2016) 6:39250. doi: 10.1038/srep39250
37. Silva-Sanchez A, Meza-Perez S, Flores-Langarica A, Donis-Maturano L, Estrada-Garcia I, Calderon-Amador J, et al. ESAT-6 targeting to DEC205+ Antigen presenting cells induces specific-T cell responses against ESAT-6 and reduces pulmonary infection with virulent *Mycobacterium tuberculosis*. *PLoS ONE.* (2015) 10:e0124828. doi: 10.1371/journal.pone.0124828
38. Trumpfheller C, Caskey M, Nchinda G, Longhi MP, Mizenina O, Huang Y, et al. The microbial mimic poly IC induces durable and protective CD4+ T cell immunity together with a dendritic cell targeted vaccine. *Proc Natl Acad Sci USA.* (2008) 105:2574–9. doi: 10.1073/pnas.0711976105
39. Apostolico JS, Lunardelli VA, Yamamoto MM, Souza HF, Cunha-Neto E, Boscardin SB, et al. Dendritic cell targeting effectively boosts T cell responses elicited by an HIV multiepitope DNA vaccine. *Front Immunol.* (2017) 8:101. doi: 10.3389/fimmu.2017.00101
40. Gurer C, Strowig T, Brilot F, Pack M, Trumpfheller C, Arrey F, et al. Targeting the nuclear antigen 1 of Epstein-Barr virus to the human endocytic receptor DEC-205 stimulates protective T-cell responses. *Blood.* (2008) 112:1231–9. doi: 10.1182/blood-2008-03-148072
41. Dhodapkar MV, Sznol M, Zhao B, Wang D, Carvajal RD, Keohan ML, et al. Induction of antigen-specific immunity with a vaccine targeting NY-ESO-1 to the dendritic cell receptor DEC-205. *Sci Transl Med.* (2014) 6:232ra251. doi: 10.1126/scitranslmed.3008068
42. Griffiths EA, Srivastava P, Matsuzaki J, Brumberger Z, Wang ES, Kocent J, et al. NY-ESO-1 vaccination in combination with decitabine induces antigen-specific T-lymphocyte responses in patients with myelodysplastic syndrome. *Clin Cancer Res.* (2018) 24:1019–29. doi: 10.1158/1078-0432.CCR-17-1792
43. Thompson BS, Chilton PM, Ward JR, Evans JT, Mitchell TC. The low-toxicity versions of LPS, MPL adjuvant and RC529, are efficient adjuvants for CD4+ T cells. *J Leukoc Biol.* (2005) 78:1273–80. doi: 10.1189/jlb.0305172
44. Mata-Haro V, Cekic C, Martin M, Chilton PM, Casella CR, Mitchell TC. The vaccine adjuvant monophosphoryl lipid A as a TRIF-biased agonist of TLR4. *Science.* (2007) 316:1628–32. doi: 10.1126/science.1138963
45. Gandhapudi SK, Chilton PM, Mitchell TC. TRIF is required for TLR4 mediated adjuvant effects on T cell clonal expansion. *PLoS ONE.* (2013) 8:e56855. doi: 10.1371/journal.pone.0056855
46. Garcon N, Di Pasquale A. From discovery to licensure, the adjuvant system story. *Hum Vaccin Immunother.* (2017) 13:19–33. doi: 10.1080/21645515.2016.1225635
47. Hemmi H, Kaisho T, Takeda K, Akira S. The roles of Toll-like receptor 9, MyD88, and DNA-dependent protein kinase catalytic subunit in the effects of two distinct CpG DNAs on dendritic cell subsets. *J Immunol.* (2003) 170:3059–64. doi: 10.4049/jimmunol.170.6.3059
48. Mutwiri GK, Nichani AK, Babiuk S, Babiuk LA. Strategies for enhancing the immunostimulatory effects of CpG oligodeoxynucleotides. *J Control Release.* (2004) 97:1–17. doi: 10.1016/j.jconrel.2004.02.022
49. Barry M, Cooper C. Review of hepatitis B surface antigen-1018 ISS adjuvant-containing vaccine safety and efficacy. *Expert Opin Biol Ther.* (2007) 7:1731–7. doi: 10.1517/14712598.7.11.1731
50. Shirota, H., and Klinman, D. M. (2017). "CpG Oligodeoxynucleotides as adjuvants for clinical use," in *Immunopotentiators in Modern Vaccines,* eds V.Schijns, and D. O'Hagan (Cambridge, MA: Academic Press), 167–198.
51. Longhi MP, Trumpfheller C, Idoyaga J, Caskey M, Matos I, Kluger C, et al. Dendritic cells require a systemic type I interferon response to mature and induce CD4+ Th1 immunity with poly IC as adjuvant. *J Exp Med.* (2009) 206:1589–602. doi: 10.1084/jem.20090247
52. Antonialli R, Sulczewski FB, Amorim K, Almeida BDS, Ferreira NS, Yamamoto MM, et al. CpG oligodeoxinucleotides and flagellin modulate the immune response to antigens targeted to CD8alpha(+) and CD8alpha(-) conventional dendritic cell subsets. *Front Immunol.* (2017) 8:1727. doi: 10.3389/fimmu.2017.01727
53. Apostolico Jde S, Boscardin SB, Yamamoto MM, de Oliveira-Filho JN, Kalil J, Cunha-Neto E, et al. HIV envelope trimer specific immune response is influenced by different adjuvant formulations and heterologous prime-boost. *PLoS ONE.* (2016) 11:e0145637. doi: 10.1371/journal.pone.0145637
54. Rosa DS, Ribeiro SP, Almeida RR, Mairena EC, Postol E, Kalil J, et al. A DNA vaccine encoding multiple HIV CD4 epitopes elicits vigorous polyfunctional, long-lived CD4+ and CD8+ T cell responses. *PLoS ONE.* (2011) 6:e16921. doi: 10.1371/journal.pone.0016921
55. Bonifaz LC, Bonnyay DP, Charalambous A, Darguste DI, Fujii S, Soares H, et al. *In vivo* targeting of antigens to maturing dendritic cells via the DEC-205 receptor improves T cell vaccination. *J Exp Med.* (2004) 199:815–24. doi: 10.1084/jem.20032220
56. Dudziak D, Kamphorst AO, Heidkamp GF, Buchholz VR, Trumpfheller C, Yamazaki S, et al. Differential antigen processing by dendritic cell subsets *in vivo*. *Science.* (2007) 315:107–11. doi: 10.1126/science.1136080
57. Kwissa M, Kasturi SP, Pulendran B. The science of adjuvants. *Expert Rev Vaccines.* (2007) 6:673–84. doi: 10.1586/14760584.6.5.673
58. Apostolico Jde S, Lunardelli VA, Coirada FC, Boscardin SB, Rosa DS. Adjuvants: classification, modus operandi, and licensing. *J Immunol Res.* (2016) 2016:1459394. doi: 10.1155/2016/1459394
59. Cheong C, Choi JH, Vitale L, He LZ, Trumpfheller C, Bozzacco L, et al. Improved cellular and humoral immune responses *in vivo* following targeting of HIV Gag to dendritic cells within human anti-human DEC205 monoclonal antibody. *Blood.* (2010) 116:3828–38. doi: 10.1182/blood-2010-06-288068
60. Flynn BJ, Kastenmuller K, Wille-Reece U, Tomaras GD, Alam M, Lindsay RW, et al. Immunization with HIV Gag targeted to dendritic cells followed by recombinant New York vaccinia virus induces robust T-cell immunity in nonhuman primates. *Proc Natl Acad Sci USA.* (2011) 108:7131–6. doi: 10.1073/pnas.1103869108
61. Idoyaga J, Lubkin A, Fiorese C, Lahoud MH, Caminschi I, Huang Y, et al. Comparable T helper 1 (Th1) and CD8 T-cell immunity by targeting HIV gag p24 to CD8 dendritic cells within antibodies to Langerin, DEC205, and Clec9A. *Proc Natl Acad Sci USA.* (2011) 108:2384–9. doi: 10.1073/pnas.1019547108
62. Ruane D, Do Y, Brane L, Garg A, Bozzacco L, Kraus T, et al. A dendritic cell targeted vaccine induces long-term HIV-specific immunity within the gastrointestinal tract. *Mucosal Immunol.* (2016) 9:1340–52. doi: 10.1038/mi.2015.133
63. Baumgartner CK, Malherbe LP. Regulation of CD4 T-cell receptor diversity by vaccine adjuvants. *Immunology.* (2010) 130:16–22. doi: 10.1111/j.1365-2567.2010.03265.x
64. Marrack P, Kappler J, Mitchell T. Type I interferons keep activated T cells alive. *J Exp Med.* (1999) 189:521–30.
65. Curtsinger JM, Valenzuela JO, Agarwal P, Lins D, Mescher MF. Type I IFNs provide a third signal to CD8 T cells to stimulate clonal expansion and differentiation. *J Immunol.* (2005) 174:4465–9.
66. Havenar-Daughton C, Kolumam GA, Murali-Krishna K. Cutting edge: the direct action of type I IFN on CD4 T cells is critical for sustaining clonal expansion in response to a viral but not a bacterial infection. *J Immunol.* (2006) 176:3315–9. doi: 10.4049/jimmunol.176.6.3315

67. Wiesel M, Kratky W, Oxenius A. Type I IFN substitutes for T cell help during viral infections. *J Immunol.* (2011) 186:754–63. doi: 10.4049/jimmunol.1003166
68. Wiesel M, Crouse J, Bedenikovic G, Sutherland A, Joller N, Oxenius A. Type-I IFN drives the differentiation of short-lived effector CD8+ T cells *in vivo*. *Eur J Immunol.* (2012) 42:320–9. doi: 10.1002/eji.201142091
69. Precopio ML, Betts MR, Parrino J, Price DA, Gostick E, Ambrozak DR, et al. Immunization with vaccinia virus induces polyfunctional and phenotypically distinctive CD8(+) T cell responses. *J Exp Med.* (2007) 204:1405–16. doi: 10.1084/jem.20062363
70. Gaucher D, Therrien R, Kettaf N, Angermann BR, Boucher G, Filali-Mouhim A, et al. Yellow fever vaccine induces integrated multilineage and polyfunctional immune responses. *J Exp Med.* (2008) 205:3119–31. doi: 10.1084/jem.20082292
71. Harari A, Petitpierre S, Vallelian F, Pantaleo G. Skewed representation of functionally distinct populations of virus-specific CD4 T cells in HIV-1-infected subjects with progressive disease: changes after antiretroviral therapy. *Blood.* (2004) 103:966–72. doi: 10.1182/blood-2003-04-1203
72. Kannanganat S, Kapogiannis BG, Ibegbu C, Chennareddi L, Goepfert P, Robinson HL, et al. Human immunodeficiencyvirus type 1 controllers but not noncontrollers maintain CD4 T cells coexpressing three cytokines. *J Virol.* (2007) 81:12071–6. doi: 10.1128/JVI.01261-07
73. McElrath MJ, Haynes BF. Induction of immunity to human immunodeficiency virus type-1 by vaccination. *Immunity.* (2010) 33:542–54. doi: 10.1016/j.immuni.2010.09.011
74. Sahay B, Nguyen CQ, Yamamoto JK. Conserved HIV epitopes for an effective HIV vaccine. *J Clin Cell Immunol.* (2017) 8:518. doi: 10.4172/2155-9899.1000518
75. Wilson NA, Keele BF, Reed JS, Piaskowski SM, MacNair CE, Bett AJ, et al. Vaccine-induced cellular responses control simian immunodeficiency virus replication after heterologous challenge. *J Virol.* (2009) 83:6508–21. doi: 10.1128/JVI.00272-09
76. Teixeira D, Ishimura ME, Apostolico JS, Viel JM, Passarelli VC, Cunha-Neto E, et al. *Propionibacterium acnes* enhances the immunogenicity of HIVBr18 human immunodeficiency virus-1 vaccine. *Front Immunol.* (2018) 9:177. doi: 10.3389/fimmu.2018.00177
77. Akondy RS, Monson ND, Miller JD, Edupuganti S, Teuwen D, Wu H, et al. The yellow fever virus vaccine induces a broad and polyfunctional human memory CD8+ T cell response. *J Immunol.* (2009) 183:7919–30. doi: 10.4049/jimmunol.0803903
78. Wang M, Tang ST, Lund O, Dziegiel MH, Buus S, Claesson MH. High-affinity human leucocyte antigen class I binding variola-derived peptides induce CD4+ T cell responses more than 30 years post-vaccinia virus vaccination. *Clin Exp Immunol.* (2009) 155:441–6. doi: 10.1111/j.1365-2249.2008.03856.x
79. Martin M, Michalek SM, Katz J. Role of innate immune factors in the adjuvant activity of monophosphoryl lipid A. *Infect Immun.* (2003) 71:2498–507. doi: 10.1128/IAI.71.5.2498-2507.2003
80. Edwards AD, Diebold SS, Slack EM, Tomizawa H, Hemmi H, Kaisho T, et al. Toll-like receptor expression in murine DC subsets: lack of TLR7 expression by CD8 alpha+ DC correlates with unresponsiveness to imidazoquinolines. *Eur J Immunol.* (2003) 33:827–33. doi: 10.1002/eji.200323797

3

CD169$^+$ Macrophages Capture and Dendritic Cells Instruct: The Interplay of the Gatekeeper and the General of the Immune System

*Joanna Grabowska†, Miguel A. Lopez-Venegas†, Alsya J. Affandi and Joke M. M. den Haan**

Department of Molecular Cell Biology and Immunology, Amsterdam University Medical Center, Cancer Center Amsterdam, Amsterdam Infection and Immunity Institute, Vrije Universiteit Amsterdam, Amsterdam, Netherlands

***Correspondence:**
Joke M. M. den Haan
j.denhaan@vumc.nl

†These authors share first authorship

Since the seminal discovery of dendritic cells (DCs) by Steinman and Cohn in 1973, there has been an ongoing debate to what extent macrophages and DCs are related and perform different functions. The current view is that macrophages and DCs originate from different lineages and that only DCs have the capacity to initiate adaptive immunity. Nevertheless, as we will discuss in this review, lymphoid tissue resident CD169$^+$ macrophages have been shown to act in concert with DCs to promote or suppress adaptive immune responses for pathogens and self-antigens, respectively. Accordingly, we propose a functional alliance between CD169$^+$ macrophages and DCs in which a division of tasks is established. CD169$^+$ macrophages are responsible for the capture of pathogens and are frequently the first cell type infected and thereby provide a confined source of antigen. Subsequently, cross-presenting DCs interact with these antigen-containing CD169$^+$ macrophages, pick up antigens and activate T cells. The cross priming of T cells by DCs is enhanced by the localized production of type I interferons (IFN-I) derived from CD169$^+$ macrophages and plasmacytoid DCs (pDCs) that induces DC maturation. The interaction between CD169$^+$ macrophages and DCs appears not only to be essential for immune responses against pathogens, but also plays a role in the induction of self-tolerance and immune responses against cancer. In this review we will discuss the studies that demonstrate the collaboration between CD169$^+$ macrophages and DCs in adaptive immunity.

Keywords: CD169, siglec-1, sialoadhesin, macrophages, dendritic cells, T cell, antigen, cross-presentation

INTRODUCTION

While the first recognized characteristic of macrophages was their excellent capacity to phagocytose, dendritic cells (DCs) were acknowledged for their superior ability to stimulate naïve T cell responses. However, ever since tissue macrophages and DCs showed overlapping expression of several markers and were both generated from monocytes in *in vitro* models, it has been debated whether these cell types were closely related and had equivalent functions. The introduction of unbiased single cell multi-parameter analyses on the protein and RNA level, and the generation of cell-type specific and inducible genetically modified mouse models has enabled a new understanding of the generation and functions of both macrophages and DCs, and has even led to a new nomenclature (1). The current view is that the two cell types have very different functions in the immune system. However, this viewpoint potentially overlooks functional collaborations between the two cell types. In this review we will focus on the interactions between lymphoid tissue resident CD169$^+$ macrophages and DCs and how these support the activation of adaptive immune responses.

DCs and Macrophages Are Different Cell Types With Different Functions

The generation of macrophages is dependent on the growth factor M-CSF and occurs in three waves [reviewed by (2, 3)]. First, during early embryonic development, yolk sac-derived progenitors seed several peripheral tissues, such as the brain and the epidermis. A second wave of progenitors derive from the fetal liver and seed lungs and liver. These two types of macrophages are characterized by high expression of F4/80 and in general reconstitute autonomously. Additionally, they are thought to have a long half-life and exhibit local proliferation. After birth, monocytes develop from hematopoietic stem cells in the bone marrow and tissues, such as the intestines and the skin that continuously receive monocytes to generate macrophages. The latter macrophages generally express low levels of F4/80.

Macrophages form a very heterogeneous population of cells and their diversity in phenotype and function is a reflection of the variety of the tissues in which they reside [reviewed by (4, 5)]. They are best known for their capacity to phagocytose and eliminate pathogens and to alarm the immune system. In addition to this important function in immunosurveillance, they are essential for the clearance of apoptotic cells and suppression of (auto) immune responses and mediate resolution of inflammatory responses and tissue repair. Furthermore, depending on their tissue of residence, macrophages have important specialized functions in development, homeostasis and metabolism [discussed in more detail in (4, 6)]. The general view is that macrophages exert their functions locally in the tissues and that in steady state tissue resident macrophages do not migrate to secondary lymph nodes to activate naïve T cells. This latter function is attributed to DCs that also reside in tissues, but upon pathogen recognition, upregulate CCR7 and travel to the lymphoid organs. However, upon inflammation monocyte-derived macrophages or DCs may also acquire the capacity to travel to the lymph nodes and stimulate T cells, which is a matter that has to be further clarified (7).

Currently, three types of DCs are being recognized [reviewed by (8, 9)]. Conventional or classical DCs (cDCs) are continuously generated in the bone marrow and require Flt3L for their generation. Pre-cDCs seed the tissues and the lymphoid organs and have a half-life of 5–7 days. Upon activation and upregulation of CCR7, tissue cDCs migrate to the lymph nodes and can activate T cells. Within cDCs two subsets can be identified. The cDC1 is more specialized in the uptake of dying cells, cross-presentation and activation of CD8$^+$ T cells, while cDC2 has a more important role in CD4$^+$ T cell activation and B cell responses. The generation of these two subsets is dependent on different transcription factors. While cDC1 requires Batf3, Id2 and Irf8, cDC2 development depends on Irf4 and RelB and requires additional Notch2 and vitamin A signals (10). With regard to the surface phenotype, cDC1 can be identified by XCR1 and CLEC9A, and additionally by CD8α in lymphoid organs and by CD103 in peripheral tissues. On the other hand, Sirpα, CD11b and CD4 expression marks the cDC2 subset. Next to cDCs, pDCs form another class of DCs that also develop in a Flt3L-dependent manner. This lineage splits from the cDC lineage before the separation in cDC1 and cDC2. They can be identified by CD123, BDCA2, and BDCA4 in humans and by high expression of BST2 and Siglec-H and by low expression of CD11c and B220 in the mouse. Recent studies have indicated further heterogeneity in CD123-expressing pDCs (11, 12). While early studies indicate that pDCs can take up antigens and stimulate T cells upon activation, recent studies suggest that very pure pDC populations only produce IFN-I and are not able to activate T cells unless they are pre-treated with CD40L and IL-3 (13). This suggests a limited function for pDC in T cell activation.

Next to these two Flt3L-dependent DC subsets, DCs can differentiate from monocytes during inflammatory conditions (7). The function of these DCs in the regulation of adaptive immune responses remains to be elucidated.

Antigen Cross-Presentation by Macrophages and Dendritic Cells

Both macrophages and DCs process antigens via the classical endogenous and exogenous pathways and present these on their MHC class I and II molecules, respectively, but they differ in their capacity to cross-present exogenous antigens in MHC class I and to cross-prime CD8$^+$ T cells. Cross-presentation was first described in 1976 by Bevan as the process in which CD8$^+$ T cell responses were initiated against donor antigens restricted by recipient MHC molecules (14). This process is thought to be essential in the activation of anti-viral and anti-tumor specific CD8$^+$ T cell responses. While a number of studies have shown that exogenous antigens can be cross-presented by different cell types including macrophages (15), the mouse cDC1 subset exhibits a higher capacity to cross-present and is especially equipped for the uptake of dead cells and the cross-presentation of cell-associated antigens (16–19). However, depending on the antigen and activation stimuli, mouse cDC2 and several human DC subsets are also able to cross-present (17, 20). There are two main routes of antigen processing exist that leads to cross-presentation. In the cytosolic route, antigens are transported from the endosomal/phagosomal pathway to the cytoplasm and this pathway depends on proteasomes and TAP. In the vacuolar route, antigens are degraded in the endosomal/phagosomal pathway and bind to recycling MHC class I molecules. This pathway relies on the activity of cathepsin S. DCs mainly utilize the cytosolic route, while macrophages and monocyte-derived DCs have been shown to use the vacuolar route of cross-presentation (21, 22). Recent studies have identified a number of molecules involved in vesicular trafficking that play a role in cross-presentation [see for more details reviews (15, 23, 24)]. One of the important factors for cross-presentation is the rate of antigen degradation. Macrophages are more proteolytically active than DCs, which impairs their capacity to cross-present (25). DCs prevent the acidification of their phagosomes and thereby inhibit proteolysis by the activity of NADPH oxidase 2 (NOX2) enzyme [reviewed in (26)]. The NOX2 enzyme may also contribute to the translocation of antigens to the cytosol by disrupting the phagosomal membrane. The longer preservation of antigens in DCs and stronger phagosome-cytotosol translocation compared to macrophages may be responsible for the more prominent role of DCs in cross-priming.

Generation of CD169$^+$ Macrophages and Their Innate Functions

Macrophages expressing high levels of CD169, also known as Siglec-1 or sialoadheasin, constitute a minor macrophage population present in lymphoid tissues (27, 28). While several macrophage populations in tissues have low levels of CD169, which can be upregulated upon exposure to IFN-I, this lymphoid resident population has a very high constitutive expression of CD169. CD169$^+$ macrophages are situated on top of B cell follicles bordering the marginal sinus in the spleen and the subcapsular sinus (SCS) in the lymph nodes and are also known as metallophilic marginal zone macrophages and SCS macrophages, respectively. The presence of B cells is necessary for the generation of CD169$^+$ macrophages, which is mediated by their production of LTα1β2 (29, 30). In addition, they require RANK, LXR, and M-CSF signals and their survival is further promoted by TNF-α (31–34). Currently it is unclear which precursor gives rise to CD169$^+$ macrophages, although their low level of F4/80 expression would suggest that they are not derived from yolk sac precursors. After elimination, they are repopulated from monocytes (34).

The strategic position of CD169$^+$ macrophages at the entry site of lymphoid tissues determines their function. CD169$^+$ macrophages are the first cell type in the spleen and lymph nodes to bind particulate antigens and pathogens and they function as a filter to remove foreign particles from the lymph fluid and blood. When these cells are deleted by clodronate liposomes in an experimental setting, pathogens can disseminate to other organs as has been demonstrated for several viral, bacterial and parasitic infections (35–39). This particular observation coined the term "gatekeeper" to describe CD169$^+$ macrophages. This first line of defense, capturing invading viruses and limiting their spread to other organs, is not only mediated via the physical binding and capture of pathogens. CD169$^+$ macrophages also exert their protective functions by the production of cytokines, such as IFN-I, IL-1, and IL-18. This cytokine secretion not only prevents subsequent infection of other cells and activates innate lymphocytes that help to contain the early infection (40–42), but also acts on DCs and stimulate adaptive immune responses.

Model Systems to Study CD169$^+$ Macrophages

Due to their low abundance and sensitivity to manipulation, CD169$^+$ macrophages are quite an enigmatic and technically challenging subset to study. Although it is feasible to extract these cells from spleen or lymph nodes by combination of mechanistic dissociation and enzymatic digestion, they rapidly die and form apoptotic blebs that bind to interacting cells (41, 43, 44). This feature greatly hampers the purification of CD169$^+$ macrophages using fluorescence-activated cell sorting (FACS) for *in vitro* analysis. Unfortunately, available *in vitro* models do not offer a satisfactory method to investigate this macrophage population. *In vitro* cultured macrophages can be treated with IFN-α, which induces CD169 expression on the cell surface, but it is not clear whether these cells exhibit other characteristics of the CD169$^+$ macrophages present *in vivo*. Most studies investigating CD169$^+$ macrophages take advantage of cell ablation tools, either chemical using clodronate liposomes or genetic using diphtheria toxin receptor (DTR) systems. Despite representing a very effective method for transient depletion of macrophages, clodronate liposomes lack specificity. This apoptosis-inducing agent is toxic for all phagocytosing cells including monocytes and DCs (45). Noteworthy, the treatment with clodronate liposomes affects the anatomy of the surrounding tissue and induces off-target effects on B cells (46). In comparison to clodronate liposomes, DTR-mediated cell ablation allows for conditional and targeted depletion of a cell subset engineered to express DTR. CD11c-DTR and CD169-DTR are two DTR transgenic mouse strains that deplete CD169$^+$ macrophages (47, 48). Although the CD11c-DTR model mainly depletes cells with high expression of CD11c, thus DCs, it does not spare macrophages that express low levels of this DC marker (49). The CD169-DTR model, on the other hand provides a more specific approach to study CD169$^+$ macrophages, leaving the DC population unaffected. The only other population affected by DT treatment in CD169-DTR model, are SIGN-R1$^+$ marginal zone macrophages that express low levels of CD169 (47). Similarly, the LXR-α KO lack both CD169$^+$ and SIGNR1$^+$ splenic marginal zone macrophage subsets (34). More recently, CD169-Cre mice have been generated and when crossed to the ROSA26-YFP mice generate reporter mice (50). The CD169-Cre mice will allow the generation of CD169-specific conditional KO mice and is therefore expected to provide a wealth of new insights for this macrophage population.

CD169$^+$ MACROPHAGES AND IFN-I PRODUCTION

Upon encounter with pathogens, such as viruses, CD169$^+$ macrophages regulate pathogen spread and induce immune responses by producing IFN-I. IFN-I consist of a single IFN-β and several subtypes of IFN-α, that signal through IFN-I receptor, a shared receptor expressed in almost all cell types (51). The importance of IFN-I signaling is 2-fold: (1) IFN-I can induce intracellular antiviral responses to suppress viral replication in the infected cells (52), and (2) IFN-I can regulate both innate and adaptive immune responses that are required to clear pathogens. However, depending on the type of pathogen, the outcome of IFN-I actions can play both protective and detrimental roles to the host (53, 54).

Viral Infection of CD169+ Macrophages Results in IFN-I Production

CD169+ macrophages rapidly produce IFN-I after infection and thereby restrict the spread of a variety of viruses including mouse cytomegaloviruses (CMV), herpesvirus, and lymphocytic choriomeningitis virus (LCMV) (55–58). Several studies using neurotropic vesicular stomatitis virus (VSV) infection show that IFN-I signaling is necessary for the survival of the mice. Upon VSV infection, IFN-I was shown to be largely produced by CD169+ macrophages and this prevented VSV from entering the central nervous system (38). Similarly, during experimental infection with recombinant modified vaccinia virus Ankara (MVA), CD169+ macrophages were found to be the main IFN-I producers (59). In this model, CD169+ macrophages recruited and activated NK cells upon MVA infection, which was dependent on the production of IFN-I by CD169+ macrophages. Additionally, MVA infection also induced inflammasome activation by CD169+ macrophages that led to pyroptotic cell death, cytokine burst, and recruitment of inflammatory cells (60).

CD169+ Macrophages Recruit and Prime IFN-I Production by pDCs

Next to CD169+ macrophages, pDCs are well-known for their capacity to produce IFN-I. They express TLR7 and TLR9 and high basal levels of IRF7 that allows them to detect intracellular nucleic acids and to produce IFN-α immediately upon encounter with pathogens (61). pDCs are located mainly in the lymphoid organs, such as bone marrow, spleen, and lymph nodes, but not in non-lymphoid tissues. In steady state, pDCs can be found in the T cell zone and peri-follicular area of the lymph node. Upon infection with pathogens, such as VSV, pDCs migrate to the SCS and medulla, areas rich in CD169+ macrophages (38). pDCs were reported to account for half of the IFN-I produced upon VSV infection, which was dependent on the presence of CD169+ macrophages. In a another study, the migration of pDCs to SCS was shown to be mediated by CXCR3, chemokine receptor of CXCL9, CXCL10, amongst others (62). It was suggested that viral particles from the infected CD169+ macrophages could activate these migrating pDCs. However, the direct interaction between SCS CD169+ macrophages and pDCs and its consequences are still unclear.

In a malaria infection model, pDCs accounted for the majority of IFN-I produced which led to lethal outcomes of infected mice (63). Spaulding et al. reported that after infection with malaria, CD169+ macrophages sustained prolonged interaction with pDCs in the bone marrow and primed them to produce IFN-I. Thus, this study provides evidence of an active interaction between CD169+ macrophages and pDCs that may also occur in other lymphoid organs.

However, pDC-derived IFN-I may be dispensable in some situations. In a study that exploited an MCMV footpad infection model, pDC depletion using αBST2 antibodies led to an increase in MCMV escape from SCS and spread to other tissues (55). Nevertheless, this effect was moderate when compared to blocking IFN-I using anti-IFN-I receptor antibodies. In another MCMV model where MCMV was administered intraperitoneally, depletion of pDCs also resulted in an increase of viral spread and dissemination, but only when a low dose was used (64). pDCs were also demonstrated dispensable for survival of the mice upon infection with VSV and *Plasmodium* (38, 63). Thus, upon pathogen encounter by CD169+ macrophages, pDCs are recruited to amplify IFN-I signaling, however this is not always essential for pathogen clearance or mice survival. Nevertheless, pDC-derived IFN-I may still contribute to other aspects of immune responses.

IFN-I Augments cDCs to Initiate Adaptive Immune Responses

The initiation of adaptive immune response by cDCs involves multiple mechanisms including antigen presentation, co-stimulatory/inhibitory molecules, and immunomodulation by cytokines. Next to its role in inhibiting viral replication, IFN-I has been demonstrated to augment NK cell function, B cell isotype switching, and T cell survival and activation (65). IFN-I is also critical for the function of cDCs to fully activate naïve T cells as it stimulates the expression of co-stimulatory molecules, enhances responses to TLR-ligands and increases antigen presentation capacity (66–69). cDC1, in particular, require the presence of IFN-I for antigen cross-presentation and subsequent CD8+ T cell activation (70). Several reports have demonstrated IFN-activated cDC1 to be important for generating CD8+ T cell responses against tumor or viral infections (71–73). In fact, IFN-I signaling induced by viruses could enhance the development of CD8+ T cell-mediated anti-tumor responses as a vaccination strategy (70, 74, 75).

Studies have been performed to identify the source of IFN-I required for the maturation of cDCs. In a vaccination system using tumor protein antigen and an iNKT cell ligand α-GalCer, splenic pDCs produced high amounts of IFN-I (76). Importantly, prior to cDC1 trafficking to the white pulp for T cell stimulation, pDCs were found to cluster with cDC1s in the CD169+ macrophage-rich marginal zone and red pulp area of the spleen. It was further shown that abolishing IFN-I signaling in CD11c+ cells led to an impaired memory T cell formation. This was in line with a previous study, where pDCs were reported to promote the generation and survival of antigen-specific CD8+ T cells upon VSV infection (64). More recently, Brewitz and colleagues have demonstrated pDC-derived IFN-I to be important for CD8+ T cell activation by cDC1 when mice were exposed to MVA (62). After MVA infection, pDCs, cDC1s, and CD8+ T cells formed superclusters in the interfollicular area of the lymph node. This event was required for CD8+ T cell responses. Additionally, in a vaccination strategy using TLR7 agonist as an adjuvant, pDC-derived IFN-I was crucial for *in vivo* CD8+ T cell killing (77). These observations suggest an important cross-talk between IFN-I-producing pDCs and CD8+ XCR1+ cDC1 for an optimal CD8+ T cell activation in vaccination or viral infection.

The effect of IFN-I derived from CD169$^+$ macrophages and pDCs on the function of cDCs is not limited to CD8$^+$ T cell activation. Upon infection with *S. mansoni* eggs, IFN-I was needed for an optimal cDC activation, migration and induction of Th2 immune responses *in vivo* (78). In a DC-targeting vaccination using HIV gag-protein and poly(I:C) as an adjuvant, CD4$^+$ Th1 responses were abolished upon interference with IFN-I signaling (79). Next to T cells, IFN-I signaling on DCs could also mediate B cell function including antibody production, isotype switching and the development of T follicular helper cells (80, 81). Thus, IFN-I stimulated DCs have an enhanced capacity to activate both humoral and cell-mediated adaptive immune responses.

A similar priming effect of IFN-I on cross-presentation has also been shown in human DCs (82, 83). In humans, the level of IFN-I is highly elevated and has been suggested to contribute to the break of tolerance in many autoimmune diseases (84). For example in systemic lupus erythematosus (SLE), the increased level of IFN-I produced by pDCs directly induced cDCs maturation and CD4$^+$ T cell activation (85). In psoriasis, pDC-derived IFN-I was sufficient to drive T cells infiltration and psoriatic plaque lesion formation (86). Interestingly, the numbers of CD169-expressing monocytes/macrophages were increased in the circulation and affected tissues of patients with systemic sclerosis and multiple sclerosis (87, 88). More investigation is needed to clarify the intricate cross-talk of CD169$^+$ macrophage and pDC-derived IFN-I, cDC1, and T cell immunity in human diseases.

Suppressive Effects of IFN-I

Of note, the role of IFN-I during an infection is largely context-dependent and can also result in immunosuppression. A sustained IFN-I production can lead to increase of IL-10 and a higher expression of PD-L1. In a model of a persistent infection using LCMV strain Docile, upregulation of PD-L1 expression by CD169$^+$ macrophages was important to promote CD8$^+$ T cell exhaustion and prevented lethal immunopathology (58). The increased expression of PD-L1 in CD169$^+$ macrophages was also observed in infection model with other LCMV strains (89). In addition, chronic infection with LCMV led to a sustained IFN-I production that prevented mice from mounting immune responses to a secondary infection by VSV (90). This was due to a reduced viral replication in CD169$^+$ macrophages and subsequent impaired antigen presentation and lack of adaptive immune responses, rather than immunosuppression. However, using a model of *E. coli*-induced septic shock and subsequent systemic challenge with ovalbumin (OVA)-containing viruses, Schwandt et al. demonstrated that mice with sepsis had reduced antigen-specific CD8$^+$ T cell responses. This suppression was mediated by macrophage-derived IFN-I that hampered cDC1 function to activate CD8$^+$ T cells (91). Together these studies indicate that during chronic infections IFN-I production by CD169$^+$ macrophages inhibits activation of immune responses toward secondary infections.

In conclusion, the production of IFN-I by CD169$^+$ macrophages, potentially amplified by pDC-derived IFN-I, can strongly stimulate cDC function and the activation of immune responses, but may also result in immunosuppression.

CD169$^+$ MACROPHAGES EFFICIENTLY CAPTURE PATHOGENS AND MEDIATE ANTIGEN TRANSFER

Their strategic location in spleen and in lymph nodes endows CD169$^+$ macrophages with the capacity to capture blood- and lymph-borne pathogens. In fact, CD169$^+$ macrophages appear to be extremely efficient in this process, as showed by multiple groups using various infection models (37, 38, 40, 92–96). Having acquired viral antigens, CD169$^+$ macrophages were reported to transfer antigen to DCs and B cells mainly contributing to the infection control but also to virus dissemination in some cases.

CD169$^+$ Macrophages Enable Containment of Viral Infection and Localized Production of Antigen

The role of CD169$^+$ macrophages as efficient gatekeepers has been demonstrated in a large number of viral infections, such as adenovirus, vaccinia virus, West Nile virus, and VSV (37, 92, 97). Additionally, experiments with human immunodeficiency virus (HIV) and murine leukemia virus (MLV) models confirmed prompt and potent virus capture by these gatekeeping macrophages (93). Deletion of splenic CD169$^+$ macrophages was reported to cause rapid dissemination of LCMV and herpes virus infection (35, 98). Along the same line, local depletion of SCS macrophages resulted in higher viral titers in the spleen and other organs providing direct evidence for the protective role of CD169$^+$ macrophages in systemic viral spread (37, 38, 40) (99). This clearly demonstrated the importance of CD169$^+$ macrophages in infection containment.

Paradoxically, CD169$^+$ macrophages can also support virus replication (33, 38, 99). Enforced virus replication within CD169$^+$ macrophages endowed them with the distinct feature of being a source of viral antigen that facilitated activation of adaptive immune responses. Accordingly, increased expression of inhibitory protein Usp18 rendered splenic CD169$^+$ macrophages unresponsive to IFN-I. As a consequence, enhanced cytopathic VSV replication in these cells was facilitated (94). CD169$^+$ macrophage-mediated VSV replication mediated a strong VSV-neutralizing antibody response that rescued infected animals. Positive correlation between viral replication in CD169$^+$ macrophages and protective adaptive immune responses was also shown in LCMV infection (100).

CD169$^+$ Macrophages Transfer Antigens to DCs in Viral Infections

Apart from effective viral capture and containment of the infection, CD169$^+$ macrophages have been previously reported to directly present particulate antigens, immune complexes as well as intact virus particles to non-cognate and cognate B cells (37, 101–103). This process was shown to stimulate germinal center responses and production of high affinity antibodies (103, 104). While in these initial studies that used clodronate liposomes, B cells were still activated in the absence of SCS macrophages (38), a recent study indicated that absence of SCS macrophages led to defective B cell responses (105). This process of intact virus presentation to B cells by CD169$^+$ macrophages has also been implicated in trans-infection of B cells, contributing to the virus dissemination rather than to the virus containment (discussed in more detail in section *CD169 as a viral receptor that mediates virus capture and trans-infection*).

Despite robust evidence proving the importance of CD169$^+$ macrophages in the induction of anti-viral B cell responses, their role in the activation of T cell responses is still being elucidated. While a number of studies demonstrate that CD169$^+$ macrophages are dispensable for T cell priming (35–38, 94, 97), interaction between CD169$^+$ macrophages and cDC1s has been shown to promote anti-viral T cell responses (44, 106, 107). The study by Backer et al. indicated that CD169$^+$ macrophages could transfer antigens to cDC1s for the stimulation of CTL responses (106). In line with this, Bernhard et al. showed that antigen transfer between CD169$^+$ macrophages and cDCs also occurred in adenoviral infection. Interestingly, CD169$^+$ macrophages were also able to directly present viral antigens to T cells bypassing the need for cDCs for T cell priming. While all epitopes, including low affinity peptides, were directly presented by CD169$^+$ macrophages, cDC1s only cross-presented high affinity T cell epitopes (107).

Recently, the collaboration between CD169$^+$ and cDC1s was investigated in more detail (44). This study revealed that the CD169 receptor enabled cell-cell contact with sialylated ligands on cDCs and thereby facilitated transfer of antigen to cDCs. In addition to mediating adhesion to DCs, CD169 has also been reported to support binding of innate-like lymphocytes and neutrophils (41, 108, 109). Remarkably, even upon disintegration, CD169$^+$ SCS macrophage cell-derived blebs are able to bind to IL-17 lymphocytes and NK cells (41, 43). Apparently, CD169 acts as an adhesion receptor that facilitates the interaction of CD169$^+$ macrophages with other innate immune cells.

Interestingly, *in vivo* blockade of CD169 receptor resulted in impaired MVA-specific, but not VSV-specific CD8$^+$ T cell responses (44). This observation could be explained by the dispensability of the cross-presentation process during certain viral infections, such as VSV in which DCs are likely to be directly infected (94). Specifically, KLRG-1^{low} CD8$^+$ T cells with memory potential were negatively affected upon CD169 blocking in MVA-infected animals, indicating that CD169$^+$ macrophage-mediated antigen transfer to cDC1s might facilitate memory responses as well. In line with this, collaboration between splenic CD169$^+$ macrophages and cDC1s was important for activation of memory CD8$^+$ T cell responses in VSV infection (33).

Van Dinther et al. showed that CLEC9A/DNGR-1 expressed on cDC1 enhanced CD8$^+$ T cell cross-priming of antigens targeted to CD169$^+$ macrophages (44). CLEC9A/DNGR-1 binds to F-actin exposed on dying cells and while it does not increase antigen transfer, it enhances T cell responses toward cell-associated material and in viral infections (110–112). A number of studies have indicated the disappearance or death of CD169$^+$ macrophages induced by viral infection or other inflammatory agents (44, 60, 105). This suggests that upon infection, CD169$^+$ macrophages quickly die and thereby form a cellular substrate for antigen transfer by the cross-presenting cDC1. This process could be of particular importance in viral infections, such as MVA, that solely depend on cross-presentation as opposed to VSV where the virus directly infects DCs (44).

CD169 as a Viral Receptor That Mediates Virus Capture and Trans-infection

A decade ago, CD169 expressed on monocyte-derived DCs was found to promote HIV infection. This discovery brought a paradigm shift in the HIV field with CD169 replacing DC-SIGN as the main capture receptor responsible not only for HIV adhesion, but also for trans-infection (113–116). Following binding of CD169 to virus membrane-associated glycolipids (GM3), HIV-1 and CD169 were demonstrated to travel together to and accumulate at a non-lysosomal compartment. Consequently, the concentration of HIV-1 and CD169 at the so called infectious synapse enabled trans-infection of CD4$^+$ T cells (117). A similar trans-infection process was also shown to be important for henipavirus infection (118).

In a study that focused on MLV and HIV infection *in vivo*, CD169-mediated virus capture was also reported to occur via CD169 binding to gangliosides on the viral membrane (93). Interestingly, CD169$^+$ macrophages that had captured MLV, but were not infected themselves, were responsible for trans-infection of permissive B cells which facilitated spread of the infection. Accordingly, considerably lower numbers of virus-infected cells were detected both in peripheral lymph nodes and spleen upon blocking of CD169 and in CD169-deficient mice. This clearly illustrated the importance of CD169 for effective virus dissemination. In line with this, MLV was also demonstrated to exploit CD169 expressed on primary mouse bone marrow macrophages for trans-infection of proliferating B cells (95). Apart from aforementioned retroviral models, a study performed in a porcine reproductive and respiratory syndrome virus (PRRSV) also experimentally addressed the role of CD169 in virus anchoring (119). The authors proved that the attachment of the virus was dependent on the sialic acid binding activity of the receptor that binds to sialylated viral glycoproteins on PRRSV.

While substantial evidence from retroviral studies validates CD169 as a viral receptor that is exploited by the pathogen for its dissemination, numerous studies in viral models have demonstrated the importance of CD169 expressing macrophages for the containment of viral infection and localized production of antigen. The latter suggests that these macrophages form a reservoir of viral antigen for transfer to cDC1. A small number of studies suggest that a similar process may take place in certain bacterial infections.

CD169$^+$ Macrophages Efficiently Trap Bacteria and Allow Trans-infection of cDCs

Similar to what has been shown in viral infections, several studies using the *Listeria monocytogenes* (Lm) model confirmed CD169$^+$ macrophages as the initial cellular host that effectively traps the bacteria (36, 120–122). While as early as 2 h post-infection, the majority of Lm was detected within macrophages in the marginal zone, by 9 h $CD11c^+$ DCs were the main cell type carrying Lm (121). Two photon microscopy results showed clustering of Lm-specific T cells that associated with $CD11c^+$ DCs in periarteriolar lymphoid sheath (PALS), which was indicative of ongoing antigen presentation. At 24 h Lm-infection foci were mainly localized to PALS where Lm was shown to replicate extensively. Using a CD11c-DTR model that allows for CD11c depletion upon DT injection, the authors confirmed that Lm transport to the PALS and subsequent antigen presentation were dependent on the presence of cDCs. However, as mentioned already, CD11c-DTR model also abrogates CD11c- expressing $CD169^+$ macrophages. Therefore, only subsequent experiments performed in the $Batf3^{-/-}$ model, formally established the role of cross-presenting cDC1 in Lm delivery to the PALS (120, 122).

Recently, Perez et al. (122) also noted a shift in Lm distribution from $CD169^+$ macrophages to cDC1 over the course of infection and showed that $CD169^+$ macrophages mediate trans-infection of cDC1. Accordingly, while in wild type animals cDC1 formed clusters near Lm-infected $CD169^+$ macrophages in the marginal zone and efficiently delivered Lm to PALS, in CD169-DTR mice such clusters were not present and transport to PALS was impaired. Therefore, the presence of $CD169^+$ macrophages closely interacting with cDC1 promoted trans-infection and enabled subsequent Lm entry to the PALS.

Similar to viral infections, $CD169^+$ macrophages also control the spread of bacteria. Perez and colleagues reported increased bacterial titers in the spleen and blood of CD169-DTR mice, suggesting that these macrophages impede Lm replication and prevent Lm dissemination (122). Finally, using a CD169-DTR-$Batf3^{-/-}$ model, that allows for conditional depletion of $CD169^+$ macrophages in cDC1-deficient mice, it was demonstrated that rapid Lm capture and clearance secured by $CD169^+$ macrophages was instrumental for Lm control. Interestingly, the authors showed that cytosolic replication within $CD169^+$ macrophages due to phagosomal escape was necessary for recruitment of cDC1.

While cDC1s have been identified as replication- permissive cellular hosts for Lm, a recent study demonstrated that $CD169^+$ macrophages can have a similar role in pneumococcal septicaemia (123). Upon infecting $CD169^+$ macrophages, *Streptococcus pneumoniae* evaded phagosomal clearance, proliferated intracellularly and after causing cell lysis disseminated to the bloodstream. The authors concluded that intracellular replication within $CD169^+$ macrophages is crucial for resulting pneumococcal septicaemia.

Collectively, the findings from studies in bacterial infections, albeit almost exclusively performed in the Lm model, illustrate the importance of $CD169^+$ macrophages as the initial cellular host. By capturing the bacteria, $CD169^+$ macrophages initially mediate pathogen clearance and prevent systemic spread of the infection. However, they also serve as a bacterial reservoir that actually promotes propagation of the bacteria into the bloodstream at a later stage in the case of *Streptococcus pneumonia* or enable trans-infection of cDC1 by Lm. In addition to these two bacterial infections, the CD169 molecule has been shown to function as a receptor for bacterial uptake of pathogens rich in sialylated polysaccharides, such as *Neisseria meningitidis*, *Campylobacter jejuni*, and *Trypanosoma cruzi* (124–126). It remains to be established whether $CD169^+$ macrophages function as a bacterial and/or antigen reservoir in these infections.

Uptake and Transfer of Apoptotic Cellular Material by CD169+ Macrophages and the Implications for Tolerance and Cancer Immunity

The distinction between self and non-self is essential for the proper function of the immune system. Next to their essential role in initiating immune responses specific for pathogens, $CD169^+$ macrophages have also been shown to play a role in the induction of tolerance and anti-cancer immune responses.

Role of CD169+ Macrophages in Tolerance

Continuous and non-inflammatory removal of apoptotic cell material is essential for the maintenance of tolerance. Using a transfer model of apoptotic cells, cDC1 cells were specifically shown to take up and present these cell-associated antigens to $CD8^+$ T cells (16, 18, 19) and subsequently induce tolerance in the steady state (127). One of the first observations indicating a tolerogenic function for $CD169^+$ macrophages was made by Miyake et al., who generated CD169-DTR mice in which all marginal zone macrophages were eliminated upon injection with DT (47). Upon injection of apoptotic cells loaded with a fragment of the myelin oligodendrocyte glycoprotein peptide (MOG peptide), an accumulation of apoptotic cell content was observed in the marginal zone in wild type mice, which prevented the development of EAE. Depletion of marginal zone macrophages via DT administration in CD169-DTR mice resulted in a failure of induction of tolerance and a switch in the uptake of apoptotic cells from $CD8^+$ cDC1s to $CD8^-$ cDC2s (47).

Next to cDC2s, also red pulp macrophages, have been accounted for the defective uptake of apoptotic cells and the abrogation of tolerance in the absence of marginal zone macrophages. When marginal zone macrophages were depleted by means of clodronate liposomes, an accumulation of apoptotic cells was detected in $F4/80^+$ macrophages. This was correlated with the production of inflammatory cytokines and loss of tolerance induction (128).

In subsequent studies by McGaha et al. the interaction between $CD169^+$ macrophages and DCs was investigated. In their system, intravenous injection of apoptotic cells induced the expression of CCL22 on $CD169^+$ macrophages, which resulted in a coordinated clustering of CCR4-expressing cDC1s and regulatory T cells within the white pulp. The induction of tolerance was dependent on both $CD169^+$ macrophages and CCR4 (129). In contrast, another study reported that CCL22 is produced by the cDC1s upon injection with apoptotic cells, showing that the role of the cell type that produces CCL22 remains to be clarified (130). However, together these studies indicate that marginal zone $CD169^+$ macrophages and cDC1s are essential in the induction of tolerance via the uptake of apoptotic cells and suggest a functional collaboration in this process.

Uptake of Tumor Cell Material and Exosomes by CD169^{+} Macrophages Stimulate Anti-cancer Immunity

The previously discussed role of CD169^{+} macrophages in mediating the removal of dying cells from the circulation to induce tolerance suggests that a similar process could potentially be involved in anti-tumor immunity. In this sense, a number of factors have been proposed to shift the balance of tolerance toward immunity. Whether DCs induce immunity is a context-dependent process, influenced by environmentally provided stimuli, stage and type of cell death as well as the location where it takes place (131, 132). An example of this has been provided by Lorenzi and colleagues, who demonstrated enhanced intracellular persistence of antigenic particles in cDC1 upon injection of tumor apoptotic cells in combination with IFN-I. After exposure to IFN-I, cDC1 not only contributed to the induction of OT-I proliferation, but also exhibited an enhanced lifespan and expression of co-stimulatory molecules (133). Since CD169^{+} macrophages can produce high amounts of IFN-I, in combination with antigen this could provide the optimal stimulus for DCs to be able to cross-present cell-associated tumor antigens and to induce T cell activation.

However, the question remains whether CD169^{+} macrophages have the capacity to cross-present tumor antigens autonomously. One of the first studies exploiting subcutaneously-injected dead cells showed these cells being transported throughout the lymphatic system to the lymph nodes, where SCS macrophages cross-presented dead cell-associated antigens to CD8^{+} T cells. Mice that were lacking SCS macrophages at the moment of vaccination did not reject the tumors successfully (134). Interestingly, in this model the CD169^{+} macrophages, and not cDC1, were thought to directly cross-prime CD8^{+} T cells. This is reminiscent of the direct presentation of adenoviral antigens in the study of Bernhard et al., although the latter cannot be formally referred to as cross-presentation (107). Further studies are necessary to determine whether CD169^{+} macrophages can cross-prime CD8^{+} T cells independently or always require the collaboration with cDC1s.

In a model in which apoptotic cells were injected *in vivo* and induced CD4^{+} T cell activation, again macrophages were shown to be the main cells involved in the uptake and in their absence or the absence of cDC1 the CD4^{+} T cell activation was significantly decreased (135). Of note, an exosomal pathway was indicated to play a role in the cell-associated antigen transfer of macrophages to DCs. Exosomes are produced by many cell types and consist of small membrane vesicles that contain proteins, lipids, and nucleic acids. These vesicles can mediate transfer of such encapsulated molecules and thereby facilitate communication between cells (136). Exosomes have been found to be efficiently taken up by CD169^{+} macrophages and cDC1 in the spleen (137). McLellan and colleagues demonstrated that exosomes can express high levels of α2,3-linked sialic acids and bind abundantly to CD169^{+} macrophages in the spleen. Interestingly, CD169-deficient mice raised stronger CD8^{+} T cell responses toward antigen-pulsed exosomes than wild type mice (138). A similar suppressive role of CD169^{+} macrophages was observed in the T cell response toward tumor-derived apoptotic vesicles (139).

These studies suggest that CD169^{+} macrophages scavenge exosomes and thereby prevent their uptake by other cell types. Proof of that concept was provided by Pittet and colleagues in a mice model bearing genetically modified B16F10 melanoma tumors. The authors observed that tumor-derived exosomes drained to the lymph node and bound to CD169^{+} macrophages, which prevented the interaction with B cells that produce tumor promoting IgG. Elimination of CD169^{+} macrophages by clodronate liposomes or by DT injection in the CD169-DTR mice promoted tumor growth. In the same study, melanoma-derived material was found in macrophages residing in the cancer-free sentinel lymph node of human biopsies, hinting to the potential relevance of these findings for human cancer research (140).

Several groups have reported association of the presence of CD169^{+} macrophages in lymph nodes with good tumor prognosis in human. Ohnishi and colleagues showed a correlation between CD169^{+} macrophages and CD8^{+} T cell infiltration in colorectal cancer, improving overall survival rates. Furthermore, they observed co-localization of CD8^{+} T cells and CD169^{+} macrophages in regional lymph node section stainings (141). Similarly, more recent work from the same group demonstrated that the presence of CD169^{+} macrophages in the lymph nodes was also correlated to CD8^{+} T cell infiltration in malignant melanoma, endometrial carcinoma (where higher numbers of NK cells were also found), breast cancer and bladder cancer (142–145), all leading to a better prognosis and increased survival rates. Quite remarkably, in the study in malignant melanoma, IFN-α producing cells were detected around CD169^{+} macrophages in the lymph node sinus area. Based on their morphology and marker expression, the authors hypothesized that the source of IFN-α, supporting the action of CD169^{+} macrophages, could be CD68^{+} macrophages and pDCs (142). Altogether, these studies present robust data illustrating the importance of CD169^{+} macrophages in lymph nodes in proficient anti-tumor responses, characterized by a consistent CD8^{+} T cell infiltration that benefits patient prognosis and survival. However, while CD169^{+} macrophages where shown to co-localize with CD8^{+} T cells, no direct evidence of antigen presentation by CD169^{+} macrophages was provided at a functional level. Therefore, there might be room for other more specialized immune cells, such as cDC1 to cooperate in the process of T cell priming.

Vaccination Strategies That Target to CD169^{+} Macrophages

The presence of CD169^{+} macrophages in lymph nodes draining different tumor types and their correlation with a better patient survival, their unique capacity to screen the lymphatic and blood circulation and, finally, their capacity to collaborate with DCs, all point to CD169^{+} macrophages as appealing targets for the design of anti-cancer vaccines. Until now, several vaccination strategies targeting CD169^{+} macrophages have been evaluated experimentally.

Due to their high specificity and the restricted expression pattern of CD169, monoclonal antibodies have been tested for antigen delivery to CD169^{+} macrophages. Upon anti-CD169-specific antibody targeting of OVA, strong CTL responses were

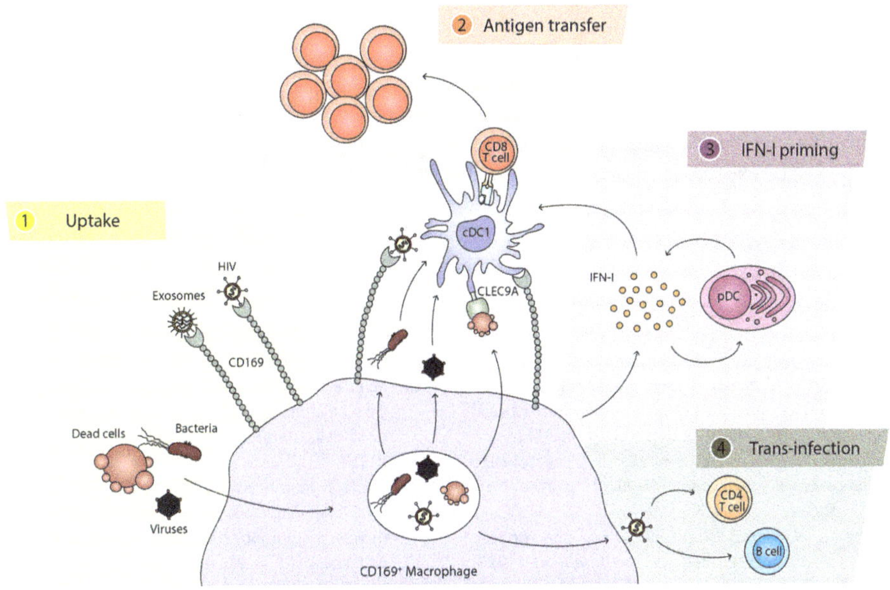

FIGURE 1 | The different functions of CD169$^+$ macrophages and their cross-talk with cDC1. (1) Uptake: CD169$^+$ macrophages capture and phagocytose pathogens, including bacteria and viruses, as well as dead cells. The CD169 molecule also directly binds to exosomes and specific pathogens, such as HIV. (2) Antigen transfer: CD169$^+$ macrophages directly interact and present antigens to cDC1s for the generation of antigen-specific CD8$^+$ T cell responses. While HIV particles are transferred via CD169, other components of bacteria and viruses can be transferred to cDC1s from the macrophages. Dead cells can stimulate cDC1s via CLEC9A expressed on the cDC1. The interaction between CD169$^+$ macrophages and cDC1s is dependent on binding of CD169 to sialic acid structures on cDC1s. (3) IFN-I priming: after encounter with bacteria, dead cells, or viruses, CD169$^+$ macrophages secrete IFN-I that is required for optimal activation of cDC1s and T cells. Subsequently, pDCs are recruited and their IFN-I production further amplifies the signal. (4) Trans-infection: in the case of HIV and MLV, CD169$^+$ macrophages can also mediate viral trans-infection to CD4 T cells and B cells.

generated mediated by antigen transfer to cDC1 (106). This effect was lost upon depletion of CD169$^+$ macrophages by the administration of clodronate liposomes and was shown to be mediated by BATF3-dependent cDC1s (44). Antibody-mediated targeting of OVA to CD169$^+$ macrophages also led to an isotype-switched and high affinity antibody production due to germinal center activity. CD169$^+$ macrophages retained intact antigen on their surface for days and upregulated costimulatory molecules for B cell interaction upon activation (103). This feature of CD169$^+$ macrophages to retain intact molecules on their membrane has been correlated with low expression of proteolytic enzymes (104).

On a different note, Delputte et al. demonstrated that monoclonal antibodies against CD169 were not only binding, but also being efficiently internalized in a clathrin-dependent manner. Immunotoxins or antigens could be delivered to CD169$^+$ macrophages via antibody targeting, leading to killing of primary porcine macrophages and the generation of anti-HSA humoral responses, respectively (146, 147). It is not clear why certain studies report internalization and others long-term presence on the cell surface with antibody targeting. Both processes could occur simultaneously, but these divergent results could also be due to antibodies binding to different regions of the CD169 molecule.

In addition, liposomes have been used to target antigens to CD169$^+$ macrophages. Chen and colleagues generated OVA-containing liposomes decorated with 3′-BPCNeuAc, a synthetic ligand of CD169, and showed that targeting of IFN-α stimulated bone marrow-derived mouse macrophages with 3′-BPCNeuAc-liposomes induced OVA specific T cell proliferation (148). Moreover, the same authors could also accomplish activation of iNKT cells by including the lipid antigen αGalCer in the 3′-BPCNeuAc-liposomes (149). CD169$^+$ macrophages seem well equipped in stimulating NKT cells via CD1d, which subsequently help B cell responses (42, 150). Liposomes with the endogenous ligand for CD169, ganglioside GM3, have also been shown to bind to CD169$^+$ monocyte-derived DCs (151). These studies indicate that also liposomal strategies could be employed to target antigens and activating agents to CD169$^+$ macrophages.

CONCLUDING REMARKS

In recent years a considerable number of studies have focused on the role that CD169$^+$ macrophages play in the SCS of the lymph node and the marginal zone of the spleen (summarized in **Figure 1**). These studies, as discussed in this review, point to CD169$^+$ macrophages as the main cell type to capture viruses, bacteria, dead cells and exosomes from the lymph fluid and the blood. This filtering capacity prevents further dissemination and enables a localized contained production of antigen that is efficiently transferred to DCs and B cells for the activation of adaptive immune responses. The collaboration between CD169$^+$ macrophages and cDC1s is especially important in the activation of CD8$^+$ T cell responses toward viral or tumor antigens. In this context, IFN-I derived from CD169$^+$ macrophages and pDCs plays a crucial role for an appropriate cDC1 activation.

However, a number of pathogens have exploited this pathway and utilize CD169$^+$ macrophages as a niche to replicate and to mediate trans-infection of other cell types. In the coming years, the role of the human equivalent of this cell type will hopefully be elucidated and the development of treatment strategies to boost or down-regulate immune responses via the actions of the CD169$^+$ macrophages may well be expected.

AUTHOR CONTRIBUTIONS

All authors listed have made a substantial, direct and intellectual contribution to the work, and approved it for publication.

ACKNOWLEDGMENTS

The authors thank D. van Dinther for critical review of the manuscript.

REFERENCES

1. Guilliams M, Ginhoux F, Jakubzick C, Naik SH, Onai N, Schraml BU, et al. Dendritic cells, monocytes and macrophages: a unified nomenclature based on ontogeny. *Nat Rev Immunol.* (2014) 14:571–8. doi: 10.1038/nri3712
2. Ginhoux F, Guilliams M. Tissue-resident macrophage ontogeny and homeostasis. *Immunity* (2016) 44:439–49. doi: 10.1016/j.immuni.2016.02.024
3. Lavin Y, Mortha A, Rahman A, Merad M. Regulation of macrophage development and function in peripheral tissues. *Nat Rev Immunol.* (2015) 15:731–44. doi: 10.1038/nri3920
4. Davies LC, Jenkins SJ, Allen JE, Taylor PR. Tissue-resident macrophages. *Nat Immunol.* (2013) 14:986–95. doi: 10.1038/ni.2705
5. Amit I, Winter DR, Jung S. The role of the local environment and epigenetics in shaping macrophage identity and their effect on tissue homeostasis. *Nat Immunol.* (2016) 17:18–25. doi: 10.1038/ni.3325
6. Mowat AM, Scott CL, Bain CC. Barrier-tissue macrophages: functional adaptation to environmental challenges. *Nat Med.* (2017) 23:1258–70. doi: 10.1038/nm.4430
7. Jakubzick CV, Randolph GJ, Henson PM. Monocyte differentiation and antigen-presenting functions. *Nat Rev Immunol.* (2017) 17:349–62. doi: 10.1038/nri.2017.28
8. Satpathy AT, Wu X, Albring JC, Murphy KM. Re(de)fining the dendritic cell lineage. *Nat Immunol.* (2012) 13:1145–54. doi: 10.1038/ni.2467
9. Mildner A, Jung S. Development and function of dendritic cell subsets. *Immunity* (2014) 40:642–56. doi: 10.1016/j.immuni.2014.04.016
10. Beijer MR, Kraal G, den Haan JM. Vitamin A and dendritic cell differentiation. *Immunology* (2014) 142:39–45. doi: 10.1111/imm.12228
11. See P, Dutertre CA, Chen J, Gunther P, McGovern N, Irac SE, et al. Mapping the human DC lineage through the integration of high-dimensional techniques. *Science* (2017) 356:eaag3009. doi: 10.1126/science.aag3009
12. Villani AC, Satija R, Reynolds G, Sarkizova S, Shekhar K, Fletcher J, et al. Single-cell RNA-seq reveals new types of human blood dendritic cells, monocytes, and progenitors. *Science* (2017) 356:eaah4573. doi: 10.1126/science.aah4573
13. Alcantara-Hernandez M, Leylek R, Wagar LE, Engleman EG, Keler T, Marinkovich MP, et al. High-dimensional phenotypic mapping of human dendritic cells reveals interindividual variation and tissue specialization. *Immunity* (2017) 47:1037–50.e6. doi: 10.1016/j.immuni.2017.11.001
14. Bevan MJ. Cross-priming for a secondary cytotoxic response to minor H antigens with H-2 congenic cells which do not cross-react in the cytotoxic assay. *J Exp Med.* (1976) 143:1283–8.
15. Cruz FM, Colbert JD, Merino E, Kriegsman BA, Rock KL. The biology and underlying mechanisms of cross-presentation of exogenous antigens on MHC-I molecules. *Annu Rev Immunol.* (2017) 35:149–76. doi: 10.1146/annurev-immunol-041015-055254
16. den Haan JM, Lehar SM, Bevan MJ. CD8(+) but not CD8(-) dendritic cells cross-prime cytotoxic T cells *in vivo*. *J Exp Med.* (2000) 192:1685–96. doi: 10.1084/jem.192.12.1685
17. Segura E, Amigorena S. Cross-Presentation in mouse and human dendritic cells. *Adv Immunol.* (2015) 127:1–31. doi: 10.1016/bs.ai.2015.03.002
18. Schulz O, Reise Sousa C. Cross-presentation of cell-associated antigens by CD8alpha$^+$ dendritic cells is attributable to their ability to internalize dead cells. *Immunology* (2002) 107:183–9. doi: 10.1046/j.1365-2567.2002.01513.x
19. Iyoda T, Shimoyama S, Liu K, Omatsu Y, Akiyama Y, Maeda Y, et al. The CD8$^+$ dendritic cell subset selectively endocytoses dying cells in culture and *in vivo*. *J Exp Med.* (2002) 195:1289–302. doi: 10.1084/jem.20020161
20. den Haan JM, Bevan MJ. Constitutive versus activation-dependent cross-presentation of immune complexes by CD8(+) and CD8(-) dendritic cells *in vivo*. *J Exp Med.* (2002) 196:817–27. doi: 10.1084/jem.20020295
21. Segura E, Albiston AL, Wicks IP, Chai SY, Villadangos JA. Different cross-presentation pathways in steady-state and inflammatory dendritic cells. *Proc Natl Acad Sci USA.* (2009) 106:20377–81. doi: 10.1073/pnas.0910295106
22. Tang-Huau TL, Gueguen P, Goudot C, Durand M, Bohec M, Baulande S, et al. Human *in vivo*-generated monocyte-derived dendritic cells and macrophages cross-present antigens through a vacuolar pathway. *Nat Commun.* (2018) 9:2570. doi: 10.1038/s41467-018-04985-0
23. Grotzke JE, Sengupta D, Lu Q, Cresswell P. The ongoing saga of the mechanism(s) of MHC class I-restricted cross-presentation. *Curr Opin Immunol.* (2017) 46:89–96. doi: 10.1016/j.coi.2017.03.015
24. Blander JM, Regulation of the cell biology of antigen cross-presentation. *Annu Rev Immunol.* (2018) 36:717–53. doi: 10.1146/annurev-immunol-041015-055523
25. Delamarre L, Pack M, Chang H, Mellman I, Trombetta ES. Differential lysosomal proteolysis in antigen-presenting cells determines antigen fate. *Science* (2005) 307:1630–4. doi: 10.1126/science.1108003
26. Alloatti A, Kotsias F, Magalhaes JG, Amigorena S. Dendritic cell maturation and cross-presentation: timing matters! *Immunol Rev.* (2016) 272:97–108. doi: 10.1111/imr.12432
27. den Haan JM, Martinez-Pomares L, Macrophage heterogeneity in lymphoid tissues. *Semin Immunopathol.* (2013) 35:541–52. doi: 10.1007/s00281-013-0378-4
28. Martinez-Pomares L, Gordon S. CD169$^+$ macrophages at the crossroads of antigen presentation. *Trends Immunol.* (2012) 33:66–70. doi: 10.1016/j.it.2011.11.001
29. Moseman EA, Iannacone M, Bosurgi L, Tonti E, Chevrier N, Tumanov A, et al. B cell maintenance of subcapsular sinus macrophages protects against a fatal viral infection independent of adaptive immunity. *Immunity* (2012) 36:415–26. doi: 10.1016/j.immuni.2012.01.013
30. Xu HC, Huang J, Khairnar V, Duhan V, Pandyra AA, Grusdat M, et al. Deficiency of the B cell-activating factor receptor results in limited CD169$^+$ macrophage function during viral infection. *J Virol.* (2015) 89:4748–59. doi: 10.1128/JVI.02976-14
31. Takahashi K, Umeda S, Shultz LD, Hayashi S, Nishikawa S. Effects of macrophage colony-stimulating factor (M-CSF) on the development, differentiation, and maturation of marginal metallophilic macrophages and marginal zone macrophages in the spleen of osteopetrosis (op) mutant mice lacking functional M-CSF activity. *J Leukoc Biol.* (1994) 55:581–8.

32. Shinde PV, Xu HC, Maney SK, Kloetgen A, Namineni S, Zhuang Y, et al. Tumor necrosis factor-mediated survival of CD169(+) cells promotes immune activation during vesicular stomatitis virus infection. *J Virol.* (2018) 92:e01637-17. doi: 10.1128/JVI.01637-17
33. Habbeddine M, Verthuy C, Rastoin O, Chasson L, Bebien M, Bajenoff M, et al. Receptor activator of NF-kappaB orchestrates activation of antiviral memory CD8 T cells in the spleen marginal zone. *Cell Rep.* (2017) 21:2515–27. doi: 10.1016/j.celrep.2017.10.111
34. A-Gonzalez N, Guillen JA, Gallardo G, Diaz M, de la Rosa JV, Hernandez IH, et al. The nuclear receptor LXRalpha controls the functional specialization of splenic macrophages. *Nat Immunol.* (2013) 14:831–9. doi: 10.1038/ni.2622
35. Seiler P, Aichele P, Odermatt B, Hengartner H, Zinkernagel RM, Schwendener RA. Crucial role of marginal zone macrophages and marginal zone metallophils in the clearance of lymphocytic choriomeningitis virus infection. *Eur J Immunol.* (1997) 27:2626–33. doi: 10.1002/eji.1830271023
36. Aichele P, Zinke J, Grode L, Schwendener RA, Kaufmann SH, Seiler P. Macrophages of the splenic marginal zone are essential for trapping of blood-borne particulate antigen but dispensable for induction of specific T cell responses. *J Immunol.* (2003) 171:1148–55. doi: 10.4049/jimmunol.171.3.1148
37. Junt T, Moseman EA, Iannacone M, Massberg S, Lang PA, Boes M, et al. Subcapsular sinus macrophages in lymph nodes clear lymph-borne viruses and present them to antiviral B cells. *Nature* (2007) 450:110–4. doi: 10.1038/nature06287
38. Iannacone M, Moseman EA, Tonti E, Bosurgi L, Junt T, Henrickson SE, et al. Subcapsular sinus macrophages prevent CNS invasion on peripheral infection with a neurotropic virus. *Nature* (2010) 465:1079–83. doi: 10.1038/nature09118
39. Gupta P, Lai SM, Sheng J, Tetlak P, Balachander A, Claser C, et al. Tissue-resident CD169(+) macrophages form a crucial front line against plasmodium infection. *Cell Rep.* (2016) 16:1749–61. doi: 10.1016/j.celrep.2016.07.010
40. Kastenmuller W, Torabi-Parizi P, Subramanian N, Lammermann T, Germain RN. A spatially-organized multicellular innate immune response in lymph nodes limits systemic pathogen spread. *Cell* (2012) 150:1235–48. doi: 10.1016/j.cell.2012.07.021
41. Zhang Y, Roth TL, Gray EE, Chen H, Rodda LB, Liang Y, et al. Migratory and adhesive cues controlling innate-like lymphocyte surveillance of the pathogen-exposed surface of the lymph node. *Elife* (2016) 5:e18156. doi: 10.7554/eLife.18156
42. Barral P, Polzella P, Bruckbauer A, van Rooijen N, Besra GS, Cerundolo V, et al. CD169(+) macrophages present lipid antigens to mediate early activation of iNKT cells in lymph nodes. *Nat Immunol.* (2010) 11:303–12. doi: 10.1038/ni.1853
43. Gray EE, Friend S, Suzuki K, Phan TG, Cyster JG. Subcapsular sinus macrophage fragmentation and CD169^{+} bleb acquisition by closely associated IL-17-committed innate-like lymphocytes. *PLoS ONE* (2012) 7:e38258. doi: 10.1371/journal.pone.0038258
44. van Dinther D, Veninga H, Iborra S, Borg EGF, Hoogterp L, Olesek K, et al. Functional CD169 on macrophages mediates interaction with dendritic cells for CD8(+) T cell cross-priming. *Cell Rep.* (2018) 22:1484–95. doi: 10.1016/j.celrep.2018.01.021
45. Van Rooijen N, Sanders A. Liposome mediated depletion of macrophages: mechanism of action, preparation of liposomes and applications. *J Immunol Methods* (1994) 174:83–93.
46. Kuka M, Iannacone M. The role of lymph node sinus macrophages in host defense. *Ann N Y Acad Sci.* (2014) 1319:38–46. doi: 10.1111/nyas.12387
47. Miyake Y, Asano K, Kaise H, Uemura M, Nakayama M, Tanaka M. Critical role of macrophages in the marginal zone in the suppression of immune responses to apoptotic cell-associated antigens. *J Clin Invest.* (2007) 117:2268–78. doi: 10.1172/JCI31990
48. Jung S, Unutmaz D, Wong P, Sano G, De los Santos K, Sparwasser T, et al. *In vivo* depletion of CD11c^{+} dendritic cells abrogates priming of CD8^{+} T cells by exogenous cell-associated antigens. *Immunity* (2002) 17:211–20. doi: 10.1016/S1074-7613(02)00365-5
49. Probst HC, Tschannen K, Odermatt B, Schwendener R, Zinkernagel RM, Van Den Broek M. Histological analysis of CD11c-DTR/GFP mice after *in vivo* depletion of dendritic cells. *Clin Exp Immunol.* (2005) 141:398–404. doi: 10.1111/j.1365-2249.2005.02868.x
50. Karasawa K, Asano K, Moriyama S, Ushiki M, Monya M, Iida M, et al. Vascular-resident CD169-positive monocytes and macrophages control neutrophil accumulation in the kidney with ischemia-reperfusion injury. *J Am Soc Nephrol.* (2015) 26:896–906. doi: 10.1681/ASN.2014020195
51. Ivashkiv LB, Donlin LT. Regulation of type I interferon responses. *Nat Rev Immunol.* (2014) 14:36–49. doi: 10.1038/nri3581
52. Yan N, Chen ZJ. Intrinsic antiviral immunity. *Nat Immunol.* (2012) 13:214–22. doi: 10.1038/ni.2229
53. Kovarik P, Castiglia V, Ivin M, Ebner F. Type I interferons in bacterial infections, a balancing act. *Front Immunol.* (2016) 7:652. doi: 10.3389/fimmu.2016.00652
54. McNab F, Mayer-Barber K, Sher A, Wack A, O'Garra A. Type I interferons in infectious disease. *Nat Rev Immunol.* (2015) 15:87–103. doi: 10.1038/nri3787
55. Farrell HE, Bruce K, Lawler C, Cardin RD, Davis-Poynter NJ, Stevenson PG. Type 1 interferons and NK cells limit murine cytomegalovirus escape from the lymph node subcapsular sinus. *PLoS Pathog.* (2016) 12:e1006069. doi: 10.1371/journal.ppat.1006069
56. Eloranta ML, Alm GV. Splenic marginal metallophilic macrophages and marginal zone macrophages are the major interferon-alpha/beta producers in mice upon intravenous challenge with herpes simplex virus. *Scand J Immunol.* (1999) 49:391–4.
57. Lawler C, Tan CS, Simas JP, Stevenson PG. Type I interferons and NK cells restrict gammaherpesvirus lymph node infection. *J Virol.* (2016) 90:9046–57. doi: 10.1128/JVI.01108-16
58. Shaabani N, Duhan V, Khairnar V, Gassa A, Ferrer-Tur R, Haussinger D, et al. CD169(+) macrophages regulate PD-L1 expression via type I interferon and thereby prevent severe immunopathology after LCMV infection. *Cell Death Dis.* (2016) 7:e2446. doi: 10.1038/cddis.2016.350
59. Garcia Z, Lemaitre F, van Rooijen N, Albert ML, Levy Y, Schwartz O, et al. Subcapsular sinus macrophages promote NK cell accumulation and activation in response to lymph-borne viral particles. *Blood* (2012) 120:4744–50. doi: 10.1182/blood-2012-02-408179
60. Sagoo P, Garcia Z, Breart B, Lemaitre F, Michonneau D, Albert ML, et al. *In vivo* imaging of inflammasome activation reveals a subcapsular macrophage burst response that mobilizes innate and adaptive immunity. *Nat Med.* (2016) 22:64–71. doi: 10.1038/nm.4016
61. Swiecki M, Colonna M. The multifaceted biology of plasmacytoid dendritic cells. *Nat Rev Immunol.* (2015) 15:471–85. doi: 10.1038/nri3865
62. Brewitz A, Eickhoff S, Dahling S, Quast T, Bedoui S, Kroczek RA, et al. CD8(+) T Cells orchestrate pDC-XCR1(+) dendritic cell spatial and functional cooperativity to optimize priming. *Immunity* (2017) 46:205–19. doi: 10.1016/j.immuni.2017.01.003
63. Spaulding E, Fooksman D, Moore JM, Saidi A, Feintuch CM, Reizis B, et al. STING-licensed macrophages prime type I IFN production by plasmacytoid dendritic cells in the bone marrow during severe plasmodium yoelii malaria. *PLoS Pathog.* (2016) 12:e1005975. doi: 10.1371/journal.ppat.1005975
64. Swiecki M, Gilfillan S, Vermi W, Wang Y, Colonna M. Plasmacytoid dendritic cell ablation impacts early interferon responses and antiviral NK and CD8(+) T cell accrual. *Immunity* (2010) 33:955–66. doi: 10.1016/j.immuni.2010.11.020
65. Fitzgerald-Bocarsly P, Feng D. The role of type I interferon production by dendritic cells in host defense. *Biochimie* (2007) 89:843–55. doi: 10.1016/j.biochi.2007.04.018
66. Simmons DP, Wearsch PA, Canaday DH, Meyerson HJ, Liu YC, Wang Y, et al. Type I IFN drives a distinctive dendritic cell maturation phenotype that allows continued class II MHC synthesis and antigen processing. *J Immunol.* (2012) 188:3116–26. doi: 10.4049/jimmunol.1101313
67. Asselin-Paturel C, Brizard G, Chemin K, Boonstra A, O'Garra A, Vicari A, et al. Type I interferon dependence of plasmacytoid dendritic cell activation and migration. *J Exp Med.* (2005) 201:1157–67. doi: 10.1084/jem.20041930
68. Kreutz M, Bakdash G, Dolen Y, Skold AE, van Hout-Kuijer MA, de Vries IJ, et al. Type I IFN-mediated synergistic activation of mouse and human DC subsets by TLR agonists. *Eur J Immunol.* (2015) 45:2798–809. doi: 10.1002/eji.201545583
69. Spadaro F, Lapenta C, Donati S, Abalsamo L, Barnaba V, Belardelli F, et al. IFN-alpha enhances cross-presentation in human dendritic cells by

modulating antigen survival, endocytic routing, and processing. *Blood* (2012) 119:1407–17. doi: 10.1182/blood-2011-06-363564
70. Le Bon A, Etchart N, Rossmann C, Ashton M, Hou S, Gewert D, et al. Cross-priming of CD8+ T cells stimulated by virus-induced type I interferon. *Nat Immunol.* (2003) 4:1009–15. doi: 10.1038/ni978
71. Diamond MS, Kinder M, Matsushita H, Mashayekhi M, Dunn GP, Archambault JM, et al. Type I interferon is selectively required by dendritic cells for immune rejection of tumors. *J Exp Med.* (2011) 208:1989–2003. doi: 10.1084/jem.20101158
72. Fuertes MB, Kacha AK, Kline J, Woo SR, Kranz DM, Murphy KM, et al. Host type I IFN signals are required for antitumor CD8+ T cell responses through CD8{alpha}+ dendritic cells. *J Exp Med.* (2011) 208:2005–16. doi: 10.1084/jem.20101159
73. Dalod M, Hamilton T, Salomon R, Salazar-Mather TP, Henry SC, Hamilton JD, et al. Dendritic cell responses to early murine cytomegalovirus infection: subset functional specialization and differential regulation by interferon alpha/beta. *J Exp Med.* (2003) 197:885–98. doi: 10.1084/jem.20021522
74. Schulz O, Diebold SS, Chen M, Naslund TI, Nolte MA, Alexopoulou L, et al. Toll-like receptor 3 promotes cross-priming to virus-infected cells. *Nature* (2005) 433:887–92. doi: 10.1038/nature03326
75. Wei J, Waithman J, Lata R, Mifsud NA, Cebon J, Kay T, et al. Influenza A infection enhances cross-priming of CD8+ T cells to cell-associated antigens in a TLR7- and type I IFN-dependent fashion. *J Immunol.* (2010) 185:6013–22. doi: 10.4049/jimmunol.1002129
76. Shimizu K, Asakura M, Shinga J, Sato Y, Kitahara S, Hoshino K, et al. Invariant NKT cells induce plasmacytoid dendritic cell (DC) cross-talk with conventional DCs for efficient memory CD8+ T cell induction. *J Immunol.* (2013) 190:5609–19. doi: 10.4049/jimmunol.1300033
77. Rajagopal D, Paturel C, Morel Y, Uematsu S, Akira S, Diebold SS. Plasmacytoid dendritic cell-derived type I interferon is crucial for the adjuvant activity of Toll-like receptor 7 agonists. *Blood* (2010) 115:1949–57. doi: 10.1182/blood-2009-08-238543
78. Webb LM, Lundie RJ, Borger JG, Brown SL, Connor LM, Cartwright AN, et al. Type I interferon is required for T helper (Th) 2 induction by dendritic cells. *EMBO J.* (2017) 36:2404–18. doi: 10.15252/embj.201695345
79. Longhi MP, Trumpfheller C, Idoyaga J, Caskey M, Matos I, Kluger C, et al. Dendritic cells require a systemic type I interferon response to mature and induce CD4+ Th1 immunity with poly IC as adjuvant. *J Exp Med.* (2009) 206:1589–602. doi: 10.1084/jem.20090247
80. Le Bon A, Schiavoni G, D'Agostino G, Gresser I, Belardelli F, Tough DF. Type I interferons potently enhance humoral immunity and can promote isotype switching by stimulating dendritic cells *in vivo*. *Immunity.* (2001) 14:461–70. doi: 10.1016/S1074-7613(01)00126-1
81. Cucak H, Yrlid U, Reizis B, Kalinke U, Johansson-Lindbom B. Type I interferon signaling in dendritic cells stimulates the development of lymph-node-resident T follicular helper cells. *Immunity.* (2009) 31:491–501. doi: 10.1016/j.immuni.2009.07.005
82. Lapenta C, Santini SM, Spada M, Donati S, Urbani F, Accapezzato D, et al. IFN-alpha-conditioned dendritic cells are highly efficient in inducing cross-priming CD8(+) T cells against exogenous viral antigens. *Eur J Immunol.* (2006) 36:2046–60. doi: 10.1002/eji.200535579
83. Lattanzi L, Rozera C, Marescotti D, D'Agostino G, Santodonato L, Cellini S, et al. IFN-alpha boosts epitope cross-presentation by dendritic cells via modulation of proteasome activity. *Immunobiology* (2011) 216:537–47. doi: 10.1016/j.imbio.2010.10.003
84. Higgs BW, Liu Z, White B, Zhu W, White WI, Morehouse C, et al. Patients with systemic lupus erythematosus, myositis, rheumatoid arthritis and scleroderma share activation of a common type I interferon pathway. *Ann Rheum Dis.* (2011) 70:2029–36. doi: 10.1136/ard.2011.1 50326
85. Blanco P, Palucka AK, Gill M, Pascual V, Banchereau J. Induction of dendritic cell differentiation by IFN-alpha in systemic lupus erythematosus. *Science* (2001) 294:1540–3. doi: 10.1126/science.10 64890
86. Nestle FO, Conrad C, Tun-Kyi A, Homey B, Gombert M, Boyman O, et al. Plasmacytoid predendritic cells initiate psoriasis through interferon-alpha production. *J Exp Med.* (2005) 202:135–43. doi: 10.1084/jem.20050500
87. York MR, Nagai T, Mangini AJ, Lemaire R, van Seventer JM, Lafyatis R. A macrophage marker, Siglec-1, is increased on circulating monocytes in patients with systemic sclerosis and induced by type I interferons and toll-like receptor agonists. *Arthritis Rheum.* (2007) 56:1010–20. doi: 10.1002/art.22382
88. Bogie JF, Boelen E, Louagie E, Delputte P, Elewaut D, van Horssen J, et al. CD169 is a marker for highly pathogenic phagocytes in multiple sclerosis. *Mult Scler.* (2018) 24:290–300. doi: 10.1177/1352458517698759
89. Zinselmeyer BH, Heydari S, Sacristan C, Nayak D, Cammer M, Herz J, et al. PD-1 promotes immune exhaustion by inducing antiviral T cell motility paralysis. *J Exp Med.* (2013) 210:757–74. doi: 10.1084/jem.20121416
90. Honke N, Shaabani N, Merches K, Gassa A, Kraft A, Ehrhardt K, et al. Immunoactivation induced by chronic viral infection inhibits viral replication and drives immunosuppression through sustained IFN-I responses. *Eur J Immunol.* (2016) 46:372–80. doi: 10.1002/eji.201545765
91. Schwandt T, Schumak B, Gielen GH, Jungerkes F, Schmidbauer P, Klocke K, et al. Expression of type I interferon by splenic macrophages suppresses adaptive immunity during sepsis. *EMBO J.* (2012) 31:201–13. doi: 10.1038/emboj.2011.380
92. Hickman HD, Takeda K, Skon CN, Murray FR, Hensley SE, Loomis J, et al. Direct priming of antiviral CD8+ T cells in the peripheral interfollicular region of lymph nodes. *Nat Immunol.* (2008) 9:155–65. doi: 10.1038/ni1557
93. Sewald X, Ladinsky MS, Uchil PD, Beloor J, Pi R, Herrmann C, et al. Retroviruses use CD169-mediated trans-infection of permissive lymphocytes to establish infection. *Science* (2015) 350:563–7. doi: 10.1126/science.aab2749
94. Honke N, Shaabani N, Cadeddu G, Sorg UR, Zhang DE, Trilling M, et al. Enforced viral replication activates adaptive immunity and is essential for the control of a cytopathic virus. *Nat Immunol.* (2011) 13:51–7. doi: 10.1038/ni.2169
95. Erikson E, Wratil PR, Frank M, Ambiel I, Pahnke K, Pino M, et al. Mouse siglec-1 mediates trans-infection of surface-bound murine leukemia virus in a sialic acid n-acyl side chain-dependent manner. *J Biol Chem.* (2015) 290:27345–59. doi: 10.1074/jbc.M115.681338
96. Akiyama H, Ramirez NP, Gibson G, Kline C, Watkins S, Ambrose Z, et al. Interferon-inducible CD169/siglec1 attenuates anti-HIV-1 effects of alpha interferon. *J Virol.* (2017) 91:e00972-17. doi: 10.1128/JVI.00972-17
97. Winkelmann ER, Widman DG, Xia J, Johnson AJ, van Rooijen N, Mason PW, et al. Subcapsular sinus macrophages limit dissemination of West Nile virus particles after inoculation but are not essential for the development of West Nile virus-specific T cell responses. *Virology* (2014) 450–51:278–89. doi: 10.1016/j.virol.2013.12.021
98. Frederico B, Chao B, Lawler C, May JS, Stevenson PG. Subcapsular sinus macrophages limit acute gammaherpesvirus dissemination. *J Gen Virol.* (2015) 96:2314–27. doi: 10.1099/vir.0.000140
99. Farrell HE, Davis-Poynter N, Bruce K, Lawler C, Dolken L, Mach M, et al. Lymph node macrophages restrict murine cytomegalovirus dissemination. *J Virol.* (2015) 89:7147–58. doi: 10.1128/JVI.00480-15
100. Duhan V, Khairnar V, Friedrich SK, Zhou F, Gassa A, Honke N, et al. Virus-specific antibodies allow viral replication in the marginal zone, thereby promoting CD8(+) T-cell priming and viral control. *Sci Rep.* (2016) 6:19191. doi: 10.1038/srep19191
101. Carrasco YR, Batista FD. B cells acquire particulate antigen in a macrophage-rich area at the boundary between the follicle and the subcapsular sinus of the lymph node. *Immunity* (2007) 27:160–71. doi: 10.1016/j.immuni.2007.06.007
102. Phan TG, Grigorova I, Okada T, Cyster JG. Subcapsular encounter and complement-dependent transport of immune complexes by lymph node B cells. *Nat Immunol.* (2007) 8:992–1000. doi: 10.1038/ni1494
103. Veninga H, Borg EG, Vreeman K, Taylor PR, Kalay H, van Kooyk Y, et al. Antigen targeting reveals splenic CD169+ macrophages as promoters of germinal center B-cell responses. *Eur J Immunol.* (2015) 45:747–57. doi: 10.1002/eji.201444983
104. Phan TG, Green JA, Gray EE, Xu Y, Cyster JG. Immune complex relay by subcapsular sinus macrophages and noncognate B cells drives antibody affinity maturation. *Nat Immunol.* (2009) 10:786–93. doi: 10.1038/ni.1745
105. Gaya M, Castello A, Montaner B, Rogers N, Reis e Sousa C, Bruckbauer A, Batista FD. Host response. Inflammation-induced disruption of SCS

macrophages impairs B cell responses to secondary infection. *Science* (2015) 347:667–72. doi: 10.1126/science.aaa1300

106. Backer R, Schwandt T, Greuter M, Oosting M, Jungerkes F, Tuting T, et al. Effective collaboration between marginal metallophilic macrophages and CD8^{+} dendritic cells in the generation of cytotoxic T cells. *Proc Natl Acad Sci USA.* (2010) 107:216–21. doi: 10.1073/pnas.0909541107
107. Bernhard CA, Ried C, Kochanek S, Brocker T. CD169^{+} macrophages are sufficient for priming of CTLs with specificities left out by cross-priming dendritic cells. *Proc Natl Acad Sci USA.* (2015) 112:5461–6. doi: 10.1073/pnas.1423356112
108. Crocker PR, Freeman S, Gordon S, Kelm S. Sialoadhesin binds preferentially to cells of the granulocytic lineage. *J Clin Invest.* (1995) 95:635–43. doi: 10.1172/JCI117708
109. van den Berg TK, Breve JJ, Damoiseaux JG, Dopp EA, Kelm S, Crocker PR, et al. Sialoadhesin on macrophages: its identification as a lymphocyte adhesion molecule. *J Exp Med.* (1992) 176:647–55.
110. Sancho D, Joffre OP, Keller AM, Rogers NC, Martinez D, Hernanz-Falcon P, et al. Identification of a dendritic cell receptor that couples sensing of necrosis to immunity. *Nature* (2009) 458:899–903. doi: 10.1038/nature07750
111. Iborra S, Izquierdo HM, Martinez-Lopez M, Blanco-Menendez N, Reis e Sousa C, Sancho D. The DC receptor DNGR-1 mediates cross-priming of CTLs during vaccinia virus infection in mice. *J Clin Invest.* (2012) 122:1628–43. doi: 10.1172/JCI60660
112. Ahrens S, Zelenay S, Sancho D, Hanc P, Kjaer S, Feest C, et al. F-actin is an evolutionarily conserved damage-associated molecular pattern recognized by DNGR-1, a receptor for dead cells. *Immunity* (2012) 36:635–45. doi: 10.1016/j.immuni.2012.03.008
113. Rempel H, Calosing C, Sun B, Pulliam L. Sialoadhesin expressed on IFN-induced monocytes binds HIV-1 and enhances infectivity. *PLoS ONE* (2008) 3:e1967. doi: 10.1371/journal.pone.0001967
114. Zou Z, Chastain A, Moir S, Ford J, Trandem K, Martinelli E, et al. Siglecs facilitate HIV-1 infection of macrophages through adhesion with viral sialic acids. *PLoS ONE* (2011) 6:e24559. doi: 10.1371/journal.pone.0024559
115. Izquierdo-Useros N, Lorizate M, Puertas MC, Rodriguez-Plata MT, Zangger N, Erikson E, et al. Siglec-1 is a novel dendritic cell receptor that mediates HIV-1 trans-infection through recognition of viral membrane gangliosides. *PLoS Biol.* (2012) 10:e1001448. doi: 10.1371/journal.pbio.1001448
116. Puryear WB, Yu X, Ramirez NP, Reinhard BM, Gummuluru S. HIV-1 incorporation of host-cell-derived glycosphingolipid GM3 allows for capture by mature dendritic cells. *Proc Natl Acad Sci USA.* (2012) 109:7475–80. doi: 10.1073/pnas.1201104109
117. Akiyama H, Ramirez NG, Gudheti MV, Gummuluru S. CD169-mediated trafficking of HIV to plasma membrane invaginations in dendritic cells attenuates efficacy of anti-gp120 broadly neutralizing antibodies. *PLoS Pathog.* (2015) 11:e1004751. doi: 10.1371/journal.ppat.1004751
118. Akiyama H, Miller C, Patel HV, Hatch SC, Archer J, Ramirez NG, et al. Virus particle release from glycosphingolipid-enriched microdomains is essential for dendritic cell-mediated capture and transfer of HIV-1 and henipavirus. *J Virol.* (2014) 88:8813–25. doi: 10.1128/JVI.00992-14
119. Delputte PL, Van Breedam W, Delrue I, Oetke C, Crocker PR, Nauwynck HJ. Porcine arterivirus attachment to the macrophage-specific receptor sialoadhesin is dependent on the sialic acid-binding activity of the N-terminal immunoglobulin domain of sialoadhesin. *J Virol.* (2007) 81:9546–50. doi: 10.1128/JVI.00569-07
120. Edelson BT, Bradstreet TR, Hildner K, Carrero JA, Frederick KE, Kc W, et al. CD8alpha(+) dendritic cells are an obligate cellular entry point for productive infection by Listeria monocytogenes. *Immunity* (2011) 35:236–48. doi: 10.1016/j.immuni.2011.06.012
121. Aoshi T, Carrero JA, Konjufca V, Koide Y, Unanue ER, Miller MJ. The cellular niche of Listeria monocytogenes infection changes rapidly in the spleen. *Eur J Immunol.* (2009) 39:417–25. doi: 10.1002/eji.200838718
122. Perez OA, Yeung ST, Vera-Licona P, Romagnoli PA, Samji T, Ural BB, et al. CD169(+) macrophages orchestrate innate immune responses by regulating bacterial localization in the spleen. *Sci Immunol.* (2017) 2:eaah5520. doi: 10.1126/sciimmunol.aah5520
123. Ercoli G, Fernandes VE, Chung WY, Wanford JJ, Thomson S, Bayliss CD, et al. Intracellular replication of Streptococcus pneumoniae inside splenic macrophages serves as a reservoir for septicaemia. *Nat Microbiol.* (2018) 3:600–610. doi: 10.1038/s41564-018-0147-1
124. Heikema AP, Koning RI, Duarte dos Santos Rico S, Rempel H, Jacobs BC, Endtz HP, et al. Enhanced, sialoadhesin-dependent uptake of Guillain-Barre syndrome-associated Campylobacter jejuni strains by human macrophages. *Infect Immun.* (2013) 81:2095–103. doi: 10.1128/IAI.01437-12
125. Jones C, Virji M, Crocker PR. Recognition of sialylated meningococcal lipopolysaccharide by siglecs expressed on myeloid cells leads to enhanced bacterial uptake. *Mol Microbiol.* (2003) 49:1213–25. doi: 10.1046/j.1365-2958.2003.03634.x
126. Monteiro VG, Lobato CS, Silva AR, Medina DV, de Oliveira MA, Seabra SH, et al. Increased association of *Trypanosoma cruzi* with sialoadhesin positive mice macrophages. *Parasitol Res.* (2005) 97:380–5. doi: 10.1007/s00436-005-1460-1
127. Liu K, Iyoda T, Saternus M, Kimura Y, Inaba K, Steinman RM. Immune tolerance after delivery of dying cells to dendritic cells *in situ*. *J Exp Med.* (2002) 196:1091–7. doi: 10.1084/jem.20021215
128. McGaha TL, Chen Y, Ravishankar B, van Rooijen N, Karlsson, MCI. Marginal zone macrophages suppress innate and adaptive immunity to apoptotic cells in the spleen. *Blood* (2011) 117:5403–12. doi: 10.1182/blood-2010-11-320028
129. Ravishankar B, Shinde R, Liu H, Chaudhary K, Bradley J, Lemos HP, et al. Marginal zone CD169^{+} macrophages coordinate apoptotic cell-driven cellular recruitment and tolerance. *Proc Natl Acad Sci USA.* (2014) 111:4215–20. doi: 10.1073/pnas.1320924111
130. Hao S, Han X, Wang D, Yang Y, Li Q, Li X, et al. Critical role of CCL22/CCR4 axis in the maintenance of immune homeostasis during apoptotic cell clearance by splenic CD8alpha(+) CD103(+) dendritic cells. *Immunology* (2016) 148:174–86. doi: 10.1111/imm.12596
131. Griffith TS, Ferguson TA. Cell death in the maintenance and abrogation of tolerance: the five Ws of dying cells. *Immunity* (2011) 35:456–66. doi: 10.1016/j.immuni.2011.08.011
132. Garg AD, Agostinis P. Cell death and immunity in cancer: from danger signals to mimicry of pathogen defense responses. *Immunol Rev.* (2017) 280:126–48. doi: 10.1111/imr.12574
133. Lorenzi S, Mattei F, Sistigu A, Bracci L, Spadaro F, Sanchez M, et al. Type I IFNs control antigen retention and survival of CD8alpha(+) dendritic cells after uptake of tumor apoptotic cells leading to cross-priming. *J Immunol.* (2011) 186:5142–50. doi: 10.4049/jimmunol.1004163
134. Asano K, Nabeyama A, Miyake Y, Qiu CH, Kurita A, Tomura M, et al. CD169-positive macrophages dominate antitumor immunity by crosspresenting dead cell-associated antigens. *Immunity* (2011) 34:85–95. doi: 10.1016/j.immuni.2010.12.011
135. Xu Y, Liu Y, Yang C, Kang L, Wang M, Hu J, et al. Macrophages transfer antigens to dendritic cells by releasing exosomes containing dead-cell-associated antigens partially through a ceramide-dependent pathway to enhance CD4(+) T-cell responses. *Immunology* (2016) 149:157–71. doi: 10.1111/imm.12630
136. Tkach M, Thery C. Communication by extracellular vesicles: where we are and where we need to go. *Cell* (2016) 164:1226–32. doi: 10.1016/j.cell.2016.01.043
137. Morelli AE, Larregina AT, Shufesky WJ, Sullivan ML, Stolz DB, Papworth GD, et al. Endocytosis, intracellular sorting, and processing of exosomes by dendritic cells. *Blood* (2004) 104:3257–66. doi: 10.1182/blood-2004-03-0824
138. Saunderson SC, Dunn AC, Crocker PR, McLellan AD. CD169 mediates the capture of exosomes in spleen and lymph node. *Blood* (2014) 123:208–16. doi: 10.1182/blood-2013-03-489732
139. Black LV, Saunderson SC, Coutinho FP, Muhsin-Sharafaldine MR, Damani TT, Dunn AC, et al. The CD169 sialoadhesin molecule mediates cytotoxic T cell responses to tumour apoptotic vesicles. *Immunol Cell Biol.* (2015) 94:430–38. doi: 10.1038/icb.2015.111
140. Pucci F, Garris C, Lai CP, Newton A, Pfirschke C, Engblom C, et al. SCS macrophages suppress melanoma by restricting tumor-derived vesicle-B cell interactions. *Science* (2016) 352:242–6. doi: 10.1126/science.aaf1328
141. Ohnishi K, Komohara Y, Saito Y, Miyamoto Y, Watanabe M, Baba H, et al. CD169-positive macrophages in regional lymph nodes are associated with a favorable prognosis in patients with colorectal carcinoma. *Cancer Sci.* (2013) 104:1237–44. doi: 10.1111/cas.12212

142. Saito Y, Ohnishi K, Miyashita A, Nakahara S, Fujiwara Y, Horlad H, et al. Prognostic significance of CD169^{+} lymph node sinus macrophages in patients with malignant melanoma. *Cancer Immunol Res.* (2015) 3:1356–63. doi: 10.1158/2326-6066.CIR-14-0180
143. Ohnishi K, Yamaguchi M, Erdenebaatar C, Saito F, Tashiro H, Katabuchi HT, et al. Prognostic significance of CD169-positive lymph node sinus macrophages in patients with endometrial carcinoma. *Cancer Sci.* (2016) 107:846–52. doi: 10.1111/cas.12929
144. Shiota T, Miyasato Y, Ohnishi K, Yamamoto-Ibusuki M, Yamamoto Y, Iwase H, et al. The clinical significance of CD169-positive lymph node macrophage in patients with breast cancer. *PLoS ONE* (2016) 11:e0166680. doi: 10.1371/journal.pone.0166680
145. Asano T, Ohnishi K, Shiota T, Motoshima T, Sugiyama Y, Yatsuda J, et al. CD169-positive sinus macrophages in the lymph nodes determine bladder cancer prognosis. *Cancer Sci.* (2018) 109:1723–30. doi: 10.1111/cas.13565
146. Delputte PL, Van Gorp H, Favoreel HW, Hoebeke I, Delrue I, Dewerchin H, et al. Porcine sialoadhesin (CD169/Siglec-1) is an endocytic receptor that allows targeted delivery of toxins and antigens to macrophages. *PLoS ONE* (2011) 6:e16827. doi: 10.1371/journal.pone.0016827
147. Ooms K, Van Gorp H, Botti S, Van Gaever T, Delputte PL, Nauwynck HJ. Evaluation of viral peptide targeting to porcine sialoadhesin using a porcine reproductive and respiratory syndrome virus vaccination-challenge model. *Virus Res.* (2013) 177:147–55. doi: 10.1016/j.virusres.2013.07.019
148. Chen WC, Kawasaki N, Nycholat CM, Han S, Pilotte J, Crocker PR, et al. Antigen delivery to macrophages using liposomal nanoparticles targeting sialoadhesin/CD169. *PLoS ONE* (2012) 7:e39039. doi: 10.1371/journal.pone.0039039
149. Kawasaki N, Vela JL, Nycholat CM, Rademacher C, Khurana A, van Rooijen N, et al. Targeted delivery of lipid antigen to macrophages via the CD169/sialoadhesin endocytic pathway induces robust invariant natural killer T cell activation. *Proc Natl Acad Sci USA.* (2013) 110:7826–31. doi: 10.1073/pnas.1219888110
150. Gaya M, Barral P, Burbage M, Aggarwal S, Montaner B, Warren Navia A, et al. Initiation of antiviral B cell immunity relies on innate signals from spatially positioned NKT cells. *Cell* (2018) 172:517–33.e20. doi: 10.1016/j.cell.2017.11.036
151. Yu X, Feizpour A, Ramirez NG, Wu L, Akiyama H, Xu F, et al. Glycosphingolipid-functionalized nanoparticles recapitulate CD169-dependent HIV-1 uptake and trafficking in dendritic cells. *Nat Commun.* (2014) 5:4136. doi: 10.1038/ncomms5136

4

Structure-Function Relationship of XCL1 Used for *in vivo* Targeting of Antigen into XCR1$^+$ Dendritic Cells

Arthur L. Kroczek[1,2,3], *Evelyn Hartung*[1], *Stephanie Gurka*[1], *Martina Becker*[1], *Nele Reeg*[1], *Hans W. Mages*[1], *Sebastian Voigt*[4], *Christian Freund*[2] *and Richard A. Kroczek*[1*]

[1] Molecular Immunology, Robert Koch-Institute, Berlin, Germany, [2] Protein Biochemistry, Institute for Biochemistry, Free University of Berlin, Berlin, Germany, [3] Institute of Biochemistry, Charité University Medicine Berlin, Berlin, Germany, [4] Virology, Robert Koch-Institute, Berlin, Germany

***Correspondence:**
Richard A. Kroczek
kroczek@rki.de

XCL1 is the ligand for XCR1, a chemokine receptor uniquely expressed on cross-presenting dendritic cells (DC) in mouse and man. We are interested in establishing therapeutic vaccines based on XCL1-mediated targeting of peptides or proteins into these DC. Therefore, we have functionally analyzed various XCL1 domains in highly relevant settings *in vitro* and *in vivo*. Murine XCL1 fused to ovalbumin (XCL1-OVA) was compared to an N-terminal deletion variant lacking the first seven N-terminal amino acids and to several C-terminal (deletion) variants. Binding studies with primary XCR1$^+$ DC revealed that the N-terminal region stabilizes the binding of XCL1 to its receptor, as is known for other chemokines. Deviating from the established paradigm for chemokines, the N-terminus does not contain critical elements for inducing chemotaxis. On the contrary, this region appears to limit the chemotactic action of XCL1 at higher concentrations. A participation of the XCL1 C-terminus in receptor binding or chemotaxis could be excluded in a series of experiments. Binding studies with apoptotic and necrotic XCR1-negative cells suggested a second function for XCL1: marking of stressed cells for uptake into cross-presenting DC. *In vivo* studies using CD8$^+$ T cell proliferation and cytotoxicity as readouts confirmed the critical role of the N-terminus for antigen targeting, and excluded any involvement of the C-terminus in the uptake, processing, and presentation of the fused OVA antigen. Together, these studies provide basic data on the function of the various XCL1 domains as well as relevant information on XCL1 as an antigen carrier in therapeutic vaccines.

Keywords: dendritic cells, XCR1, XCL1, cross-presentation, antigen targeting

INTRODUCTION

Murine XCL1 is a chemokine of 93 amino acids, and has been originally identified as lymphotactin by Kelner et al. (1), while human XCL1 was found by us (2), and by Yoshida et al. (3). Mature murine XCL1 exhibits a high degree of homology to human XCL1 (also 93 aa), with 61% identity and 84% similarity, and both homologs have an identical structure [for alignment please refer to Geyer et al. (4)]. The XCL1/XCR1 chemokine ligand-receptor pair exhibits some special structural and functional features.

XCL1 is secreted by activated NK cells, activated Th1-polarized CD4+ T cells, and activated CD8+ T cells, and co-secreted with IFN-γ, MIP-1α, MIP-1β, and RANTES and is thus part of the Th1 immune defense (5, 6). XCR1 is the only receptor for XCL1, and XCL1 is the only ligand of this receptor (7, 8). Thus, this ligand/receptor pair is monogamous, a rare feature in the world of around 50 chemokines.

The receptor XCR1 is exclusively expressed on a subset of dendritic cells (DC), the "cross-presenting" DC (and not elsewhere in the body), in the mouse, the rat, and the human (4, 9–13). This narrow expression spectrum is another unusual feature of the XCL1/XCR1 axis. XCR1+ DC, earlier designated as CD8+ DC in the mouse, were demonstrated to be particularly efficient in the uptake of cells stressed by (intracellular) infection (14–16). Moreover, CD8+ DC have consistently been shown to excel in antigen "cross-presentation," in which exogenous antigen is not presented in the context of MHC class II to CD4+ T cells, but instead shunted into the MHC class I pathway of antigen presentation to CD8+ T cells (17–19). Given the secretion profile of XCL1, XCR1+ DC can be regarded as a DC population closely cooperating with NK cells, Th1-polarized CD4+ T cells, and CD8+ T cells in the surveillance of stressed/ transformed cells for "danger" (16). The cross-presenting XCR1+ DC are now also commonly referred to as cDC1.

In the past, we have employed this highly specific expression of XCR1 to target antigens into cross-presenting DC *in vivo*. In these experiments, ovalbumin (OVA), recombinantly fused to the C-terminal portion of murine XCL1 ("XCL1-OVA"), was highly efficient in inducing antigen-specific CD8+ T cell cytotoxicity, when compared to untargeted OVA (20). These experiments demonstrated that XCL1 can be employed as a carrier for therapeutic vaccines intended to elicit potent antigen-specific T cell cytotoxicity *in vivo*.

Because of this therapeutic potential, we are interested in the structure-function relationship of various domains of XCL1. Like classical chemokines, XCL1 has a free N-terminus of around 10 amino acids (aa), which is followed by a structured core domain of around 60 aa containing a three-stranded antiparallel beta-sheet and a C-terminal alpha-helix (classical "chemokine fold"). The C-terminal portion of XCL1 of around 20 aa is, typical for chemokines, again unstructured (21). The C-terminus is highly conserved between mouse, rat, and human XCL1, and of unknown function.

XCL1 is the only chemokine with one disulphide bridge, while all other chemokines stabilize their tertiary structure by two disulphide bridges. Kuloglu et al. (22) have demonstrated *in vitro* that due to the lack of this second disulphide bridge, XCL1 can assume at some more extreme conditions (45°C, no salt) an alternative conformation (which is exceptional in the chemokine world), which could imply a second function. This unusual feature raised the question whether the various domains of XCL1 functionally differ from classical chemokines or whether XCL1 has more than one function.

Abbreviations: DC, dendritic cells; OVA, ovalbumin; MFI, mean fluorescence intensity.

To fully understand the usefulness of XCL1 as a vector system for protein vaccines, we set out to systematically test the contribution of XCL1-domains on receptor binding, its chemotactic function, and on antigen processing and presentation to CD8+ T cells *in vivo*. To this end, N-terminal and C-terminal deletion variants of XCL1-OVA (which we have previously used for antigen targeting *in vivo* [Hartung et al. (20), see above] were generated. Further, we also replaced the entire C-terminal domain of XCL1 with the C-terminal domain of viral XCL1 (vXCL1), a rat cytomegalovirus-encoded XCL1 homolog, which we have recently identified and characterized (4). vXCL1, which can be assumed to interfere with the immune defense, has a fully intact chemotactic activity on cross-presenting DC and mainly differs in its C-terminal portion from its rat homolog. We thus utilized the viral C-terminus in order to determine whether this domain in some ways contributes to the function of XCL1.

MATERIALS AND METHODS

Cloning, Expression, and Purification of XCL1-OVA and Its Structural Variants

The DNA fragments coding for the various XCL1-OVA constructs with a C-terminal Strep-tag (IBA, Germany) were cloned into the drosophila expression vector pRmHa-3 (23) by standard procedures. XCL1-OVA encoding plasmids were electroporated together with the plasmid phshs.PURO into drosophila Schneider SL-3 cells (24) using a Bio-Rad Gene Pulser (450 V and 500 mF). The phshs.PURO plasmid (kindly provided by M. McKeown, Salk Institute) allows selection of positive transfectants by puromycin. Clones from limiting dilution cultures of transfected SL-3 cells were induced with 1 mM $CuSO_4$ and analyzed for high protein production using either XCL1- or Strep-tag-specific ELISA. Positive clones were expanded in Insect-XPRESS medium (Lonza) on a shaker platform (100 rpm) in normal air at 27°C. XCL1-OVA proteins were purified from supernatants using Strep-Trap HP columns from GE Healthcare according to the manufacturer's instructions. Protein concentration was determined by measuring OD_{280} using a Nanodrop ND-1000 (Thermo Scientific). LPS content in all protein samples was <0.5 EU/mg protein.

Mice

C57BL/6 mice (8–12 week old) were used for experiments and cell isolation, unless indicated otherwise. B6.XCR1-lacZ (The Jackson Laboratory) are XCR1-deficient mice in which the XCR1 gene has been replaced by the β-Gal reporter gene; these mice were fully backcrossed (>10x) onto the C57BL/6 background. OT-I TCR-transgenic mice were crossed onto the B6.PL background to allow identification of CD8+ T cells using the CD90.1 marker. All mice were bred under specific pathogen-free conditions in the animal facility of the Federal Institute for Risk Assessment (Berlin, Germany). All animal experiments were performed according to state guidelines and approved by the local animal welfare committee.

Cell Isolation

Splenocytes were obtained by mashing spleens through 70 μm cell sieves into PBS, followed by erythrocyte lysis with ACK Buffer (155 mM NH_4Cl, 10 mM $KHCO_3$, 0.1 mM EDTA).

Chemotaxis

To obtain sufficient DC for chemotaxis assays, C57BL/6 mice were injected s.c. at 2 sites, each site with 1.5×10^6 B16 cells secreting Flt3 ligand (25) for 9 days. DC were then enriched by cutting spleens into small pieces followed by digestion with Collagenase D (500 μg/ml) and DNase I (20 μg/ml, both Roche) for 25 min at 37°C in RPMI 1640 containing 2% FCS (low endotoxin, Biochrom); EDTA (10 mM) was added for additional 5 min and cells were filtered through a 70 μm nylon sieve (BD Falcon). DC were further enriched by centrifugation over a 1.073 g/ml density gradient (NycoPrep, Axis-Shield). For chemotaxis assays, 1×10^6 DC (purity ~70%) were suspended in 100 μl chemotaxis medium (RPMI 1,640, 1% BSA, 50 mM β-ME, 100 mg/ml penicillin/streptomycin) and placed into the upper chamber of a 24-well Transwell system (6.5 mm diameter, 5-μm pore polycarbonate membrane; Corning Costar). The lower chamber was filled with chemotaxis medium to which recombinant XCL1-OVA or the XCL1-variants were added. After incubation in 5% CO_2 for 2 h at 37°C, the number of migrated DC was determined by counting cells in the lower chamber using a flow cytometer. DC were identified by staining for XCR1, CD8, CD11c, and MHC II after gating out cells expressing B220 and CD3. The percentage of migrated cells was calculated by dividing the number of cells in the lower chamber by the number of input cells (number migrated cells/number input cells × 100).

In vivo Proliferation of OT-I T Cells

Recipient C57BL/6 mice were adoptively transferred with splenocytes containing 1×10^6 OT-I ($CD8^+$) resting T cells (negative for CD25, CD69, and ICOS). For proliferation analysis, OT I cells were labeled with 5 μM CFSE (Invitrogen) before transfer and analyzed 48 h after immunization using the CFSE dilution assay. Detection of OT-I T cells after adoptive transfer was with mAb to CD8 and CD90.1 after gating out $CD4^+$ T cells and $B220^+$ cells.

In vivo Cytotoxicity Assay

Animals were immunized with the indicated amounts of either XCL1-OVA or the respective variants together with 3 μg of LPS (Sigma), which was mixed with the protein variants before injection i.v.. 6 days later, 10×10^6 syngeneic splenocytes were pulsed with SIINFEKL peptide (GenScript) and labeled with 10 μM CFSE ($CFSE^{high}$) *in vitro*, while 10×10^6 splenocytes were left unpulsed and labeled with 1 μM CFSE ($CFSE^{low}$). Both preparations were injected together i.v. into immunized and control animals, and the CFSE signal was determined by flow cytometry 18 h later. Specific lysis was calculated using the following formula: specific lysis (%) = 100–([$CFSE^{high}$ immunized/$CFSE^{low}$ immunized]/[$CFSE^{high}$ control/$CFSE^{low}$ control]) × 100.

Antibodies and Staining Reagents

Hybridomas producing mAb recognizing CD4 (clone YTS 191.1), CD8 (53–6.72), CD11c (N418), CD44 (IM7.8.1), CD45R (B220 clone RA3-6B2), CD62L (MEL-14), Ly6G/C (RB6-8C5), and MHC class II (M5/114.15.2) were obtained from ATCC, CD90.1 (OX-7) from ECACC. Mab to CD69 (H1.2F3) was from Biolegend, mAb PD-1 (J43) from eBioscience. Anti-CD3 (KT3) was generously provided by H. Savelkoul, anti-CD25 (2E4) by E. Shevach. Generation of anti-XCR1 mAb MARX10 (13) and anti-ICOS mAb [MIC-280 (26)] has been described before. Mab MTAC-311 detects the C-terminal part of murine XCL1 (unpublished antibody and data). Generation of XCL1-StrepTag is described in Hartung et al. (20). The non-agonistic mAb MARX10 (mouse IgG2b, in the recombinant version IgG1) does not block the binding of XCL1 to XCR1. OT-I T cells were identified with mAbs to Vα2-TCR (B20.1, eBioscience) and Vβ5-TCR (MR9-4, BD Biosciences). StrepMAB Immo conjugated to Oyster 645 was from IBA Lifesciences.

Flow Cytometry

Antibodies were titrated for optimal signal-to-noise ratio. To block unspecific binding to Fc-receptors, cells were pre-incubated with 100 μg/ml 2.4G2 mAb. Standard staining with mAb was in PBS, 0.25% BSA, 0.1% NaN_3 for 25 min on ice. For exclusion of dead cells 4′,6-diamidino-2-phenylindole (DAPI) was added 5 min before measurement. Doublets and autofluorescent cells were excluded from the analysis. Data were acquired on a LSRII cytometer (BD Biosciences), and analyzed using FlowJo (Tree Star Inc.). DC were defined as $CD11c^+$ MHC-II^+ Lin^- cells.

Stressed Cells Assay

P3X63Ag8.653 myeloma cells (ATCC) were cultured at a density of 2×10^6 cell/ml in complete RMPI1640 medium. Some cells were exposed to heat shock (52°C for 15 min) and thereafter cultured at a density of 2×10^6 cells/ml in a 6-well plate overnight at 37°C and 5% CO_2. Then, 0.5×10^6 cells were transferred into 24-well culture plate wells and 1 μg or 2 μg of wt XCL1-OVA or one of its variants were added for the last hour of culture. The cells were washed and stained with mAb StrepMAB Immo conjugated to Oyster 645 (to detect bound XCL1-OVA) and Annexin V-Cy5 (BD Pharmingen) in a binding buffer (10 mM Hepes, 140 mM NaCl, 2,5 mM CaCl2, 1% NaN3). After a further washing step, cells taken up in binding buffer and were analyzed by flow cytometry, DAPI was added just before analysis.

RESULTS

Generation of XCL1-OVA and the Structural Variants Del-N7, Del-C7, Del-C17, and vCterm

Various formats of XCL1 recombinantly fused to OVA were generated in order to test for the impact of the various domains (i) on the function of murine XCL1, (ii) on the ability of XCL1 to target the antigen OVA into $XCR1^+$ DC *in vivo*, and (iii) on the capacity of $XCR1^+$ DC to process and cross-present the attached antigen. The design, production, and *in vivo* targeting capacity and specificity of XCL1-OVA, used here as the standard for comparison, has been described earlier (20). Del-N7 XCL1 is a variant lacking the first seven N-terminal amino acids (aa) of XCL1, but is otherwise identical to XCL1-OVA (**Figure 1A**). Del-C7 XCL1 lacks the C-terminal 7 aa, Del-C17 the C-terminal 17 aa of XCL1; in both deletion variants a glycine-serine linker (GGGGS) was introduced C-terminally in order to (partially) compensate for any size/positional effects (**Figure 1B**). vCterm XCL1 is a variant in which the 17 C-terminal aa of murine XCL1 were replaced by the 20 C-terminal aa of a rat cytomegalovirus-encoded XCL1 homolog (4). All constructs contained a C-terminal Strep-tag to allow detection of the bound protein variants to XCR1. The various constructs are represented schematically in **Figure 1A**. For clarity, the C-terminal sequences of the XCL1-variants are also shown (**Figure 1B**). The constructs were used to express the protein in Schneider cells.

The N-Terminus of XCL1 Is Critical for Binding to XCR1

The binding of XCL1-OVA and its structural variants to its receptor XCR1 was determined by incubating splenocytes with carefully titrated concentrations of each reagent for 25 min on ice, followed by washing. The bound protein variants on XCR1$^+$ DC were then detected using an anti-Strep-tag mAb and flow cytometry. Some of the results (incubation of the cells at 2.5, 0.625, 0.16, and 0.04 μg/ml) are represented in histograms in **Figure 2A**. **Figure 2B** summarizes experimental data points obtained with all concentrations of the respective protein variants. Small concentrations of XCL1-OVA (0.04 μg/ml) sufficed to achieve substantial binding, and saturation was achieved at around 0.5 μg/ml. The Del-C7 and Del-C17 structural variants showed a binding pattern comparable to wildtype XCL1-OVA (**Figures 2A,B**). In contrast, the Del-N7 variant only bound at high concentrations of protein. At 2.5 μg/ml, the binding efficiency of Del-N7 was comparable to binding of XCL1-OVA at around 0.05 μg/ml, and thus was diminished around 50-fold. Incubation with vCterm XCL1 resulted in clearly stronger binding signals, when compared to XCL1-OVA (**Figures 2A,B**).

To control for unspecific signals, the binding experiments were repeated with cells from XCR1-deficient (XCR1$^{-/-}$) mice on the same C57BL/6 background. As can be seen from **Figure 2C**, all variants exhibited a similar XCR1-unspecific binding (only at this high concentration, data not shown), with the exception of the Del-C17 variant.

These experiments determined that the first seven N-terminal aa of XCL1 have a major influence on the binding of XCL1 to its receptor, which can be partially compensated at high protein concentrations by other structural elements of XCL1. At the same time, the experiments excluded any significant contribution of the C-terminal 17 aa to the binding of XCL1 to XCR1. Binding studies with XCR1$^{-/-}$ dendritic cells further demonstrated that all binding of XCL1 to the DC is mediated by XCR1; the unspecific signals obtained at higher protein concentrations (2.5 μg) are apparently mediated by the C-terminal portion of XCL1 and are most likely of no major relevance *in vivo*.

Effects of the Structural Variants on Chemotaxis

In order to determine the functional capacity of the XCL1-OVA structural variants, DC were enriched from splenocytes and tested at various concentrations of the variants for chemotaxis in a transwell system. All of the cells which have migrated into the lower chamber were quantitatively analyzed using flow cytometry; therefore the intensity of the dot-plots truly represents the number of migrated cells. The DC in the input cell population were composed of around 70% of XCR1$^+$ DC and 30% XCR1$^-$ DC (**Figure 3A**, leftmost dotplot in upper panel). Virtually no migration into the lower chamber was observed in the medium control, while both XCR1$^+$ and XCR1$^-$ DC migrated equally well to the chemokine CCL21, which was used as a positive control (**Figure 3A**, upper panels). Essentially only XCR1$^+$ DC migrated in response to the various XCL1-OVA constructs, with virtually no response of T cells, B cells or other XCR1$^-$ cells (data not shown). The migration of XCR1$^+$ DC to various concentrations of the XCL1-OVA standard (1 ng/ml−10,000 ng/ml) exhibited the bell-shaped curve typical for chemokines, with maximal chemotactic activity at 100 ng/ml (**Figures 3A,B**). A similar pattern was observed for Del-C7, Del-C17, and also for vCterm (**Figures 3A,B**). With Del-N7, barely any chemotaxis was observed up to 100 ng/ml and even at 1,000 ng/ml the efficiency did not reach the maximum seen with wt XCL1-OVA. Interestingly, by further increasing the concentration of Del-N7 to 10,000 ng/ml in the lower chamber, Del-N7 was chemotactically active above the levels seen with optimal amounts (100 ng/ml) of wt XCL1-OVA (**Figures 3A,B**). This was a consistent phenomenon throughout the experiments.

The results obtained in this functional experiment were congruent with the previous binding studies. All XCL1-OVA versions exhibiting good binding also induced effective chemotaxis. Since the Del-C17 variant was similarly active compared to XCL1-OVA, it can be concluded that the C-terminal 17 aa of XCL1 do not participate in the induction of chemotaxis and thus must have other function(s). The positive functional data obtained with Del-N7 XCL1 at very high concentrations indicate that the core domain of XCL1 between aa 8 and 76 contains all necessary structural elements to induce chemotaxis. The first 7 N-terminal aa apparently play a major role in the stabilization of ligand binding to the receptor for induction of chemotaxis. Interestingly, for unknown reason, this N-terminal stretch of XCL1 seems also to limit the signaling at high ligand concentrations.

Binding of XCL1-OVA and Its Variants Del-N7, Del-C7, Del-C17, and vCterm to Apoptotic and Necrotic Cells

As outlined in the introduction, XCL1 is an integral part of the Th1-defense. Given the secretion of XCL1 by activated NK cells, Th1-polarized CD4$^+$ T cells, and by activated CD8$^+$ T cells, we tested the hypothesis that secreted XCL1 could "mark" stressed cells and thus facilitate their uptake by cross-presenting DC. To test this hypothesis, we examined the binding of wt XCL1-OVA and its structural variants to stressed

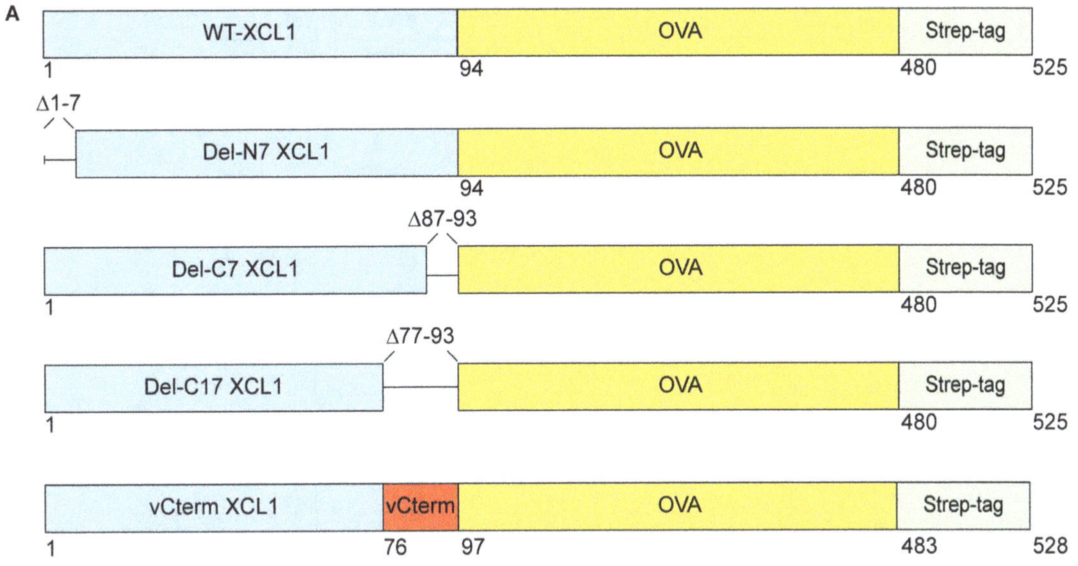

B

WT-XCL1	....**VKAAIKTVDGRASTRKNMAETVPTGAQRSTSTAITLTG-OVA-Strep-tag**
Del-N7	....**VKAAIKTVDGRASTRKNMAETVPTGAQRSTSTAITLTG-OVA-Strep-tag**
Del-C7	....**VKAAIKTVDGRASTRKNMAETVPTGAQRSTSGGGGSGGGGS-OVA-Strep-tag**
Del-C17	....**VKAAIKTVDGRASTRKNMAET-------GGGGSGGGGS-OVA-Strep-tag**
vCterm	....**VKAAIKTVDGRASTRKNMAETTTVIPTQVPVSTNETTTVYG-OVA-Strep-tag**

FIGURE 1 | XCL1-OVA and its variants Del-N7, Del-C7, Del-C17, and vCterm. **(A)** Schematic representation of XCL1-OVA and its variants. Del-N7 lacks the first seven amino acids (aa), in Del-C7 and Del-C17, the final 7 and 17 C-terminal aa were deleted, respectively. In vCterm, the 17 C-terminal aa were replaced by the 20 C-terminal aa of murid herpesvirus 8-encoded XCL1. **(B)** C-terminal aa sequences of XCL1 in the respective protein variants.

cells. To this end, P3X63Ag8.653 myeloma cells obtained from standard culture (and thus without stress signals) were double-stained with DAPI and Annexin V and arbitrarily subdivided into populations designated as "live" (Annexin V^- $DAPI^-$), "apoptotic" (Annexin V^+ $DAPI^{low}$), "necrotic" (Annexin V^+ $DAPI^+$), and "dead" (Annexin V^- $DAPI^+$) (**Figure 4A**). While live and dead cells did not exhibit a strong binding of the various reagents, apoptotic and necrotic cells bound each reagent to a substantial degree, with a rather uniform staining pattern (**Figure 4B**, background staining with StrepMAB-Immo in gray). When the P3X cells were subjected to thermal stress (52°C for 15 min, followed by overnight culture), again both necrotic and apoptotic cells bound the various reagents in an uniform fashion (**Figures 4C,D**). To determine which component(s) of the constructs was responsible for the observed binding, additional experiments were performed. Live, apoptotic, necrotic, and dead cells were reacted with XCL1 or with XCL1-StrepTag and any bound reagent detected with a mAb directed to murine XCL1 (**Figure 4E**). Only apoptotic and necrotic cells gave the characteristic signal pattern, after incubation with either XCL1 or XCL1-StrepTag. Since both reagents gave a staining pattern similar to the other constructs (**Figure 4B**), any significant binding of StrepTag or OVA to stressed cells could be excluded. Together, these experiments determined that XCL1 was responsible for binding to stressed cells. Furthermore, it could be concluded that the structured core region of XCL1 was responsible for the binding to stressed cells, with no obvious contribution of the free N-terminal or C-terminal regions. Altogether, the data were compatible with the notion that XCL1 marks stressed cells.

Induction of $CD8^+$ T Cell Proliferation and Cytotoxic Capacity After *in vivo* Targeting of Antigen With XCL1-OVA and Its Variants Del-N7, Del-C7, Del-C17, and vCterm

In the next experiments we tested whether the various structural elements of XCL1 influence targeting of antigen *in vivo*. To this end, fluorescently labeled OT-I T cells were adoptively transferred into syngeneic C57BL/6 mice. One day later, mice were immunized i.v. with various amounts (0.1 μg, 0.3 μg, 1 μg) of wt XCL1-OVA, or alternatively with equal amounts of its variants Del-N7, Del-C7, Del-C17, and vCterm without adjuvant; PBS was used as negative control. After 48 h, spleens were removed and the proliferation of the OT-I T cells determined through dilution of the fluorescence signal using flow cytometry. In two independent experiments, Del-C17 induced higher proliferation of the OT-I $CD8^+$ T cells at lower dosages, possibly reflecting its higher binding capacity

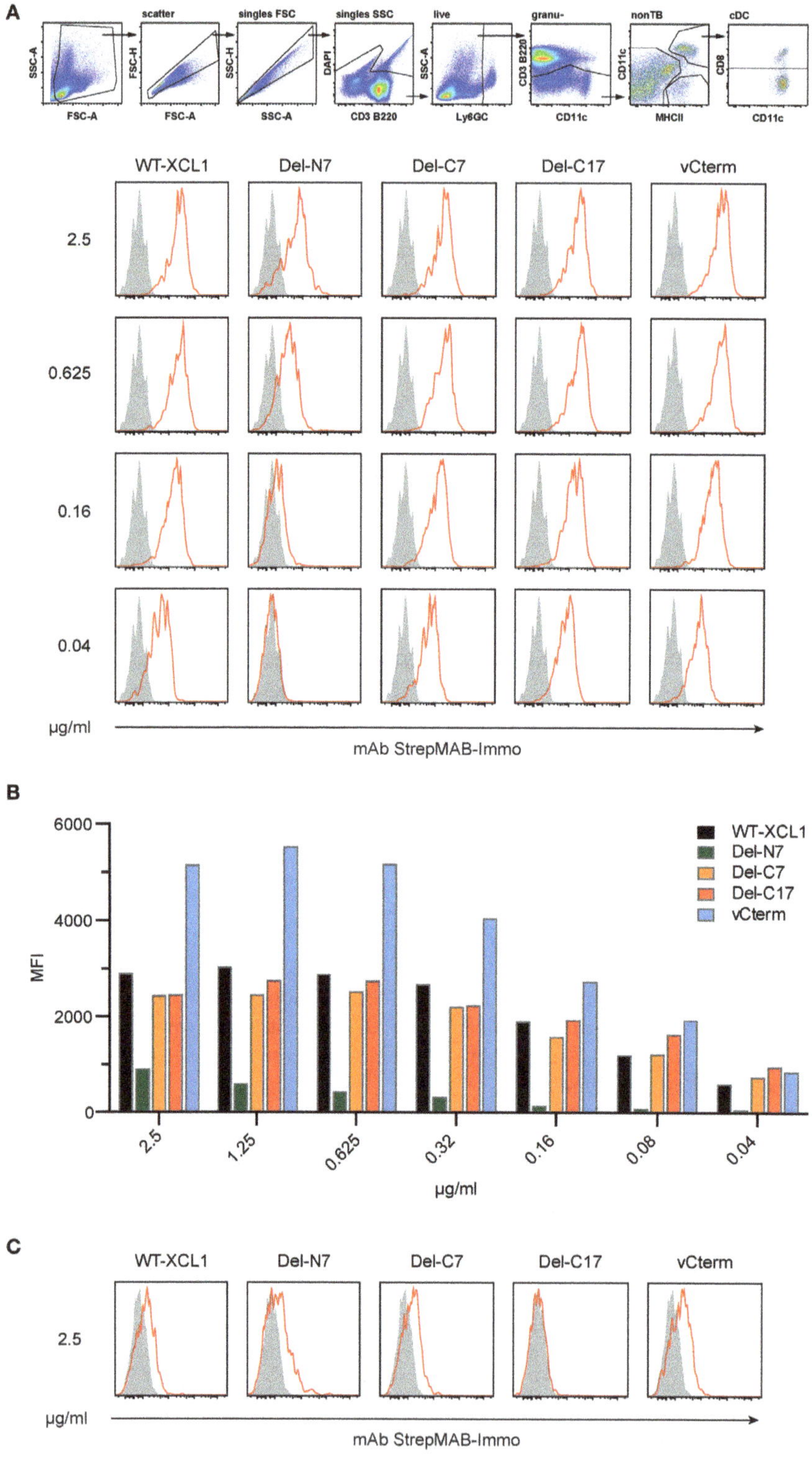

FIGURE 2 | Binding of XCL1 and the structural variants Del-N7, Del-C7, Del-C17, and vCterm to XCR1 expressed on primary dendritic cells. Splenocytes were incubated with carefully titrated (0.04, 0.08, 0.16, 0.315, 0.625, 1.25, and 2.5 µg/ml) concentrations of all XCL1-OVA protein variants (all concentrations are given based on the XCL1-component of the constructs) for 25 min on ice, washed, and the bound protein was detected on Ly6G/C$^-$ CD3$^-$ B220$^-$ CD8$^+$ CD11c$^+$ MHC-II$^+$ cells using an anti-Strep-tag mAb StrepMAB-Immo and flow cytometry (red histograms). Background staining, without pre-incubation, using StrepMAB-Immo is shown in gray. **(A)** Signals obtained with XCL1-variants at 0.04, 0.16, 0.625, and 2.5 µg/ml. **(B)** Graphical representation of the mean fluorescence intensity (MFI) obtained in flow cytometry with all protein concentrations of the XCL1-OVA variants used. **(C)** Signals (shown for 0.625 and 2.5/µg/ml) obtained on CD8$^+$ DC lacking XCR1. Data are representative of 3 independent experiments.

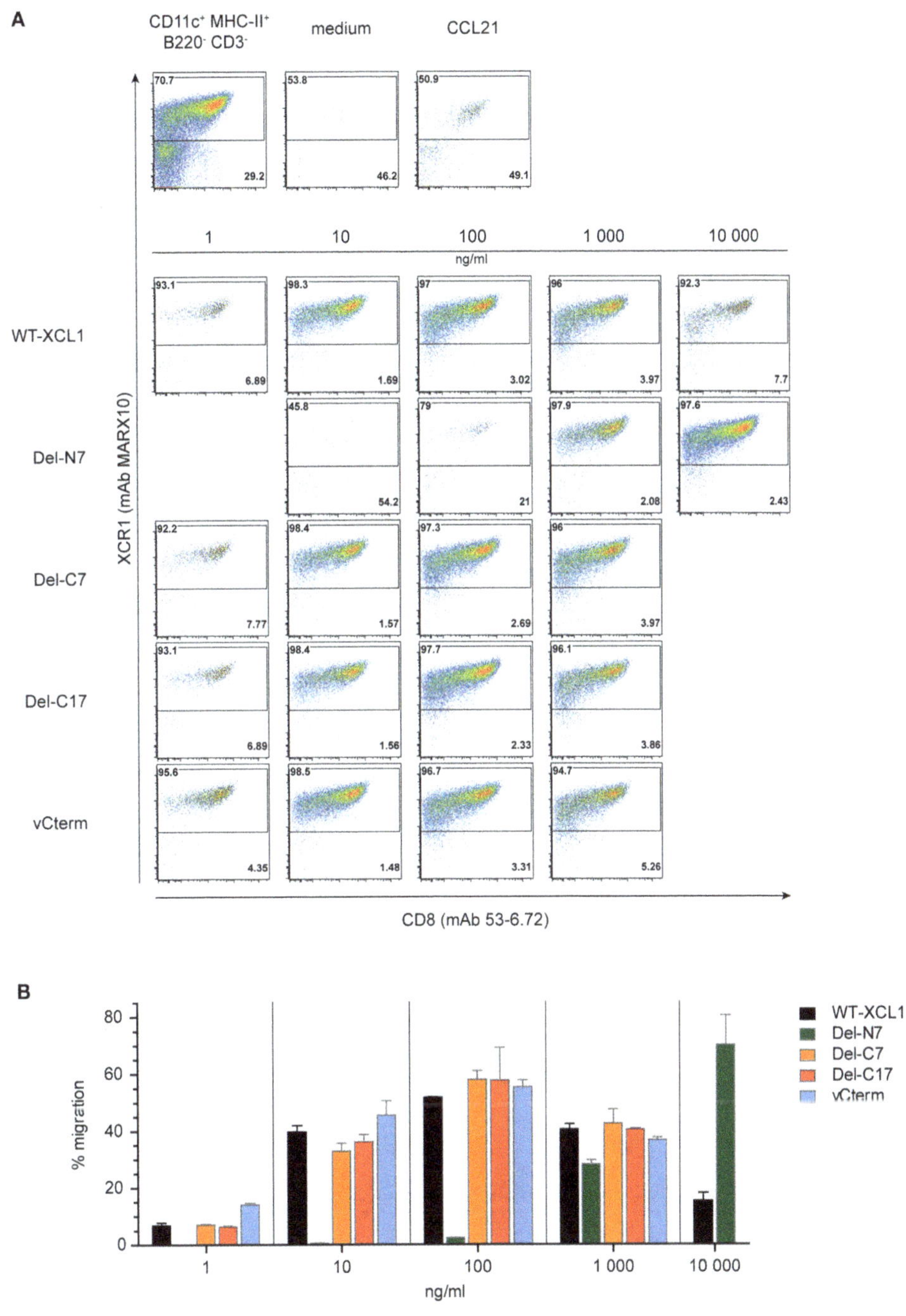

FIGURE 3 | Chemotaxis induced by XCL1-OVA and its variants Del-N7, Del-C7, Del-C17, and vCterm. **(A)** DC enriched from splenocytes by density gradient centrifugation were placed in the upper chamber of a transwell system, the composition of input DC is shown in the leftmost dotplot in the upper pannel. Various concentrations of wt XCL1-OVA and the structural variants were established in the lower chamber and migration of cells was allowed for 2 h. All concentrations are given based on the XCL1-component of the constructs. Thereafter, all cells from the lower chambers were quantitatively analyzed by flow cytometry after staining for XCR1 (mAb MARX10 binds to XCR1 independent of XCL1) and CD8 (mAb 53-6.2). Therefore, the number of events in the dot plots directly represent the number of cells detected. The effect of the negative (medium) and the positive controls (CCL21) is shown in the upper pannels of dot plots. **(B)** Quantitave evaluation of migrated $XCR1^+$ DC expressed as percentage of input $XCR1^+$ DC of the experiment shown in **(A)**. One experiment representative of 2 independent experiments (each independent experiment was done in duplicate on the same day and the data were combined (mean ± SEM).

(see **Figure 2**). vCterm was somewhat less effective, while Del-C7 was comparable to the wt XCL1-OVA standard regarding $CD8^+$ T cell proliferation (**Figures 5A,B**). Del-N7 gave at 1 μg a very subtle proliferation signal (**Figure 5B**). This experiment demonstrated a comparably effective targeting of XCL1-OVA *in vivo* into DC by all XCL1-OVA variants with comparable

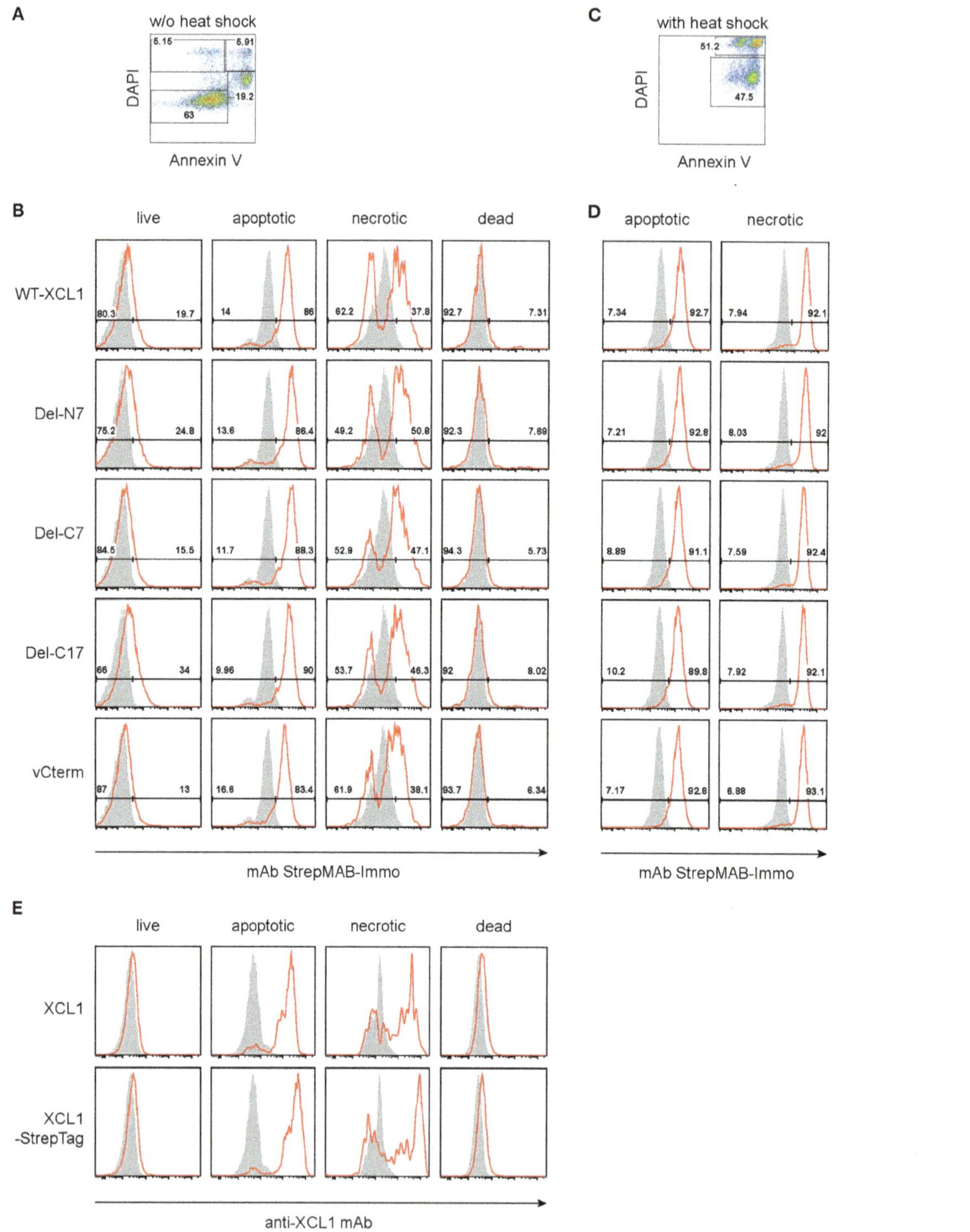

FIGURE 4 | Binding of XCL1-OVA and its variants Del-N7, Del-C7, Del-C17, and vCterm to apoptotic and necrotic cells. P3X63Ag8.653 cells were either **(A,B,E)** cultured at standard conditions without stress, or **(C,D)** subjected to thermal stress (52°C for 15 min, followed by culture overnight). For the last hour of culture, 1 μg of wt XCL1-OVA or one of its variants were added to the culture. For analysis, the cells were washed, and stained with DAPI and AnnexinV to subdivide the cells into "live" (Annexin$^-$DAPI$^-$), "apoptotic" (AnnexinV$^+$DAPI^{low}), "necrotic" (Annexin$^+$DAPI$^+$), and "dead" (Annexin$^-$DAPI$^+$) cells. **(A) G**ating and **(B)** staining of cells without thermal stress, **(C)** gating and **(D)** staining of cells after thermal stress, using anti-StrepMAB-Immo for signal detection (red histograms); background staining with StrepMAB-Immo without any preincubation is shown in gray histograms. **(E)** P3X63Ag8.653 cells were cultured under identical conditions, without thermal stress. For the last hour of culture, 1 μg of wt XCL1 or XCL1-StrepTag were added to the culture. Washing of cells and gating with DAPI and AnnexinV was as described above. Signal was detected with mAb MTAC-311 specific for murine XCL1 (red histograms), background signals with MTAC-311, without any preincubation, are shown in gray. Concentrations of XLC1-variants are based on the XCL1-component of the respective construct.

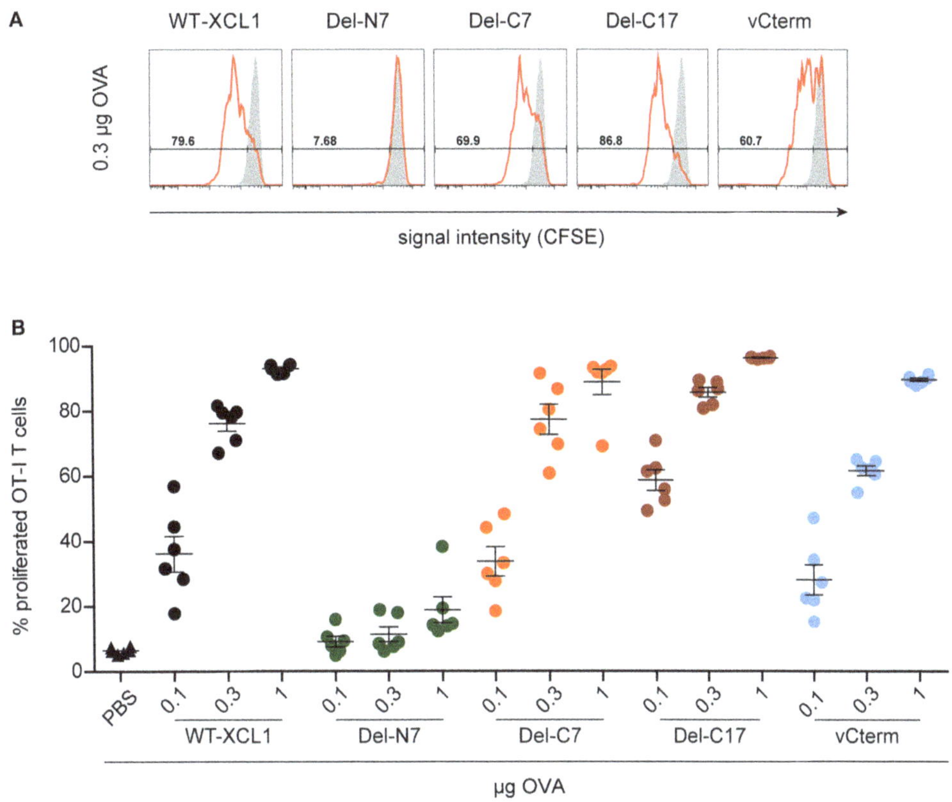

FIGURE 5 | Induction of CD8$^+$ T cell proliferation after *in vivo* targeting of antigen using XCL1-OVA and its variants Del-N7, Del-C7, Del-C17, and vCterm. Fluorescently labeled OT-I T cells (1×10^6) were adoptively transferred into syngeneic C57BL/6 mice. One day later the animals were immunized with the indicated amounts (based on the content of OVA) of wt XCL1-OVA and its structural variants (w/o adjuvant). Two days after immunization, the spleens were removed and the percentage of proliferated OT-I T cells was determined using the CSFE dilution assay in flow cytometry. **(A)** Exemplary histograms of the fluorescence signal obtained with 0.3 µg of each protein reagent. **(B)** Percentage of proliferated OT-I T cells after immunization with 0.1, 0.3, and 1 µg of each protein reagent. Combined data from 2 independent experiments are shown (mean ± SEM).

binding capacity *in vitro*. This observation excluded a major effect of the C-terminal portion of XCL1 on OVA processing and presentation.

Induction of Cytotoxic Capacity After *in vivo* Targeting of Antigen With XCL1-OVA and Its Variants Del-N7, Del-C7, Del-C17, and vCterm

To further test the *in vivo* functional capacity of T cells induced by the various formats of targeted antigen, C57BL/6 mice were immunized i.v. with titrated amounts of wt XCL1-OVA and its variants, which were injected together with 3 µg LPS. On day 6, an *in vivo* cytotoxicity assay was performed. As can be seen from **Figure 6**, Del-C7, Del-C17, and vCterm were similarly effective in inducing cytotoxicity as XCL1-OVA. The Del-N7 variant, at 3.3 µg, also induced modest cytotoxic activity. The cytotoxicity results were thus congruent with the proliferation data of OT-I T cells obtained earlier and excluded a major effect of the C-terminal portion of XCL1 on the induction of cytotoxicity *in vivo*.

DISCUSSION

Structures of many chemokines have been solved by NMR and X-ray crystallography. These studies revealed that despite low sequence homology, chemokines adopt a remarkably conserved tertiary structure consisting of a disordered N-terminus of 6–10 aa, a structured core region (chemokine fold), and a disordered C-terminus of variable length (27, 28). From a great number of structure-function studies a general concept evolved which assumes an initial specific binding of the chemokine fold-domain to the N-terminus of the receptor. In a second step, this initial interaction is stabilized by a subsequent integration of the N-terminal disordered domain of the ligand into the orthosteric pocket of the receptor. Additional studies suggested that this N-terminal domain of the chemokine ligand has signaling capacity. For example, an N-terminal deletion variant of MCP-1_{9-76} bound to its receptor with similar strength compared to the wild-type version MCP-1_{1-76}, but had lost all chemotactic activity (29). Based on many experiments of this type, the disordered N-terminal region of chemokines is generally regarded as a key signaling domain (27, 28).

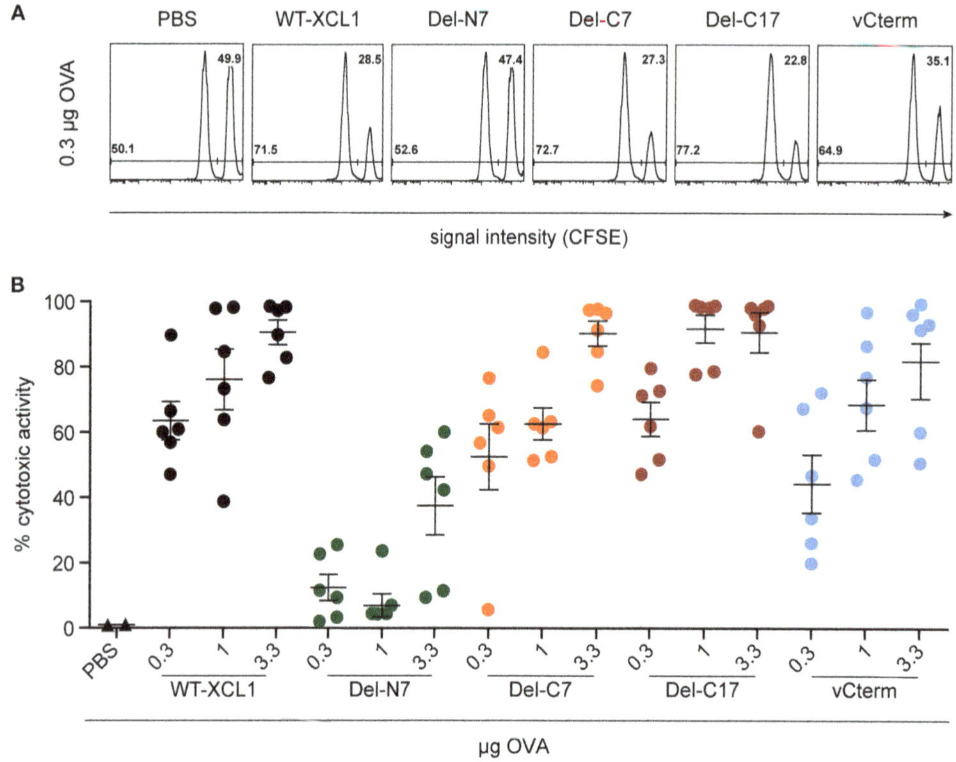

FIGURE 6 | Induction of cytotoxic capacity after *in vivo* targeting of antigen with XCL1-OVA and its variants Del-N7, Del-C7, Del-C17, and vCterm. C57BL/6 mice were immunized with the indicated amounts of wt XCL1-OVA and its variants (based on the content of OVA) together with 3 µg LPS on day 0. On day 6, the animals were injected with CFSE-labeled target cells to quantitate the induced cytotoxicity *in vivo* (for details, see Materials and Methods). **(A)** Exemplary flow cytometry histograms of the data obtained with 0.3 µg of each reagent. **(B)** Percentage of specific lysis obtained with 0.3, 1 and 3.3 µg of each reagent (mean ± SEM).

In our work, the N-terminal deletion variant Del-N7 ($XCL1_{8-93}$) reduced the binding of murine XCL1 to its receptor XCR1 approximately 50-fold. This reduction in binding was accompanied by a similar reduction in chemotaxis. The capacity of XCL1 to bind to its receptor was thus directly correlated to its chemotactic action. These data are compatible with a stabilization of the ligand-receptor interaction and thus with the general concept. However, we also made the surprising observation that at very high concentrations (approximately 100-fold of the presumed physiological concentration), this N-terminal deletion variant still exhibited fully preserved chemotactic action. Thus, with murine XCL1 there is no indication of an important signaling element in the N-terminal disordered domain which would be required for chemotaxis, as suggested by the general concept. Interestingly, at these supra-physiological concentrations (10,000 ng/ml) the N-terminal deletion variant consistently induced higher chemotaxis, when compared to the wild-type XCL1 at its optimal concentration (100 ng/ml). This observation indicates that the chemokine fold of XCL1 contains all necessary structures to induce chemotaxis. Finally, wild-type XCL1 at the same supra-physiological concentrations (10,000 ng/ml), exhibited largely reduced chemotaxis compared to its optimum at 100 ng/ml (as is typical for chemokines). This observation suggest that the disordered N-terminal region of XCL1 in some ways limits the functional activity of XCL1 at high concentrations.

When we analyzed the functional contribution of the C-terminal portion of murine XCL1, the deletion variants Del-C7 ($XCL1_{1-86}$) and Del-C17 ($XCL1_{1-76}$) did not show any functional effects on receptor binding or chemotaxis. Thus, we can exclude a major contribution of this region to the chemotactic function of murine XCL1. This conclusion clearly differs from the findings of a study utilizing human $XCL1_{1-72}$ (30), where a complete loss of calcium activity was observed. However, this particular C-terminal deletion variant was 4 aa shorter than Del-C17 ($XCL1_{1-76}$) which was used in the present study. Our results are fully compatible with data on a series of C-terminally truncated variants of human XLC1 (1–68, 1–72, 1–78, and 1–85), which all elicited normal calcium signals in XCR1-transfected HEK-293 cells (31).

Regarding the structure-function relationship of murine XCL1, our data can be summarized as follows. The core domain of XCL1 contains all necessary structural elements to specifically bind to XCR1 and to elicit chemotaxis. This observation differs from the general concept for chemokines, which assumes a critical signal contribution of the N-terminal domain for chemotaxis (27, 28). The first 7 aa of the N-terminal domain stabilize the binding of XCL1 to its receptor and thus certainly optimize chemotaxis. At the same time, and apparently paradoxically, the first 7 aa appear to limit the chemotactic effect of supra-physiological concentrations of murine XCL1, suggesting some type of negative regulatory role of the N-terminus at high XCL1 concentrations. A contribution of the disordered C-terminus of XCL1 to chemotaxis can clearly be ruled out.

These conclusions were reached with binding and chemotaxis assays using primary cells expressing the native XCR1 receptor. This is in contrast to the very few studies on the structure-function relationship of XCL1, which were conducted with XCR1-transfectants and mainly based on calcium mobilization studies.

Since XCL1 is secreted by activated NK cells, we pursued the hypothesis that in addition to its chemotactic function, XCL1 could "decorate" stressed cells recognized by NK cells. In such a scenario bound XCL1 could mark these stressed cells for phagocytosis by DC specialized for uptake of such cells (16). Using a murine myeloma line as an *in vitro* model system and also employing heat-shock experiments, we consistently observed binding of XCL1 to cells characterized as "necrotic" or "apoptotic," based on the use of Annexin V and DAPI. This binding was clearly mediated by the chemokine fold of XCL1, with no apparent contribution of the disordered N-terminal or C-terminal regions. It is unclear at present, to which structural elements present on apoptotic and necrotic cells XCL1 binds. Therefore, it remains to be determined whether this binding is specific or mediated by structural elements common to many chemokines, e.g., domains capable to mediate binding to glycosaminoglycans (present in the core domain of chemokines, also with XCL1). Preliminary studies with primary cells gave similar results as with the myeloma line, but turned out to be less reproducible, and therefore more work is needed to reach firm conclusions here. In particular, *in vivo* work will be required to generate essential data in order to support or reject the "decoration" hypothesis.

We are interested to use XCL1 as a carrier to transport proteins or peptides into cross-presenting DC. Therefore, all experiments were performed with XCL1 variants which were C-terminally fused to full-length OVA. We wanted to determine whether the various domains of XCL1 exert any influence on the targeting of the model protein to $XCR1^+$ DC *in vivo*. As independent and very sensitive readouts for $CD8^+$ T cell activation we used both induction of proliferation (response by adoptively transferred OT-I T cells) as well as induction of cytotoxic activity (by endogenous $CD8^+$ T cells). Since $CD8^+$ T cells *in vivo* become activated through cross-presentation of the soluble antigen OVA (17–19), we assume that these readouts measure cross-presentation of OVA-derived peptide SIINFEKL by $XCR1^+$ DC *in vivo*. They thus reflect the combined effects of antigen uptake, efficiency of antigen processing, and antigen presentation on the cell surface of the DC. Previous experiments which demonstrated that targeting of OVA using either XCL1 or an antibody directed to murine XCR1 drastically reduces the amount of antigen necessary to elicit $CD8^+$ T cell responses *in vivo* (20) support this assumption.

Several conclusions can be reached from our experiments regarding the use of XCL1 as antigen carrier. First, an intact N-terminus is required to efficiently target any peptide/protein cargo to $XCR1^+$ DC. Second, attachment of a relatively large protein cargo of around 40 kDa to the C-terminus does not sterically inhibit binding of XCL1 to its receptor. Third, attachment of protein cargo does not influence chemotaxis of $XCR1^+$ DC (chemotaxis was identical when compared with native XCL1 without OVA, data not shown). Since a chemotactic signal usually induces internalization of the chemokine receptor 27, 28), we assume that fusion of protein cargo to XCL1 does not influence the uptake of the protein into $XCR1^+$ DC. Fourth, the disordered C-terminus can be eliminated from XCL1, if necessary, when using protein cargo without any obvious deficits in antigen uptake and presentation. The last conclusion is supported by exchanging the natural C-terminus of XCL1 with the C-terminal domain of murid herpesvirus 8-encoded XCL1, which also did not show any changes in antigen presentation.

The conclusions on the capacity of XCL1 as an antigen carrier were reached with the model antigen OVA. Since this particular antigen is ideal in that it is highly soluble and shows little interaction with other proteins, there may be some limitations to the conclusions reached. Other proteins prone to binding to other structures in the body may not as efficiently be transported to $XCR1^+$ DC as OVA. Other cargo proteins may also interact with XCL1 in an intra- or intermolecular fashion. In spite of these potential limitations, our data clearly demonstrate the usefulness of XCL1 as a carrier to directly target large proteins or peptides to $XCR1^+$ cross-presenting DC. Such an antigen carrier system appears attractive for induction of antigen-specific cytotoxicity in anti-tumor therapeutic vaccines.

AUTHOR CONTRIBUTIONS

ALK performed all experiments and wrote parts of the manuscript. EH, NR, MB, and SG assisted in some of the biological experiments. HWM assisted in the molecular biology experiments. SV contributed information on the viral XCL1. CF and RAK designed the experiments. RAK wrote the manuscript.

ACKNOWLEDGMENTS

ALK thanks Prof. Elke Krüger (Charité) for continuing interest and support.

REFERENCES

1. Kelner GS, Kennedy J, Bacon KB, Kleyensteuber S, Largaespada DA, Jenkins NA, et al. Lymphotactin: a cytokine that represents a new class of chemokine. *Science* (1994) 266:1395–9. doi: 10.1126/science.7973732
2. Müller S, Dorner B, Korthäuer U, Mages HW, D'Apuzzo M, Senger G, et al. Cloning of ATAC, an activation-induced, chemokine-related molecule exclusively expressed in $CD8^+$ T lymphocytes. *Eur J Immunol.* (1995) 25:1744–8. doi: 10.1002/eji.1830250638
3. Yoshida T, Imai T, Kakizaki M, Nishimura M, Yoshie O. Molecular cloning of a novel C or γ type chemokine, SCM-1. *FEBS Lett.* (1995) 360:155–9. doi: 10.1016/0014-5793(95)00093-O
4. Geyer H, Hartung E, Mages HW, Weise C, Beložić R, Vugrek O, et al. Cytomegalovirus expresses the chemokine homologue vXCL1 capable of attracting $XCR1^+$ $CD4^-$ dendritic cells. *J. Virol.* (2014) 88:292–302. doi: 10.1128/JVI.02330-13
5. Dorner BG, Scheffold A, Rolph MS, Hüser MB, Kaufmann SH, Radbruch A, et al. MIP-1α, MIP-1β, RANTES, and ATAC/lymphotactin function together with IFN-γ as type 1 cytokines. *Proc Natl Acad Sci USA.* (2002) 99:6181–6. doi: 10.1073/pnas.092141999
6. Kroczek RA, Henn V. The Role of XCR1 and its ligand XCL1 in antigen cross-presentation by murine and human dendritic cells. *Front Immunol.* (2012) 3:14. doi: 10.3389/fimmu.2012.00014
7. Yoshida T, Izawa D, Nakayama T, Nakahara K, Kakizaki M, Imai T, et al. Molecular cloning of mXCR1, the murine SCM-1/ lymphotactin receptor. *FEBS Lett.* (1999) 458:37–40.
8. Shan L, Qiao X, Oldham E, Catron D, Kaminski H, Lundell D, et al. Identification of viral macrophage inflammatory protein (vMIP)-II as a ligand for GPR5/XCR1. *Biochem Biophys Res Commun.* (2000) 268:938–41. doi: 10.1006/bbrc.2000.2235
9. Dorner BG, Dorner MB, Zhou X, Opitz C, Mora A, Güttler S, et al. Selective expression of the chemokine receptor XCR1 on cross-presenting dendritic cells determines cooperation with $CD8^+$ T cells. *Immunity* (2009) 31:823–33. doi: 10.1016/j.immuni.2009.08.027
10. Bachem A, Güttler S, Hartung E, Ebstein F, Schaefer M, Tannert A, et al. Superior antigen cross-presentation and XCR1 expression define human $CD11c^+CD141^+$ cells as homologues of mouse $CD8^+$ dendritic cells. *J Exp Med.* (2010) 207:1273–81. doi: 10.1084/jem.20100348
11. Crozat K, Guiton R, Contreras V, Feuillet V, Dutertre CA, Ventre E, et al. The XC chemokine receptor 1 is a conserved selective marker of mammalian cells homologous to mouse $CD8\alpha^+$ dendritic cells. *J Exp Med.* (2010) 207:1283–92. doi: 10.1084/jem.20100223
12. Crozat K, Tamoutounour S, Vu Manh TP, Fossum E, Luche H, Ardouin L, et al. Cutting edge: expression of XCR1 defines mouse lymphoid-tissue resident and migratory dendritic cells of the $CD8\alpha^+$ type. *J Immunol.* (2011) 187:4411–5. doi: 10.4049/jimmunol.1101717
13. Bachem A, Hartung E, Güttler S, Mora A, Zhou X, Hegemann A, et al. Expression of XCR1 characterizes the Batf3-dependent lineage of dendritic cells capable of antigen cross-presentation. *Front Immunol.* (2012) 3:214. doi: 10.3389/fimmu.2012.00214
14. Iyoda T, Shimoyama S, Liu K, Omatsu Y, Akiyama Y, Maeda Y, et al. The $CD8^+$ dendritic cell subset selectively endocytoses dying cells in culture and in vivo. *J Exp Med.* (2002) 195:1289–302. doi: 10.1084/jem.200 20161
15. Schulz O, Reis e Sousa C. Cross-presentation of cell-associated antigens by $CD8\alpha^+$ dendritic cells is attributable to their ability to internalize dead cells. *Immunology* (2002) 107:183–9. doi: 10.1046/j.1365-2567.2002.0 1513.x
16. Shortman K, Heath WR. The $CD8^+$ dendritic cell subset. *Immunol Rev.* (2010) 234:18–31. doi: 10.1111/j.0105-2896.2009.00870.x
17. Kurts C, Kosaka H, Carbone FR, Miller JF, Heath WR. Class I-restricted cross-presentation of exogenous self-antigens leads to deletion of autoreactive $CD8^+$ T cells. *J Exp Med.* (1997) 186:239–45. doi: 10.1084/jem.186. 2.239
18. den Haan JM, Lehar SM, Bevan MJ. $CD8^+$ but not $CD8^-$ dendritic cells cross-prime cytotoxic T cells in vivo. *J Exp Med.* (2000) 192:1685–96. doi: 10.1084/jem.192.12.1685
19. Pooley JL, Heath WR, Shortman K. Cutting edge: intravenous soluble antigen is presented to CD4 T cells by $CD8^-$ dendritic cells, but cross-presented to CD8 T cells by $CD8^+$ dendritic cells. *J Immunol.* (2001) 166:5327–30. doi: 10.4049/jimmunol.166.9.5327
20. Hartung E, Becker M, Bachem A, Reeg N, Jäkel A, Hutloff A, et al. Induction of potent CD8 T cell cytotoxicity by specific targeting of antigen to cross-presenting dendritic cells in vivo via murine or human XCR1. *J Immunol.* (2015) 194:1069–79. doi: 10.4049/jimmunol.1401903
21. Kuloglu ES, McCaslin DR, Kitabwalla M, Pauza CD, Markley JL, Volkman BF. Monomeric solution structure of the prototypical 'C' chemokine lymphotactin. *Biochemistry* (2001) 40:12486–96. doi: 10.1021/bi011106p
22. Kuloglu ES, McCaslin DR, Markley JL, Volkman BF. Structural rearrangement of human lymphotactin, a C chemokine, under physiological solution conditions. *J Biol Chem.* (2002) 277:17863–70. doi: 10.1074/jbc.M200402200
23. Wallny H. Production of MHC class II molecules in drosophila melanogaster Schneider cells. In: Lefkovits editor. *Immunological Methods Manual Volume 1*, San Diego, CA: Academic Press (1997), 51–59.
24. Schneider I. Cell lines derived from late embryonic stages of Drosophila melanogaster. *J Embryol Exp Morphol.* (1972) 27:353–65.
25. Mach N, Gillessen S, Wilson SB, Sheehan C, Mihm M, Dranoff G. Differences in dendritic cells stimulated in vivo by tumors engineered to secrete granulocyte-macrophage colony-stimulating factor or Flt3-ligand. *Cancer Res.* (2000) 60:3239–46.
26. Löhning M, Hutloff A, Kallinich T, Mages HW, Bonhagen K, Radbruch A, et al. Expression of ICOS in vivo defines $CD4^+$ effector T cells with high inflammatory potential and a strong bias for secretion of interleukin 10. *J Exp Med.* (2003) 197:181–93. doi: 10.1084/jem.20020632
27. Allen SJ, Crown SE, Handel TM. Chemokine: receptor structure, interactions, and antagonism. *Ann Rev Immunol.* (2007) 25:787–820. doi: 10.1146/annurev.immunol.24.021605.090529
28. Bachelerie F, Ben-Baruch A, Burkhardt AM, Combadiere C, Farber JM, Graham GJ, et al. International union of basic and clinical pharmacology. [corrected] LXXXIX Update on the extended family of chemokine receptors and introducing a new nomenclature for atypical chemokine receptors. *Pharmacol Rev.* (2014) 66:1–79. doi: 10.1124/pr.113.007724
29. Gong JH, Clark-Lewis I. Antagonists of monocyte chemoattractant protein 1 identified by modification of functionally critical NH2-terminal residues. *J Exp Med.* (1995) 181:631–40. doi: 10.1084/jem.181.2.631
30. Marcaurelle LA, Mizoue LS, Wilken J, Oldham L, Kent SB, Handel TM, et al. Chemical synthesis of lymphotactin: a glycosylated chemokine with a C-terminal mucin-like domain. *Chemistry* (2001) 7:1129–32. doi: 10.1002/1521-3765(20010302)7:53.0.CO;2-W
31. Tuinstra RL, Peterson FC, Elgin ES, Pelzek AJ, Volkman BF. An engineered second disulfide bond restricts lymphotactin/XCL1 to a chemokine-like conformation with XCR1 agonist activity. *Biochemistry* (2007) 46:2564–73. doi: 10.1021/bi602365d

5

Importance of EMT Factor ZEB1 in cDC1 "MutuDC Line" Mediated Induction of Th1 Immune Response

Shuchi Smita [1,2†], Abdul Ahad [1,2†], Arup Ghosh [1,3], Viplov K. Biswas [1,3], Marianna M. Koga [4], Bhawna Gupta [3], Hans Acha-Orbea [4] and Sunil K. Raghav [1,2,3]*

[1] Immuno-genomics and Systems Biology Laboratory, Institute of Life Sciences (ILS), Bhubaneswar, India, [2] Manipal Academy of Higher Education, Manipal, India, [3] Department of Biotechnology, Kalinga Institute of Industrial Technology (KIIT), Bhubaneswar, India, [4] Department of Biochemistry CIIL, University of Lausanne (UNIL), Epalinges, Switzerland

***Correspondence:**
Sunil K. Raghav
sunilraghav@ils.res.in;
raghuvanshi2010@yahoo.co.in

† These authors have contributed equally to this work

The role of Epithelial to Mesenchymal Transition (EMT) factor Zeb1 is well defined in metastasis and cancer progression but it's importance in dendritic cells (DCs) is unexplored until now. For the first time we report here that Zeb1 controls immunogenic responses of CD8α$^+$ conventional Type-I (cDC1) DCs. We found that ZEB1 expression increases significantly after TLR9 stimulation and its depletion impairs activation, co-stimulation and secretion of important cytokines like IL-6, IL-10 and IL-12 in cDC1 MutuDC line. We further confirmed our findings in primary cDC1 DCs derived from bone marrow. Co-culture of these Zeb1 knock down (KD) DCs with OT-II CD4$^+$ T helper cells skewed their differentiation toward Th2 subtype. Moreover, adoptive transfer of activated Zeb1 KD DCs cleared intestinal worms in helminth infected mice by increasing Th2 responses *in vivo*. Integrative genomic analysis showed Zeb1 as an activator of immune response genes in cDC1 MutuDCs as compared to other pathway genes. In addition, differentially regulated genes in Zeb1 KD RNA-seq showed significant enrichment of Th2 activation pathways supporting our *in vitro* findings. Mechanistically, we showed that decreased IL-12 secreted by Zeb1 KD DCs is the plausible mechanism for increased Th2 differentiation. Collectively our data demonstrate that Zeb1 could be targeted in DCs to modulate T-cell mediated adaptive immune responses.

Keywords: ZEB1, cDC1 dendritic cells, integrative genomics, Th2 response, ChIP-seq, RNA-seq, helminth infection, immune modulation

INTRODUCTION

Dendritic cells (DCs) are potent antigen presenting cells that play a pivotal role in developing immune responses as they govern both the initiation and polarization of adaptive immunity (1–5). The complex classification and nomenclature of DCs has now been refined into two levels, conventional or classical DCs comprising cDC1 (CD8α$^+$ and CD103$^+$) and cDC2 (CD11b$^+$ and CD172a$^+$ DCs) depending on their distinct developmental pathways, and the plasmacytoid DCs (pDCs) (6–8). Genetic and functional studies have revealed that CD8α$^+$ (Lymphoid-resident DCs) and CD103$^+$ (Non-lymphoid tissue resident migratory DCs) DCs are specialized in antigen cross-presentation and polarization of Th cells into Th1 subset in response to stimulation via Toll Like receptor (TLR) ligands such as CpG for TLR9 and poly-IC for TLR3 (6, 7, 9–12). Upon pathogen encounter, DCs are activated leading to their maturation and migration toward secondary lymph nodes where they instruct T helper (Th) cell differentiation into different subtypes in a signal dependent manner (13–19). Among the many Th cell subsets, Th1 cells are critical for host defense against intracellular pathogens, while Th2 cells defend extracellular parasites (12, 15–17). Priming of Th cells toward Th1 requires inflammatory cytokine IL-12 whereas Th17 subtype depends on IL-6 and IL-23 cytokines produced by DCs (20, 21). In contrast, it has been widely accepted that DCs do not produce the Th2 speciation cytokines like IL-4 and IL-13. Therefore, decreased secretion of Th1 or Th17 promoting cytokines by DCs could induce the Th2 cell differentiation as a default outcome (22–24). Besides, considerable evidences suggest that DCs are required for optimal Th2 cell priming *in vivo* and expression of co-stimulatory molecules like OX40L or the Notch ligand Jagged-1 by DCs promotes Th2 cell priming (25, 26). On the other hand, it is explicitly known that cDC1 are prone to induce Th1 responses whereas cDC2 cells provide cooperative signal for Th2 responses where the IL-4 cytokine remains the key-determining factor for their polarization (27–29). Interestingly, there are several reports showing upregulation of Th2 transcription factor GATA3 through IL-4 by activating STAT5 and STAT6 transcription factors (TFs), but few of them indicate that GATA3 expression can be independent of IL-4 as well (28, 30). Apart from signaling molecules, it has been reported that IRF4 depleted DCs are unable to induce Th2 differentiation (28, 31, 32), whereas increased KLF2 in DCs negatively regulates Th2 induction (33).

E-Box motif binding TF Zeb1 is a member of Zinc finger TF family, a known EMT master regulator. TGFβ signaling is one of the main mechanisms promoting EMT and is known to induce Zeb1 through SMAD signaling which in turn is well documented to repress E-cadherin (Cdh1) expression in epithelial cells (34, 35). The mir200 family members are predominantly present in epithelial cells and fine-tune the transcript expression of Zeb1 through feedback regulation (34, 36). In breast cancer cells, knock down of Zeb1 inhibits pro-inflammatory cytokines including IL-6 and IL-8 (37). Similarly, it has been widely reported that EMT in tumors is positively induced by inflammation (36, 38–41). In contrast, Zeb1 has been reported to repress IL-2 by recruiting CTBP2 at its proximal promoter in T-cells irrespective of activation (42). There are reports suggesting higher expression of Zeb1 in migratory Langerhans cells, pertinent for their migration to secondary lymph nodes to present antigens to Th cells (43). This indicated that Zeb1 might be playing an important role in cDC1 axis of immune biology beyond just migratory properties. A forward genetic screen also revealed Zeb1 requirement for marginal zone of peritoneal B-1 B-cell development, T-cell development, germinal center formation, and memory B-cell responses (44). Though Zeb1 has been widely studied in cancer biology, few evidences with immunity and inflammation make it a potential candidate to look upon for its role in cDCs trajectory.

Here in this study, we investigated the role of Zeb1 in CD8α$^+$ cDC1 DCs and found it to be pertinent for their activation, co-stimulation and secretion of important immune response cytokines like IL-10 and IL-12. As a result, Zeb1 depleted DCs generated a strong Th2 phenotype *ex vivo* and *in vivo*, independent of IL-4 cytokine. Integrative genomic analysis demonstrated that Zeb1 has an indirect control on important cDC1 response cytokines and it does not act as a global repressor of immune response genes in DCs.

METHODS

Dendritic Cell (DC) Culture

Here in this study we have used CD8α$^+$ cDC1 MutuDC line recently developed by Prof. Hans Acha-Orbea's group. They have extensively characterized and compared these DC lines with primary CD8α$^+$ cDC1 DCs and reported that they perfectly mimic *ex vivo* immature CD8α$^+$ DCs isolated from spleen of C57BL/6 mice (9). The DCs were grown in IMDM-glutamax (GIBCO) buffered with $NaHCO_3$ and supplemented with 8–10% heat inactivated FCS (tested for endotoxin toxicity toward DC cultures), 10 mM HEPES (GIBCO 15630), 50 μM β-Mercaptoethanol (GIBCO 31350), and 50 U/mL of penicillin and 50 μg/mL streptomycin (GIBCO 15070). The cells were maintained at 37°C in a humidified incubator with 5% CO_2. These DCs were dissociated with short incubation in non-enzymatic, 5 mM EDTA-based cell dissociation buffer (5 mM EDTA in 20 mM HEPES-PBS) at 37°C.

For *in vitro* experiments, the DCs were plated in 6-well plates at a density of 5×10^5 cells/ml overnight. The cells were then challenged with different activation media containing TLR9 agonist CpG-B (Invivogen, cat no. tlrl-1826), TLR3 agonist pIC (Invivogen, cat no. tlrl-pic) and CpG+pIC for 2, 6, and 12 h. For performing RT-qPCR analysis the cells were washed in the plate once with PBS followed by addition of RNA-later (LBP) lysis buffer (Macherey-Nagel) for lysis of cells. The plates were then stored at −80°C until further RNA isolation and processing of samples.

Generation of Stable Zeb1 KD CD8α$^+$ MutuDCs

For generating stable Zeb1 knockdown and corresponding control DCs, lentiviral vector pLKO.1 (Sigma) containing three different Zeb1-specific shRNAs or control shRNA were used. Viral particles packaged with shRNA expressing transfer plasmids were produced in 293T cells using Cal-Phos ($CaPO_4$) mammalian transfection kit (Clontech) according to an optimized protocol (45). 293T cells were transfected with transfer plasmids containing three different Zeb1 shRNAs or control shRNAs along with packaging plasmids (pCMVR8.74 and pMD2G). After 12–14 h the culture medium was replenished and supernatant containing viral particles were collected after 24 h in 50 ml conical tubes. Viral particle-containing culture supernatant was filtered through 0.45 μm syringe filters (PES filters) and preserved at −80°C in small aliquots. For transduction of shRNA containing viruses in CD8α$^+$ cDC1 MutuDC lines, the cells were plated at a density of 1.5×10^5 cells/well of 12 well plate followed by transduction with virus particles containing supernatant. The media was replaced with fresh media after 12 h of virus incubation with DCs followed by addition of 1 μg/ml puromycin selection medium after 72 h of media replacement. The cells were puromycin selected for 2–3 weeks to get stable

Zeb1 KD cells. The cells were also transduced with control shRNA-containing viruses to develop control cells for analysis comparisons. Efficiency of Zeb1 KD was quantified using Zeb1 gene specific primers by RT-qPCR (**Supplementary Table 8**). The shRNA that showed significant and maximum decrease in Zeb1 gene transcript levels compared to control transduced cells were used for further detailed study.

RNA Isolation and RT-qPCR

The cells preserved in LBP lysis buffer for RT-qPCR experiments were first taken out from −80°C and thawed by placing the plates/tubes on ice. Total RNA was isolated using NucleoSpin RNA Plus kit (Machery-Nagel) according to manufacturer's protocol. RNA concentration was estimated by nanodrop (Thermo) and then 1 μg of total RNA was used to prepare cDNA using High capacity cDNA Reverse Transcriptase kit (Applied biosystems). Quantiative PCR was performed using SYBR Green master mix (Roche) and PCR amplification was monitored in real-time using LightCycler-480 Instrument (Roche). Primer oligonucleotides for qPCR were designed using universal probe library assay design system (Roche) and the primer pairs used are listed in **Supplementary Table 8**. Primers were optimized for linear and single product amplification by performing standard curve assays.

Flow Cytometry (FACS)

Flow cytometric analyses of *in vitro* and *ex vivo* cultured cells were performed using well established protocol for FACS staining and analysis. For surface and intracellular (IC) staining $5*10^5$ and $1.5*10^6$ cells were seeded respectively and stimulated with CpG, pIC and CpG + pIC for 12 h. After dissociation from plates, the cultured cells were washed with FACS buffer (3% FCS in PBS, 5 mM EDTA) followed by re-suspension in surface staining buffer. After washing, fluorochrome conjugated antibodies for proteins of interest were added to the cells as a cocktail (**Supplementary Table 8**). For intracellular (IC) staining of cytokines the cells were first fixed with 2% paraformaldehyde followed by permeabilisation using 1x permeabilisation buffer (eBiosciences). The fixed cells were then resuspended in intracellular staining buffer and stained with fluorochrome tagged antibodies for selected cytokines. For optimal staining the cells were incubated with antibodies for 30 min in dark at 4°C. After incubation the cells were washed twice with FACS wash buffer and then acquired for differential expression analysis using LSRII fortessa flow cytometer (BD Biosciences). The acquired data was analyzed using FlowJo-X software (Treestar).

We used single color antibody stained cells as controls using pooled cells from all untreated and treated conditions for compensation and gating of positive population. In one of the biological replicates for immune profiling experiments, we used Florescence Minus One controls (FMO) to gate cells and for compensation. We found that single color stained and unstained negative control cells were giving similar results and therefore we didn't include FMOs in all our further experiments. From live cell population (high GFP positive cells) first we removed doublet cell population and then similar gates were employed for both control and Zeb1 KD DCs to observe any percentage cell population differences in surface markers and intracellular cytokines. Unstimulated DCs do not secrete cytokines therefore we used these cells stained with similar cocktail of antibodies for gating the cytokine positive cell population. In addition, we also analyzed for Median Florescence Intensity (MFI) shifts for each population in replicates to observe overall activation/co-stimulation markers and cytokines in control and Zeb1 depleted DCs.

Bio-Plex Assay for Cytokine Quantitation From Cell Culture Supernatants

Bio-Plex assay (multiplex ELISA) was used to estimate the cytokine levels secreted in the cell culture supernatants of Zeb1 KD and control DCs after 12 h of CpG stimulation. After culture, the supernatants were stored at −80°C in small aliquots until analysis. Cytokine levels were estimated using 23-plex-mouse cytokine assay kit following the vendor recommended protocol (Biorad).

Generation of Bone Marrow Derived DCs (BMDCs) for *ex-vivo* Studies

Six to eight-week-old female C57BL/6 mice were killed by cervical dislocation and disinfected using 75% ethanol. The tibias and femurs were removed under sterile conditions, then soaked in RPMI-1640 medium supplemented with 10% FBS. Both ends of the bone were cut off with scissors, and the needle of a 1-mL syringe was inserted into the bone cavity to rinse the bone marrow out of the cavity into a sterile culture dish with RPMI-1640 medium (46). The cell suspension in the dish was collected and centrifuged at 350 g for 5 min, and the supernatant was discarded. The cell pellet was suspended with 1X RBC lysis buffer (Tonbo: TNB-4300) to lyse the RBCs and incubated for 5–10 min on ice. Cell clumps were then passed through a 70 μm strainer to obtain single cell suspensions. The lysed cells were washed once with RPMI-1640, counted and used for differentiation into DCs.

We followed a well-established protocol for differentiation of BMDCs with slight modifications (47). The cells, suspended in RPMI-1640 medium supplemented with 10% FBS, were distributed into 6-well plates at a density of 1×10^6 cell/ml/well. Subsequently, 1μl/ml of FLT3L containing sera (derived from Flt3L expressing mice, gift from Hans Acha-Orbea, UNIL, Lausanne, Switzerland) was added into the medium. The cells were cultured at 37°C in an incubator containing 5% CO_2 and left untouched for 5 days. On day 5, the suspended and loosely attached cells were collected, washed and counted. The cells were plated into 24-well plate for lentiviral transduction using concentrated viruses at a density of $0.4*10^6$ cells/well for each Zeb1 shRNA and Control shRNA. After 72 h the cells were stimulated with CpG for 12 h and then immune-profiling was done at protein level using flow cytometry for observed markers that were found to be differentially regulated in $CD8\alpha^+$ cDC1 cells *in vitro*. The antibodies used for staining were same as used for *in vitro* experiments.

Co-culture of DCs With CD4+ T Cells for Assessing T-Cell Proliferation and Differentiation

DC-T cell co-culture experiments were performed as described before (9). Naïve $CD4^+$ T cells were purified from spleen of TCR-transgenic OT-II mice using $CD4^+$ T cell isolation kit (EasySepTM Mouse $CD4^+$T cells isolation Kit, Stem Cell Technologies). Zeb1 KD and control $CD8\alpha^+$ cDC1 DCs were seeded at a density of 10,000 cells/well in round bottom 96 well plates followed by pulsing with OVA peptide (aa 323-339) and CpG for 2 h. After 2 h, purified OT-II T cells were added at the density of 100,000 cells/well (1:10 ratio) (48). Then T-cell proliferation and differentiation into distinct Th subtypes Th1, Th2, Th17 and Tregs were analyzed by FACS. Proliferation was measured using an amine based dye (eFluor 670). The rate of T-cell proliferation was inversely proportional to the Median Fluorescence Intensity (MFI) measured in FACS after 72 h of co-culture. For Th cell differentiation profiling after 96 h, the co-cultured T cells were re-stimulated with PMA (10 ng/mL) and Ionomycin (500 ng/mL) and followed by Brefeldin-A (10 µg/mL) treatment for 5 h to block the intracellular cytokines from being secreted. After 5 h, fluorochrome conjugated antibodies specific to different T cell subtypes were used to profile T cells into Th1 (Tbet and IFNγ), Th2 (GATA3, IL-13), Tregs (CD25, FoxP3) and Th17 (IL-17) (49). For gating effector T cells we used CD44 as a marker (see **Supplementary Table 8** for details of antibodies).

To confirm the default Th2 program recombinant IL-12 (5 ng/ml) and anti-IL4 (5 µg/ml) was used in OT-II co-culture experiments to confirm any perturbation in Th subtype differentiation using similar antibodies for various subtypes.

Chromatin Immuno-Precipitation (ChIP) for Zeb1

The ChIP for Zeb1 was performed according to the methods optimized previously by Raghav and Meyer's lab (50, 51). For ChIP assays, $30{*}10^6$ $CD8a^+$ cDC1 MutuDCs were seeded in 15 cm^2 plates and prepared for ChIP by 10 min cross-linking with 1% formaldehyde (sigma) at room temperature followed by quenching using 2.5 M glycine (sigma) for 10 min. The plates were placed on ice and the cells were scraped and collected in 50 ml conical tubes. The cells were then washed three times using cold 1x PBS at 2,000 rpm for 10 min at 4°C and the cell pellets were stored at −80°C. At the day of the ChIP experiment, the cells were thawed on ice followed by lysis using nuclei extraction buffer (50 mM HEPES-NaOH pH 7.5, 140 mM NaCl, 1 mM EDTA pH 8.0, 10% glycerol, 0.5% NP-40, 0.25% Triton-X100) supplemented with protease and phosphatase inhibitors (Roche) for 10 min at 4°C on rocker shaker. The prepared nuclei were then washed using protein extraction buffer (200 mMNaCl, 1 mM EDTA pH 8.0, 0.5 mM EGTA pH 8.0, 10 mM Tris-Cl pH 8.0) supplemented with a protease and phosphatase inhibitors (Roche) at room temperature for 10 min. Washed nuclei were resuspended in chromatin extraction buffer (1 mM EDTA pH 8.0, 0.5 mM EGTA pH 8.0, 10 mM Tris-Cl pH 8.0 and 1% TritonX-100) supplemented with protease and phosphatase inhibitors (Roche) and incubated for 20 min on ice for equilibration. The chromatin was fragmented using a Bioruptor (Diagenode) sonicator for 30 min using high amplitude and 30s ON & 30s OFF cycles to obtain 200-500 bp size fragments. A cooling unit was used to circulate the cold water during sonication to avoid de-crosslinking because of overheating. After sonication, chromatin length was checked in agarose gel. The fragmented chromatin was centrifuged at 10,000 rpm for 5 min and then clear supernatant was collected in 15 ml conical tubes. The DNA concentration of the chromatin was estimated using a Nano-Drop (Thermo) and the chromatin was diluted with ChIP dilution buffer (1 mM EDTA pH 8.0, 10 mM Tris-Cl pH 8.0 and 1% TritonX-100 containing protease and phosphatase inhibitors) to use 150 µg/ml of chromatin for each IP. BSA and ssDNA (Salmon Sperm DNA) preblocked protein-A sepharose (80 µl/IP) beads were added to the samples on ice and incubated for 2 h to remove non-specific-binding chromatin. To the supernatant, 25 µl of rabbit polyclonal anti-Zeb1 (Santa Cruz H-102) were added to immunoprecipitate the chromatin complex at 4°C overnight on rocker shaker. After the overnight incubation, 50 µl blocked beads were added to each sample and incubated for 2.5 h at 4°C to pull down the respective antibody-chromatin complexes. The beads were then washed three times with low salt wash buffer (20 mM Tris-Cl pH 8.0, 150 mM NaCl, 2 mM EDTA pH 8.0, 0.1% SDS, 1% TritonX-100) followed by two washes with high salt wash buffer (20 mM Tris-Cl pH 8.0, 500 mM NaCl, 2 mM EDTA pH 8.0, 0.1% SDS, 1% TritonX- 100), lithium chloride wash buffer (10 mM Tris-Cl pH 8.0, 0.25 M LiCl, 1 mM EDTA pH 8.0, 1% NP-40, 1% sodium deoxycholate) and Tris-EDTA (TE) buffer (10 mM Tris-Cl pH 8.0, 1 mM EDTA pH 8.0). After removing the wash buffer completely, protein-bound chromatin complexes were eluted from beads for 30 min using elution buffer (100 mM $NaHCO_3$ and 1% SDS in milli-Q water). The eluted chromatin was then reverse crosslinked by incubating the eluted supernatant at 65°C overnight on a heat block after adding 8 µl of 5 M NaCl. Next day DNA was purified from the reverse cross-linked chromatin by proteinase-K and RNase digestion followed by purification using PCR purification kit (Qiagen). The purified DNA was eluted in 40 µl of elution buffer.

ChIP-/RNA-seq Library Preparation for Next Generation Sequencing (NGS)

The RNA-seq library preparation was performed for Zeb1 KD and control cDC1 MutuDCs at 0, 6, and 12 h after CpG activation. As we did time kinetics we included two independent biological replicates to identify the Zeb1 depletion mediated global transcriptome changes. For RNA-seq library preparation 2 µg of total RNA was used to isolate mRNA through magnetic beads using mRNA isolation kit (PolyA mRNA isolation Module, NEB) followed by RNA-seq library preparation using mRNA library preparation kit (NEB) strictly following the vendor recommended protocol. After library preparation concentration of libraries were estimated using qubit 2.0 (Invitrogen) and the recommended fragmentation sizes were confirmed by Bio-analyzer (Agilent). For ChIP-seq library preparation, 30 µl of ChIP-DNA was processed for library preparation according to ChIP-seq library preparation recommended protocol (NEB).

After library preparation and quality check using Bio-analyzer, the libraries were send to NGS service provider for Illumina sequencing using Hiseq-2500 instrument.

Western Blotting

Cells were collected in RIPA buffer (0.5 M EDTA, 1 M Tris-Cl pH7.5, 1 M NaCl, 200 mM PMSF, 10% NP-40, 10% SDS, 5% sodium deoxycholate, 1 M sodium orthovanadate and 1X Roche protease inhibitor) before and after CpG stimulation at different time points (0, 1, 2, 6, & 12 h). Cells were lysed completely by sonicating the samples in Bioruptor (Diagenode) for 10 min using high amplitude and 30s ON & 30s OFF cycles. Protein concentrations were measured in 96 well plate using BCA protein assay kit (BioRad).

Adoptive Transfer of DCs in Helminth (*Heligmosomoides polygyrus)* Infection Mice Model

For DC Adoptive transfer experiments we took 6–8 week old female C57BL/6 mice and infected them with 200 infective L3 larvae/mice in PBS though oral gavage. Prof. Nicola Harris from EPFL (École Polytechnique Fédérale de Lausanne), Lausanne, Switzerland, provided the infective L3 larvae. The larvae were hatched from fecal charcoal cultures at day 7 after collection (52). After 7 days of infection, mice were treated with 100 μl of anti-CD8b antibody/mice followed by adoptive transfer of 10^*10^6 CpG pulsed Zeb1 KD and control $CD8\alpha^+$ cDC1 MutuDCs in sterile PBS intra-peritoneally (IP). Two booster doses of 5^*10^6 cells pulsed with CpG were adoptively transferred consequtively after 48 h. After adoptive transfer of DCs the feces from infected animals were collected for worm eggs counting after every 24 h time period till day 31 using a well-optimized protocol. After observing a significant difference in egg count between Zeb1 KD DC treated and control animals, four mice from each group were sacrificed for detailed T cell profiling from mesenteric lymph nodes and the helminth worm counting from the intestine of the dissected animals. The intestines were longitudinally opened and flipped to count the worms and to take pictures. The T cell differentiation into Th1, Th2, Tregs, and Th17 subtypes was assessed using FACS as detailed above. This mouse experiment was performed following the institutional animal ethics guidelines after taking due approval from the institutional animal ethics committee at ILS, Bhubaneswar, India.

Mixed Lymphocyte Reaction (MLR)

MLR setup was performed following well-documented protocol with slight modifications (49). The Zeb1 KD and control DCs were co-cultured with allogenic T cells from spleen of Balb/C mice. The Zeb1 KD and control $CD8\alpha^+$ DCs were seeded at a density of 20,000 cells/well in a round bottom 96 well plates followed by challenge with CpG for 2 h. After 2 h, splenocytes containing mostly T cells from 6–8 week old Balb/C mice were added at the density of 200,000 cells/well (1:10 ratio). After 4 days (96 h) of co-culture, T-cell differentiation was assessed using same method as for OT-II co-culture.

NGS ANALYSIS

Quality Control & Preprocessing

The quality of RNA-seq and ChIP-seq reads from all sequencing experiments were determined using FastQC v0.11.5 (https://www.bioinformatics.babraham.ac.uk/projects/fastqc/) tool. Reads having Phred Score(Q) <30 and over-represented sequences i.e. primer sequences, adapter sequences were removed using Trimmomatic (53) (http://www.usadellab.org/cms/?page=trimmomatic) from both pairs. For binding events comparison, PU.1 (0 h) and Irf4 (0 and 2 h) ChIP-seq data of bone marrow-derived dendritic cell (BMDC) provided with LPS stimulation were accessed form GSE36104 (54).

RNA-seq Analysis

Filtered reads from transcriptome data were aligned with Tophat2 (55) using mm10 mouse genome assembly and Gencode M17 (GRCm38.p6) as reference transcript file. Rest of the alignment parameters remained same as Tophat2 is optimized for mammalian sequence alignment by default. Cufflinks v2.2.1 was used to calculate the abundance of transcripts from aligned files in terms of fragments per kilobase per million of reads (FPKM) and also generated the assembly file for differential expression using CuffDiff. All the assembly files from biological replicates were merged using Cuffmerge command from the same tool. Genes/transcripts form differential expression analysis having $p < 0.05$(significance) and $q < 0.05$ (false discovery rate) were classified as significant.

ChIP-seq Analysis

Alignment of ChIP-seq data was aligned with Bowtie2 (56) using mm10 mouse genome assembly as reference genome and—no-mixed,—no-discordant options to avoid unpaired read alignments. Aligned reads were deduplicated using Samtools (57) and randomly down-sampled to 22 million reads using Picard tool (https://broadinstitute.github.io/picard/). Peak calling was done using find Peaks tool form Homer suite (58) using a threshold of 4-fold change against input control and–factor option. Transcription factor motifs in −100/+100 region of the peaks were searched using findMotifsGenome.pl, and peaks were annotated to nearby gene using annotated Peaks.pl. Motifs obtained from both "*De novo*" and "Known Motifs" (having highest motif score) search having $p <$ 10-20 were considered significant. Aligned reads from BMDC PU.1 and Irf4 ChIP-seq were compared with Zeb1 ChIP-seq data using SeqMiner (59) k-means clustering. To validate the ChIP-seq results we randomly selected Zeb1 peaks found in ChIP-seq to confirm the enrichment using two independent ChIP-qPCR experiments.

Pathway Analysis

Ingenuity Pathway Analysis (IPA) software from Qiagen was used throughout the analysis process and p-value cutoff of 0.05 was considered significant. All the raw results of pathway analysis are attached as **Supplementary Files**.

Visualization

Gene expression scatter plot, pathway bar plots and other sequencing data representing bar graphs were generated using

Ggplot2 (https://cran.r-project.org/web/packages/ggplot2/index.html) R package. The heatmap was generated using Complex Heatmap R package with row-wise clustering option (60).

RESULTS

EMT Factor Zeb1 KD Suppresses Activation, Co-stimulation and Cytokine Production in CD8α$^+$cDC1 DCs

In this study, we have used a CD8α$^+$ cDC1 MutuDC line recently developed and well characterized by Fuertes Maracco and colleagues (9). They showed that this DC line mimic remarkably the primary lymphoid resident cDC1 responses isolated from spleen. While analyzing an unpublished RNA-seq data from these cDC1 cells, we found that Zeb1 transcript is constitutively expressed in cDC1 and upon TLR9 stimulation by CpG the expression increased significantly (**Supplementary Figures 1A,B**). To characterize the functional role of Zeb1 in cDC1, we generated a stable Zeb1 KD in cDC1 MutuDC line using lentiviral shRNA transduction followed by puromycin selection. We used three different shRNAs targeting different regions of Zeb1 transcript and found that two of them showed significant depletion of Zeb1 transcript (**Supplementary Table 8**). For downstream analyses we moved ahead with one shRNA sequence i.e., shRNA3, which showed higher Zeb1 depletion. We obtained 55–80% reduction of Zeb1 transcript in stable KD DCs and a concomitant decreased ZEB1 protein levels before and after 0.5, 2, 6, and 12 h after CpG activation as evident from western blotting analysis (**Figures 1A**). The western blot analysis demonstrated low levels of ZEB1 expression in unstimulated cells and a prominently increased expression within first few hours of CpG challenge that was decreased at later time points i.e., 6 and 12 h (**Figures 1A,B**).

After confirming the Zeb1 KD at transcript and protein level in stable KD DCs, we analyzed the impact of its depletion on DC activation and concomitant cytokine expression in CD8α$^+$ cDC1 MutuDCs. We performed detailed immune profiling of these stable Zeb1 KD DCs before and after 2, 6, and 12 h of CpG stimulation. It has been well established that Zeb1 directly represses Cdh1 gene and therefore first we analyzed the transcript expression of Cdh1 gene and found it to be significantly increased after Zeb1 depletion in cDC1 DCs confirming the impact of Zeb1 depletion (**Figure 1B**). Then we investigated the impact of Zeb1 KD on DC activation and co-stimulation along with expression of cytokine genes 12 h after CpG challenge using qPCR, flow cytometry (FACS) and multiplex ELISA (Bioplex) to profile the Zeb1 mediated immune-modulations. We found that Zeb1 KD DCs showed significantly reduced transcript expression of important DC response cytokines Il-10 and Il-27, while Il-12 (subunit p40) showed significant and sustained increase after 12 h of CpG stimulation in Zeb1 KD DCs (**Figure 1B**). Moreover, the Il-12p35 subunit of IL-12 cytokine showed significantly decreased expression after Zeb1 KD (**Figure 1B**). We did not observe any significant change in the mRNA expression of Cd80 and Cd86 activation markers upon Zeb1 KD before and after CpG activation (**Figure 1B**). FACS analysis showed significantly decreased expression of CD80 and CD86 in Zeb1 KD unstimulated DCs as compared to control cells, but no significant differences were observed after CpG stimulation (**Figure 1C**). The MFI analysis showed a significant increase in CD86 in CpG condition, whereas percent positive cells showed an insignificant increasing trend as CpG activation makes nearly 99–100 percent cells positive for CD86 (**Figure 1C**). The CD40 expression was unchanged in Zeb1 KD as compared to control DCs, whereas MHC-I and MHC-II percent positive cells showed a significant decrease in unstimulated condition (**Figures 1C,D**). In addition, the MFI shifts depicted a significant MHC-II decrease before and after CpG activation with a decreasing trend for MHCI (**Figures 1C,D**). Consequently the intracellular levels of IL-10 and IL-27 cytokines were significantly decreased in Zeb1 KD DCs after CpG activation (**Figures 2A,B**). Moreover, the MFI analysis (bar-plots and histograms) also showed similar trends (**Figures 1C,D, 2A**). The cytokine IL-6 showed insignificant but decreasing trend (**Figure 2A**). Besides, the IL-12p40 levels were significantly increased in 12 h CpG activated Zeb1 KD DCs. At early time points (2 and 6 h) of CpG activation, we did not observe any significant change in the IL-12p40 expression (data not shown). Furthermore to estimate the secreted cytokine levels, we performed multiplex ELISA i.e., Bio-plex analysis, which demonstrated a significant decrease in IL-6, IL-10, IL-12p70, and IFNγ cytokine levels in CpG activated Zeb1 KD DCs (**Figure 2B** and **Supplementary Figure 1F**). We observed significantly decreased levels of IL-12p70 in the culture supernatants of 12 h CpG activated Zeb1 KD DCs in contrast to a significant increase we found for IL-12p40, an important subunit of this cytokine (**Figure 2B**). This may be due to significantly decreased IL-12p35 subunit, which is an exclusive subunit of bioactive inflammatory cytokine IL-12. Other important DC markers like PDL1 and IL-27 also showed a significant decrease after Zeb1 depletion as compared to control DCs (**Figures 1C, 2A**). These results showed that Zeb1 depletion suppressed DC activation and co-stimulation leading to decreased secretion of important DC response cytokines.

The cDC1 MutuDCs that we employed in our study express high levels of both TLR3 and TLR9 receptors (9). Therefore, we also treated Zeb1 KD and control DCs with TLR3 ligand pIC and CpG + pIC simultaneously to activate both TLR3 and TLR9 receptors together. We found that pIC resulted in weak activation of DCs as compared to CpG whereas simultaneous CpG + pIC activation resulted in strong activation as evident from CD80 and CD86 expression and synergistic expression of cytokines like IL-6, IL-10, and IL-12p40 (**Supplementary Figures 1C,D**). We found that Zeb1 depletion resulted in similar decrease in activation, co-stimulation and cytokine genes as we found after CpG activation. These results further confirmed that Zeb1 KD results in suboptimal activation of DCs leading to decreased expression of pro- and anti-inflammatory cytokines in cDC1 DCs, irrespective of any strong antigenic challenge.

To validate our *in vitro* findings, we generated primary cDC1 DCs from the bone marrow precursor cells using fms-like tyrosine kinase 3 ligand (FLT3L) supplemented medium (see Methods for details) (47). Bone marrow culture with FLT3L is the recent method that allow the generation of both cDCs

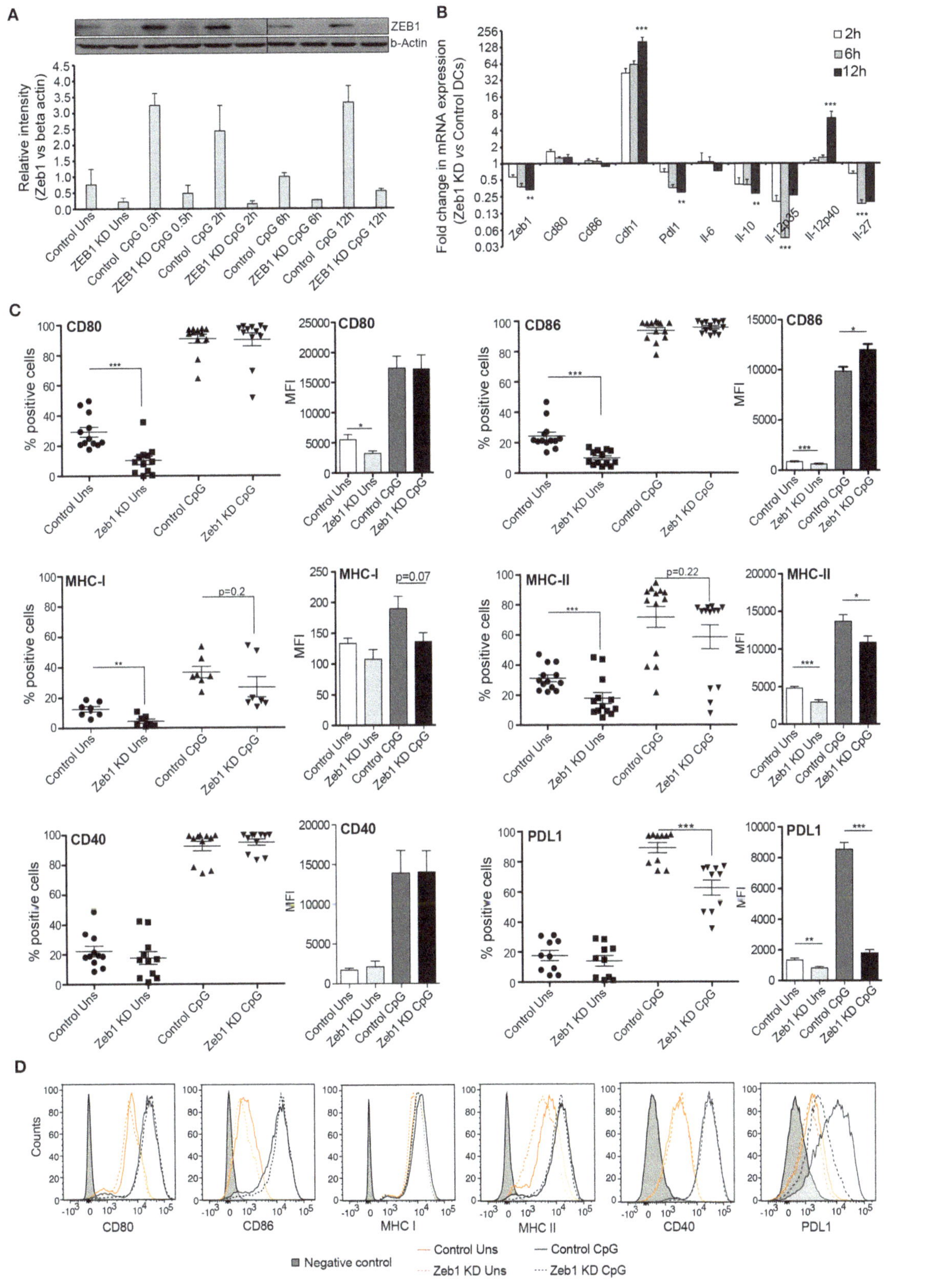

FIGURE 1 | Zeb1 transcription factor KD suppresses activation and co-stimulation of CD8α$^+$ cDC1 MutuDCs. **(A)** Western blot and its densitometric analysis showing the ZEB1 protein expression kinetics and its KD by shRNA at 0, 0.5, 2, 6, and 12 h after CpG activation in CD8α$^+$ cDC1 DCs $n = 2$. **(B)** Bar-plot demonstrating the fold changes in the transcript expression of DC activation/co-stimulation markers and selected cytokine genes in Zeb1 KD DCs compared to control cells using

(Continued)

FIGURE 1 | qPCR $n = 3$. **(C)** Scatter-plots showing the percentage positive cells for cell-surface expression of activation and co-stimulatory markers CD80, CD86, MHC-I, MHC-II, CD40, and PDL1 on Zeb1 KD cDC1 MutuDCs compared to control cells before and after 12 h CpG activation. The corresponding panels with bar plots depict the Median Florescence Intensity (MFI) shifts for the respective genes $n = 6–12$. **(D)** Representative histogram plots demonstrating the MFI shift observed for the activation/co-stimulatory markers and cytokines. p-values are calculated using two tailed unpaired student's t-test, error bars represent SEM. $^{*}\leq 0.05$, $^{**}\leq 0.01$, $^{***}\leq 0.001$.

and pDCs. In purview of published reports, which suggests that FLT3L derived DCs (FL-DCs) are $CD11c^{hi}CD24^{hi}$ and $CD11b^{low}$, are putative of $CD8\alpha^{+}$ cDC1 equivalent (47, 61), therefore we gated $CD11c^{+}CD24^{+}MHCII^{+}$ population in FACS to analyze the impact of Zeb1 transient depletion on cDC1 activation and cytokine expression. We found that transient KD of Zeb1 in primary cDC1 cells using Zeb1 shRNA reduced their activation, co-stimulation and production of cytokines like IL-6, IL-10, IL-12p40, and IL-27 as compared to control KD DCs (**Figures 3A–D** and **Supplementary Figure 2A**). In contrast to Zeb1 KD MutuDCs, IL-12p40 showed decreased expression in BMDCs. This could be due to transient Zeb1 KD, differential expression kinetics of IL-12p40 in BMDCs or due to cell heterogeneity of BMDCs. We also found that Zeb1 is expressed at similar levels in different primary DC subsets cDC1, cDC2, and pDCs isolated from spleen of FLT3L transgenic mice. Here we have focused on the role of Zeb1 in cDC1 DCs but it would be further intriguing to explore its importance in other DC subsets as well (**Supplementary Figure 2F**).

OT-II T Helper Cells Co-cultured With Zeb1 KD DCs Enhanced Th2 Responses

As we found a consistent decrease in all the measured cytokines in Zeb1 KD DCs we were interested to identify if Zeb1 KD cDC1 MutuDCs would functionally interfere in T-helper (Th) cell differentiation. For the same, Zeb1 KD and control DCs were pulsed with OTII peptide with or without CpG for 2 h. Then, $CD4^{+}$ Th cells isolated from spleen of OT-II transgenic mice were labeled with a proliferation dye efluor 670 followed by co-culture with these DCs for 72 h. Upon priming by DCs, the naïve T helper cells first undergo several rounds of clonal amplification and then polarization into various effector subtypes depending upon the DC responses (62, 63). We found that Zeb1 KD DCs induced higher antigen-specific $CD4^{+}$ Th cell proliferation compared to control DCs (**Figure 4A**). This was also observed when DCs had been previously stimulated with CpG, which induced even higher T cell proliferation after 3 days of co-culture (**Figures 4A,B**). As we observed a decrease in activation and co-stimulation markers in Zeb1 KD DCs the increased proliferation of T cells was puzzling and therefore we looked into expression of IL-2 in cell culture supernatants of Zeb1 KD and control cells by Bio-plex. We found increased IL-2 cytokine after CpG activation in Zeb1 KD DC supernatants as compared to control cells (**Supplementary Figure 2E**). In addition, we looked into T cell differentiation profiles of these co-cultured Th cells. We found significantly increased differentiation of Zeb1 KD DCs primed Th cells toward Th2 subtype marked by increased number of GATA3 and $GATA3^{+}IL\text{-}13^{+}$ expressing Th cells (**Figures 4C,D**). At the same time the $Tbet^{+}IFN\gamma^{+}$ expressing Th1 cells were majorly decreased in CpG activated Zeb1 KD condition (**Supplementary Figures 2B,C**). We did not observe any significant difference in the Treg differentiation marker FoxP3 (**Supplementary Figure 2D**) In unstimulated conditions we did not found any significant increase in $GATA3^{+}$ alone or $GATA3^{+}IL\text{-}13^{+}$ double positive Th cells (**Figures 4C,D**) and on the contrary the $Tbet^{+}IFN\gamma^{+}$ population was increased (**Supplementary Figures 2B,C**)

Moreover we also performed allogeneic mixed lymphocytic reaction (MLR) assay to confirm the induction of Th2 responses by Zeb1 KD DCs (**Supplementary Figure 3A**). We found that the $CD3^{+}CD4^{+}CD44^{+}$ effector Th cells showed enhanced Th2 responses as evidenced by significantly increased GATA3 and IL-4 expression in T cells primed by CpG pulsed Zeb1 KD compared to control DCs (**Supplementary Figure 3B**). On the other hand, the Th1 subtype polarization marker Tbet and its signature cytokine $IFN\gamma$ showed insignificant but decreasing trend (**Supplementary Figure 3C**). These analyses demonstrated that Zeb1 has the potential to modulate T helper cell differentiation toward Th2 subtype by modulating DC responses. We also looked into the impact of Zeb1 KD cDC1 on $CD8^{+}$ T cell function by gating them separately from $CD4^{+}$ Th cells (**Supplementary Figure 3D**). We found that the effector $CD8^{+}$ T cells generated in co-culture with Zeb1 KD DCs produced significantly less Granzyme and Perforin as compared to $CD8^{+}$ T cells cultured with control DCs (**Supplementary Figures 3D,E**) suggesting Zeb1 as important factor for inducing optimal T cell cytotoxic responses.

Adoptive Transfer of Zeb1 Depleted DCs Enhanced Helminth Clearance in Mice

After confirming that Zeb1 KD cDC1 MutuDCs enhanced Th2 cell development *in vitro*, we were interested in determining if these DCs were able to affect Th2 responses in an *in vivo* parasite infected animal model. Helminth (*Heligmosomoides polygyrus*) infection mice model is considered as one of the best-characterized disease models where it has been established that perturbation of Th cell subtype responses modulates the worm load in the intestine (64–67). Besides that the penetrance of pathogenesis is quite uniform in this disease model. Therefore, we performed adoptive transfer of CpG pulsed control and Zeb1 KD MutuDCs in *H. polygyrus* infected mice to identify its physiological impact on disease burden. The egg load in the feces were calculated starting from day 9 (D9) till 1 month after adoptive transfer of DCs to get an idea about the mature worm abundance in the intestine of infected animals. At D9, there were no eggs observed in both Zeb1 KD and control DC treated animals. This observation is consistent with the previous reports that worms get mature and move to intestinal lumen on the

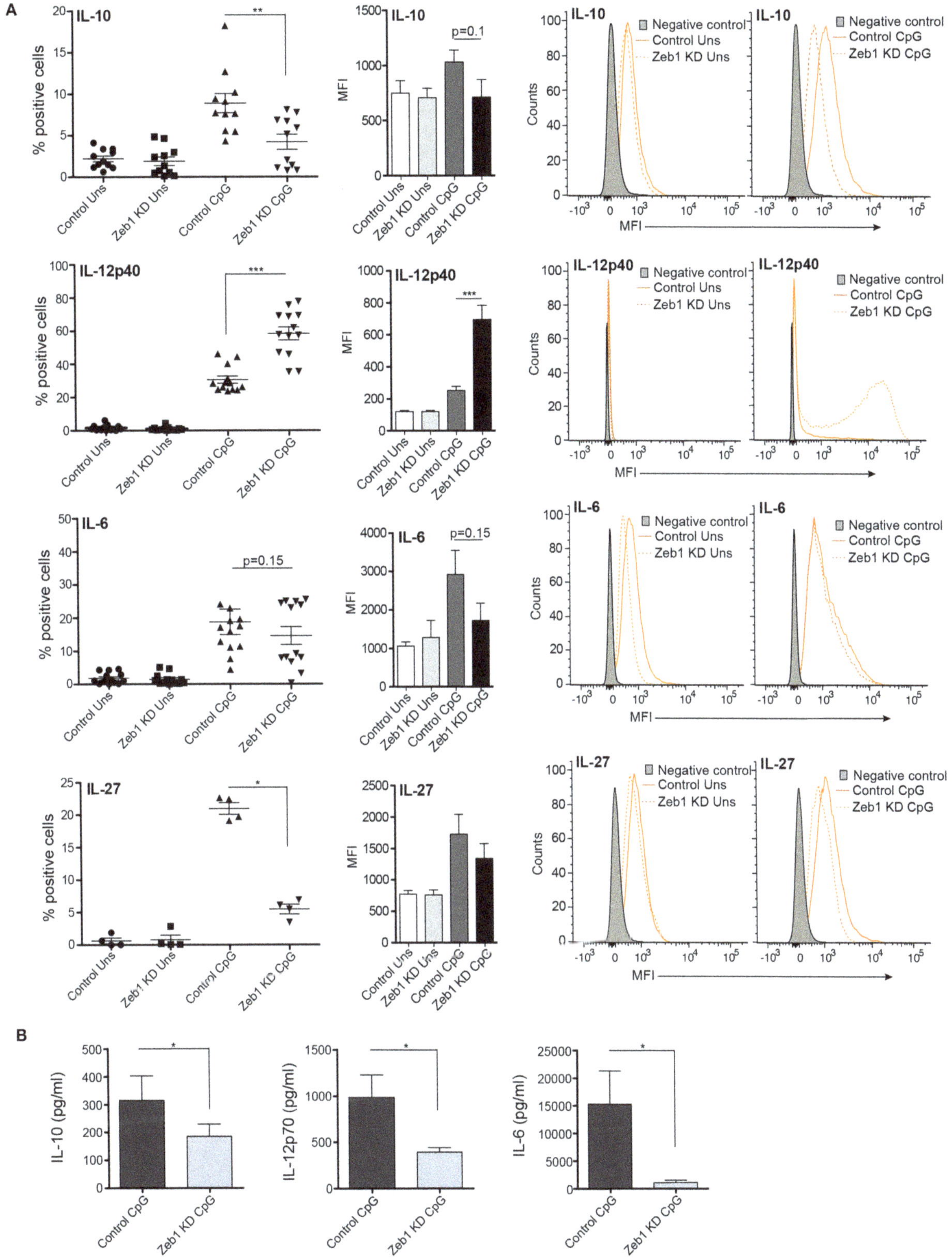

FIGURE 2 | EMT factor Zeb1 KD suppresses expression of important DC response cytokines in cDC1 MutuDCs. **(A)** Scatter-plots showing the percentage positive cells for intracellular cytokines IL-10, IL-12p40, IL-6, and IL-27 in Zeb1 KD cDC1 MutuDCs compared to control cells before and after 12 h CpG activation. The corresponding bar plots and representative histograms in each panel depicting the MFI shifts for these cytokines in Zeb1 KD as compared to control DCs $n = 8$–12. **(B)** Bar-plots demonstrating the Bio-plex based quantitation of IL-10, IL-12p70, and IL-6 cytokines secreted in the supernatants of 12 h CpG activated Zeb1 KD and control DCs $n = 5$. p-values are calculated using two tailed unpaired student's t-test, error bars represent SEM. $^{*}\leq 0.05$, $^{**}\leq 0.01$, $^{***}\leq 0.001$.

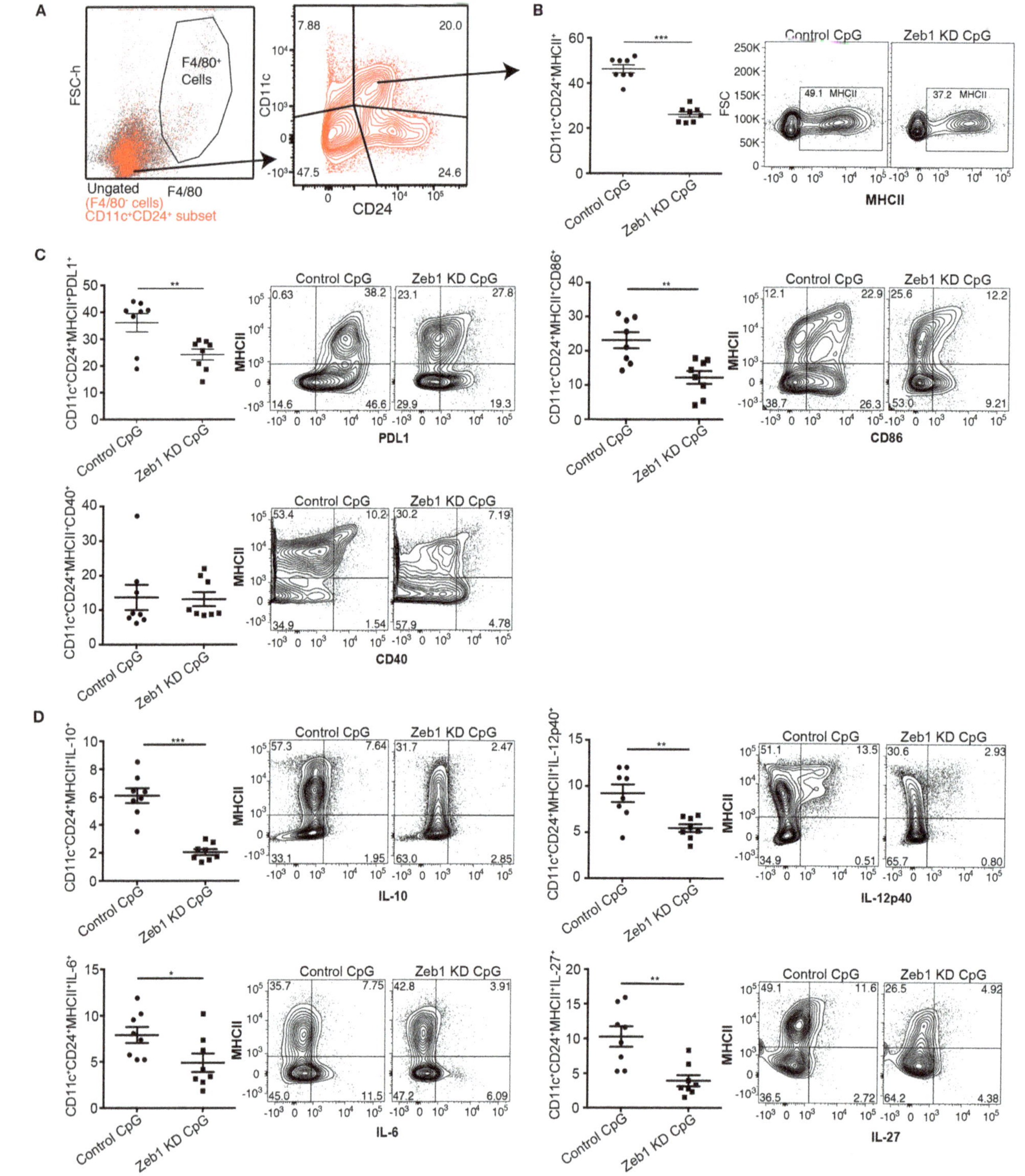

FIGURE 3 | Zeb1 depletion in bone-marrow derived primary cDC1 DCs showed decreased DC activation, co-stimulation and cytokine secretion $n = 6$–8. **(A)** FACS contour-plot showing the gating strategy used to remove F4/80 positive macrophage population from the $CD11c^+$ DCs to analyze the impact of Zeb1 KD on $CD11c^+CD24^+MHCII^+$ DC population. High $CD11c^+CD24^+$ double positive DCs were considered as cDC1 DCs for analysis. **(B)** Scatter-plot and representative contour plots depicting the percentage of MHCII positive cells in $F4/80^-CD11c^+CD24^+$ gated BMDCs treated with control and Zeb1 shRNA3 followed by 12 h CpG stimulation $n = 6$–8. **(C)** Scatter-plots and representative contour plots depicting the percentage positive cells for cell surface markers PDL1, CD86, and CD40 in $F4/80^-CD11c^+CD24^+$ gated BMDCs treated with control and Zeb1 shRNA3 followed by 12 h CpG stimulation $n = 6$–8. **(D)** Scatter-plots showing the percentage positive cells for intracellular cytokines IL-10, IL-12p40, IL-6, and IL-27 in $F4/80^-CD11c^+CD24^+MHCII^+$ gated BMDCs treated with control and Zeb1 shRNA3 followed by 12 h CpG stimulation $n = 6$. *p*-values were calculated using two tailed unpaired student's *t*-test, error bars represent SEM. $^*\leq 0.05$, $^{**}\leq 0.01$, $^{***}\leq 0.001$.

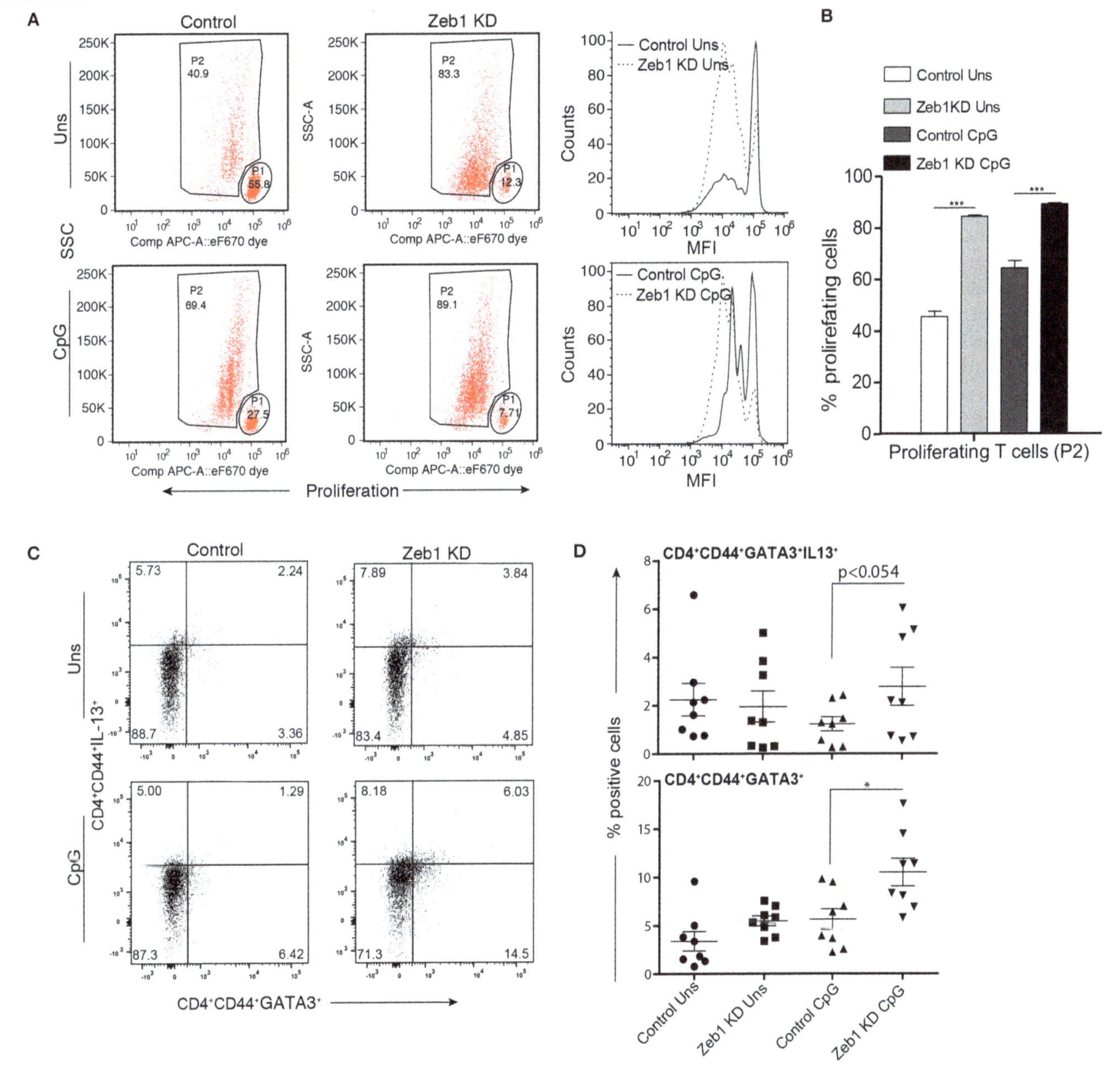

FIGURE 4 | OT-II T helper cells co-cultured with CpG activated Zeb1 KD cDC1 MutuDCs showed enhanced proliferation and differentiation toward Th2 phenotype. **(A)** Representative FACS dot-plots showing gated parent population (P1) and proliferating cell population (P2) depicting the changes in proliferation rate of OT-II Th cells co-cultured for 72 h with Zeb1 KD cDC1 MutuDCs as compared to control DCs with or without CpG pulsing. The corresponding panel shows the histogram showing the MFI shifts for the proliferation of T cells. $n = 3$. **(B)** Bar-plot depicting the percentage of proliferating Th cells (P2) in $CD4^+$ T cells co-cultured with unstimulated and CpG activated Zeb1 KD and control DCs $n = 3$. **(C)** FACS dot-plots showing the percentage positive $CD4^+CD44^+GATA3^+IL\text{-}13^+$ Th cells in Th cells co-cultured with unstimulated and CpG pulsed Zeb1 KD and control cDC1 MutuDCs for 96 h $n = 8$. **(D)** Scatter-plots showing the percentage of double positive cells for $GATA3^+IL\text{-}13^+$ and single positive $GATA3^+$ cells in effector $CD4^+CD44^+$ Th cell population $n = 8$. p-values are calculated using two tailed unpaired student's t-test, error bars represent SEM. $^*\leq 0.05$, $^{***}\leq 0.001$.

D10 and reproduce, resulting in release of eggs in feces (68). Interestingly at D10, we found that Zeb1 KD DC treated animals showed less egg counts in their feces compared to control DC treated animals even after injecting them with equal number of L3 stage larvae at D0 (**Figure 5A**). In addition, in Zeb1 KD DCs treated mice the intestines were almost clear of helminth infection as no or only few worms were found in the intestine depicted by the drastically reduced number of eggs on D31 (**Figure 5B**). Five animals from each group were dissected at D14 and D31 to estimate the worm load in the intestines. We found that animals treated with CpG activated Zeb1 KD DCs showed a significant decrease in intestinal helminth load as compared to control DC treated animals at D14 (**Figure 5C**). Besides, at D31 insignificant differences were observed in intestinal helminth count in animals treated with unstimulated Zeb1 KD and control DCs as clear from similar egg counts found at D31 (data not shown). However, the animals treated with CpG pulsed Zeb1 KD DCs were almost free of helminth infection in the intestine as compared to control DC treated mice at D31 (**Figure 5D**).

Furthermore to identify the impact of CD8α^+ cDC1 MutuDCs adoptive transfer on Th cell polarization in animals leading to the observed phenotype, we performed detailed Th cell subtype profiling from mesenteric lymph nodes (MLNs) of all the infected and treated animals at D14 and D31. We found that in CpG pulsed Zeb1 KD DC treated animals at D14 presented increased number of Th2 effector CD4$^+$CD44$^+$ cells with significantly higher expression of GATA3 and IL-5 as compared to control DC treated animals (**Figure 5E**). The cytokine IL-13 also showed an insignificant but increasing trend (**Figure 5E**). We also observed mice that were treated with CpG pulsed Zeb1 depleted DCs had reduced Tbet and IFNγ positive cells in the MLNs. FoxP3, a Treg marker showed an increase in Zeb1 KD cells, which is well reported to be elevated during Th2 response (**Figure 5E**). At D31, we found a significant increase of IL-5 and IL-10. The cytokine IL-13 showed increasing trend, whereas IFNγ was significantly increased (**Supplementary Figure 4**), which could be the reason for increased Tregs. Increased Th2 cells in MLNs of helminth infected animals by treating animals with Zeb1 KD DCs strongly suggested that Zeb1 depletion in CD8α^+ cDC1 could potentiate Th2 responses *in vivo*, affecting helminth clearance.

Transcriptome Analysis of Zeb1 KD DCs Showed an Enrichment of Th2 Pathway

To understand mechanisms underlying the control of Zeb1 mediated DC responses we performed RNA-seq analysis of control and Zeb1 KD cDC1 MutuDCs at 0, 6, and 12 h after CpG stimulation. First we confirmed the significantly decreased transcript levels of Zeb1 and a concomitant significant increase in Cdh1 expression in RNA-seq datasets at all the analyzed time points (**Supplementary Table 1**). Downstream analysis and manual curation of the genes that were differentially expressed (corrected p-value ≤ 0.05) in Zeb1 KD DCs showed a significant down-regulation of cytokines like Il-6, Il-10, and Il-27 along with several C-type lectin receptors (CLRs) such as Clec1a, Clec4a1, Cleca7A (Dectin-1), Clec9a and Clec12a as compared to control cells (**Figures 6A,B** and **Supplementary Table 1**). It has been reported that CLRs present on DCs act in a pathogen/antigen dependent manner to control Th cell differentiation. Whereas one of the CLR i.e., DC-SIGN (Cd209c, Cd209f, Cd209g) showed significant and highest increase in 6 h as well as 12 h CpG activated Zeb1 KD DCs as compared to control cells (**Figures 6A–C** and **Supplementary Table 1**). We found that there were more upregulated genes after Zeb1 KD as compared to down-regulated ones at all the time points suggesting toward global repressive function of Zeb1 (**Figure 6D**). There were 229, 308, and 396 genes upregulated after Zeb1 KD at 0, 6 and 12 h time point, whereas 113, 212, and 234 genes were down regulated respectively (**Figure 6D** and **Supplementary Table 1**). Moreover, the major anti-inflammatory or tolerogenic cytokine Il-10 was also significantly decreased at both 6 and 12 h time points in Zeb1 depleted cells (**Figure 6C** and **Supplementary Table 2**). Ultimately to identify the biological pathways that were enriched for the genes differentially expressed in Zeb1 KD DCs after 6 and 12 h CpG activation, we performed Ingenuity pathway analysis (IPA). We found that at both the time points there was enrichment of "Dendritic cell maturation," "Receptors for bacterial/virus recognition," "Th2 pathways," "Th cell differentiation," and "STAT3 pathways" (**Figure 6E, Supplementary Figures 5A,B** and **Supplementary Table 3**).

Zeb1 Chip-seq Identified Its Direct and Indirect Target Genes in CD8α^+ cDC1 MutuDCs

We performed ChIP-seq for Zeb1 in unstimulated DCs to identify the genes that were directly bound and regulated by Zeb1. The major aim was to correlate the Zeb1 binding in ChIP-seq with RNA-seq to identify the genes that were directly controlled by Zeb1 in DCs. We found ~3400 genomic regions bound by Zeb1 in unstimulated CD8α^+ cDC1 (**Supplementary Table 4**). Upon overlap of genes bound in ChIP-seq with RNA-seq list we found 76, 130, and 141 genes to be directly regulated by Zeb1 (**Figure 7A**). Out of these genes 52, 85, and 95 were upregulated, whereas 24, 45 and 46 genes were down regulated at 0, 6, and 12 h respectively after Zeb1 KD (**Figure 7A**). To identify the Zeb1 bound genomic regions with respect to transcription start site (TSS), we did GREAT analysis and found that majority of Zeb1 bindings were distal (775 peaks in ±5 KB, 1576 peaks in > ±5 KB and < ±50 K region) and far from TSS (**Figure 7B**). Then, to identify if Zeb1 DNA binding motif is enriched on these bound peaks we did *de novo* motif analysis using HOMER and found 42% of bound regions showed canonical Zeb1 motif whereas other Zeb1 bound genomic regions showed significant enrichment of DNA motifs for IRF, ETS (PU.1), E2A and ETS-IRF (PU.1-IRF) TFs (**Figure 7C**). To experimentally validate it, we performed ChIP-seq for PU.1, and the SeqMINER overlap with Zeb1 peaks showed that indeed PU.1 overlaps strongly at Zeb1 bound genomic regions (**Figure 7D**). We also overlapped publicly available IRF4 ChIP-seq data from unstimulated and 2 h LPS stimulated BMDCs with Zeb1 and found that IRF4 also showed similar percentage of overlap as predicted in our *de novo* motif analysis (**Figures 7C,D** and **Supplementary Table 5**). Moreover, Th1 and Th2 pathways are enriched for genes annotated to Zeb1-PU1-IRF4 overlapping genomic regions (**Supplementary Figure 5C**). Although Zeb1 is a known transcriptional repressor and there are more upregulated genes as compared to down regulated genes in RNA-seq data, we observed that most of the DC immune response genes were down regulated after Zeb1 depletion in our *in vitro* and *ex vivo* immune-profiling experiments. To understand it better, we divided all the Zeb1 KD differentially regulated genes into two groups based on gene ontology, i.e., immune response pathway and the other pathway genes and

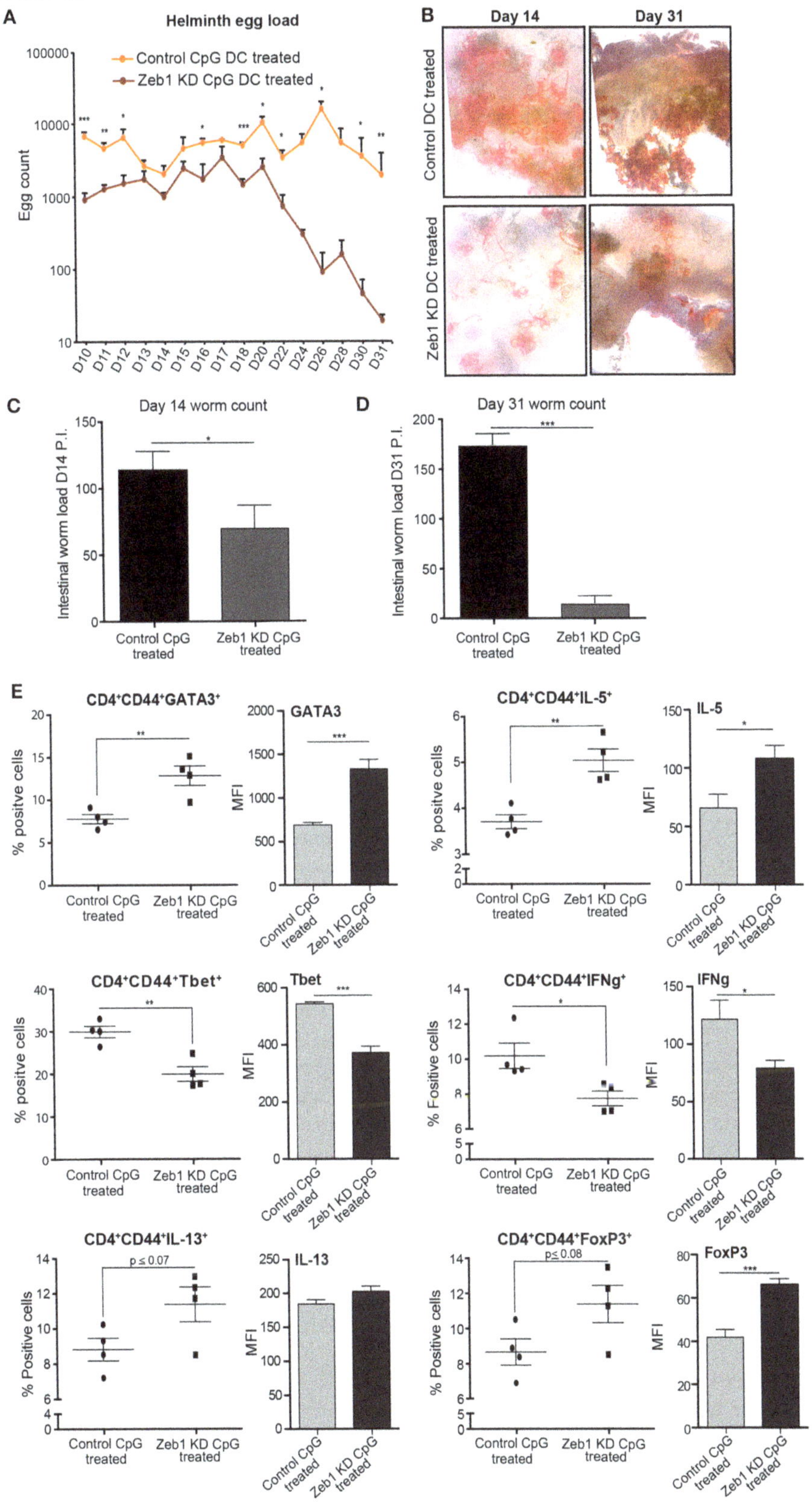

FIGURE 5 | Adoptive transfer of CpG activated Zeb1 KD cDC1 MutuDCs in helminth-infected mice enhances worm clearance by increasing Th2 responses. **(A)** Line-graphs depicting the Helminth egg counts in the feces of CpG pulsed Zeb1 KD CD8α$^+$ cDC1 MutuDCs and control DC treated mice from D10 to D31. The mice were infected with *H. polygyrus* larvae at D0 and treated with CpG pulsed control and Zeb1 KD CD8α$^+$ cDC1 cells consecutively at D7, D9, and D11. The egg

(Continued)

FIGURE 5 | counting was started from D10 till D31. At day 9 there were no eggs detected in feces of animals $n = 10$. **(B)** Representative intestinal sections of helminth infected mice at D14 and D31 after helminth infection and treatment with CpG pulsed Zeb1 KD and control DC treated animals $n = 5$. **(C)** Intestinal worm load at day 14 in mice adoptively treated with CpG activated Zeb1 KD and control DCs $n = 5$. **(D)** Intestinal worm load in mice adoptively treated with CpG activated Zeb1 KD and control DCs at day 31 after infection $n = 5$. **(E)** Scatter-plots for Th1, Th2, and Treg markers like GATA3, IL-5, Tbet, IFNγ, IL-13, and FoxP3 from detailed immune profiling of $CD4^+CD44^+$ effector Th cells isolated form mesenteric lymph nodes of helminth infected animals and treated with activated Zeb1 KD and control DCs. The corresponding panels also depict bar plots for MFI shifts for each marker in $CD4^+CD44^+$ effector Th cell population $n = 5$. p-values are calculated using two tailed unpaired student's t-test, error bars represent SEM. $^*\leq 0.05$, $^{**}\leq 0.01$, $^{***}\leq 0.001$.

looked for any preferential Zeb1 bindings differences in these two groups. Surprisingly, the ratio of Zeb1 unbound vs. bound regulated genes was ≥2.5 for both the gene groups. Then, we analyzed the number of up- vs. down-regulated genes in immune response and other pathway group and interestingly we found that similar number of immune response genes were differentially regulated (ratio of ∼1.0 for up- vs. down genes) whereas for other pathways gene group there were more upregulated genes (ratio ≥ 1.6–2.5) (**Figures 7E,F** and **Supplementary Table 6**). This suggested that Zeb1 does not appear to be a global transcriptional repressor for immune response genes. Ultimately we analyzed the pathways enriched for the genes directly bound and regulated by Zeb1 using IPA. We found "T helper cell differentiation" and "Th2 pathway" to be significantly enriched for genes differentially regulated at 12 h time point (**Figure 7G** and **Supplementary Table 7**). It was interesting to find that even with such a low number of direct target genes we found T cell differentiation and Th2 pathway as highly enriched pathways.

Decreased IL-12 Cytokine Secretion by Zeb1 KD DCs Leads to Th2 Development

Though we found in our genomic analysis that CLRs were significantly down regulated along with IL-10, IL-6, and IL-12p70 cytokines, we were unable to pinpoint specific molecular mediator leading to the induction of Th2 responses by Zeb1 KD DCs. It has been reported extensively that decreased secretion of inflammatory IL-12p70 cytokine by DCs results in default polarization of T cells toward Th2 subtype (22, 28, 31, 69). Therefore we decided to confirm if Zeb1 KD DCs upon supplementation with recombinant IL-12 (rIL-12) containing medium decreased the polarization of Th cells toward Th2 with a concomitant increased Th1 subtype. We found that OT-II Th cells co-cultured with Zeb1 KD DCs supplemented with 5 ng/ml rIL-12 resulted into significantly increased IFNγ expressing Th1 cells comparable to control DCs (**Figure 8A** and **Supplementary Figure 6A**). On the contrary there was a significantly decreased expression of $GATA3^+$ Th2 cells in Zeb1 KD DCs after rIL-12 supplementation (**Figure 8B** and **Supplementary Figure 6B**). The MFI analysis of Tbet, Th1 inducing factor also demonstrated significant increase after rIL-12 addition in Zeb1 KD DCs whereas GATA3 showed insignificant ($p = 0.09$) but decreasing trend (**Figures 8C,D**). This lead us to conclude that decreased IL-12p70 secreted by activated Zeb1 KD DCs leads to default development of Th2 phenotype. As Il-12p35 is an exclusive subunit of bioactive IL-12 cytokine whereas Il-12p40 subunit is used as a dimerization partner for other cytokines, we suspected that the decreased IL-12 in Zeb1 KD DCs may be due to decreased Il-12p35. Besides, in our RNA-seq data as well we identified that FPKM of IL12p35 gene was ≥2-fold decreased in Zeb1 KD DCs as compared to control cells after 2 h CpG activation (**Supplementary Figure 5D**). Furthermore, we found IRF4 transcription factor to be significantly increased in Zeb1 KD DCs, which is well reported to repress inflammatory cytokines in DCs to increase Th2 development (**Supplementary Figures 6C,D**). Moreover, it would be difficult to exclude the effect of other molecules such as CLRs, Stat5b and other cytokines that are differentially regulated in Zeb1 KD DCs and are reported to impact Th cell polarization intoTh2 subtypes.

DISCUSSION

Dendritic cells (DCs) are one of the major sentinels of the immune system that determines the fate of T cell dependent adaptive responses. Recently it has been proposed that altering the DC responses can be exploited to affect Th cell subtype development and hence the diseases phenotypes (70, 71). In this study, for the first time, we explored the role of EMT factor Zeb1 in DC function and found that Zeb1 depletion has immune-modulatory effects which skews the Th cells toward the Th2 subtype. Besides that, adoptive transfer of Zeb1 KD cDC1 MutuDCs clears helminth infection by inducing IL-13 and IL-5 secreting Th2 cells in MLNs of infected animals. Moreover, we identified that Zeb1 KD suppresses wide-variety of inflammatory response genes including several CLRs. We concluded that decreased secretion of Th1 inducing inflammatory cytokine IL-12 by Zeb1 KD cDC1 resulted into increased Th2 differentiation. Although the impact of other important factors that were differentially expressed in Zeb1 KD DCs cannot be ignored (24).

Zeb1 is a well-known EMT master regulator that induces mesenchymal properties in cancer cells by increasing N-cadherin and Vimentin levels making it more invasive and metastatic. It directly controls the expression of E-cadherin (Cdh1) by binding to its proximal promoter (72–74). We identified that Zeb1 decrease in our $CD8a^+$ DCs cDC1 correlated with the levels of Cdh1 and the cells appeared less migratory and smaller in size *in vitro* as compared to control DCs (data not shown). The impact on Cdh1 was so robust that in all our experiments including RNA-seq we used Cdh1 expression as an indicative of Zeb1 levels. It has been reported that decreased activation and co-stimulation of DCs marked by CD80, CD86, MHC-I and MHC-II resulted into suppression of cytokine secretion (21–23, 28, 31). Besides, these moderately activated

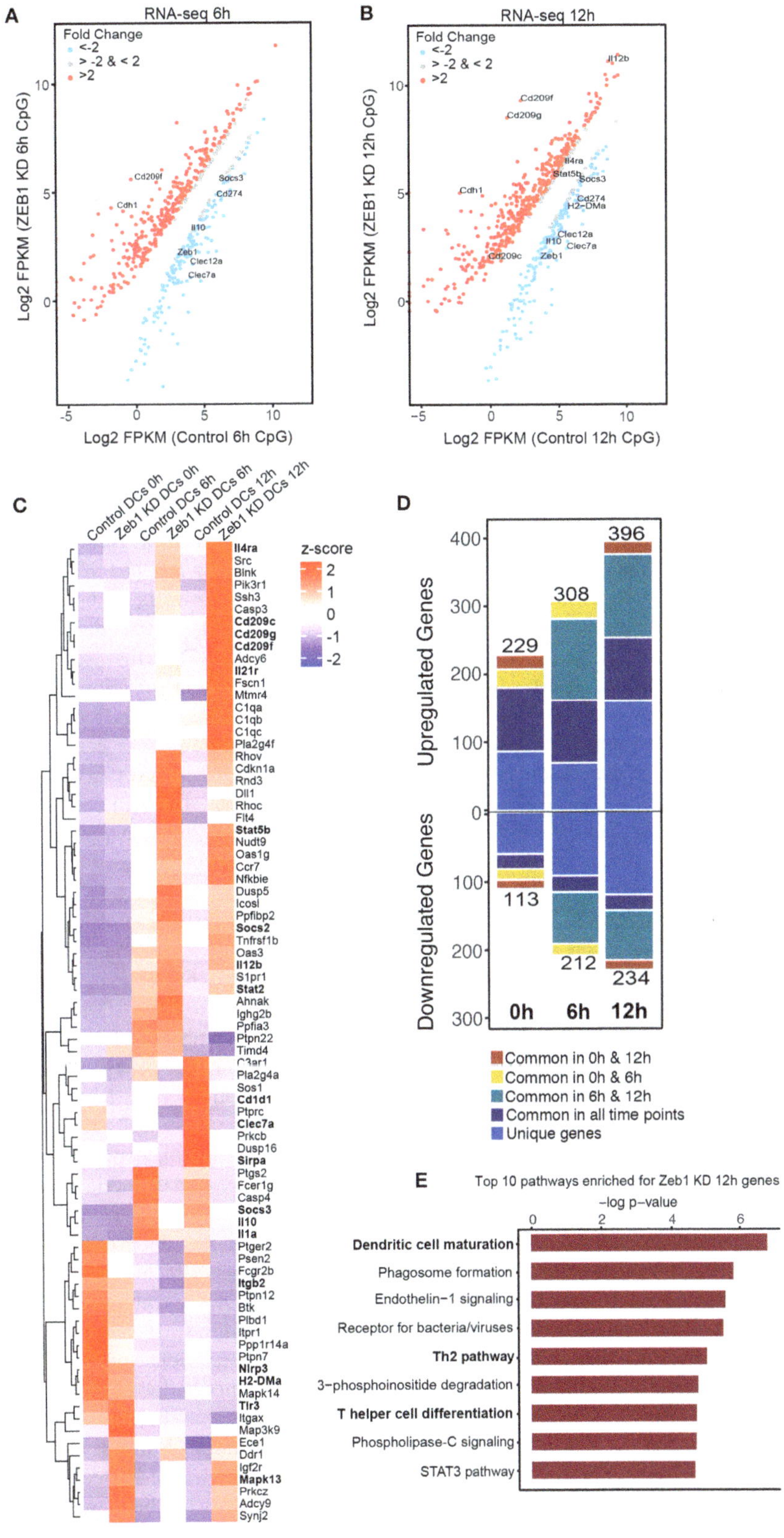

FIGURE 6 | Global transcriptome analysis of Zeb1 KD cDC1 MutuDCs showed enrichment of pathways involved in T helper cell differentiation and Th2 pathways. Two independent biological replicates with three time points (0, 6, 12 h) were used for this analysis. **(A)** RNA-seq scatter-plot showing the differentially regulated genes in Zeb1 KD cDC1 MutuDCs as compared to control DCs at 6 h after CpG activation $n = 2$. **(B)** Scatter-plot showing the differentially regulated genes in Zeb1

(Continued)

FIGURE 6 | KD cDC1 MutuDCs as compared to control DCs at 12 h after CpG activation $n = 2$. **(C)** Heat-map generated from a list of manually curated genes identified from differentially regulated gene list in Zeb1 KD RNA-seq data, which includes the genes that are reported to induce Th2 responses upon activation by DCs. Major DC response genes found to be predominantly regulated after Zeb1 KD are highlighted in bold. To generate this bar-graph Z-score was calculated for each gene from normalized FPKM values to demonstrate the differential regulation of genes in control and Zeb1 KD DCs at 0, 6, and 12 h after CpG activation. **(D)** Bar-plot depicting the number of genes differentially regulated in Zeb1 KD DCs at 0, 6, and 12 h CpG activation as compared to control DCs. Different color codes indicate the genes that are unique or similar in the list of differentially regulated genes at different time points (0, 6, and 12 h). **(E)** Bar-plot depicting the biological pathways that were significantly enriched for the genes that differentially regulated after Zeb1 KD in 6 and 12 h CpG activation as compared to control cells. Ingenuity Pathway Analysis (IPA) was used to perform pathway enrichment analysis.

DCs are either immune-suppressive leading to development of anergic T cells or immune-modulatory resulting into Th2 phenotype, which depends on the extent of DC activation (21, 75, 76). We observed a significantly decreased activation of DCs in Zeb1 KD DCs both before and after CpG activation. This resulted into decreased cytokine levels in our Zeb1 depleted DCs at both transcript and protein levels. Moreover we cannot exclude the weak TCR strength in this context with low CD80, CD86 and MHCII for triggering a Th2 phenotype.

We know that DCs educate naïve Th cells to differentiate into different subtypes (Th1, Th2, Th17 or Tregs) which depends on the state of DC activation and the extracellular milieu containing a cytokine cocktail majorly of IL-4, IL-10, IL-12p70, IL-6, TGFβ along with others (21, 77). The cDC1 DCs are reported to induce strong Th1 effector response as compared to their counterpart cDC2 DCs which have the inherent property of inducing Th2 responses (78). We observed constitutive expression of Zeb1 in DCs, which could be important to maintain the cDC1-mediated induction of Th1 cell differentiation. Th1 subtype is generated if there is higher concentration of inflammatory cytokine IL-12 in the milieu whereas increased IL-10 or TGFβ with IL-6 leads to Tregs or Th17 phenotype respectively (22, 28). Moreover, IL-12p40 is also reported to form dimer in the absence of IL-12p35 subunit, which is a potent inhibitor of IL-12p70 activity (79). In contrast the cytokine IL-4 is considered pertinent for Th2 subtype development but it is not secreted by DCs in general, therefore the mode of Th2 generation is considered as a default subtype in the absence or decreased secretion of IL-12 along with absence of other T cell differentiation modulators (21–23, 28, 30, 31, 77). In addition to cytokine milieu, the cell surface receptors like CLRs such as CLEC7a, CLEC4a, DC-SIGN are also reported to skew speciation of Th subtypes in a pathogen/antigen dependent manner (24, 80, 81). These reports supported the development of the Th2 phenotype by our Zeb1 KD cDC1 MutuDCs as we observed a significant decrease in Th1 and Th17 polarizing CLRs along with inflammatory cytokine IL-12p70 in Zeb1 KD DCs. It has also been reported that DC-SIGN interacts with ICAM-1 on T cells and enhances the activation and proliferation of T cells (82). In addition, the cytokine IL-27 that is reported to suppress Th2 differentiation was significantly decreased in our Zeb1 KD DCs (83). This further adds up as a plausible mechanism of Th2 polarization after Zeb1 depletion.

It has been extensively reported that Th subtype balance i.e., Th1 and Th2 controls the helminth *H. polygyrus* infection in animals. In Balb/C mice that are Th2 prone, the worms are cleared from intestine much faster i.e., 8 weeks as compared to in C57BL/6 animals where the inherent Th1 behavior sustains the worm infection levels for more than 15–20 weeks (66, 68). Therefore we performed adoptive transfer of activated Zeb1 KD cDC1 MutuDCs in C57BL/6 mice to identify if at physiological level Zeb1 KD DCs could skew the Th subtype toward Th2 and thereby leading to increased worm clearance from intestine. We found that treatment of the helminth infected mice with CpG pulsed Zeb1 KD cDC1 MutuDCs cleared the intestinal worms by D31. Even at D10 the egg counts were lower in Zeb1 KD DC treated mice, though we infected all the animals with equal number of larva at D0. We speculate that it was due to adoptive transfer of CpG pulsed Zeb1 KD DCs that secrete suboptimal inflammatory cytokines, at D7 after infection. Furthermore, we also observed that wild type $CD8\alpha^+$ cDC1 treated animals showed 4- to 5-fold higher egg counts as compared to PBS treated animals due to their inherent property of inducing Th1 responses *in vivo*. Collectively, this depicted that ZEB1 expression in DCs is pertinent for initial activation of DCs leading to outburst of cytokines important for development of optimal inflammatory Th1 subtypes.

At the mechanistic level it has been demonstrated that Zeb1 acts as a global transcriptional repressor in pre-adipocytes, $CD8^+$ T cells and mesenchymal to epithelial transition (MET) process (84). In contrast to its role as transcriptional repressor there are studies indicating Zeb1 as a co-activator, for example, in complex with Yap1 it activates metastatic inducer genes (85). In addition, Gene Set Enrichment Analysis (GSEA) of Zeb1 depleted breast cancer cells showed its activating role in the expression of inflammatory response genes IL-6, IL-8, and IL-1α (37). Though our transcriptome analysis showed Zeb1 as a global repressor with higher number of upregulated genes at all the time points, we observed down-regulation of most of the immunogenic genes including CLRs, IL-6, IL-10, IL-12, and IL-27 in Zeb1 KD DCs as compared to control cells. We also showed here by integrating ChIP-seq and RNA-seq data that Zeb1 does not act as transcriptional repressor for immune response gene cluster as for other pathway genes group. It further substantiates and suggests that Zeb1 forms some differential complex to control the immune response genes or Zeb1 mostly regulates them indirectly at transcript level. Even in the cases of EMT and immune evasion it has been widely reported that EMT process coincides well with the increased inflammatory environment (86–88). It might be possible that Zeb1 upregulation during EMT also results in increased inflammation in the tumor microenvironment.

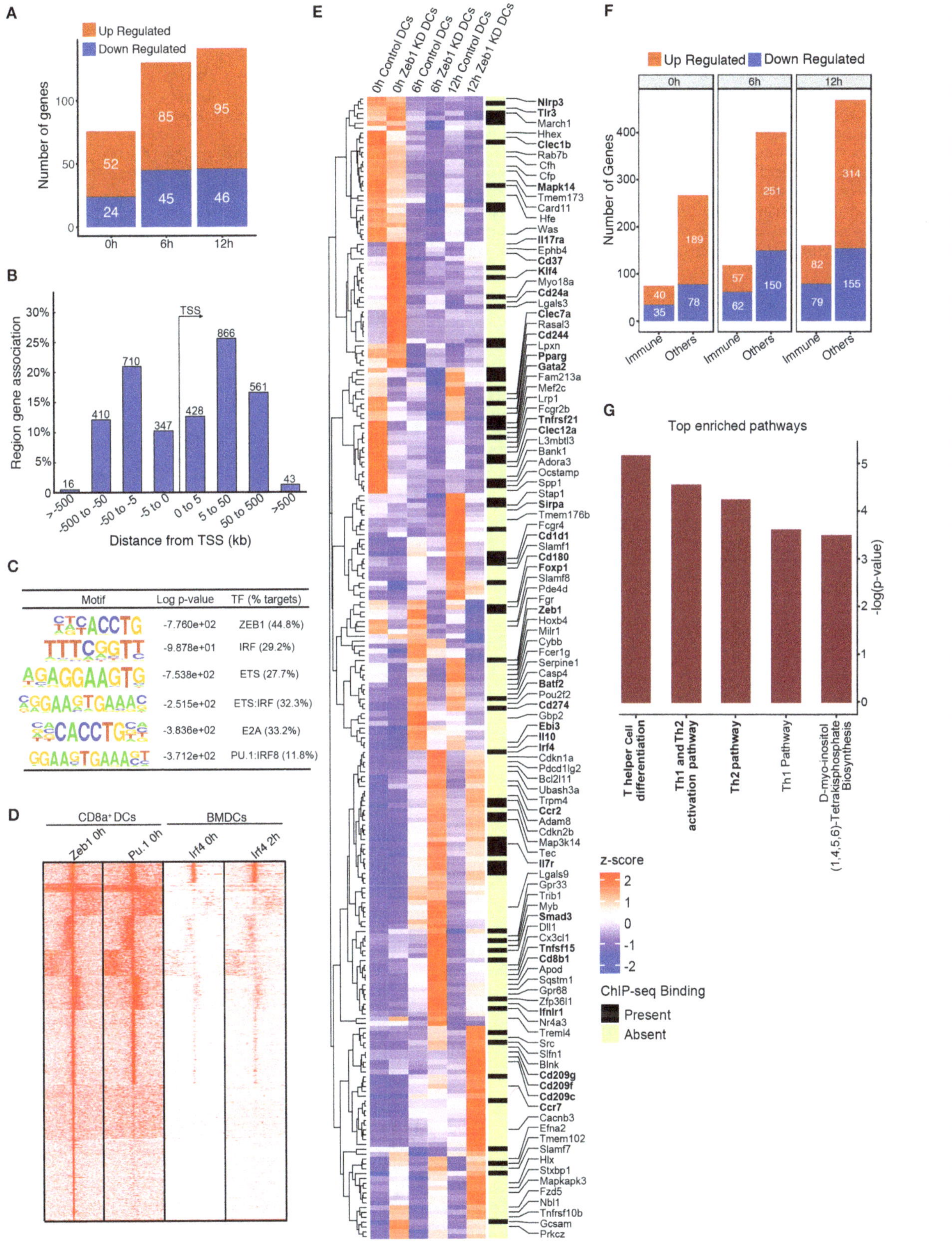

FIGURE 7 | Integrative genomic analysis using ChIP-seq and RNA-seq identified that Zeb1 does not act as global repressor of immune response genes. **(A)** Bar-plot depicting the genes that were directly regulated (upregulated and down-regulated) by Zeb1 KD at 0, 6, and 12 h after CpG activation in cDC1 DCs. The direct target genes of Zeb1 were identified by correlating the gene list from Zeb1 KD RNA-seq and Zeb1 ChIP-seq binding analysis. **(B)** Genomic Regions Enrichment of

(Continued)

FIGURE 7 | Zeb1 ChIP-seq bound peaks by annotations tool GREAT showing the genomic locations of Zeb1 bound regulatory regions with respect to gene transcription start sites (TSS). **(C)** List of top *de-novo* motifs significantly enriched at the Zeb1 bound peaks in unstimulated DCs and their annotated TFs. Zeb1 motif was found to be the top highly enriched motif. **(D)** SeqMINER clustering demonstrating the overlap of Zeb1 bound peaks in unstimulated CD8α^+ cDC1 with PU.1 bound genomic regions in similar condition. The peaks were also overlapped with IRF4 ChIP-seq publicly available data of control and LPS stimulated primary BMDCs. **(E)** Heat-map demonstrating the immune response pathway genes that were differentially regulated after Zeb1 KD 0, 6, and 12 h after CpG activation as compared to control cells. The ChIP-seq binding was also overlapped to identify if Zeb1 directly regulates immune response genes. All the immune response genes that were differentially regulated (>2-fold up or down-regulated) are listed. The genes that were reported and are important in Th cell polarization through DCs are highlighted in bold. To generate this bar-graph Z-score was calculated for each gene from normalized FPKM values to demonstrate the differential regulation of genes in control and Zeb1 KD DCs at 0, 6, and 12 h after CpG activation. **(F)** Bar-plot depicting the differential regulated genes in Zeb1 KD DCs at 0, 6, and 12 h after CpG activation. The genes were classification into two different groups based on GO annotation i.e., immune response genes (immune) and other pathway genes (others). It was observed that in immune response gene group there is preferential upregulation of genes after Zeb1 KD whereas in the other group there was higher number of upregulated genes (>1.6- to 2.5-fold) compared to down-regulated ones. **(G)** Bar-plot showing the IPA pathways significantly enriched for the genes that were directly bound and regulated by Zeb1 at 12 h after CpG activation.

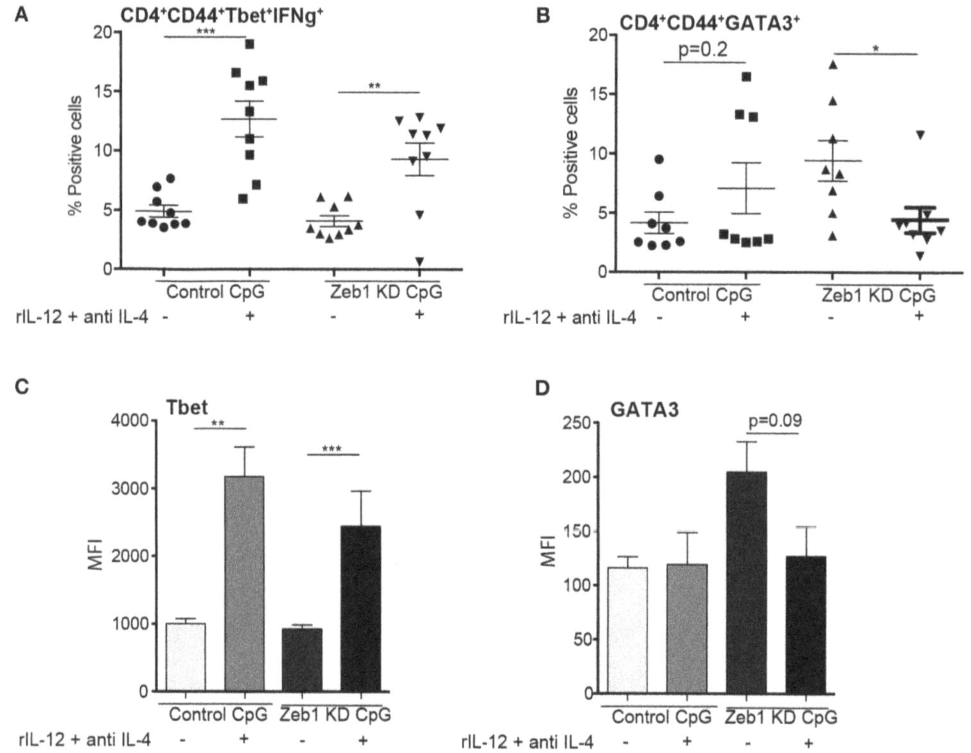

FIGURE 8 | Decreased IL-12 secreted by Zeb1 KD cDC1 DCs is responsible for inducing Th2 differentiation $n = 8$–10. **(A)** Scatter-plot depicting an increase in percentage positive cells for Th1 markers Tbet$^+$ IFNγ^+ in Zeb1 KD DCs upon supplementation of recombinant IL-12 and anti-IL4 cytokine in the culture media during DC -T cell co-culture $n = 8$–10. **(B)** Scatter-plot depicting a significant decrease in percentage positive cells for Th2 marker GATA3$^+$ in Zeb1 KD DCs upon addition of recombinant IL-12 cytokine and anti-IL4 in the culture media during DC-T cell co-culture $n = 8$–10. **(C)** Bar-plot representing the MFI for Th1 marker Tbet$^+$ in Zeb1 KD DCs upon supplementation of rIL12 and anti-IL4 cytokine in the culture media during DC -T cell co-culture $n = 8$–10. **(D)** Bar-plot representing the MFI for Th2 marker GATA3$^+$ in Zeb1 KD DCs upon supplementation of rIL12 and anti-IL4 cytokine in the culture media during DC -T cell co-culture $n = 8$–10. *p*-values are calculated using two tailed unpaired student's *t*-test, error bars represent SEM. *≤0.05, **≤0.01, ***≤0.001).

We would like to conclude with a message that expression of TF Zeb1 is pertinent for CD8α^+ cDC1 activation leading to immunogenic response generation. It regulates activation and thereby secretion of cytokines by CD8α^+ cDC1 DCs that are pertinent to induce pathogen/signal specific T cell responses.

AUTHOR CONTRIBUTIONS

SS, AA, BG, HA-O and SR designed the study. SS, AA, VB, MK performed the experiments SS, AA, BG, HA-O and SR did interpretation of the results. AG, SR performed the computational/bio-informatics analysis. SS, HA-O and SR wrote the manuscript. SS, AA, AG, BG, MK, HA-O and SR edited the manuscript.

ACKNOWLEDGMENTS

We thank Nicola Harris lab at EPFL, Lausanne for providing the helminth larvae. Christine Lavenchy and Vanessa Mack for excellent technical help. Thanks to Ton Rolink for providing the FLT3L transgenic mice. Atimukta Jha for editing the manuscript. SS and AG is supported by ILS fellowship. AA is supported by DBT-SRF. VB is supported by SERB grant.

REFERENCES

1. Steinman RM. The control of immunity and tolerance by dendritic cell. *Pathol Biol.* (2003) 51:59–60. doi: 10.1016/S0369-8114(03)00096-8
2. Steinman RM. Linking innate to adaptive immunity through dendritic cells. *Novartis Found Symp.* (2006) 279:101–9. doi: 10.1002/9780470035399.ch9
3. Steinman RM, Hemmi H. Dendritic cells: translating innate to adaptive immunity. *Curr Top Microbiol Immunol.* (2006) 311:17–58. doi: 10.1007/3-540-32636-7_2
4. Banchereau J, Steinman RM. Dendritic cells and the control of immunity. *Nature* (1998) 392:245–52. doi: 10.1038/32588
5. Steinman RM. Lasker basic medical research award. dendritic cells: versatile controllers of the immune system. *Nat Med.* (2007) 13:1155–9. doi: 10.1038/nm1643
6. Schlitzer A, Sivakamasundari V, Chen J, Sumatoh HR, Schreuder J, Lum J, et al. Identification of cDC1- and cDC2-committed DC progenitors reveals early lineage priming at the common DC progenitor stage in the bone marrow. *Nat Immunol.* (2015) 16:718–28. doi: 10.1038/ni.3200
7. Guilliams M, Ginhoux F, Jakubzick C, Naik SH, Onai N, Schraml BU, et al. Dendritic cells, monocytes and macrophages: a unified nomenclature based on ontogeny. *Nat Rev Immunol.* (2014) 14:571–8. doi: 10.1038/nri3712
8. Collin M, Bigley V. Human dendritic cell subsets: an update. *Immunology* (2018) 154:3–20. doi: 10.1111/imm.12888
9. Fuertes Marraco SA, Grosjean F, Duval A, Rosa M, Lavanchy C, Ashok D, et al. Novel murine dendritic cell lines: a powerful auxiliary tool for dendritic cell research. *Front Immunol.* (2012) 3:331. doi: 10.3389/fimmu.2012.00331
10. Reis e Sousa, C. Activation of dendritic cells: translating innate into adaptive immunity. *Curr Opin Immunol.* (2004) 16:21–5. doi: 10.1016/j.coi.2003.11.007
11. Takeuchi O, Akira S. Pattern recognition receptors and inflammation. *Cell* (2010) 140:805–20. doi: 10.1016/j.cell.2010.01.022
12. Reizis B. Intracellular pathogens and CD8(+) dendritic cells: dangerous liaisons. *Immunity* (2011) 35:153–5. doi: 10.1016/j.immuni.2011.08.003
13. Leon B, Ardavin C. Monocyte-derived dendritic cells in innate and adaptive immunity. *Immunol Cell Biol.* (2008) 86:320–4. doi: 10.1038/icb.2008.14
14. Belz GT. Getting together: dendritic cells, T cells, collaboration and fates. *Immunol Cell Biol.* (2008) 86:310–1. doi: 10.1038/icb.2008.18
15. Romagnani S. Th1/Th2 cells. *Inflamm Bowel Dis.* (1999)5:285–94.
16. Akbulut HH, Kilic SS, Bulut V, Ozden M. Determination of intracellular cytokines produced by Th1 and Th2 cells using flow cytometry in patients with brucellosis. *FEMS Immunol Med Microbiol.* (2005) 45:253–8. doi: 10.1016/j.femsim.2005.04.001
17. Yang F, Wang D, Li Y, Sang L, Zhu J, Wang J, et al. Th1/Th2 Balance and Th17/Treg-mediated immunity in relation to murine resistance to dextran sulfate-induced colitis. *J Immunol Res.* (2017) 2017:7047201. doi: 10.1155/2017/7047201
18. Kapsenberg ML. Dendritic-cell control of pathogen-driven T-cell polarization. *Nat Rev Immunol.* (2003) 3:984–93. doi: 10.1038/nri1246
19. Hochweller K, Wabnitz GH, Samstag Y, Suffner J, Hammerling GJ, Garbi N. Dendritic cells control T cell tonic signaling required for responsiveness to foreign antigen. *Proc Natl Acad Sci USA.* (2010) 107:5931–6. doi: 10.1073/pnas.0911877107
20. Satpathy AT, Murphy KM, Kc W. Transcription factor networks in dendritic cell development. *Semin Immunol.* (2011) 23:388–97. doi: 10.1016/j.smim.2011.08.009
21. Kaiko GE, Horvat JC, Beagley KW, Hansbro PM. Immunological decision-making: how does the immune system decide to mount a helper T-cell response? *Immunology* (2008) 123:326–38. doi: 10.1111/j.1365-2567.2007.02719.x
22. MacDonald AS, Maizels RM. Alarming dendritic cells for Th2 induction. *J Exp Med.* (2008) 205:13–7. doi: 10.1084/jem.20072665
23. MacDonald AS, Straw AD, Dalton NM, Pearce EJ. Cutting edge: Th2 response induction by dendritic cells: a role for CD40. *J Immunol.* (2002) 168:537–40. doi: 10.4049/jimmunol.168.2.537
24. Geijtenbeek TB. Gringhuis SI. C-type lectin receptors in the control of T helper cell differentiation. *Nat Rev Immunol.* (2016) 16:433–48. doi: 10.1038/nri.2016.55
25. Besnard AG, Togbe D, Guillou N, Erard F, Quesniaux V, Ryffel B. IL-33-activated dendritic cells are critical for allergic airway inflammation. *Eur J Immunol.* (2011) 41:1675–86. doi: 10.1002/eji.201041033
26. Ito T, Wang YH, Duramad O, Hori T, Delespesse GJ, Watanabe N, et al. TSLP-activated dendritic cells induce an inflammatory T helper type 2 cell response through OX40 ligand. *J Exp Med.* (2005) 202:1213–23. doi: 10.1084/jem.20051135
27. Skokos D, Nussenzweig MC. CD8- DCs induce IL-12-independent Th1 differentiation through Delta 4 Notch-like ligand in response to bacterial LPS. *J Exp Med.* (2007) 204:1525–31. doi: 10.1084/jem.20062305
28. Pulendran B, Tang H, Manicassamy S. Programming dendritic cells to induce T(H)2 and tolerogenic responses. *Nat Immunol.* (2010) 11:647–55. doi: 10.1038/ni.1894
29. Na H, Cho M, Chung Y. Regulation of Th2 cell immunity by dendritic cells. *Immune Netw.* (2016) 16:1–12. doi: 10.4110/in.2016.16.1.1
30. Zhu J, Yamane H, Paul WE. Differentiation of effector CD4 T cell populations (*). *Annu Rev Immunol.* (2010) 28:445–89. doi: 10.1146/annurev-immunol-030409-101212
31. Walker JA, McKenzie ANJ. TH2 cell development and function. *Nat Rev Immunol.* (2018) 18:121–33. doi: 10.1038/nri.2017.118
32. Williams JW, Tjota MY, Clay BS, Vander Lugt B, Bandukwala HS, Hrusch CL, et al. Transcription factor IRF4 drives dendritic cells to promote Th2 differentiation. *Nat Commun.* (2013) 4:2990. doi: 10.1038/ncomms 3990
33. Xiong Y, Lingrel JB, Wuthrich M, Klein BS, Vasudevan NT, Jain MK, et al. Transcription factor KLF2 in dendritic cells downregulates Th2 programming via the HIF-1alpha/Jagged2/Notch Axis. *MBio* (2016) 7:e00436-16. doi: 10.1128/mBio.00436-16
34. Gregory PA, Bert AG, Paterson EL, Barry SC, Tsykin A, Farshid G, et al. The miR-200 family and miR-205 regulate epithelial to mesenchymal transition by targeting ZEB1 and SIP1. *Nat Cell Biol.* (2008) 10:593–601. doi: 10.1038/ncb1722
35. Shirakihara T, Saitoh M, Miyazono K. Differential regulation of epithelial and mesenchymal markers by deltaEF1 proteins in epithelial mesenchymal transition induced by TGF-beta. *Mol Biol Cell* (2007) 18:3533–44. doi: 10.1091/mbc.e07-03-0249
36. Cohen EN, Gao H, Anfossi S, Mego M, Reddy NG, Debeb B, et al. Inflammation mediated metastasis: immune induced epithelial-to-mesenchymal transition in inflammatory breast cancer cells. *PLoS ONE* (2015) 10:e0132710. doi: 10.1371/journal.pone.0132710
37. Katsura A, Tamura Y, Hokari S, Harada M, Morikawa M, Sakurai T, et al. ZEB1-regulated inflammatory phenotype in breast cancer cells. *Mol Oncol* (2017) 11:1241–62. doi: 10.1002/1878-0261.12098
38. Dominguez C, David JM, Palena C. Epithelial-mesenchymal transition and inflammation at the site of the primary tumor. *Semin Cancer Biol.* (2017) 47:177–84. doi: 10.1016/j.semcancer.2017.08.002
39. Leibovich-Rivkin T, Liubomirski Y, Bernstein B, Meshel T, Ben-Baruch A. Inflammatory factors of the tumor microenvironment induce plasticity in nontransformed breast epithelial cells: EMT, invasion, and collapse of normally organized breast textures. *Neoplasia* (2013) 15:1330–46. doi: 10.1593/neo.131688

40. Ricciardi M, Zanotto M, Malpeli G, Bassi G, Perbellini O, Chilosi M, et al. Epithelial-to-mesenchymal transition (EMT) induced by inflammatory priming elicits mesenchymal stromal cell-like immune-modulatory properties in cancer cells. *Br J Cancer* (2015) 112:1067–75. doi: 10.1038/bjc.2015.29
41. Suarez-Carmona M, Lesage J, Cataldo D, Gilles C. EMT and inflammation: inseparable actors of cancer progression. *Mol Oncol.* (2017) 11:805–23. doi: 10.1002/1878-0261.12095
42. Wang J, Lee S, Teh CE, Bunting K, Ma L, Shannon MF. The transcription repressor, ZEB1, cooperates with CtBP2 and HDAC1 to suppress IL-2 gene activation in T cells. *Int Immunol.* (2009) 21:227–35. doi: 10.1093/intimm/dxn143
43. Konradi S, Yasmin N, Haslwanter D, Weber M, Gesslbauer B, Sixt M, et al. Langerhans cell maturation is accompanied by induction of N-cadherin and the transcriptional regulators of epithelial-mesenchymal transition ZEB1/2. *Eur J Immunol.* (2014) 44:553–60. doi: 10.1002/eji.201343681
44. Arnold CN, Pirie E, Dosenovic P, McInerney GM, Xia Y, Wang N, et al. A forward genetic screen reveals roles for Nfkbid, Zeb1, and Ruvbl2 in humoral immunity. *Proc Natl Acad Sci USA.* (2012) 109:12286–93. doi: 10.1073/pnas.1209134109
45. Salmon P, Trono D. Production and titration of lentiviral vectors. *Curr Protoc Hum Genet.* (2007) Chapter 12:Unit 12 10. doi: 10.1002/0471142905.hg1210s54.
46. Pedersen CD, Fang JJ, Pedersen AE. A comparative study of transfection methods for RNA interference in bone marrow-derived murine dendritic cells. *Scand J Immunol.* (2009) 70:447–56. doi: 10.1111/j.1365-3083.2009.02320.x
47. Naik SH, Proietto AI, Wilson NS, Dakic A, Schnorrer P, Fuchsberger M, et al. Cutting edge: generation of splenic CD8+ and CD8- dendritic cell equivalents in Fms-like tyrosine kinase 3 ligand bone marrow cultures. *J Immunol.* (2005) 174:6592–7. doi: 10.4049/jimmunol.174.11.6592
48. Hopken UE, Lehmann I, Droese J, Lipp M, Schuler T, Rehm A. The ratio between dendritic cells and T cells determines the outcome of their encounter: proliferation versus deletion. *Eur J Immunol.* (2005) 35:2851–63. doi: 10.1002/eji.200526298
49. Yu Q, Kovacs C, Yue FY, Ostrowski MA. The role of the p38 mitogen-activated protein kinase, extracellular signal-regulated kinase, and phosphoinositide-3-OH kinase signal transduction pathways in CD40 ligand-induced dendritic cell activation and expansion of virus-specific CD8+ T cell memory responses. *J Immunol.* (2004) 172: 6047–56. doi: 10.4049/jimmunol.172.10.6047
50. Raghav SK, Waszak SM, Krier I, Gubelmann C, Isakova A, Mikkelsen TS, et al. Integrative genomics identifies the corepressor SMRT as a gatekeeper of adipogenesis through the transcription factors C/EBPbeta and KAISO. *Mol Cell* (2012) 46:335–50. doi: 10.1016/j.molcel.2012.03.017
51. Kilpinen H, Waszak SM, Gschwind AR, Raghav SK, Witwicki RM, Orioli A, et al. Coordinated effects of sequence variation on DNA binding, chromatin structure, and transcription. *Science* (2013) 342:744–7. doi: 10.1126/science.1242463
52. Massacand JC, Stettler RC, Meier R, Humphreys NE, Grencis RK, Marsland BJ, et al. Helminth products bypass the need for TSLP in Th2 immune responses by directly modulating dendritic cell function. *Proc Natl Acad Sci USA.* (2009) 106:13968–73. doi: 10.1073/pnas.0906367106
53. Bolger AM, Lohse M, Usadel B. Trimmomatic: a flexible trimmer for Illumina sequence data. *Bioinformatics* (2014) 30:2114–20. doi: 10.1093/bioinformatics/btu170
54. Garber M, Yosef N, Goren A, Raychowdhury R, Thielke A, Guttman M, et al. A high-throughput chromatin immunoprecipitation approach reveals principles of dynamic gene regulation in mammals. *Mol Cell.* (2012) 47:810–22. doi: 10.1016/j.molcel.2012.07.030
55. Kim D, Pertea G, Trapnell C, Pimentel H, Kelley R, Salzberg SL. TopHat2: accurate alignment of transcriptomes in the presence of insertions, deletions and gene fusions. *Genome Biol.* (2013) 14:R36. doi: 10.1186/gb-2013-14-4-r36
56. Langmead B, Salzberg SL. Fast gapped-read alignment with Bowtie 2. *Nat Methods* (2012) 9:357–9. doi: 10.1038/nmeth.1923
57. Li H, Handsaker B, Wysoker A, Fennell T, Ruan J, Homer N, et al. The sequence alignment/map format and SAMtools. *Bioinformatics* (2009) 25:2078–9. doi: 10.1093/bioinformatics/btp352
58. Heinz S, Benner C, Spann N, Bertolino E, Lin YC, Laslo P, et al. Simple combinations of lineage-determining transcription factors prime cis-regulatory elements required for macrophage and B cell identities. *Mol Cell* (2010) 38:576–89. doi: 10.1016/j.molcel.2010.05.004
59. Ye T, Krebs AR, Choukrallah MA, Keime C, Plewniak F, Davidson I, et al. seqMINER: an integrated ChIP-seq data interpretation platform. *Nucleic Acids Res.* (2011) 39:e35. doi: 10.1093/nar/gkq1287
60. Gu Z, Eils R, Schlesner M. Complex heatmaps reveal patterns and correlations in multidimensional genomic data. *Bioinformatics* (2016) 32:2847–9. doi: 10.1093/bioinformatics/btw313
61. Ruckwardt TJ, Morabito KM, Bar-Haim E, Nair D, Graham BS. Neonatal mice possess two phenotypically and functionally distinct lung-migratory CD103(+) dendritic cell populations following respiratory infection. *Mucosal Immunol.* (2018)11:186–98. doi: 10.1038/mi.2017.28
62. Pennock ND, White JT, Cross EW, Cheney EE, Tamburini BA, Kedl RM. T cell responses: naive to memory and everything in between. *Adv Physiol Educ.* (2013) 37:273–83. doi: 10.1152/advan.00066.2013
63. Mogensen TH. Pathogen recognition and inflammatory signaling in innate immune defenses. *Clin Microbiol Rev.* (2009) 22:240–73. doi: 10.1128/CMR.00046-08
64. Everts B, Smits HH, Hokke CH, Yazdanbakhsh M. Helminths and dendritic cells: sensing and regulating via pattern recognition receptors, Th2 and Treg responses. *Eur J Immunol.* (2010) 40:1525–37. doi: 10.1002/eji.200940109
65. Hussaarts L, Yazdanbakhsh M, Guigas B. Priming dendritic cells for th2 polarization: lessons learned from helminths and implications for metabolic disorders. *Front Immunol.* (2014) 5:499. doi: 10.3389/fimmu.2014.00499
66. Mendez-Samperio P. Molecular events by which dendritic cells promote Th2 immune protection in helmith infection. *Infect Dis.* (2016) 48:715–20. doi: 10.1080/23744235.2016.1194529
67. Taylor MD, van der Werf N, Maizels RM. T cells in helminth infection: the regulators and the regulated. *Trends Immunol.* (2012) 33:181–9. doi: 10.1016/j.it.2012.01.001
68. Filbey KJ, Grainger JR, Smith KA, Boon L, van Rooijen N, Harcus Y, et al. Innate and adaptive type 2 immune cell responses in genetically controlled resistance to intestinal helminth infection. *Immunol Cell Biol.* (2014) 92:436–48. doi: 10.1038/icb.2013.109
69. Kim B, Kim TH. Fundamental role of dendritic cells in inducing Th2 responses. *Korean J Intern Med.* (2018) 33:483–9. doi: 10.3904/kjim.2016.227
70. Ganguly D, Haak S, Sisirak V, Reizis B. The role of dendritic cells in autoimmunity. *Nat Rev Immunol.* (2013) 13:566–77. doi: 10.1038/nri3477
71. Schnorrer P, Behrens GM, Wilson NS, Pooley JL, Smith CM, El-Sukkari D, et al. The dominant role of CD8+ dendritic cells in cross-presentation is not dictated by antigen capture. *Proc Natl Acad Sci USA.* (2006) 103:10729–34. doi: 10.1073/pnas.0601956103
72. Lamouille S, Xu J, Derynck R. Molecular mechanisms of epithelial-mesenchymal transition. *Nat Rev Mol Cell Biol.* (2014) 15:178–96. doi: 10.1038/nrm3758
73. Liu Y, El-Naggar S, Darling DS, Higashi Y, Dean DC. Zeb1 links epithelial-mesenchymal transition and cellular senescence. *Development* (2008) 135:579–88. doi: 10.1242/dev.007047
74. Serrano-Gomez SJ, Maziveyi M, Alahari SK. Regulation of epithelial-mesenchymal transition through epigenetic and post-translational modifications. *Mol Cancer* (2016) 15:18. doi: 10.1186/s12943-016-0502-x
75. Sallusto F, Lanzavecchia A. The instructive role of dendritic cells on T-cell responses. *Arthritis Res.* (2002) (4 Suppl 3):S127–32. doi: 10.1186/ar567
76. Schmidt SV, Nino-Castro AC, Schultze JL. Regulatory dendritic cells: there is more than just immune activation. *Front Immunol.* (2012) 3:274. doi: 10.3389/fimmu.2012.00274

77. Xie ZX, Zhang HL, Wu XJ, Zhu J, Ma DH, Jin T. Role of the immunogenic and tolerogenic subsets of dendritic cells in multiple sclerosis. *Mediators Inflamm.* (2015) 2015:513295. doi: 10.1155/2015/513295
78. Price JD, Tarbell KV. The role of dendritic cell subsets and innate immunity in the pathogenesis of type 1 diabetes and other autoimmune diseases. *Front Immunol.* (2015) 6:288. doi: 10.3389/fimmu.2015.00288
79. Mattner F, Ozmen L, Podlaski FJ, Wilkinson VL, Presky DH, Gately MK, et al. Treatment with homodimeric interleukin-12 (IL-12) p40 protects mice from IL-12-dependent shock but not from tumor necrosis factor alpha-dependent shock. *Infect Immun.* (1997) 65:4734–7.
80. Gringhuis SI, den Dunnen J, Litjens M, van der Vlist, M, Geijtenbeek TB. Carbohydrate-specific signaling through the DC-SIGN signalosome tailors immunity to *Mycobacterium tuberculosis*, HIV-1 and Helicobacter pylori. *Nat Immunol.* (2009) 10:1081–8. doi: 10.1038/ni.1778
81. van Vliet SJ, Garcia-Vallejo JJ, van Kooyk Y. Dendritic cells and C-type lectin receptors: coupling innate to adaptive immune responses. *Immunol Cell Biol.* (2008) 86:580–7. doi: 10.1038/icb.2008.55
82. Geijtenbeek TB, Kwon DS, Torensma R, van Vliet SJ, van Duijnhoven GC, Middel J, et al. DC-SIGN, a dendritic cell-specific HIV-1-binding protein that enhances trans-infection of T cells. *Cell* (2000) 100:587–97. doi: 10.1016/S0092-8674(00)80694-7
83. McHedlidze T, Kindermann M, Neves AT, Voehringer D, Neurath MF, Wirtz S. IL-27 suppresses type 2 immune responses *in vivo* via direct effects on group 2 innate lymphoid cells. *Mucosal Immunol.* (2016) 9:1384–94. doi: 10.1038/mi.2016.20
84. Gubelmann C, Schwalie PC, Raghav SK, Roder E, Delessa T, Kiehlmann E, et al. Identification of the transcription factor ZEB1 as a central component of the adipogenic gene regulatory network. *Elife* (2014) 3:e03346. doi: 10.7554/eLife.03346
85. Lehmann W, Mossmann D, Kleemann J, Mock K, Meisinger C, Brummer T, et al. ZEB1 turns into a transcriptional activator by interacting with YAP1 in aggressive cancer types. *Nat Commun.* (2016) 7:10498. doi: 10.1038/ncomms10498
86. Brekken RA, Wnuk-Lipinska K. Drivers of EMT and Immune Evasion. In: Akslen LA, and Watnick RS, editors. *Biomarkers of the Tumor Microenvironment: Basic Studies and Practical Applications.* Cham: Springer International Publishing (2017). p. 221–39.
87. Chen HH, Su WC, Lin PW, Guo HR, Lee WY. Hypoxia-inducible factor-1alpha correlates with MET and metastasis in node-negative breast cancer. *Breast Cancer Res Treat* (2007) 103:167–75. doi: 10.1007/s10549-006-9360-3
88. Datar I, Schalper KA. Epithelial-mesenchymal transition and immune evasion during lung cancer progression: the chicken or the egg? *Clin Cancer Res.* (2016) 22:3422–4. doi: 10.1158/1078-0432.CCR-16-0336

6

NH36 and F3 Antigen-Primed Dendritic Cells Show Preserved Migrating Capabilities and CCR7 Expression and F3 is Effective in Immunotherapy of Visceral Leishmaniasis

Dirlei Nico[1], Fernanda Martins Almeida[2,3], Juliana Maria Motta[4], Fellipe Soares dos Santos Cardoso[2], Celio Geraldo Freire-de-Lima[5], Leonardo Freire-de-Lima[6], Paula Melo de Luca[7], Ana Maria Blanco Martinez[2], Alexandre Morrot[7,8] and Clarisa Beatriz Palatnik-de-Sousa [1,9]*

[1] Departamento de Microbiologia Geral, Instituto de Microbiologia Paulo de Góes, Universidade Federal do Rio de Janeiro, Rio de Janeiro, Brazil, [2] Programa de Pós Graduação em Anatomia Patológica, HUCFF, Universidade Federal do Rio de Janeiro, Rio de Janeiro, Brazil, [3] Programa de Graduação de Histologia, Instituto de Ciências Biomédicas, Universidade Federal do Rio de Janeiro, Rio de Janeiro, Brazil, [4] Programa de Glicobiologia, Instituto de Bioquímica Médica Leopoldo De Meis, Universidade Federal do Rio de Janeiro, Rio de Janeiro, Brazil, [5] Programa de Imunobiologia, Instituto de Biofísica Carlos Chagas Filho, Universidade Federal do Rio de Janeiro, Rio de Janeiro, Brazil, [6] Programa de Medicina Regenerativa, Instituto de Biofísica Carlos Chagas Filho, Universidade Federal do Rio de Janeiro, Rio de Janeiro, Brazil, [7] Laboratório de Imunoparasitologia, Instituto Oswaldo Cruz (IOC), Rio de Janeiro, Brazil, [8] Centro de Pesquisas em Tuberculose, Faculdade de Medicina, Universidade Federal do Rio de Janeiro, Rio de Janeiro, Brazil, [9] Instituto Nacional de Ciência e Tecnologia de Investigação em Imunologia, São Paulo, Brazil

***Correspondence:**
Clarisa Beatriz Palatnik-de-Sousa
immgcpa@micro.ufrj.br

Physical contact between dendritic cells (DCs) and T cell lymphocytes is necessary to trigger the immune cell response. CCL19 and CCL21 chemokines bind to the CCR7 receptor of mature DCs, and of T cells and regulate DCs migration to the white pulp (wp) of the spleen, where they encounter lymphocytes. In visceral leishmaniasis (VL), cellular immunosuppression is mediated by impaired DC migration due to the decreased chemokine secretion by endothelium and to the reduced DCs CCR7 expression. The *Leishmania (L.) donovani* nucleoside hydrolase NH36 and its C-terminal domain, the F3 peptide are prominent antigens in the generation of preventive immunity to VL. We assessed whether these vaccines could prevent the migrating defect of DCs by restoring the expression of CCR7 receptors. C57Bl6 mice were vaccinated with NH36 and F3 and challenged with *L. (L.) infantum chagasi*. The F3 vaccine induced a 100% of survival and a long-lasting immune protection with an earlier $CD4^+$Th1 response, with secretion of higher IFN-γ and TNF-α/IL-10 ratios, and higher frequencies of $CD4^+$ T cells secreting IL-2^+, TNF-α^+, or IFN-γ^+, or a combination of two or the three cytokines (IL-2^+TNF-α^+IFN-γ^+). The $CD8^+$ T cell response was promoted earlier by the NH36-vaccine, and later by the F3-vaccine. Maximal number of F3-primed DCs migrated *in vitro* in response to CCL19 and showed a high expression of CCR7 receptors (26.06%). Anti-CCR7 antibody treatment inhibited DCs migration *in vitro* (90%) and increased parasite load *in vivo*. When transferred into 28-day-infected mice, only 8% of DCs from infected, 59%

of DCs from NH36-vaccinated, and 84% of DCs from F3-vaccinated mice migrated to the wp. Consequently, immunotherapy of infected mice with F3-primed DCs only, promoted increases in corporal weight and reductions of spleen and liver parasite loads and relative weights. Our findings indicate that vaccination with F3-vaccine preserves the maturation, migration properties and CCR7 expression of DCs, which are essential processes for the generation of cell-mediated immunity. The F3 vaccine is more potent in reversing the migration defect that occurs in VL and, therefore, more efficient in immunotherapy of VL.

Keywords: visceral leishmaniasis, dendritic cells defective migration, CCR7 expression, nucleoside hydrolase, NH36, F3 domain, *Leishmania donovani*, *Leishmania infantum chagasi*

INTRODUCTION

Leishmaniasis is still considered one of the most neglected diseases in the world (1). Approximately, 350 million people are at risk, and about two million new cases are registered annually (2). More than 20 *Leishmania* species are involved in the transmission of Leishmaniasis. The parasites are transferred to humans by hematophagous phlebotomine sandflies (3). *Leishmania (L.) donovani*, *L. (L.) infantum*, and *Leishmania (L.) infantum chagasi* are the agents of visceral leishmaniasis (VL). While the disease is anthroponotic in India and East Africa, in the Americas, North Africa, Asia, and the Mediterranean, VL is a canid zoonosis (4). Clinical signs of human VL, include fever, malaise, anorexia, cachexia, hypergammaglobulinemia, hepato- and splenomegaly, anemia, and progressive suppression of the cellular immune response. Currently, the annual incidence reaches 400 thousands cases and 30 thousands deaths worldwide (5). Ninety percent of VL cases are registered in India, Ethiopia, South Sudan, Bangladesh, Sudan, and Brazil. Although the VL control programs in South-East Asia are reducing the human incidence of the disease, and the number of VL cases declined in Bangladesh, India, and Nepal (3), recurrent outbreaks of VL in and Sudan, Kenya, Ethiopia, and South Sudan are raising concern.

The development of the cellular immune response requires that T cell lymphocytes make contact with dendritic cells (DCs) in the spleen and lymph nodes (6, 7). When the spleen is chronically infected with *Leishmania* parasites, the structural design of the B cell follicles and the marginal zone (MZ) are disrupted (8–10). This disorder determines an insufficient antigen presentation to T cells. In fact, splenic T cells and DCs move from the MZ to the periarteriolar lymphoid sheath (PALS), where there are increased concentrations of chemokines (11). CCL19 and CCL21 chemokines produced by endothelium venules (12) bind to CCR7 receptor. These chemokines are attractants to T cell naïve lymphocytes, mature DCs, and a subset of memory T cells (12, 13). Therefore, although the number of splenic DCs increases after *L. (L.) donovani* infection (11), they fail to migrate to PALS, due to the reduced chemokine secretion by PALS, and to the inhibition of CCR7 expression on DCs (11). This spatial separation of T lymphocytes and DCs impedes their physical contact and is one of the reasons of the suppression of cellular immune response in VL (11).

Confirming the results obtained by Ato et al. (11) who studied the *L. (L.) donovani* infections, we recently demonstrated that mice chronically infected with *L. (L.) infantum chagasi* also show an increased spleen relative weight, correlated to a DCs hyperplasia, and to an increased spleen parasite load (14). In contrast, mice vaccinated with the nucleoside hydrolase (NH36) recombinant antigen, or with its C-terminal moiety (F3) and saponin, showed a strong reduction in spleen parasite load and prevented the hyperplasia of spleen DCs and an increase in spleen relative weight (14).

NH36 is a promising vaccine antigen, which protects mice and dogs from VL infection (15–18). NH36 domains and epitopes are recognized by PBMC of subclinical and cured human patients from Brazil (19) and from Spain (20). F3 holds the most important NH36-epitopes for antibodies and MHC class II receptors of mice and induces a $CD4^+$ T-cell-mediated protection against VL, correlated with an enhanced TNF-α and strong decrease of IL-10 secretion (15, 21).

No human vaccine against VL has been licensed until now and chemotherapy shows toxicity and failure issues (22, 23). Leishmaniasis remains as one of the main parasitic diseases of major impact on humanity and the search for isolated, combined, or alternative therapies that are safe, effective, and easily administered for the treatment of VL remains a promising target study. In this investigation, we take a step further in the study of the efficacy of the NH36 and F3 vaccines against murine VL and demonstrate that, besides preventing the increase of the numbers of DCs, they also prevent the migration dysfunction of DCs by restoring their CCR7 receptor expression. Additionally, we show that immunotherapy of infected mice with DCs derived from animals vaccinated with the F3 domain is a potential tool to assist in the treatment of the VL.

MATERIALS AND METHODS

Ethical Statement and Biosafety Measures

Protocol design of the experiments was approved by the Comissão de Ética no Uso de Animais of the Universidade Federal do Rio de Janeiro (CEUA protocol IMPPG040-07/16), in agreement with Brazilian laws for animal safety and the guidelines of National Institute of Health (15). Animals were maintained at the Instituto de Microbiologia Paulo de Góes, which is part of Universidade Federal do Rio de Janeiro (UFRJ) facilities, given water and food *ad libitum*, with a 12 h light/dark cycles and controlled temperature (15). We aimed to reduce any animal suffering to a minimum.

In this investigation, we worked with genetically modified *Escherichia coli* BL21 and DH5 strains cloned with the pET28b plasmid expressing the NH36 and F3 recombinant proteins. These bacterial clones used in this investigation are considered OGM risk level 1 (CQB 0108/99 IMPG-UFRJ) because they are not associated with disease in adults. We also manipulated non-genetically modified *Leishmania* parasites for which the CTNBio biosafety level is 2. Following the Brazilian Ministry of Health Biosafety regulations for Biomedical and Microbiology laboratories we performed the following biosafety measures: use of apron, gloves, masks, and protective glasses, decontamination of infected biological material and animal cases before washing and limited access to, security block and signalizing of the risk area. Additionally, we used laminar flow, aseptic chambers, automatic pipetters, and reservoirs with sterilizing solutions. On the day of the experiments with the bacterial clones, no other manipulation of microorganisms occurred. All the non-disposable material and surgery tools are autoclaved. A separated manipulation room with an ultraviolet and exhaust chamber was used when necessary. Carcasses were incinerated.

Recombinant NH36 Antigen and F3 Domain

NH36 is composed of 314 amino acids. The NH36 sequence is deposited in SWISS-PROT (accession code Q8WQX2), EMBL (AY007193), GenBank™ and DDJB (AAG02281.1) data bases (15, 20). F3 is composed of the amino acids 199–314 of NH36. The sequences of the NH36 and F3 were cloned in the pET28b plasmid system, expressed in *E. coli* Bl21DE3 cells and purified by affinity chromatography (Ni-NTA, Qiagen), as described before (15, 20). The presence or absence of LPS was confirmed using the LAL QCL-1000 kit (Lonza). The levels of LPS were lower than the sensitivity range of the Limulus amebocyte lysate test, which is 0.1–1.0 EU/ml. Therefore, there was no need for endotoxin removal.

Vaccination and Challenge With *L. (L.) infantum chagasi*

Eight-week-old C57BL/6 female mice, obtained from the Fiocruz-Cecal facilities (Rio de Janeiro, Brazil) were vaccinated subcutaneously, with three doses of 100 µg of NH36 or F3 formulated with 100 µg of saponin (SIGMA), at weekly intervals (15). Control mice received only saline. On week 4, mice were challenged with an intravenous injection in the tail vain of 3×10^7 *L. (L.) infantum chagasi* amastigotes (strain IOC-L 3324) isolated from infected hamsters' as described before (24, 25). On day 28 after infection, euthanasia was performed and the variation in total body weight and relative liver/body weight were recorded (15). The parasite load in the livers was determined by microscopic observation of Giemsa-stained impression smears. The parasite burden was assessed as LDU values (number of amastigotes per 1,000 of organ cell nuclei/mg of organ weight) (11, 15, 16, 18, 25). Alternatively, the parasite burden was assessed by a limiting dilution assay (LDA) of the aseptically removed liver fragments suspended in a 1/5 serial dilution in Schneider's medium, and incubated at 26°C. Promastigotes present in the last well containing visible parasites were quantified in a hemocytometer (21). Two-independent experiments were performed with $n = 7$ mice per treatment in each treatment.

Assessment of the Intradermal Response to Leishmanial Antigen (IDR)

IDR against *L. (L.) donovani* lysate was measured in the footpads on day 7 after immunization and on day 25 after challenge (15, 26). The right hind footpads were injected intradermally with 10^7 freeze–thawed *L. (L.) donovani* promastigotes at the stationary phase (15, 26–28). Before, and at 24 and 48 h after injection the swelling was assessed with a Mitutoyo apparatus. Each animal received only 0.1 ml saline in the left hind footpad as control. Values of the saline control were subtracted from the reaction due to *Leishmania* antigen, at each measurement (15, 26). Two-independent experiments were performed with $n = 6$–7 C57BL/6 mice per treatment in each experiment.

DCs Isolation and Migration Tests *In Vitro* and *In Vivo*

Dendritic cells was isolated from spleens of vaccinated mice, 28 days after challenge, following the instructions of the magnetic beads manufacturer (Miltenyi Biotec, USA). Briefly, spleens were collected, shredded, and incubated with collagenase, at 1 mg/ml, and DNAse (Sigma) at 20 µg/ml concentration (29), respectively, for 20 min, at room temperature (Figure S1 in Supplementary Material). After that, the spleens were macerated and the splenocytes passed through a cell mesh. Also an ACK solution was used for erythrocyte lysis. Magnetic microbeads conjugated with anti-mouse CD11c were added to the preparation and then incubated for an additional 30 min. After that, the DCs were purified using MACS magnetic columns (Miltenyi Biotec, Germany) (11) and labeled with anti-mouse CD11c antibody conjugated to fluorescein isothiocyanate (FITC), clone N418 (eBiosciense, USA). Cells were additionally incubated with allophycocyanin (APC)-conjugated to anti-CCR7 (eBioscense) (two experiments with $n = 5$ mice per treatment for each experiment) (Figure S1 in Supplementary Material). The cytometry analysis was performed using a FACSCalibur apparatus (Becton Dickinson).

The *in vitro* migration assays used DCs purified from C57BL/6 naïve, *L. (L.) infantum chagasi* infected and NH36 or F3 vaccinated and infected mice. The DCs (5×10^5 per well) were suspended in RPMI containing 1% fetal calf serum and placed into the upper chamber of Transwell inserts (5 µm pore size, Coaster, Corning). The inserts were further positioned in plates containing RPMI, with or without the addition of 100 ηM CCL19 (R&D Systems). After 2 h of incubation at 37°C, the cells in the lower wells of the inserts were collected and counted in a hemocytometer chamber. For the purity analysis, cells which migrated were stained with anti-mouse CD11c antibody, and analyzed by flow cytometry. Two-independent experiments were performed, each one of them with $n = 5$–6 mice per treatment. In order to prove that the DCs migration is due to the sensitivity of CCR7 receptors to the CCL19 chemokine gradient, blocking experiments were performed by incubating the DCs obtained from infected or

F3sap-vaccinated mice with anti-CCR7 antibody (e Bioscience) at 1/50 dilution for 30 min at 4°C, before the migration assay in transwell plates, as described.

The migration assays *in vivo* used DCs purified from spleens of *L. (L.) infantum chagasi* infected and NH36 or F3-vaccinated, or from infected mice. Isolation and purification of DCs were performed using magnetic beads as described for the *in vitro* assays (Figure S1 in Supplementary Material). Additionally, the DCs were stained with two drops/ml (6 μg/ml) of Hoescht 33342 (Life Technologies), for 20 min at 37°C, protected from light. After that, 10^6 labeled DCs were injected intravenously into the infected receptors, on day 28 after infection, as described by Ato et al. (11). Spleens of receptors were removed 24 h after the DCs transfer and immersed in paraformaldehyde, followed by cryoprotection in an increasing sucrose gradient (10, 20, and 30%). Cryostat sections (16 μm) were performed and mounted in Fluoromount and observed under a confocal microscope (LeicaTCS SP5). Sections from three mice of each treatment were chosen randomly and analyzed for the presence of labeled DCs in the white pulp (wp) or in the red pulp (rp) or in the MZ. Approximately 1,000 stained DCs were recorded and the differences between the proportions detected in the wp, and the rp, were analyzed by the Fischer exact test for comparison of proportions (https://www.graphpad.com/quickcalcs/contingency2/). Two-independent experiments were performed, each one of them with $n = 3$ receptor mice per treatment.

DCs Immunotherapy

Splenic DCs from *L. (L.) infantum chagasi*-infected mice, and from NH36 or F3-vaccinated and challenged mice, were purified on day 28 after infection. The total amount of purified DCs obtained from the spleens from the different experimental groups varied from 1 to 2.6×10^6. For the immunotherapy experiments, 10^6 DCs of each group of mice were injected intravenously into *L. (L.) infantum chagasi*-infected C57BL/6 recipients on day 28 post infection. The parasite loads in spleen and livers, the spleen and liver/corporal relative weights, and the variation in body weights were recorded in the recipient mice 7 days later by LDU. Two-independent experiments were performed with $n = 5$ mice per treatment in each experiment. As a control, blocking experiments to prove that migration of DC is critical for the protection in mice were performed using DCs obtained from normal, infected, and NH36, and F3-vaccinated and infected mice, that were pre-incubated with anti-CCR7 antibody and further transferred to infected receptors.

Cytokine-Secretion Assay in Vaccinated Mice

Spleens were aseptically removed and splenocyte suspensions were prepared as described before (21). Purified DCs were also obtained. Cells were distributed into 96-well plate (10^6 cell/well) and incubated with 5 μg/ml NH36 or lysate of stationary phase *L. (L.) infantum chagasi* promastigotes, or with no addition for 72 h *in vitro*, at 37°C with 5% CO_2. After that, supernatants were harvested and assayed using the Mouse IFN gamma, TNF-α, and IL10 ELISA Ready-SET-Go! (e-Biosciences, USA). The sensitivity of the assay was established with a range of 10–1,000 pg/ml for TNF-α, 100–1,000 pg/ml for, and of 15–2,000 pg/ml for IFN-γ. Reactions were developed using biotinylated anti-cytokine antibodies, streptavidin (SAv-HRP) enzymatic reagent, and TMB (Zymed, USA). Absorbances were monitored in a BioRad ELISA reader at 655 ηm. Two-independent experiments ($n = 5$ mice per treatment in each experiment) were performed.

Intracellular Cytokine Staining in Vaccinated Mice

The analysis of the T cell response used splenocytes stimulated *in vitro* with 5 μg/ml NH36 or lysate of stationary phase *L. (L.) infantum chagasi* promastigotes or with no addition for 24 h at 37°C with 5% CO_2, as described (21), and with incubation with Brefeldin A (SIGMA). After that, the splenocytes were stained with rat anti-mouse-CD4FITC (clone GK1.5) and -CD8FITC (clone 53-6.7) monoclonal antibodies (eBioscience), fixed, washed, treated with 0.5% saponin-FACS buffer, and stained with IFN-γAPC, IL-2-PerCP-Cy5.5, and TNF-αPE monoclonal antibodies (eBioscience). A total of 100,000 events were acquired. Gating for $CD4^+$ ad $CD8^+$ T cells was performed using a FACSCalibur apparatus (Becton Dickinson). Data analysis was performed with the Flow-jo program (Treestar, USA). Two-independent experiments were performed with $n = 5$ mice per treatment in each experiment.

Statistical Analysis

Means were compared using the Kruskal–Wallis and Mann–Whitney non-parametrical tests. Correlation coefficients were established by the Pearson's two-tailed correlation test (GraphPad Prism 6 software) as described (21). Also compared the survival distribution of individuals in infected controls and vaccinated and challenged mice were compared using the Log-rank (Mantel–Cox) and the Gehan–Breslow–Wilcoxon tests (GraphPad Prism 6 software).

RESULTS

Vaccination With F3 and NH36 Prevents Dysfunctional DCs Migration and Decreased CCR7 Expression

In the present investigation, we aimed to assess whether DCs from vaccinated mice preserve their correct migrating capabilities in response to CCL19 chemokine, and if this fact is related to their normal sustained expression of the CCR7 receptor.

As a source of DCs we used normal, infected, and NH36 and F3-vaccinated and challenged mice. Initially, we confirmed that the vaccine-induced protection in the these mice by assessing the achievement of enhanced IDR responses, reduced liver parasite loads and liver relative weights, and sustained corporal weights (**Figure 1**). In fact, vaccination with both, the F3 and the NH36 vaccines, significantly increased the IDR after complete immunization (**Figures 1A,C**), and after challenge (**Figures 1B,D**) above the levels detected in normal control mice, at all tested times (24 and 48 h after injection). Remarkably, after infection, the F3 vaccine was 74 and 79% stronger than controls, at 24 and

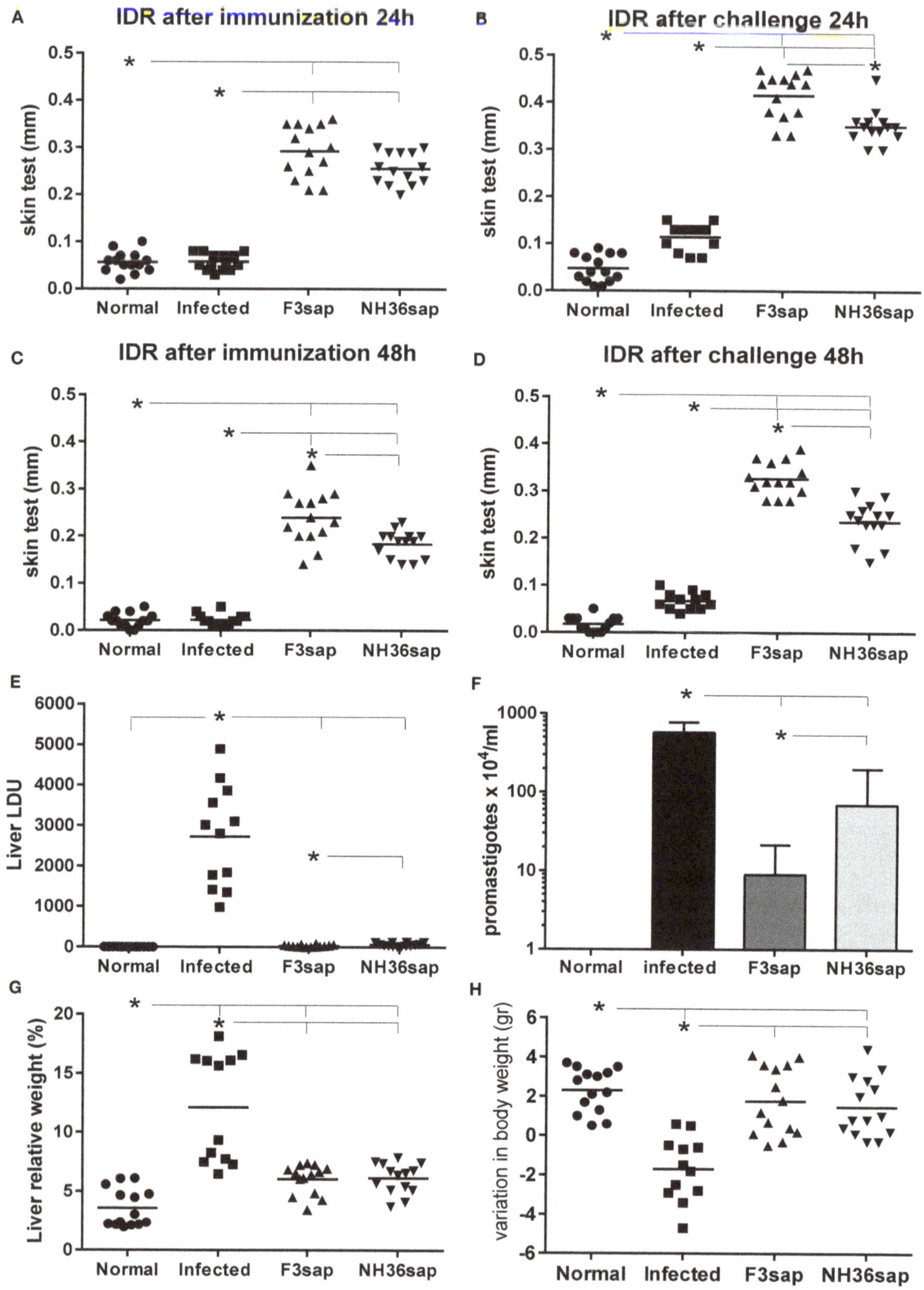

FIGURE 1 | F3 and NH36-vaccinated dendritic cells donor mice showed enhanced IDR and reduced clinical and parasitological impact of infection. IDR to the leishmanial antigen was measured at 24 h **(A,B)** and 48 h **(C,D)** after complete immunization with the F3 (F3sap) and the NH36 (NH36sap) vaccines, and after immunization and challenge. Parasite load in liver is expressed as LDU values **(E)** and total promastigotes/ml, in *in vitro* cultures of livers as determined by the limiting dilution assay method **(F)**. Liver relative weight **(G)**, and gain in corporal weight in grams **(H)** were recorded after euthanasia. Results represent the individual values of two-independent experiments (n = 6–7 C57BL/6 mice per treatment for each experiment). Horizontal full lines represent the mean values. Asterisks and horizontal lines show significant differences between treatments as disclosed by Mann–Whitney non-parametrical test.

48 h, respectively and 27% stronger ($p < 0.0001$) than the NH36 vaccine (**Figures 1B,D**).

IDR values correlated negatively with the liver/body relative weight after immunization ($p < 0.0001$, $R = -0.5768$, $R^2 = 0.3327$ at 24 h and $p < 0.0001$, $R = -0.5833$, $R^2 = 0.3402$ at 48 h after injection) and after challenge ($p < 0.0001$, $R = -0.5989$, $R^2 = 0.3587$ at 24 h and $p < 0.0001$, $R = -0.6334$, $R^2 = 0.4012$ at 48 h after injection).

Notably, both vaccines strongly reduced the liver LDU values compared to those of infected mice ($p < 0.0001$) (**Figure 1E**). Compared to infected controls, F3 vaccine produced a 98.8% reduction, and the NH36 vaccine, a 97.6% of reduction of the parasite load ($p = 0.0318$) (**Figure 1E**). F3 vaccine reduced the LDUs values by 50% in comparison to the NH36 vaccine. The reduction of the parasite load determined by both vaccines was also confirmed by the LDA method (**Figure 1F**). The F3 vaccine induced 98% ($p < 0.079$), and the NH36 vaccine only 88% reduction ($p < 0.0079$) ($p < 0.05$) of the number of promastigote in liver culture. Additionally, the F3 vaccine reduced the promastigotes counts by 87% ($p < 0.05$) in comparison to the NH36 vaccine (**Figure 1F**). The LDU and LDA values for the liver parasite loads were positively correlated ($p < 0.026$, $R = 0.496$, $R^2 = 0.2464$).

The increases in IDR after infection were strong correlates of protection regarding the liver LDU values. In fact, LDU values were negatively correlated with IDR after immunization, at 24 h ($p < 0.0001$, $R = -0.7875$, $R^2 = 0.6202$) and at 48 h ($p < 0.0001$, $R = -0.7674$, $R^2 = 0.5890$) and after challenge, at 24 h ($p < 0.0001$, $R = -0.7796$, $R^2 = 0.6077$) and at 48 h ($p < 0.0001$, $R = -0.7543$, $R^2 = 0.5690$).

Increases in liver/body relative weight were also significantly higher in infected control animals than in normal uninfected controls and in F3 and NH36-vaccinated and challenged mice ($p < 0.0001$ for all comparisons) (**Figure 1G**). In addition, only infected controls lose corporal weight (**Figure 1H**) in comparison to normal, F3 and NH36-vaccinated mice ($p < 0.0001$ for all comparisons). Vaccinated and normal mice showed similar gain in corporal weight. Besides, IDR was positively correlated to corporal weight gain after immunization ($p = 0.0009$, $R = 0.5055$, $R^2 = 0.2556$, at 24 h and $P = 0.0002$, $R = 0.5504$, $R^2 = 0.3030$, at 48 h after injection) and after challenge ($p < 0.0001$, $R = 0.5888$, $R^2 = 0.3467$, at 24 h and $p < 0.0001$, $R = 0.6532$, $R^2 = 0.4267$, at 48 h after injection).

Once the generation of a protective response was confirmed, we further studied the migrating capabilities of DCs obtained from these vaccinated, naïve controls, and infected mice on day 28 after challenge. In **Figure 2**, we represent the results as boxes and whiskers. The whiskers show the maximal and minimum values and the top and bottom of the bars show, respectively, the 75th and 25th percentiles. The 75th percentile is the value below which 75% of observations in a group of observations fall. **Figure 2A** shows that the number of total splenocytes isolated was, as expected, higher in infected mice than in the two vaccinated groups. FACS cytometry analysis of the affinity chromatography purified $CD11c^+$ DCs preparations disclosed 90–100% rates of purity. We further observed that the number of DCs purified from total splenocytes was higher in infected and F3-vaccinated, than in normal mice (**Figure 2B**).

Additionally, none of the DCs migrated toward the medium containing no additions (**Figure 2C**). In contrast, while DCs of normal controls and of F3 and NH36-vaccinated mice migrated toward the CCL19 gradient, DCs of infected animals did not ($p < 0.008$ for all comparisons). The maximal number of migrated DCs was 11,496 for the F3, and 9,152 for the NH36 vaccine (**Figure 2C**). Accordingly, 75% of the migrated DCs count of the F3 vaccine group fall below 8,596, while 75% of the NH36 vaccine counts fall only below 6,130 DCs counts. Therefore, although the differences in the generation of the DC migrating capabilities of the two vaccines were not statistically significant, the maximal values and 75th percentiles suggest the superiority of the F3 vaccine. As a blocking control, we incubated DCs obtained from either infected or F3sap-vaccinated and challenged mice, with anti-CCR7 antibody, in the presence of CCL19 stimulus (**Figure 2D**). The anti-CCR7 antibody blocked 90% of the *in vitro* migrating capabilities of the DCs obtained from the F3sap-vaccinated mice.

Our results indicate that protective immunity against the F3 and NH36 antigens, not only restores the DCs migrating dysfunction of mice infected with *L. (L.) infantum chagasi*, but it also potentiates this capability above the levels found in normal naïve mice (**Figure 2**). In agreement with the parasitological results, which indicated that the F3 vaccine was the most protective, the superiority of the F3 vaccine is reinforced by the finding of a higher number of purified DCs, higher maximal counts of migrated DCs, and strong inhibition of these migrating capabilities by treatment with anti-CCR7 antibody.

In VL, abnormal DC migration is partially due to the reduced expression of their CCR7 receptor, which is sensitive to the CCL19 chemokine. In order to evaluate whether the restored DCs migrating capabilities of vaccinated mice were related to a preserved CCR7 expression on DCs. With that aim, we analyzed the CCR7 protein expression on the surface of purified splenic DCs using APC-conjugated anti-CCR7 antibody and flow cytometry analysis. Based on our findings (**Figure 3**), vaccination with F3sap and NH36 upregulated the expression of CCR7 receptor on DCs. CCR7 expression was low in normal mice (1.56%) (**Figure 3A**), extremely reduced in infected mice (0.37%) (**Figure 3B**), and much stronger in animals treated with the F3 vaccine (26.06%) (**Figure 3C**) than in those vaccinated with NH36 (5.29%) (**Figure 3D**).

Therefore, vaccination with F3 and NH36 stimulates IDR, protects mice from clinical VL, restores and enhances DCs migrating capabilities probably due to the increase in CCR7 expression on DCs. Our findings of the reduced liver parasite load, increased IDR and enhancement of the CCR7 expression highlight the stronger immunogenic effect of the F3 vaccine.

Immunotherapy With DCs

In order to confirm the DC migration *in vivo*, DCs from infected, or NH36- or F3-vaccinated and *L. (L.) infantum chagasi*-challenged mice, were stained with Hoescht 33342 *in vitro*, and further injected into infected mice. Twenty four hours after injection, the spleens of receptors were removed and frozen, and the transferred DCs were observed by fluorescence microscopy in the wp or rp of the frozen sections (**Figure 4**). Fluorescent DCs were counted

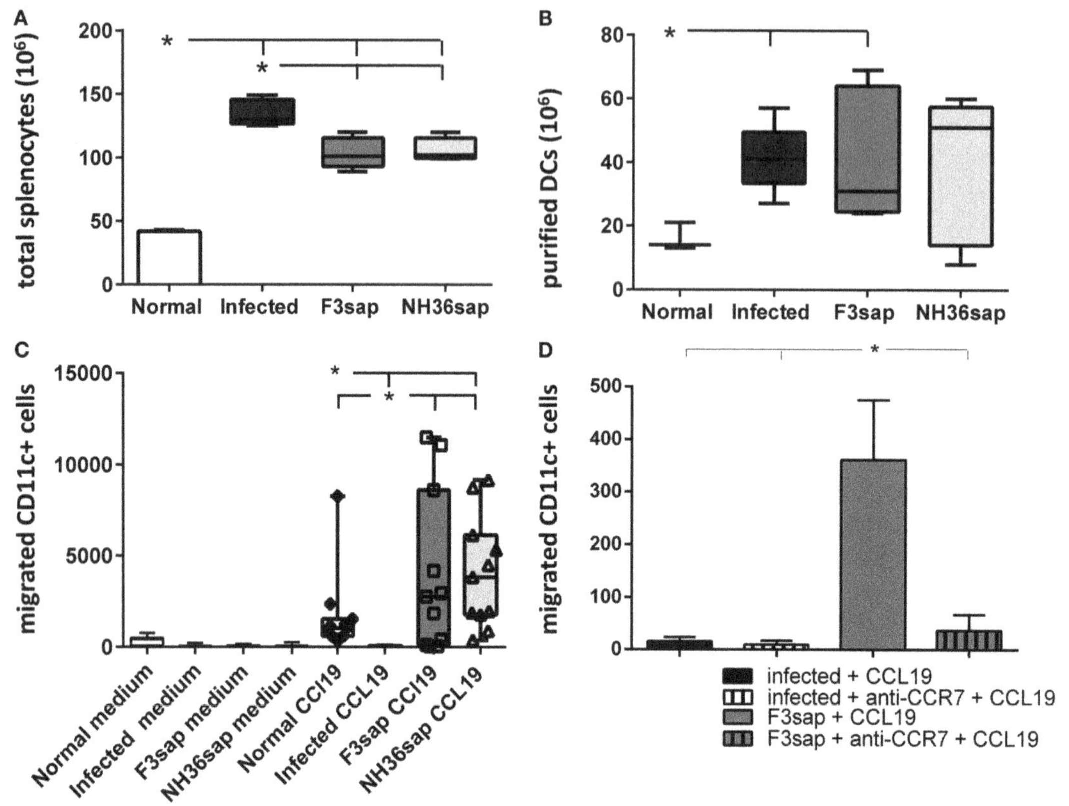

FIGURE 2 | F3- and NH36-primed dendritic cells (DCs) show enhanced migration response to CCL19 chemokine. Splenic DCs were purified from, normal, infected and F3, and NH36-vaccinated and *Leishmania infantum chagasi*-challenged mice. DCs were isolated at day 28 after challenge. The whiskers show the maximal and minimum values, and the top and bottom of the bars show respectively, the 75th and 25th percentiles. The 75th percentile is the value below which 75% of observations in a group of observations fall. **(A)** Total splenocytes. **(B)** Number of DCS purified by magnetic beads-affinity chromatography. **(C)** The chemotactic responses to 100 ηM CCL19 were assessed using a transwell system. After 2 h of incubation, migrated DCs were collected, stained using fluorescein isothiocyanate-conjugated anti-CD11c antibody, and counted by flow cytometry in a FacsCalibur apparatus (Becton Dickinson). In the boxes, the individual results for migrating DCs counts of normal mice (diamonds), F3-vaccinated (squares), and NH36-vaccinated mice (triangles). **(D)** Number of DCs from infected or F3-vaccinated and challenged mice, pre-incubated with anti-CCR7 antibody or no addition, which migrated toward CCL19. Results represent two-independent experiments (n = 5–6, mice per treatment in each experiment). Asterisks and horizontal lines show significant differences between treatments as disclosed by Mann–Whitney non-parametrical test.

in a total of 19–21 sections of each treatment and representative images are shown in **Figures 4A–C**. Additionally, the records are represented as proportions of DCs from donors distributed either in the white or rps of infected receptor spleens. On day 28 of the infection of recipients, DCs from infected donors remained mostly in the rp (92%) (**Figure 4A**) and, only minor proportions migrated to the MZ of the wp (8%; $p < 0.001$). DCs from NH36-vaccinated mice are equally distributed between the white (59%) and the rp (41%; $p = 0.1144$) (**Figure 4B**). Remarkably, 84% of DCs from F3-vaccinated mice preferentially migrated to the wp and its MZ (**Figure 4C**), while only 16% remained in the rp ($p < 0.0001$).

In order to study the potential use of F3 and NH36 antigen-primed DCs in the immunotherapy of VL we transferred DCs from infected, and from vaccinated and challenged mice, into recipient mice infected with *L. (L.) infantum chagasi* 28 days before. Seven days after the DCs transfer, the impact on the parasitological and clinical cure was assessed. While infected animals lost 1.54 g of corporal weight, the weight loss was 79% lower in mice that received F3-primed DCs (0.32 g), and 91% lower in mice treated with NH36-primed DCs (0.14 g) (**Figure 5A**). Additionally, only the F3-primed DCs were able to alter the impact of the infection on mice, by reducing the parasite load in the spleen ($p < 0.007$) (**Figure 5B**), the spleen/body relative weight (**Figure 5C**), the liver/body relative weight ($p < 0.05$) (**Figure 5D**), and the liver LDU values ($p < 0.05$) (**Figure 5E**). Therefore, the results of immunotherapy with DCs correlate with the results of the preventive vaccination, thus demonstrating that the F3 vaccine is more potent than the NH36 vaccine. The immunotherapeutic effect of F3-primed DCs (**Figure 5F**), but not of the NH36-primed DCs (not shown) was blocked by pre-incubation with anti-CCR7 antibody, and a 43 and 52% increased parasite load was observed in spleens and livers, respectively of the recipient mice. These results indicate that the increased migrating capabilities of DCs from F3-vaccinated mice, both *in vitro* and *in vivo* (**Figures 2D, 4C** and **5F**) are related to the enhanced CCR7 receptor expression (**Figure 3**), which contributes to the cure of VL.

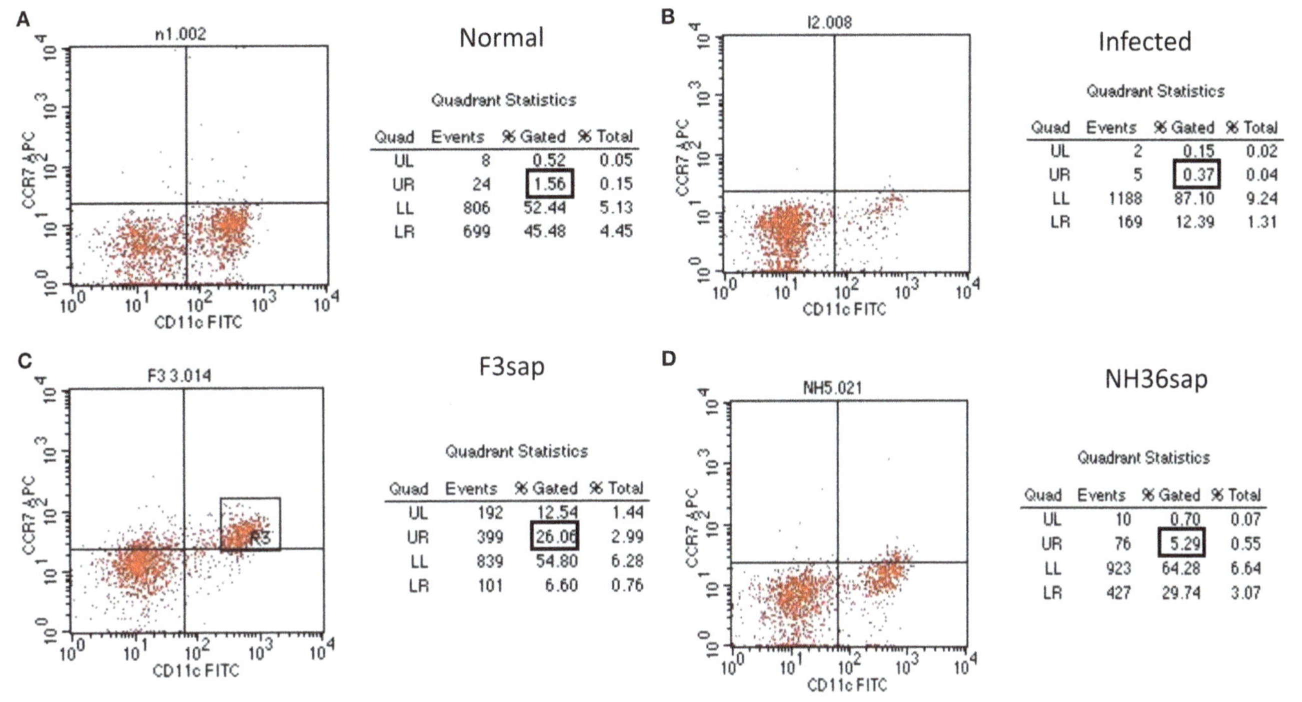

FIGURE 3 | Enhanced CCR7+ expression in F3 and NH36-primed dendritic cells (DCs). DCs from normal **(A)**, infected **(B)**, and F3 **(C)** or NH36 **(D)** vaccinated and challenged C57BL/6 mice were purified and analyzed by flow cytometry. DCs CD11c+ populations were gated and analyzed for CCR7 expression using anti-CCR7-allophycocyanin antibody. Results are representative of the individual percentages gated of two experiments (*n* = 5 per treatment for each experiment).

Evolution of the Cellular Immune Response of Vaccinated DC Donor Mice Secreted Cytokines and Survival

We assessed the profile of IFN-γ, TNF-α, and IL-10 secretion along the time, in the supernatants of splenocytes of mice vaccinated with F3 or NH36 vaccines and further challenged (**Figure 6**). We monitored the cytokine secretion of splenocytes in response to NH36 or to the *L. (L.) infantum chagasi* lysate antigen. On day 15 after challenge, when the parasite load was maximal in livers (**Figure 6C**), the F3-vaccine enhanced the IFN-γ and TNF-α secretion in response to NH36, five times more than the NH36 vaccine (**Figures 6A,D**). The F3-vaccine also enhanced by a factor of 1.4–5, the respective IFN-γ and TNF-α levels when compared to infected controls (**Figures 6A,D**). On the other hand, IL-10 secretion was reduced more by the F3 than by the NH36 vaccine (**Figure 6G**). The IFN-γ/IL-10 and TNF-α/IL-10 ratios (**Figure 6I**), that were also higher for the F3 vaccine (10 and 2.9, respectively) than for the NH36 vaccine (6.5 and 1.7, respectively) suggest the superiority of the F3sap vaccine in the induction of a probable Th1 response. The *Leishmania* lysate promoted a similar response with superiority of the F3 vaccine although with a lower IFN-γ on day 15 and higher IL-10 secretion on day 28 (**Figures 6B,G**). Globally, the pro-inflammatory cytokine response of splenocytes was maximal (**Figures 6A,B,D,E**) since the early infection, when vaccine protection was already registered in spleens (**Figure 6F**). Levels of IFN-γ and TNF-α decreased until day 28, when, in contrast, IL-10 secretion was maximal. This pike in IL-10 secretion is coincident with the maximal parasite load detected in spleens. However, the vaccine efficacy was also long-lasting until day 28, when the parasite load was higher in spleens. In fact, while 90% of the parasite load reduction was induced by the F3 vaccine on day 15, protection was maximal (94%) on day 28 after infection (**Figure 6F**).The survival Kaplan–Meier curve analysis represented in **Figure 7**, confirmed that protection generated by the F3sap vaccine is long-lasting. In fact, while all mice from the infected control group died between day 29 and day 40 after infection, a 100% of mice vaccinated with F3sap survived until euthanasia on day 45, confirming the longevity of the vaccine immune response. In contrast, 80% of NH36-vaccinated mice survived until day 29 and only 40% of them were alive on day 45 (**Figure 7**).We also studied the cytokine response *in vitro*, in the supernatants of DCs obtained from infected, and vaccinated and infected DC donors, on day 28, before transfer to infected mice (**Figure 8**). Although the total splenocyte cytokine response was lower on day 28, than on day 15 (**Figures 6A,B,D,E,G,H**), the DCs of F3-vaccinated mice secreted enhanced levels of IFN-γ, in response to NH36 and lysate (**Figure 8A**) and of TNF-α, in response to lysate only (**Figure 8B**). No significant differences in IL-10 levels were observed in response to the antigens (**Figure 8C**).

Intracellular Expression of Cytokines

The Figure S2 in Supplementary Material, summarized the strategy used for the analysis of multifunctional T cell response

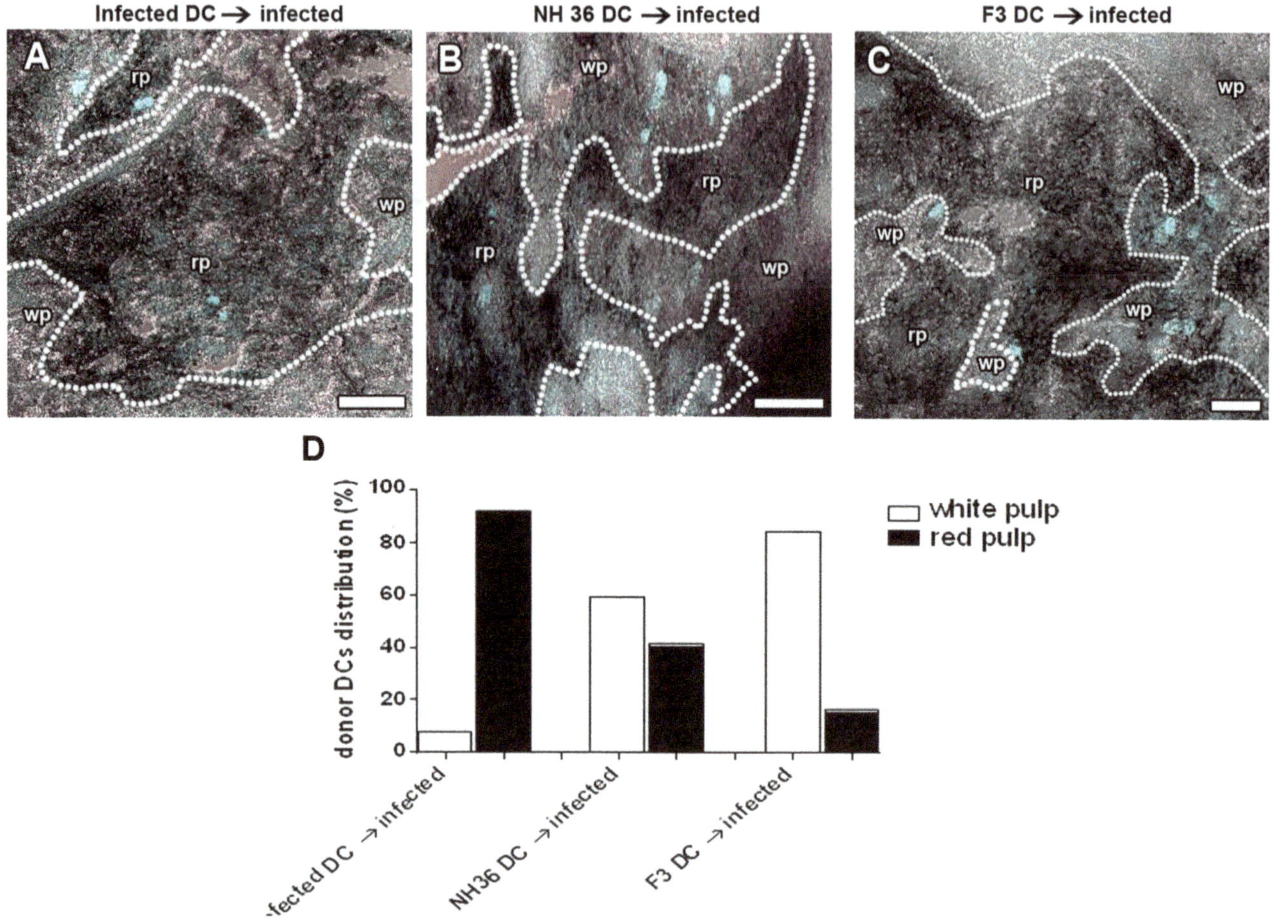

FIGURE 4 | F3-primed dendritic cells (DCs) migrate to the spleen white pulp (wp) of infected mice. DCs of day 28-infected mice and F3- and NH36-primed and -challenged mice were labeled with Hoescht nuclear fluorescent stain, and injected into 28-day-infected mice. Recipient mice were euthanized 24 h after injection. Spleens were fixed and frozen and the distribution of stained DCs was assessed in cryostat sections to confirm the *in vivo* migration of DCs. We show the image overlay of cryostat sections from bright field to evidence spleen morphology, and confocal image to show Hoescht labeled cells in blue. The dotted lines indicate the marginal zone (MZ) which separates the red pulp (rp) from the wp. It is possible to observe the localization of the labeled DCs in mice that received DCs from infected **(A)**, NH 36- **(B)**, or F3-vaccinated donors **(C)** as well as the distribution of these cells **(D)**. Scale bar = 120 μm. Data are representative of one experiment with three mice per treatment. DCs from infected donors remain mostly in the rp (92%; $p < 0.001$). DCs from NH36-vaccinated mice are equally distributed between the white and the rp ($p = 0.1144$) while 84% ($p < 0.0001$) of DCs from F3-vaccinated mice migrated to the wp and its MZ **(C)**.

using a four-color flow cytometry panel to simultaneously analyze multiple cytokines at the single-cell level in splenocytes cultures. After analyzing the total production of each cytokine by CD4$^+$ or CD8$^+$ cells, the Boolean gates (or combinatorial analysis) tool of the FlowJo program was used to determine the frequencies of the possible seven combinations of cytokine-producing cells.

In correlation with the cytokine secretion to supernatants by splenocytes (**Figure 6**), the intracellular expression of cytokines by CD4$^+$ T lymphocytes in response to NH36, was more intense on day 15 than on day 28 after infection (**Figure 9**). On both days, the F3sap vaccine was superior to the NH36 formulation enhancing all types of CD4$^+$ T cells secreting one cytokine (IL-2$^+$, TNF-α$^+$, or IFN-γ$^+$) (**Figures 9A,D,G**), the combination of two (IL-2$^+$TNF-α$^+$, TNF-α$^+$IFN-γ$^+$, or IL-2$^+$IFN-γ$^+$) (**Figures 9B,E,H**), or the three cytokines simultaneously (IL-2$^+$TNF-α$^+$IFN-γ$^+$) (**Figure 9C**). The only exception was detected in CD4$^+$TNF-α$^+$ (**Figure 9D**) and CD4$^+$TNF-α$^+$IFN-γ$^+$ T cells (**Figure 9H**) which were increased more, in the infected controls than in the F3-vaccinated mice, only on day 15.

Additionally, the global proportions of CD4$^+$ T lymphocytes were lower in infected, than in normal mice (**Figure 9F**), although the F3 vaccine sustained higher CD4$^+$ T cells counts than the NH36 vaccine, even despite the advancement of spleen infection on day 28 (**Figure 6F**).

In contrast to the IFN-γ and TNF-α splenocyte secretion to supernatants (**Figure 6**), which were slightly higher in response to NH36 than to the lysate (**Figure 6**), the intracellular expression of cytokines in CD4$^+$ T cells was similar, in response to both antigens (**Figure 9**; Figure S3 in Supplementary Material). In fact, the *Leishmania* lysate stimulus also increased the frequencies of CD4$^+$-secreting T cells, more on day 15 than on day 28 after

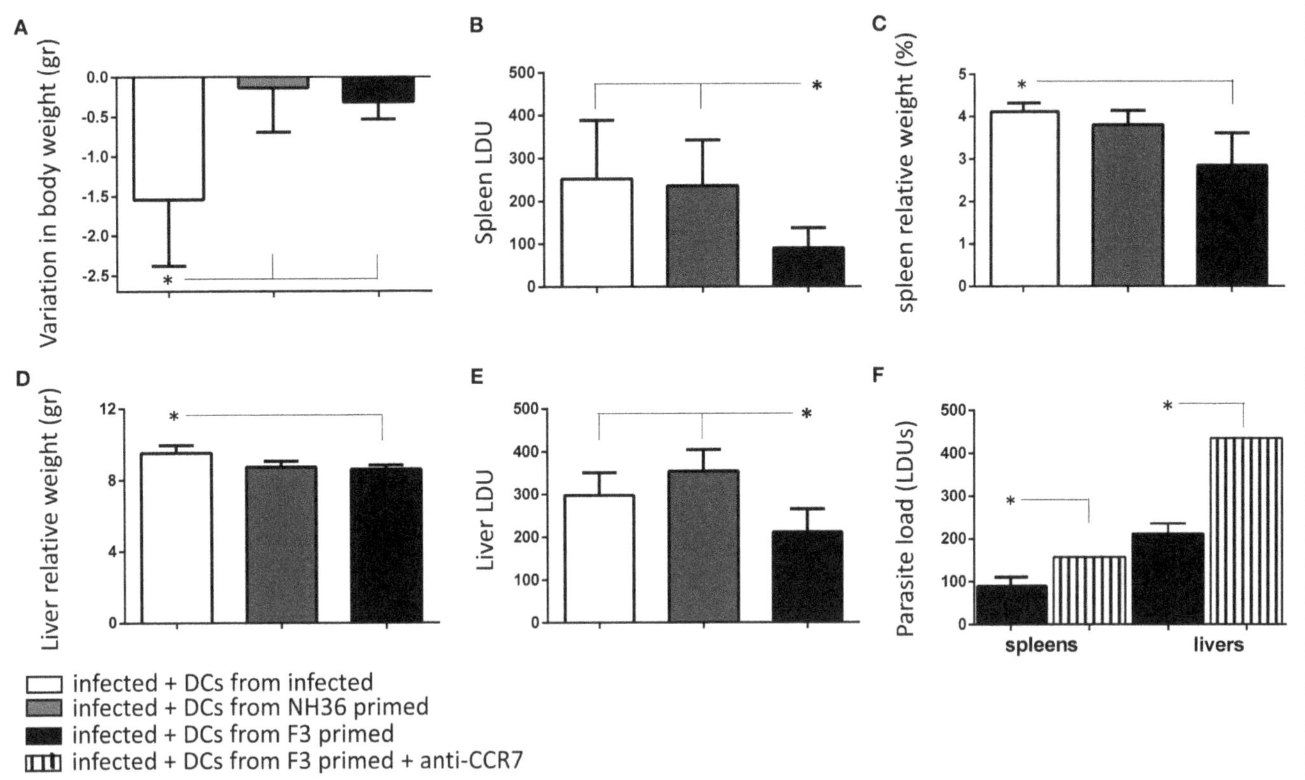

FIGURE 5 | Immunotherapy with F3-primed dendritic cells (DCs) reduces parasite and clinical signs of visceral leishmaniasis. DCs (10^6) purified from *Leishmania (L.) infantum chagasi*-infected mice, or mice treated with the F3 or the NH36 vaccines and challenged, were injected into infected mice on day 28 after infection. Recipient mice were euthanized after 7 days after DC transfer and the variation in corporal weight **(A)**, spleen LDU **(B)**, spleen/body relative weight **(C)**, liver LDU **(D)**, and liver/body relative weight **(E)** were calculated. As a control we also showed the increase of the parasite load of spleens and livers of day 28-infected mice that received an injection of F3-primed DCs pre-incubated with anti-CCR7 antibody **(F)**. The results are compared with the parasite load of infected mice that received F3-primed DCs with no previous incubation. Bars represent the mean + SE values of two-independent experiments (n = 5 mice per treatment in each experiment). Asterisks and horizontal lines show significant differences between treatments as disclosed by Mann–Whitney non-parametrical test.

infection. The F3 vaccine was stronger than the NH36 vaccine for all types of CD4$^+$ T cells (Figure S3 in Supplementary Material). Also, and as detected after stimulation with NH36, the frequencies of CD4$^+$TNF-α$^+$ and CD4$^+$TNF-α$^+$IFN-α T cells were still higher in infected controls and only increased by the F3-vaccine, on day 28 after infection (Figures S3D,E in Supplementary Material).

Regarding the cytotoxic immunity in response to NH36, the NH36-vaccine was the strongest enhancer of the proportions of CD8$^+$IL-2$^+$ and CD8$^+$TNF-α$^+$IFN-α$^+$ on day 15 (**Figures 10A,E**) and of CD8$^+$IL-2$^+$TNF-α$^+$IFN-γ$^+$ lymphocytes on day 28 (**Figure 10C**). In contrast, on day 28, the F3-vaccine was the most potent enhancer of the frequencies of CD8$^+$IL-2$^+$ (**Figure 10A**), IFN-γ$^+$ (**Figure 10G**), TNF-α$^+$IL-2$^+$ (**Figure 10B**), TNF-α$^+$IFN-γ$^+$ (**Figure 10E**), and IL-2$^+$IFN-γ$^+$-secreting T cells (**Figure 10H**). The F3-vaccine superiority for TNF-α$^+$IL-2$^+$ enhancement was already evident on day 15 (**Figure 10B**).

Additionally, when stimulated with lysate stronger frequencies of CD8$^+$IL-2$^+$, CD8$^+$TNF-α$^+$IL-2$^+$, CD8$^+$TNF-α$^+$IFN-γ$^+$, and CD8$^+$IL-2$^+$TNF-α$^+$IFN-γ$^+$ T cells were observed, on day 15 (Figure S4 in Supplementary Material) in mice vaccinated with the NH36 vaccine. In contrast, the F3-vaccine was superior for the proportions of CD8$^+$IFN-γ$^+$ and CD8$^+$IL-2$^+$IFN-γ$^+$ T cells, both on days 15 and 28, and of CD8$^+$IL-2$^+$ and CD8$^+$IL-2$^+$IFN-γ$^+$ T cells, on day 28. Similar to what was detected for CD4$^+$ T cell whole frequencies (**Figure 9F**) the CD8$^+$ T cell proportions were reduced in all challenged mice, but in this case, no preventive effective was induced by any of the vaccines (Figure S4F in Supplementary Material).

DISCUSSION

Although no human vaccine is available for human VL yet, there are four veterinary vaccines that have been developed for prophylaxis of canine VL (30–33). FML, a complex glycoprotein antigen of *L. (L.) donovani* and saponin, are the components of Leishmune®, the first licensed canine vaccine against leishmaniasis (33–35). The Leishmune® dog vaccination has decreased the incidence of canine and human leishmaniasis in endemic areas (33). Leishmune® is a transmission blocking vaccine (27, 34) and vaccinated dogs remained non-infective to insect vectors (35). NH36 is the main antigen of FML (27, 36) and F3 is its C-terminal domain (15). The F3-vaccine induced a significantly higher decrease in parasite load (95%) and splenomegaly (49%) in C57Bl6 mice infected with *L. (L.) infantum chagasi* (14) than

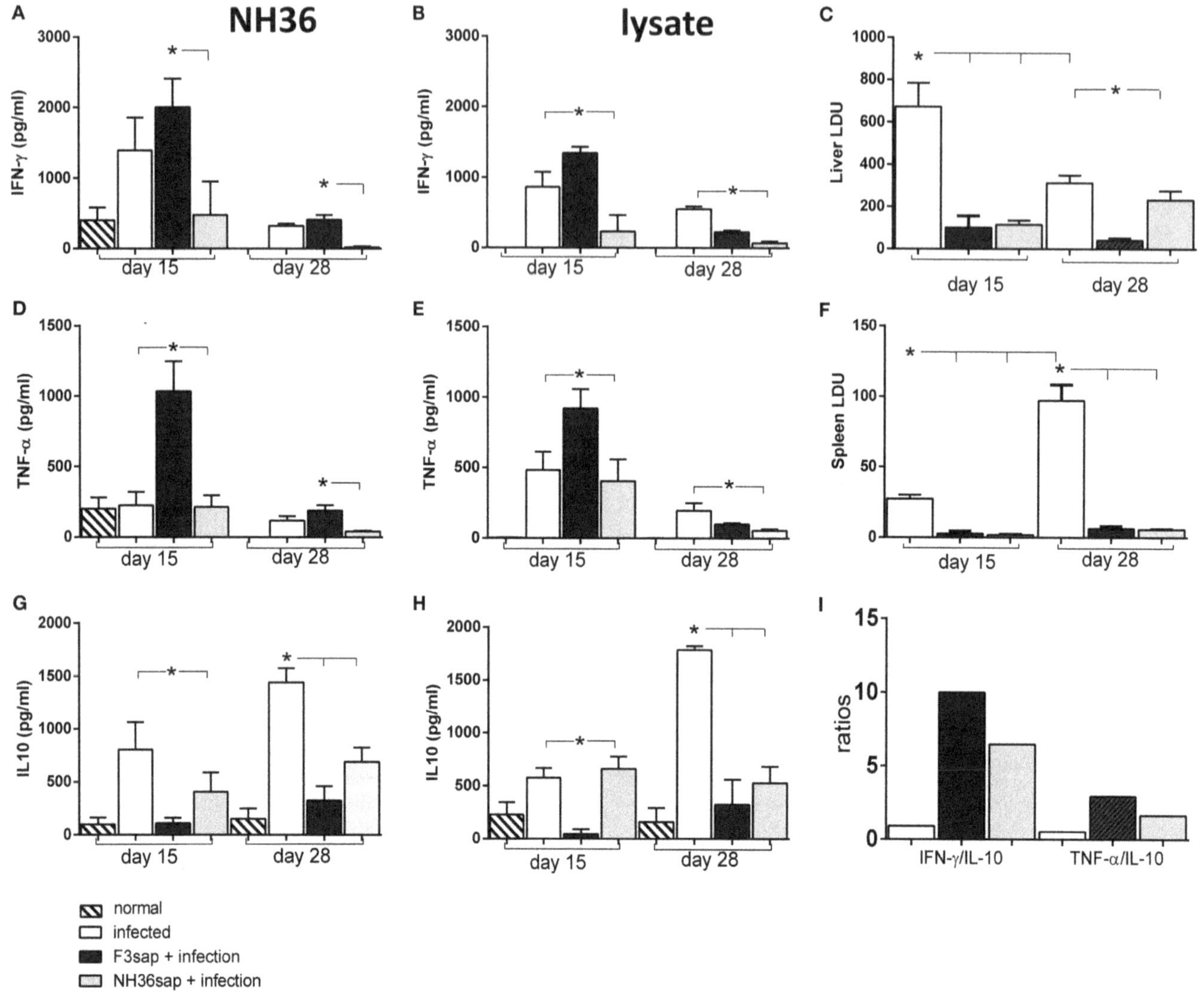

FIGURE 6 | Cytokines secreted by splenocytes along the infection. Splenocyte secretion of IFN-γ **(A,B)**, TNF-α **(D,E)**, and IL-10 **(G,H)** were measured in supernatants of *in vitro* cultures of infected, F3sap and NH36sap vaccinated and infected, in response to NH36 or *Leishmania (L.) infantum chagasi* lysate antigens, both on days 15 and 28 after infection. LDU values show that the parasite load is maximal in livers at day 15 **(C)** and in spleens, only on day 28 **(F)**. Bars represent the mean + SE values of two-independent experiments (n = 5 mice per treatment in each experiment). Asterisks and horizontal lines show significant differences between treatments as disclosed by Mann–Whitney non-parametrical test. IFN-γ/IL-10 and TNF-α/IL-10 ratios in response to NH36 were calculated on day 15 **(I)**.

the NH36 vaccine, which in contrast, reduced the parasite load and relative weight by 87 and 39%, respectively (14). Both vaccines, however, prevented, to a similar extent, the increase in total counts of DCs and severe splenomegaly due to *L. (L.) infantum chagasi* infection (14), both of which were also previously observed during infections with *L. (L) donovani* in BALB/c and C57BL/6 mice (11).

In this investigation, we demonstrate that both NH36 and F3 vaccines increased the IDR, strongly reduced the parasite load in livers and the liver/body relative weight and promoted a gain in corporal weight. We also showed that IDR was also a strong correlate of protection against VL (15). Noteworthy, F3 was more potent than the NH36-vaccine in IDR after *L. (L.) infantum chagasi* challenge and also in reducing the liver parasite load of C57Bl6 mice. The importance of NH36 in immune prevention against VL has been extensively proven in mice (15, 16, 18, 21), dogs (17), and suggested for humans (19, 20, 37). Nonetheless, we also demonstrated that the F3 domain is the responsible for the $CD4^+$ T cell-mediated protection induced by NH36 (15). In fact, F3 was 37% more powerful than the NH36 cognate protein in the increase of antibodies, frequencies of $CD4^+$ T lymphocytes, levels of secreted IFN-γ, and ratios of $CD4^+$ and $CD8^+$ T lymphocytes producing IFN-γ and IL-10 (15) and holds the most potent antibody (15, 38) and MHC class II restricted epitopes (15, 21). In that investigation (15), IDR and ratios of TNFα/IL-10 producing $CD4^+$ T cells were strong correlates of protection. Further, *in vivo* depletion with anti-CD4 and anti-CD8 monoclonal antibodies confirmed protection, which

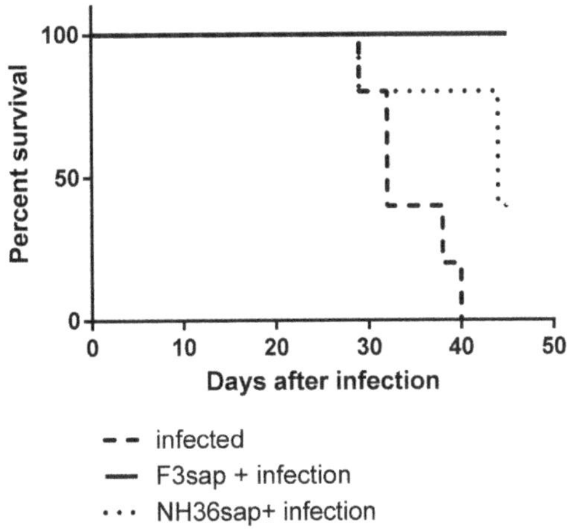

FIGURE 7 | Longevity of vaccine efficacies. The survivability of infected, F3sap, and NH36sap vaccinated and infected mice were recorded and represented using a Kaplan–Meir curve. Comparison of the survival distribution of infected controls and vaccinated and challenged mice, using the Log-rank Mantel–Cox and the Gehan–Breslow–Wilcoxon tests disclosed significant differences for the F3sap vaccine ($p = 0.0018$ and $p = 0.0039$, respectively). Differences between controls and the NH36sap vaccine were, however, only detected by the Log-rank Mantel–Cox ($p = 0.0277$).

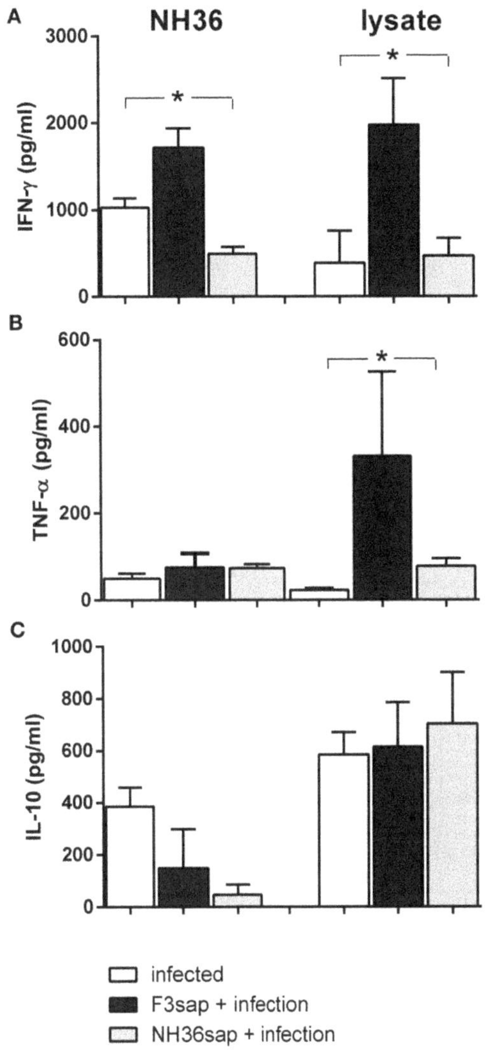

FIGURE 8 | Cytokines secreted by dendritic cells (DCs) on day 28 after challenge. Secretion of IFN-γ **(A)**, TNF-α **(B)**, and IL-10 **(C)** were measured in supernatants of *in vitro* cultures of purified DCs obtained from infected, F3sap, and NH36sap vaccinated and infected in response to NH36 or *Leishmania (L.) infantum chagasi* lysate antigens, on day 28 after infection. Bars represent the mean + SE values of two-independent experiments ($n = 5$ mice per treatment in each experiment). Asterisks and horizontal lines show significant differences between treatments as disclosed by Mann–Whitney non-parametrical test.

was also, long-lasting. The F3 domain was also responsible for the $CD4^+$ T cell-mediated protection against mice infection by *L. (L.) amazonensis* (21).

In this investigation, our results confirm the superior efficacy of the F3-vaccine in inducing a Th1 response against *L. (L.) infantum chagasi* infection in C57Bl6 mice, which includes the generation of long-lasting protection. The F3 vaccine induced an earlier protective T cell response (day 15) with multifunctional $CD4^+IL\text{-}2^+TNF\text{-}\alpha^+IFN\text{-}\gamma^+$ T cells, while the NH36 vaccine promoted a $CD8^+IL\text{-}2^+TNF\text{-}\alpha^+IFN\text{-}\gamma^+$ T cell response, which started later (day 28). Besides the multifunctional T cells, the F3 vaccine also increased the proportions of $CD4^+$ T cell secreting IL-2 or IL-2 and TNF-α, and the NH36 vaccine enhanced the frequencies of $CD8^+$ T cell secreting IL-2 or IL-2 and TNF-α. These cells have been considered as a reservoir of memory T cells that have also effector potential and that can, together with the multifunctional T cells, promote optimal protection (39).

Additionally, the response of $CD4^+$-secreting T cells was slightly higher for the NH36 than to the lysate stimulus, indicating that the NH36 is an important and predominant antigen of *Leishmania* promastigotes. The cytotoxic response, in contrast, is more stimulated by the lysate than by the NH36 antigen, and stronger in mice vaccinated with the NH36, than with the F3 vaccine. These results suggest that the CD8 response is directed to epitopes of NH36, which are not located in the F3 domain. As a matter of fact, the most important epitope for MHC class I molecules of NH36 is the YPPEFKTKL epitope of the F1 domain, which was also shown to be responsible for IL-10 secretion (21). In this way, this F1 domain-epitope contributes to the lowest IFN-γ and TNF-α/IL-10 ratios found in supernatants of splenocytes of NH36-vaccinated mice.

Some of the evidence gathered in this investigation pointed out the superiority of the F3 vaccine, which correlated with the parasitological results. Among them, we can consider the findings of: (1) higher numbers of purified DCs in F3-vaccinated mice; (2) higher maximal counts of migrated DCs; (3) stronger inhibition of these migrating capabilities *in vitro* and *in vivo* by treatment with anti-CCR7 antibody, and (4) higher expression of CCR7, detected on DCs of vaccinated mice. This shows why, the F3 vaccine protects mice from the defective migration of DCs. The higher expression of CCR7 receptors on DCs and the stronger migration of DCs to the splenic wp, induced by the F3-vaccine, explain the

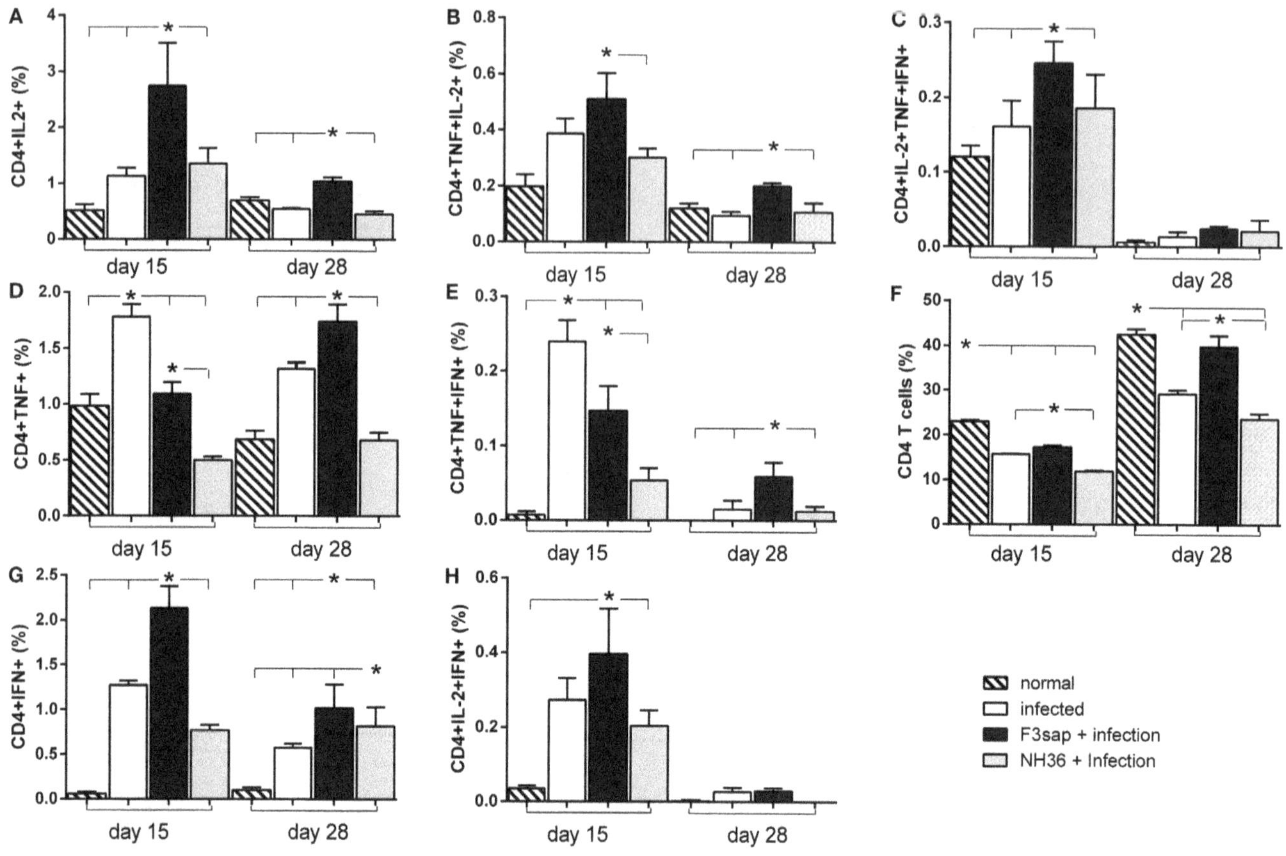

FIGURE 9 | Cytokines expressed by CD4$^+$ T lymphocytes in response to NH36. Effect of the F3 and NH36-vaccines on the frequencies of CD4$^+$IL-2$^+$ **(A)**, TNF-α$^+$ **(D)**, IFN-γ$^+$ **(G)**, TNF-α$^+$IL-2$^+$ **(B)**, TNF-α$^+$IFN-γ$^+$ **(E)**, IL-2$^+$IFN-γ$^+$ **(H)**, and IL-2$^+$TNF-α$^+$IFN-γ$^+$-secreting T cells **(C)** in response to the NH36 antigen, on day 15 and 28 post challenge. The total CD4$^+$ T cell frequencies are also represented **(F)**. Bars represent the mean + SE values of two-independent experiments (n = 5 mice per treatment in each experiment). Asterisks and horizontal lines show significant differences between treatments as disclosed by Mann–Whitney non-parametrical test.

triggering of the most potent CD4-Th1 immune response. This immune response determines the cure of VL, as evidenced by the significant reduction of spleen and liver parasite load and spleen and liver/relative weights, the long-lasting immunity and 100% of survival. On the other hand, NH36-primed DCs, which showed lower expression of CCR7 receptors and consequently lower migration capabilities (11), did not show an effective cure of VL. However, the direct effect of protection offered by F3 vaccination *via* DC-mediated mechanism against other *Leishmania* species, agents of visceral or cutaneous leishmaniasis, has not yet been investigated and this is a limitation.

The CCR7 expression on the surfaces of DCs is mandatory to ensure their correct movement toward lymph nodes. The geographical encounter of DCs and naive T lymphocytes occurs in secondary lymphoid organs (40). This important event is compromised in VL. The main mechanism that promotes the defective localization of DCs is dependent on the IL-10-mediated inhibition of the CCR7 expression. IL-10 reduced migration of DCs by 47% and decreased the DCs CCR7 expression, in *L. (L.) donovani*-infected mice (11). Treatment with anti-IL-10 monoclonal antibody even restored DC migration (11). We recently showed in BALB/c mice that, in contrast to the high IL-10 secretion observed in infected animals, F3-vaccinated and challenged mice showed absolutely no secretion of IL-10 (15, 21). In fact, we described that the FRYPRPKHCHTQVA and KFWCLVIDALKRIG CD4-epitopes of F3, promoted the secretion of TNF-α, but not of IL-10 (21). In the present investigation, secretion of IL-10 was present in infected animals, but was more reduced by the F3 than by the NH36 vaccine, as observed by their respective IFN-γ/IL-10 and TNF-α/IL-10 ratios, which characterize a Th1 response against the infection. These results can partially explain the sustained high CCR7 expression on DCs of thr F3-vaccinated mice and their correct migration capabilities.

In VL, the protective response to VL is compromised by the functional impediment of DCs, which no longer move toward the areas of secondary lymphoid organs, where T cells are located (11). This defect restricts the initial specific-T cell response to *Leishmania* infection (41). Immunization with NH36 and F3 were able to restore the functional impairment of CD11c$^+$ DCs by inducing CCR7/CCL19-mediated responses and protective immunity in VL. We explored the possible use of mature DCs obtained from mice previously immunized with the C-terminal F3 or the NH36 antigens, to recover protective responses in

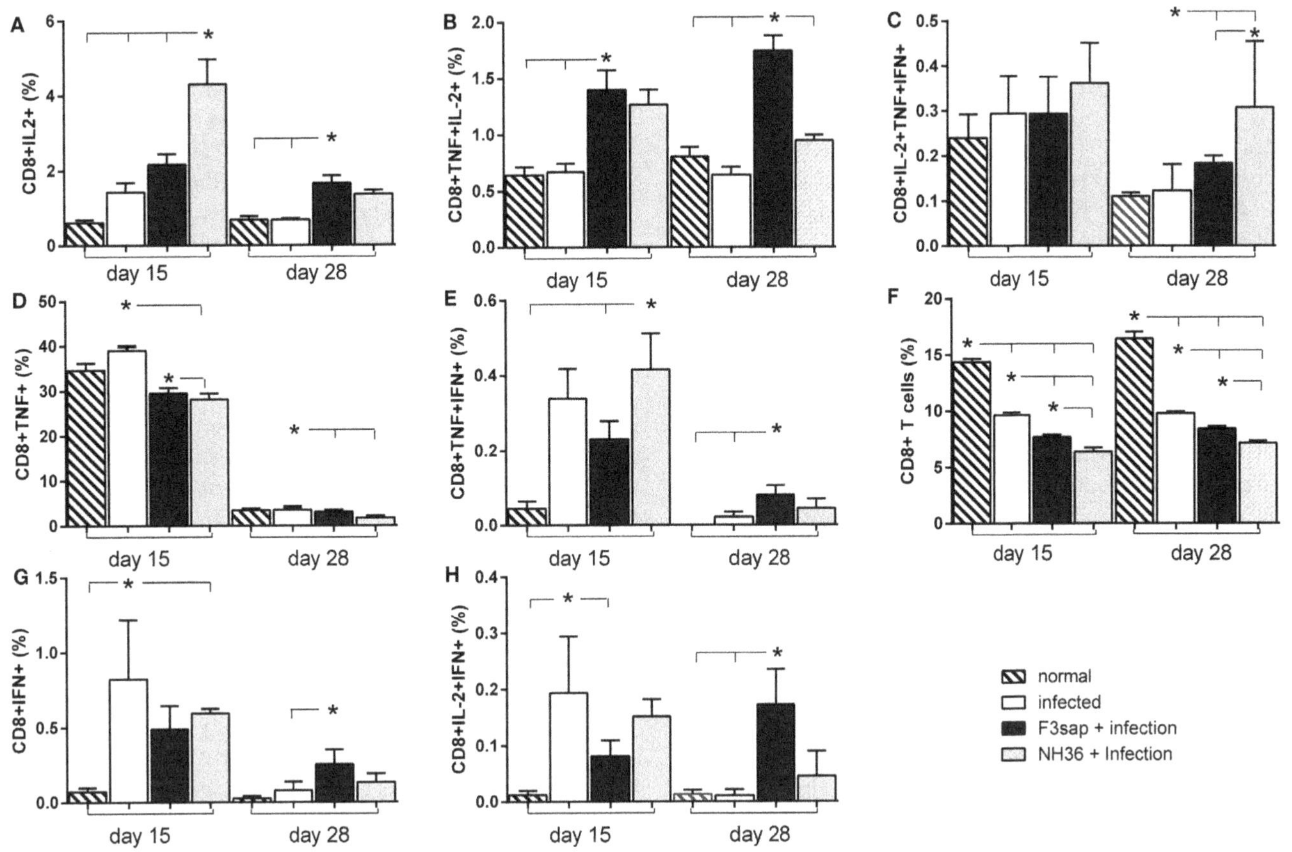

FIGURE 10 | Cytokines expressed by $CD8^+$ T lymphocytes in response to NH36. Effect of the F3 and NH36-vaccines on the frequencies of $CD8^+IL\text{-}2^+$ **(A)**, $TNF\text{-}\alpha^+$ **(D)**, $IFN\text{-}\gamma^+$ **(G)**, $TNF\text{-}\alpha^+IL\text{-}2^+$ **(B)**, $TNF\text{-}\alpha^+IFN\text{-}\gamma^+$ **(E)**, $IL\text{-}2^+IFN\text{-}\gamma^+$ **(H)**, and $IL\text{-}2^+TNF\text{-}\alpha^+IFN\text{-}\gamma^+$-secreting T cells **(C)** in response to the NH36 antigen, on day 15 and 28 post challenge. The total $CD8^+$ T cell frequencies are also represented **(F)**. Bars represent the mean + SE values of two-independent experiments (n = 5 mice per treatment in each experiment). Asterisks and horizontal lines show significant differences between treatments as disclosed by Mann–Whitney non-parametrical test.

L. (L.) infantum chagasi-infected mice. Our results indicate a clear immunotherapeutic effect in mice receiving the F3 antigen-primed DCs.

The work of Ato et al. (11), showed that normal naïve DCs preserve their migration capabilities and, in this way, help in immunotherapy of VL. However, they used DCs pre-pulsed with LPS and/or antigen to obtain a reduction of the spleen parasite load (11). We now showed that DCs of F3-vaccinated mice enhanced by 58% the migrating capabilities of DCs from normal mice *in vitro,* and without antigen or LPS pre-incubation, and also determined a 65% of reduction of spleen parasite load *in vivo.* While only 70% of DCs of normal naïve mice migrate to the wp of *L (L.) donovani*-infected mice (11), we demonstrated that 84% of DCs from F3-vaccinated mice preferentially migrated to the wp of *L. (L.) infantum chagasi*-infected mice. These effects explain the F3-vaccine usefulness and its higher efficacy in immunotherapy of VL, long-lasting preventive immune response and the 100% survival.

NH36 is a recombinant protein that was first described as the main native glycoprotein GP36 of the FML extract (42). The GP36-glycidic moiety is composed of short chains of 4-O-mannopyranose alternating with 3-O and 4-O-substituted fucopyranose residues (27) and its antigenicity is abolished by treatment with sodium m-periodate (27, 42). We, and others, further identified and cloned the NH36 gene and described its peptide sequence (36, 43). NH36 recombinant protein is a very strong and specific protein diagnostic antigen for human and canine VL (36, 44) and is recognized by mice antibodies (15, 21, 26). We proved that vaccination with the NH36 recombinant protein or DNA protect mice from visceral (15, 16, 18) and cutaneous leishmaniasis (16, 21, 26, 45), and controls canine VL (17). NH36 protein sequence, obtained in *E. coli* is now considered worldwide, as a very potent *Leishmania* antigen and a good candidate for an animal and human vaccine against leishmaniasis (15–21, 26, 37, 38, 45). Recently, the NH36 sequence was analyzed and four N-glycosylation sites represented by asparagine (Q) were found (46), but only two of them of high predictive value. As expected, the further cloning in *Pichia pastoris* enhanced the expressed protein yield but also, apparent molecular weight of NH36, suggesting the presence of high mannose chains (46). However, in order to avoid the glycoside moiety interference to the peptide antigenicity, the asparagine residues were mutated, and still, the un-glycosylated NH36 remained strongly antigenic (46).

Although the GP36 antigen in its native form, exhibits a glycidic moiety (27), it is the NH36 protein that is explored as an extremely successful antigen, and is the tool developed for effective vaccination (15–21, 26, 37, 38, 45). We showed that F3 is the strongest NH36 domain to be used in vaccination and, supporting our strategy, none of the four potential sites of glycosylation of NH36 are located in the F3 domain (amino acids N39, N77, N89, and N189) (46). Therefore, there would be no influence of any carbohydrate native moiety in the native form of the F3 antigen.

Trying to assess which are the receptors for F3 on DCs we previously studied the potential contribution of G-protein-coupled kinin receptors (B2R) in the protective immunity against mice VL induced by the F3-saponin vaccine (47). $B2R^{-/-}$ and wild type C57BL/6 controls ($B2R^{+/+}$) were vaccinated with F3 and saponin, challenged with amastigotes of *Leishmania (L.) infantum chagasi* and euthanized 30 days later. The IDR to leishmanial from $B2R^{-/-}$ vaccinated mice was lower than in wild type controls. Additionally, a significant decrease of 44.7% of spleen relative weight was noted in vaccinated $B2R^{+/+}$, but not in vaccinated $B2R^{-/-}$ mice, indicating that the B2R of kinin, present on the surface of DCs cells has a partial contribution to the protection against splenomegaly, induced by the F3 vaccine (47). The G protein-coupled bradykinin type 2 receptor (B2R) may couple different classes of G proteins and simultaneously initiate different signal chains, which have extensive cross-talk. In addition, the B2R receptor can generate mitogenic signals that involve the mitogen-activated protein kinases and transactivation of receptor tyrosine kinases (48). Therefore, the signaling pathway activated after recognition of F3 deserves further studies.

Additionally, MHC class II receptors on the surface of DCs of mice are potential targets of recognition of the epitopes of NH36. We recently described the induction of a mixed Th1/Th2 immunity in response to the FMLQILDFYTKVYE of F3, and in contrast, the generation of a main Th1 response, with a predominant TNF-α production and low IL-10 secretion induced by two final CD4-predicted epitopes of F3, FRYPRPKHCHTQVA, and KFWCLVIDALKRIG (21). The FRYPRPKHCHTQVA epitope is also the more potent enhancer of the $CD4^{+}TNF\text{-}\alpha^{+}$, $\text{-}IFN\text{-}\gamma^{+}$, $\text{-}TNF\text{-}\alpha^{+}IL\text{-}2^{+}$, $\text{-}TNF\text{-}\alpha^{+}IFN\text{-}\gamma^{+}$, and $\text{-}IFN\text{-}\gamma^{+}IL\text{-}2^{+}$ T cell proportions, confirming its capability to raise a specific Th1 response. Additionally, the multifunctional $IL\text{-}2^{+}TNF\text{-}\alpha^{+}IFN\text{-}\gamma^{+}$-secreting $CD4^{+}$ T-cells were raised only, in response to the FRYPRPKHCHTQVA and FMLQILDFYTKVYE (21).

NH36 is a strong phylogenetic marker of the genus *Leishmania*, which exhibits high identity of its amino acid sequence in all studied species of *Leishmania*. Hence, vaccination with NH36 in recombinant protein or DNA forms induced strong prophylactic effect against mice VL due to *L. (L.) donovani* and *L. (L.) infantum chagasi* (15, 16) and tegumentary leishmaniasis due to *L. (L.) amazonensis* (15, 21) and *L (L.) mexicana* (16).

However, recent advances in vaccinology demonstrate that vaccine-induced protection could be enhanced by the identification of the main domains or epitopes of the whole protein. In fact, vaccines that contain the short peptides, which represent the immunogenic epitopes, are able to optimize and even exceed the protective potential induced by the whole cognate protein (15, 21, 26, 49). These short peptide vaccines can also induce universal T cell responses, which are related to many human HLA-DR allotypes and to diverse mice strains (50, 51). This is the rationale of the development of T-epitope vaccines and it was also the guide for the development of the NH36 vaccines (15, 21, 26).

In fact, although 1 M of F3 (13,100 g/l) represents only 38% of 1 M of NH36 (34,240 g/l), its sequence is the most immunogenic in the NH36 molecule. The three $CD4^{+}$ T cell epitopes of NH36: FMLQILDFYTKVYE (1,810.13 g/l), FRYPRPKHCHTQVA (1,740.01 g/l), and KFWCLVIDALKRIG (1,620 g/l) correspond to a 42 amino acid sequence totally located in F3. Taken together, 1 M of these 42 amino acids (5,180 g/l) constitutes 39% of the sequence of the F3 peptide (13,100 KDa), which is composed of the last 115 amino acids of NH36, but represents only 15% of the sequence of the whole NH36 protein (34,240 KDa), which is composed of 314 amino acids. Therefore, although the most potent epitopes are also present in NH36, in the F3 domain they are 2.6 times more concentrated. That is why the F3 vaccine exceeds the protective potential of the NH36 whole protein. The superiority of the F3 peptide domains over the NH36 vaccine in prophylaxis was previously observed in several parasitological and immunological variables before and it was calculated according to the following equation = (F3-NH36/F3) values × 100 = protective effect increment (15, 26). This is a concept related to the purification yield of an active peptide by biochemical techniques. As expected, using that calculation we found a 36% average stronger protective response induced by the F3 vaccine against mice infection by *L. (L.) infantum chagasi* (15) and a 40% enhanced response against challenge by *L. (L.) amazonensis* (26). Accordingly, in this investigation, the F3 vaccine promoted an increment of 80% in the expression of CCR7, of 42% in the migration of DCs to the wp, and of 54% in the reduction of the spleen parasite load after immunotherapy induced by the F3 vaccine.

Although it is true that F3 holds the most important epitopes of NH36, the adaptive immune response starts with the interaction of DCs with lymphocytes, and the reasons why the F3 vaccine induced a higher expression of CCR7 and stronger migration of DCs than NH36 are not yet, fully understood.

F3 epitopes not only interact more than the rest of the NH36 epitopes with the G-protein-coupled kinin receptors (BR2) (47), but they are also more expressed more by the MHC class II receptors (15, 21, 26) and induce a higher expression of CCR7. However, the CCR7 expression alone does not guarantee the correct DC migration toward CCL19 or CCL21 gradients (52). A second signal, mediated by prostaglandin E2 (PGE2), is responsible for DC migration. The PGE2–EP4 axis is involved not only in migration, but also in upregulation of co-stimulatory molecules and increased T cells activation (52), and thus is, crucial for the development of the immune response. In contrast, activation of the liver X receptor (LXR)α interferes with CCR7 expression and migration of DCs resulting in a reduced immune response. PGE2 was recently demonstrated to downregulate LXRα expression in *ex vivo* DCs, by enhancing CCR7 expression and migration of LXR-activated DCs (52). These facts indicate that the F3 peptide and its epitopes, more than the whole NH36 antigen, not only promote the upregulated expression of CCR7, but also probably the PGE2 signaling and stimulation of DCs, which triggers the Th1 immune response against *Leishmania (L.) infantum chagasi*. This hypothesis deserves further studies.

Our findings suggest that DCs can be used in efficacious antigen transportation in vaccination protocols against VL (41). Other infection models using *Mycobacterium tuberculosis* (53), *Chlamydia trachomatis* (54), and other infectious diseases and cancer (55) have shown that immunizations performed with DCs previously incubated with the antigen, as natural adjuvant, can achieve the generation of protective pathogen-specific T cell responses. Although the use of DCs in immunotherapeutic protocols has been considered a promising tool to induce effective immunity against VL (41), the limitations of using DC base therapeutic immunization and prevention have also been extensively discussed (56, 57).

The main contribution of our investigation is the description of the enhancement of CCR7 expression and the migrating DCs capabilities generated by the F3 vaccine. This vaccine property might be an important trigger of the Th1 response and of an immunotherapeutic effect against VL.

ETHICS STATEMENT

All animals studies followed the guidelines set by the National Institutes of Health, USA, and the Institutional Animal Care and Use Committee approved the animal protocols (Comissão de Ética no Uso de Animais da Universidade Federal do Rio de Janeiro, CEUA protocol IMPPG040-07/16). All animal experimentation was performed in accordance with the terms of the Brazilian guidelines for the animal welfare regulations. Animals were kept at the Instituto de Microbiologia Paulo de Góes, da Universidade Federal do Rio de Janeiro (UFRJ) facilities, with controlled temperature, 12 h light/dark cycles and given water and feed *ad libitum*. We made all efforts in order to minimize animal suffering.

AUTHOR CONTRIBUTIONS

DN, AM, FA, and JM conducted the experiments. DN, AM, CF-d-L, LF-d-L, and FC acquired data. DN, FA, PL, CP-d-S analyzed data. CP-d-S, AM, and AMBM designed research studies. DN and CP-d-S wrote the manuscript. All authors have read and approved the final manuscript.

ACKNOWLEDGMENTS

The authors would like to acknowledge Dr. Maria Alice Fusco for kindly providing C57BL/6 mice from the Instituto de Pesquisas Biomédicas – Hospital Naval Marcílio Dias and Professor Leonardo R. Andrade of the Programa de Histologia, Instituto de Ciências Biomédicas, Universidade Federal do Rio de Janeiro, for kindly giving the NucBlue™ Life Ready probes™ Reagent. We also thank David Straker for language review.

SUPPLEMENTARY MATERIAL

FIGURE S1 | Schematic representation of dendritic cells (DCs) purification method and transwell experiment. DCs of mice vaccinated with F3 and challenged with *Leishmania (L.) infantum chagasi* migrate from the upper to the lower chamber of a transwell plate, in response to the CCL19 chemokine gradient. In contrast, DCs from unvaccinated infected mice are unresponsive to CCL19 and do not migrate.

FIGURE S2 | Strategy for the analysis of multifunctional T cell response using a four-color flow cytometry panel to simultaneously analyze multiple cytokines at the single-cell level in splenocytes cultures. After single cells selection (FSC-A × FSC-H), lymphocytes from a representative mouse immunized with the F3 vaccine were selected according to a FSC-A versus SSC-A dot plot, followed by $CD4^+$ **(A)** or $CD8^+$ **(B)** gating. Afterward, $CD4^+$ or $CD8^+$ T-cell phenotypes were plotted against each cytokine individually: interferon-γ (IFN-γ), tumor necrosis factor-α (TNF-α), and interleukin (IL)-2. Boolean gating was performed to generate the frequencies of the possible seven combinations of cytokine-producing $CD4^+$ or $CD8^+$ cells using FlowJo V10 software. In this demonstrative figure, we show the results obtained with splenocytes from an animal immunized with the F3 vaccine, 15 days after infection, stimulated "*in vitro*" with the NH36 recombinant protein.

FIGURE S3 | Cytokines expressed by $CD4^+$ T lymphocytes in response to *Leishmania (L.) infantum chagasi* lysate. Effect of the F3 and NH36-vaccines on the frequencies of $CD4^+IL\text{-}2^+$ **(A)**, $TNF\text{-}\alpha^+$ **(D)**, $IFN\text{-}\gamma^+$ **(G)**, $TNF\text{-}\alpha^+IL\text{-}2^+$ **(B)**, $TNF\text{-}\alpha^+IFN\text{-}\gamma^+$ **(E)**, $IL\text{-}2^+IFN\text{-}\gamma^+$ **(H)**, and $IL\text{-}2^+TNF\text{-}\alpha^+IFN\text{-}\gamma^+$-secreting T cells **(C)** in response to the promastigote lysate, on day 15 and 28 post challenge. The total $CD4^+$ T cell frequencies are also represented **(F)**. Bars represent the mean + SE values of two-independent experiments ($n = 5$ mice per treatment in each experiment). Asterisks and horizontal lines show significant differences between treatments as disclosed by Mann–Whitney non-parametrical test.

FIGURE S4 | Cytokines expressed by $CD8^+$ T lymphocytes to *Leishmania (L.) infantum chagasi* lysate. Effect of the F3 and NH36-vaccines on the frequencies of $CD8^+IL\text{-}2^+$ **(A)**, $TNF\text{-}\alpha^+$ **(D)**, $IFN\text{-}\gamma^+$ **(G)**, $TNF\text{-}\alpha^+IL\text{-}2^+$ **(B)**, $TNF\text{-}\alpha^+IFN\text{-}\gamma^+$ **(E)**, $IL\text{-}2^+IFN\text{-}\gamma^+$ **(H)**, and $IL\text{-}2^+TNF\text{-}\alpha^+IFN\text{-}\gamma^+$-secreting T cells **(C)** in response to the promastigote lysate, on day 15 and 28 post challenge. The total $CD8^+$ T cell frequencies are also represented **(F)**. Bars represent the mean + SE values of two-independent experiments ($n = 5$ mice per treatment in each experiment). Asterisks and horizontal lines show significant differences between treatments as disclosed by Mann–Whitney non-parametrical test.

REFERENCES

1. Yamey G. The world's most neglected diseases. Ignored by the pharmaceutical industry and by public-private partnerships. *BMJ* (2002) 325:176–7. doi:10.1136/bmj.325.7357.176
2. World Health Organization (WHO). Control of the leishmaniasis. *Report of a Meeting of the WHO Expert Commitee on the Control of Leishmaniases.* Geneva: WHO Technical Report Series (2010). 28 p. no. 949 Mar 22-26.
3. WHO. *Leishmaniasis, Epidemiological Situation.* Available from: http://www.who.int/leishmaniasis/burden/en/ (Accessed: June 26, 2017).

4. Palatnik-de-Sousa CB, Day MJ. One health: the global challenge of epidemic and endemic leishmaniasis. *Parasit Vectors* (2011) 4:197. doi:10.1186/1756-3305-4-197
5. Alvar J, Velez ID, Bern C, Herrero M, Desjeux P, Cano J, et al. Leishmaniasis worldwide and global estimates of its incidence. *PLoS One* (2012) 7:e35671. doi:10.1371/journal.pone.0035671
6. Banchereau J, Steinman RM. Dendritic cells and the control of immunity. *Nature* (1998) 392:245–52. doi:10.1038/32588
7. Palucka K, Banchereau J. Dendritic-cell-based therapeutic cancer vaccines. *Immunity* (2013) 39:38–48. doi:10.1016/j.immuni.2013.07.004
8. Engwerda CR, Ato M, Cotterell SEJ, Mynott TL, Taschannerl A, Gorak-Stolinska G, et al. A role for tumor necrosis factor-α in remodeling the splenic marginal zone during *Leishmania donovani* infection. *Am J Pathol* (2002) 161:429–37. doi:10.1016/S0002-9440(10)64199-5
9. Smelt SC, Engwerda CR, McCrossen M, Kaye PM. Destruction of follicular dendritic cells during chronic visceral leishmaniasis. *J Immunol* (1997) 158(8):3813–21.
10. Engwerda CR, Ato M, Kaye PM. Macrophages, pathology and parasite persistence in experimental visceral leishmaniasis. *Trends Parasitol* (2004) 20:524–30. doi:10.1016/j.pt.2004.08.009
11. Ato M, Stager S, Engwerda CR, Kaye PM. Defective CCR7 expression on dendritic cells contributes to the development of visceral leishmaniasis. *Nat Immunol* (2002) 3:1185–91. doi:10.1038/ni861
12. Cyster JG. Chemokines and cell migration in secondary lymphoid organs. *Science* (1999) 286:2098–102. doi:10.1126/science.286.5447.2098
13. Kellermann SA, Hudak S, Oldham ER, Liu YJ, McEvoy LM. The CC chemokine receptor-7 ligands 6Ckine and macrophage inflammatory protein-3 beta are potent chemoattractants for in vitro- and in vivo-derived dendritic cells. *J Immunol* (1999) 162:3859–64.
14. Nico D, Morrot A, Palatnik-de-Sousa CB. Vaccination with nucleoside hidrolase (NH36) of *L. (L.) donovani* or its C-terminal portion (F3) in formulation with saponin prevents the increase of the proportions of spleen dendritic cells in murine experimental visceral leishmaniasis. *Procedia Vaccinol* (2014) 8:58–61. doi:10.1016/j.provac.2014.07.010
15. Nico D, Claser C, Borja-Cabrera GP, Travassos LR, Palatnik M, Soares IS, et al. Adaptive immunity against *Leishmania* nucleoside hydrolase maps its C-terminal domain as the target of the CD4+ T cell-driven protective response. *PLoS Negl Trop Dis* (2010) 4(11):e866. doi:10.1371/journal.pntd.0000866
16. Aguilar-Be I, Zardo RS, Paraguai de Souza E, Borja-Cabrera GP, Rosado-Vallado M, Mut-Martin M, et al. Cross-protective efficacy of a prophylactic *Leishmania donovani* DNA vaccine against visceral and cutaneous murine leishmaniasis. *Infect Immun* (2005) 73:812–9. doi:10.1128/IAI.73.2.812-819.2005
17. Borja-Cabrera GP, Santos FB, Nico D, Gravino AE, Manna L, Palatnik M, et al. The Leishmune®'s nucleoside hydrolase DNA vaccine as an aid in immunotherapy of canine visceral leishmaniasis. *Procedia Vaccinol* (2012) 6:64–73. doi:10.1016/j.provac.2012.04.009
18. Gamboa-León R, Paraguai de Souza E, Borja Cabrera GP, Santos FN, Miyashiro LM, Pinheiro RO, et al. Immunotherapy against visceral leishmaniasis with the nucleoside hydrolase-DNA vaccine of *L. donovani*. *Vaccine* (2006) 24:4863–73. doi:10.1016/j.vaccine.2006.03.005
19. Barbosa Santos ML, Nico D, de Oliveira FA, Barreto AS, Palatnik-de-Sousa I, Carrillo E, et al. *Leishmania donovani* nucleoside hydrolase (NH36) domains induce T-cell cytokine responses in human visceral leishmaniasis. *Front Immunol* (2017) 8:227. doi:10.3389/fimmu.2017.00227
20. Carrillo E, Fernandez L, Ibarra-Meneses AV, Santos MLB, Nico D, de Luca PM, et al. F1 domain of the *Leishmania donovani* nucleoside hydrolase promotes a Th1 response in *Leishmania infantum* cured patients and in asymptomatic individuals living in an endemic area of leishmaniasis. *Front Immunol* (2017) 8:750. doi:10.3389/fimmu.2017.00750
21. Alves-Silva MV, Nico D, Morrot A, Palatnik M, Palatnik-de-Sousa CB. A chimera containing CD4+ and CD8+ T-cell epitopes of the *Leishmania donovani*-nucleoside hydrolase NH36 optimizes cross-protection against *Leishmania amazonesis* infection. *Front Immunol* (2017) 8:100. doi:10.3389/fimmu.2017.00100
22. Moore EM, Lockwood DN. Treatment of visceral leishmaniasis. *J Glob Infect Dis* (2010) 2:151–8. doi:10.4103/0974-777X.62883
23. Maltezou HC. Drug resistance in visceral leishmaniasis. *J Biomed Biotechnol* (2010) 2010:617521. doi:10.1155/2010/617521
24. Freitas EO, Nico D, Alves-Silva MV, Morrot A, Clinch K, Evans GB, et al. Immucillins ImmA and ImmH are effective and non-toxic in the treatment of experimental visceral leishmaniasis. *PLoS Negl Trop Dis* (2015) 9:e0004297. doi:10.1371/journal.pntd.0004297
25. Bradley DJ, Kirkley J. Regulation of *Leishmania* populations within the host. I. the variable course of *Leishmania donovani* infections in mice. *Clin Exp Immunol* (1977) 30:119–29.
26. Nico D, Gomes DC, Alves-Silva MV, Freitas EO, Morrot A, Bahia D, et al. Cross-protective immunity to *Leishmania amazonensis* is mediated by CD4+ and CD8+ epitopes of *Leishmania donovani* nucleoside hydrolase terminal domains. *Front Immunol* (2014) 5:189. doi:10.3389/fimmu.2014.00189
27. Palatnik-de-Sousa CB, Barbosa Ade F, Oliveira SM, Nico D, Bernardo RR, Santos WR, et al. The FML-vaccine against canine visceral leishmaniasis: from the second generation to the synthetic vaccine. *Expert Rev Vaccines* (2008) 7:833–51. doi:10.1586/14760584.7.6.833
28. Stober CB, Jeronimo SM, Pontes NN, Miller EN, Blackwell JM. Cytokine responses to novel antigens in a peri-urban population in Brazil exposed to *Leishmania infantum chagasi*. *Am J Trop Med Hyg* (2012) 87:663–70. doi:10.4269/ajtmh.2012.12-0180
29. Matter MS, Hilmenyuk T, Claus C, Marone R, Schürch C, Tinguely M, et al. Destruction of lymphoid organ architecture and hepatitis caused by CD4+ T cells. *PLoS One* (2011) 6:e24772. doi:10.1371/journal.pone.0024772
30. Oliva G, Nieto J, Foglia Manzillo V, Cappiello S, Fiorentino E, Di Muccio T, et al. A randomised, double-blind, controlled efficacy trial of the LiESP/QA-21 vaccine in naïve dogs exposed to two *Leishmania infantum* transmission seasons. *PLoS Negl Trop Dis* (2014) 8:e3213. doi:10.1371/journal.pntd.0003213
31. Carcelén J, Iniesta V, Fernández-Cotrina J, Serrano F, Parejo JC, Corraliza I, et al. The chimerical multi-component Q protein from *Leishmania* in the absence of adjuvant protects dogs against an experimental *Leishmania infantum* infection. *Vaccine* (2009) 27:5964–73. doi:10.1016/j.vaccine.2009.07.069
32. Fernandes AP, Coelho EA, Machado-Coelho GL, Grimaldi G Jr, Gazzinelli RT. Making an anti-amastigote vaccine for visceral leishmaniasis: rational, update and perspectives. *Curr Opin Microbiol* (2012) 15:476–85. doi:10.1016/j.mib.2012.05.002
33. Palatnik-de-Sousa CB, Silva-Antunes I, Morgado Ade A, Menz I, Palatnik M, Lavor C. Decrease of the incidence of human and canine visceral leishmaniasis after dog vaccination with Leishmune in Brazilian endemic areas. *Vaccine* (2009) 27:3505–12. doi:10.1016/j.vaccine.2009.03.045
34. Saraiva EM, de Figueiredo Barbosa A, Santos FN, Borja-Cabrera GP, Nico D, Souza LO, et al. The FML-vaccine (Leishmune®) against canine visceral leishmaniasis: a transmission blocking vaccine. *Vaccine* (2006) 24:2423–31. doi:10.1016/j.vaccine.2005.11.061
35. Nogueira FS, Moreira MAB, Borja Cabrera GP, Santos FN, Menz I, Parra LE, et al. Leishmune ® vaccine blocks the transmission of canine visceral leishmaniasis. Absence of *Leishmania* parasites in blood, skin and lymph nodes of vaccinated exposed dogs. *Vaccine* (2005) 23:4805–10. doi:10.1016/j.vaccine.2005.05.011
36. Santana DM, Paraguai de Souza E, Borja-Cabrera GP, Sturm NR, Palatnik de Sousa CB, Campbell DA. Nucleoside hydrolase from *Leishmania (L.) donovani* is an antigen diagnostic for visceral leishmaniasis. *Mol Biochem Parasitol* (2002) 120:315–9. doi:10.1016/S0166-6851(02)00010-5
37. Coler RN, Duthie MS, Hofmeyer KA, Guderian J, Jayashankar L, Vergara J, et al. From mouse to man: safety, immunogenicity and efficacy of a candidate leishmaniasis vaccine LEISH-F3+GLA-SE. *Clin Transl Immunology* (2015) 4:e35. doi:10.1038/cti.2015.6
38. Costa MM, Penido M, dos Santos MS, Doro D, de Freitas E, Michalick MS, et al. Improved canine and human visceral leishmaniasis immunodiagnosis using combinations of synthetic peptides in enzyme-linked immunosorbent assay. *PLoS Negl Trop Dis* (2012) 6:e1622. doi:10.1371/journal.pntd.0001622
39. Seder RA, Darrah PA, Roederer M. T cell quality in memory and protection: implications for vaccine design. *Nat Rev Immunol* (2008) 8(4):247–58. doi:10.1038/nri2274
40. Hansson M, Lundgren A, Elgbratt K, Quiding-Järbrink M, Svennerholm AM, Johansson EL. Dendritic cells express CCR7 and migrate in response to CCL19 (MIP-3beta) after exposure to *Helicobacter pylori*. *Microbes Infect* (2006) 8:841–50. doi:10.1016/j.micinf.2005.10.007
41. Moll H, Berberich C. Dendritic cell-based vaccination strategies: induction of protective immunity against leishmaniasis. *Immunobiology* (2001) 204:659–66. doi:10.1078/0171-2985-00105

42. Palatnik de Sousa CB, Dutra HS, Borojevic R. *Leishmania donovani* surface glycoproteins GP36, is the major immunogen component of the fucose mannose ligand (FML). *Acta Trop* (1993) 53:59–72. doi:10.1016/0001-706X(93)90006-W
43. Cui L, Rajasekariah GR, Martin SK. A nonspecific nucleoside hydrolase from *Leishmania donovani*: implications for purine salvage by the parasite. *Gene* (2001) 280:153–62. doi:10.1016/S0378-1119(01)00768-5
44. Palatnik de Sousa CB, Gomes EM, de Souza EP, dos Santos WR, de Macedo SR, de Medeiros LV, et al. The FML (fucose mannose ligand) of *Leishmania donovani*. a new tool in diagnosis, prognosis, transfusional control and vaccination against human kala-azar. *Rev Soc Bras Med Trop* (1996) 29:153–63. doi:10.1590/S0037-86821996000200008
45. Souza LOP, Palatnik de Sousa CB. The Nucleoside hydrolase DNA vaccine VR1012NH36 in prophylactic vaccination against mice tegumentar leishmaniaisis. *Procedia Vaccinol* (2009) 1:120–3. doi:10.1016/j.provac.2009.07.022
46. Hudspeth EM, Wang Q, Seid CA, Hammond M, Wei J, Liu Z, et al. Expression and purification of an engineered, yeast-expressed *Leishmania donovani* nucleoside hydrolase with immunogenic properties. *Hum Vaccin Immunother* (2016) 12:1707–20. doi:10.1080/21645515.2016.1139254
47. Nico D, Feijó DF, Scharfstein J, Morrot A, Palatnik de Sousa CB. Partial contribution of the B2 receptor of the kinin inflammation pathway in protection against murine visceral leishmaniasis by the C-terminal domain of nucleoside hydrolase vaccine. *Abstract of the 5th Elsevier Vaccine and ISV Annual Global Congress*. Seattle, USA (2011).
48. Liebmann C, Böhmer FD. Signal transduction pathways of G protein-coupled receptors and their cross-talk with receptor tyrosine kinases: lessons from bradykinin signaling. *Curr Med Chem* (2000) 7:911–43. doi:10.2174/0929867003374589
49. Kao DJ, Hodges RS. Advantages of a synthetic peptide immunogen over a protein immunogen in the development of an anti-pilus vaccine for *Pseudomonas aeruginosa*. *Chem Biol Drug Res* (2009) 74:33–42. doi:10.1111/j.1747-0285.2009.00825
50. Parra-López C, Calvo-Calle M, Cameron TO, Vargas LE, Salazar LM, Patarroyo ME, et al. Major histocompatibility complex and T cell interactions of a universal T-cell epitope from *Plasmodium falciparum* circumsporozoite protein. *J Biol Chem* (2006) 281:14907–17. doi:10.1074/jbc.M511571200
51. Moreno A, Clavijo P, Edelman R, Davis J, Sztein M, Sinigaglia F, et al. CD4+ T cell clones obtained from *Plasmodium falciparum* sporozoite-immunized volunteers recognize polymorphic sequences of the circumsporozoite protein. *J Immunol* (1993) 151:489–99.
52. Bruckner M, Dickel D, Singer E, Legler DF. Converse regulation of CCR7-driven human dendritic cell migration by prostaglandin E_2 and liver X receptor activation. *Eur J Immunol* (2012) 42:2949–58. doi:10.1002/eji.201242523
53. Satake Y, Nakamura Y, Kono M, Hozumi H, Nagata T, Tsujimura K, et al. Type-1 polarised dendritic cells are a potent immunogen against *Mycobacterium tuberculosis*. *Int J Tuberc Lung Dis* (2017) 21:523–30. doi:10.5588/ijtld.16.0371
54. Su H, Messer R, Whitmire W, Fischer E, Portis JC, Caldwell HD. Vaccination against chlamydial genital tract infection after immunization with dendritic cells pulsed ex vivo with nonviable chlamydiae. *J Exp Med* (1998) 188:809–18. doi:10.1084/jem.188.5.809
55. Banchereau J, Schuler-Thurner B, Palucka AK, Schuler G. Dendritic cells as vectors for therapy. *Cell* (2001) 106:271–4. doi:10.1016/S0092-8674(01)00448-2
56. Kalinski P, Urban J, Narang R, Berk E, Wieckowski E, Muthuswamy R. Dendritic cell-based therapeutic cancer vaccines: what we have and what we need. *Future Oncol* (2009) 5:379–90. doi:10.2217/fon.09.6
57. Chen P, Liu X, Sun Y, Zhou P, Wang Y, Zhang Y. Dendritic cell targeted vaccines: recent progresses and challenges. *Hum Vaccin Immunother* (2016) 12:612–22. doi:10.1080/21645515.2015.1105415

7

Nuclear Receptor Nur77 Deficiency Alters Dendritic Cell Function

*Nina Tel-Karthaus[1], Esther D. Kers-Rebel[1], Maaike W. Looman[1], Hiroshi Ichinose[2], Carlie J. de Vries[3] and Marleen Ansems[1]**

[1] Department of Radiation Oncology, Radiotherapy & OncoImmunology Laboratory, Radboud Institute for Molecular Life Sciences, Radboud University Medical Center, Nijmegen, Netherlands, [2] School of Life Science and Technology, Tokyo Institute of Technology, Yokohama, Japan, [3] Department of Medical Biochemistry, Academic Medical Center, Amsterdam Cardiovascular Sciences, Amsterdam, Netherlands

***Correspondence:**
Marleen Ansems
marleen.ansems@radboudumc.nl

Dendritic cells (DCs) are the professional antigen-presenting cells of the immune system. Proper function of DCs is crucial to elicit an effective immune response against pathogens and to induce antitumor immunity. Different members of the nuclear receptor (NR) family of transcription factors have been reported to affect proper function of immune cells. Nur77 is a member of the NR4A subfamily of orphan NRs that is expressed and has a function within the immune system. We now show that Nur77 is expressed in different murine DCs subsets *in vitro* and *ex vivo*, in human monocyte-derived DCs (moDCs) and in freshly isolated human BDCA1$^+$ DCs, but its expression is dispensable for DC development in the spleen and lymph nodes. We show, by siRNA-mediated knockdown of Nur77 in human moDCs and by using Nur77$^{-/-}$ murine DCs, that Nur77-deficient DCs have enhanced inflammatory responses leading to increased T cell proliferation. Treatment of human moDCs with 6-mercaptopurine, an activator of Nur77, leads to diminished DC activation resulting in an impaired capacity to induce IFNγ production by allogeneic T cells. Altogether, our data show a yet unexplored role for Nur77 in modifying the activation status of murine and human DCs. Ultimately, targeting Nur77 may prove to be efficacious in boosting or diminishing the activation status of DCs and may lead to the development of improved DC-based immunotherapies in, respectively, cancer treatment or treatment of autoimmune diseases.

Keywords: dendritic cells, dendritic cell-based immunotherapy, nuclear receptors, NR4A, Nur77

INTRODUCTION

Dendritic cells (DCs) are professional antigen-presenting cells. An important function of DCs is to instruct T cells to elicit immunity or tolerance (1, 2). Many factors contribute to the way DCs are shaped to elicit this function. Important factors are the type of pathogens that DCs encounter, such as bacteria or viruses, but also different microenvironmental factors in the tissues they reside in play a crucial role. DCs can be subdivided into classical or conventional DCs (cDC), interferon-producing plasmacytoid DCs (pDC), and monocyte-derived DCs (moDC) each with their own specialized function (3–5). Because of their crucial role in the immune system, different subsets of DCs are exploited in immune therapy (6–15). So far, treatment success is limited and functional knowledge on how DCs initiate and stably steer antitumor responses *in vivo* is important (13–15). Identification of transcription factors that control DC function in both immunity and tolerance is highly relevant, as these factors may serve as targets to modulate DC activity and function for the development of more successful DC-based immunotherapies.

Different members of the nuclear receptor (NR) family of transcription factors and their ligands have been shown to affect immune cells, including DCs (16–20). NRs are ligand inducible transcription factors having among others, steroid hormones or cellular metabolites as ligands. Several members have been well studied and were shown to play an immune modulatory role in DCs. Another group of NRs are so called "orphan" NRs for which no natural ligand has been identified yet, and the existence of ligands is disputed. The NR4A subfamily of orphan receptors comprises three members, namely, Nur77 (NR4A1/TR3/NGFI-B), Nurr1 (NR4A2/NOT/TINUR), and NOR-1 (NR4A3/TEC/MINOR). Their activity appears to be primarily regulated at the expression level. The expression of the NR4As can be induced by a diverse range of signals, including fatty acids, stress, growth factors, cytokines, peptide hormones, and physical stimuli (21). Hallmark of this subfamily is to respond quickly to such changes in cellular environments and regulate gene expression in a ligand-independent manner.

Members of this subfamily have been shown to be involved in a wide variety of pathological conditions. They have been shown to be dysregulated in multiple cancer types and promote or suppress tumors depending on specific cellular and tissue context, subcellular localization, external stimuli, protein–protein interactions, and post-translational modifications in cancer cells [reviewed in Ref. (22)]. In addition, there is also increasing evidence that the NR4As play a role in neurodegenerative disorders such as Alzheimer's and Parkinson's disease by contributing to neuronal cell death *via* modulating mitochondrial function and ER stress by controlling intracellular levels of ROS and Ca^{2+} and regulating cellular autophagy (23–26). Also in autoimmune-driven central nervous system (CNS) inflammation, the NR4A NRs have been shown to play an important role (27, 28).

NR4A receptors have emerged to play an important role within the immune balance by transcriptional regulation of cytokines and growth factors in macrophages (29, 30). In addition, they have been shown to be involved in the negative selection of self-reactive T cell clones in the thymus (31, 32) and are essential for thymic regulatory T cell development (33). Studies in $Nur77^{-/-}$ mice imply that Nur77 functions as a master regulator in the differentiation and survival of $Ly\text{-}6C^{-}$ monocytes (34, 35). $Ly\text{-}6C^{+}$ and $Ly\text{-}6C^{-}$ monocytes that do express Nur77 do not develop into moDCs (36). Thus, Nur77 expression is not required for the development into moDCs but is for differentiation of $Ly\text{-}6C^{+}$ monocytes into $Ly\text{-}6C^{-}$ "patrolling" monocytes (34, 36). Moreover, Nur77 has been shown to be involved in the polarization of macrophages toward an inflammatory phenotype important in atherosclerosis (37, 38).

We and others have recently reported expression of Nur77, Nurr1, and NOR-1 in murine DCs (39–43). Nurr1 has been shown to restrict the immunogenicity of bone marrow derived DCs (BMDCs) (43) and NOR-1 leads to activation-induced cell death in DCs (39), is important in DC migration (42), and is involved in TLR-mediated activation and gene expression of DCs (44). However, so far, the role of Nur77 expression in DCs remains elusive. We here set out to assess the expression kinetics and function of Nur77 in multiple subsets of murine and human DCs and its subsequent effect on inducing T cell activation, revealing a function as activation modulator for Nur77 in DCs. Knowledge regarding the possibilities in altering the activation status of DCs may prove to be beneficial in improving DC-based vaccination strategies.

MATERIALS AND METHODS

Mice

6- to 16-week-old C57BL/6J and Balb/C mice (Charles River), $Nur77^{-/-}$ mice (45) on a C57BL/6 background, and $Nur77^{GFP}$ mice [016607; C57BL/6-Tg(Nr4a1-EGFP/cre)820Khog/J; Jackson Laboratory] were housed under specific pathogen-free conditions in individually ventilated cage units at the Central Animal Laboratory (Nijmegen, The Netherlands). Standard laboratory chow and sterile drinking water were provided *ad libitum*. All animal experiments were approved by the Radboud University's Animal Welfare Body (*Instantie voor Dierenwelzijn IvD*) and the Animal Experiment Committee (*DierExperimentenCommissie, RUDEC*) that is recognized by the CCD (Central Authority for Scientific Procedures on Animals). The experiments were performed according to institutional, national, and European guidelines as stipulated in the *Wet op de dierproeven* and in the *Dierproevenbesluit*.

In Vitro Generation of Murine DCs

DCs were generated from murine BM isolated from the femur/tibia of the mice. To obtain pDCs and cDCs, cells were cultured for 8–10 days (37°C, 10% CO_2) in RPMI 1640 supplemented with 10% fetal calf serum (Gibco-BRL Life Technologies), 0.5% antibiotic–antimycotic (Gibco/Invitrogen), 1% ultra-glutamine (Lonza), 50 µM β-mercaptoethanol (Sigma-Aldrich), and 200 ng/ml human rFlt3L (PeproTech). Pure cell populations were isolated by labeling single cell suspensions with anti-SiglecH-FITC (eBiosciences) and anti-CD11c-APC antibodies for pDCs and cDCs, respectively. pDCs were positively sorted with anti-FITC microbeads, the negative fraction was subjected to positive selection with anti-APC microbeads (both Miltenyi Biotec, Germany) to obtain cDCs as described previously (40). $CD103^{+}$ murine DCs were generated by culturing BM cells in RPMI 1640 supplemented with 10% FCS, 0.5% antibiotic–antimycotic, 1% ultra-glutamine, 50 µM β-mercaptoethanol, 5 ng/ml mGM-CSF, and 200 ng/ml human rFlt3L, fresh medium was added at day 6, and cells were replated in fresh medium at day 9. Cells were harvested and used for experiments at day 14. The purity of the isolated DC subsets was ensured by flow cytometry.

Tumor Induction

The transgenic cell line 9464D was derived from spontaneous tumors from TH-MYCN transgenic mice on C57BL/6 background and were a kind gift from Dr. Orentas (NIH, Bethesda, MD, USA). 9464D cells were cultured in DMEM containing 10% fetal calf serum, 1% non-essential amino acids, 0.5% antibiotic–antimycotic, and 50 µM β-mercaptoethanol. For induction of tumors, 1 × 10e6 9464D cells were injected s.c. in 100 µl PBS on the right flank of the mice. Tumor growth was measured every 3–4 days using calipers. Spleen and lymph nodes (LNs) of the mice were taken when the tumor was more than 5 mm in diameter.

Flow Cytometry

To obtain single cells for flow cytometric staining, murine spleen was passaged over a 100 µm cell strainer, and murine LNs were incubated in serum-free medium containing collagenase (Worthington) and DNAseI (Roche), later supplemented with 1 mM EDTA. *In vitro* generated human and murine DCs, and *ex vivo* isolated murine spleen and LN cells were stained using standard antibody staining protocols with antibodies listed in Table S1 in Supplementary Material. Cell viability was assessed by staining with fixable viability dye eFluor™ 450 (eBioscience). Samples were acquired on a FACS Verse (BD Bioscience), and data were analyzed with FlowJo software (Tree Star).

ELISA

Human and mouse IL-6, TNFα, IL-12p70, and human IFNγ present in the supernatant of DC cultures was measured using the ELISA kit (Thermo Fisher) according to the manufacturers protocol.

Murine Type I IFN Bioassay

Type I IFN activity in the supernatant of murine pDCs was measured using L929 cells transfected with an interferon-sensitive luciferase construct (ISRE-L929) (46) with reference to a recombinant mouse IFN-β standard (Sigma). In short, pDC culture supernatants were added to ISRE-L929 IFN reporter cells and incubated for 4–6 h. Then, the cells were lysed in Passive Lysis Buffer (Promega), mixed with firefly luciferin substrate (Promega), and measured on a Victor3 Luminometer.

Mixed Leukocyte Reaction (MLR) Murine DCs

After 16–24 h of stimulation with 1 µg/ml CpGB (1668, Sigma-Aldrich) or 4 µg/ml R848, pDCs, cDCs, or CD103+ DCs were washed and co-incubated with carboxyfluorescein diacetate succinimidyl ester (CFSE)-labeled allogeneic BalB/C T cells. T cells were isolated using the T cell isolation kit (EasySep). The cells were co-incubated for 3 days in round-bottom 96-well cluster plates (Corning). T cell proliferation was measured by CFSE dilution by FACS.

Generation of Human DCs

DCs were generated from cells isolated from buffy coats obtained from healthy volunteers (Sanquin, Nijmegen, The Netherlands) after written informed consent as per the Declaration of Helsinki. The study was approved by the Institutional Review Board of the Radboud University Nijmegen Medical Center, Commissie Mensgebonden Onderzoek. Peripheral blood mononuclear cells (PBMCs) were purified *via* Ficoll density gradient centrifugation (Lucron Bioproducts). moDCs were cultured as described previously (47). In short, plastic-adherent monocytes were cultured for 6 days in RPMI 1640 medium with 1% ultra-glutamine, 0.5% antibiotic–antimycotic, 10% (v/v) fetal calf serum, 300 U/ml IL4, and 450 U/ml GM-CSF (both Cellgenix). IL4 and GM-CSF were added again at day 3. To obtain fresh human myeloid dendritic cells (mDCs), CD14+ cells were depleted from the PBMCs followed by BDCA1+ DC isolation using the CD1c (BDCA1)+ Dendritic Cell Isolation Kit (Miltenyi Biotec). Purity of the freshly isolated mDCs was ensured by flow cytometry.

Small Interfering RNA-Mediated Knockdown

For Nur77 silencing in human moDCs, the ON-TARGETplus SMARTpool NR4A1 (Dharmacon) containing four different Nur77 targeting siRNA oligos each 19 nt long was used. The irrelevant siRNA ON-TARGETplus Non-Targeting siRNA#1 (Dharmacon) was used as control. moDCs were electroporated at day 4 as described before (47). Electroporated DCs were stimulated with 1 µg/ml LPS (Sigma) or 4 µg/ml R848 (Enzo Life Sciences) at day 6. Supernatant was taken 24 h later.

RNA Isolation and Quantitative PCR

Total RNA was isolated and cDNA was synthesized as described before (47). mRNA levels for the genes of interest were determined with a CFX96 sequence detection system (Bio-Rad) using the Faststart SYBR green mastermix (Roche) with SYBR Green as the fluorophore and gene-specific oligonucleotide primers. The primers for human porphobilinogen deaminase (PBGD), IL-6, TNFα, and IL-12 (47) and murine PBGD, TLR7, and TLR9 (40) were described previously. Other primers used (forward and reverse) are listed in Table S2 in Supplementary Material. Reaction mixtures and program conditions were used that were recommended by the manufacturer (Bio-Rad). Quantitative PCR data were analyzed with the CFX Manager V1.6.541.1028 software (Bio-Rad) and checked for correct amplification and dissociation of the products. As we described previously for human and murine DCs, mRNA levels of the genes of interest were normalized to mRNA levels of the housekeeping gene PBGD (19, 20, 40, 47, 48) and were calculated according to the cycle threshold method (49).

Human MLR

Human day 6 moDCs were pretreated with 1 or 10 µM 6-mercaptopurine (6-MP) (Sigma) or vehicle control (DMSO) for 8 h, before o/n stimulation with 4 µg/ml R848. At day 7, the medium was replaced with fresh DC medium, and allogeneic peripheral blood lymphocytes were added to the DCs, in a ratio of 1:10 (DCs:T cells) and cocultured for 144 h. Supernatant was taken for IFNγ measurements.

Statistical Analysis

In each experiment, at least three mice or human donors were used to be able to perform statistical testing. Each legend contains the information of the number of mice or human donors used including the statistics that was used to calculate significance. Statistical testing was performed using GraphPad Prism 5 software (GraphPad, La Jolla, CA, USA). A $P < 0.05$ was considered significant.

RESULTS

Nur77 Expression and Function in Murine DCs

As NR4A NRs are typical early response genes induced upon stimulation (29), we tested Nur77 expression in cDCs and pDCs 3 h after stimulation with a combination of the TLR7/8 ligand R848 and the TLR9 ligand CpG. DCs were differentiated from murine BM *in vitro* with FLT3L as this reflects physiologic DC development and gives rise to a mixture of both cDCs and pDCs (50). pDCs were detected as CD11c^{pos}B220^{pos}SiglecH^{pos} and cDCs were defined as CD11c^{pos}B220^{neg}SiglecH^{neg} and were sorted and stimulated as described before (40) (Figure S1A in Supplementary Material). In agreement with its classification as early response gene, Nur77 mRNA levels were strongly upregulated after 3 h of stimulation in murine pDCs as well as cDCs compared with freshly sorted cells (0 h) (**Figure 1A**). To further assess Nur77 expression kinetics, we used BM cells from transgenic Nur77 reporter mice, where the induction of the Nur77 promoter drives GFP expression (Nur77^{GFP}) (51). In line with its mRNA expression, cDCs and to a lesser extend pDCs up regulate Nur77^{GFP} already after 3 h of stimulation with CpG (**Figure 1B**). In addition to FLT3L-derived BMDCs, we tested Nur77^{GFP} in BMDCs differentiated into Batf3-dependent CD103$^+$ DCs (CD11c^{pos}B220^{neg}CD103^{pos}) when cultured with GM-CSF and FLT3L (52) (for gating strategy see Figure S1B in Supplementary Material). In CD103$^+$ DCs, there is also already prominent expression of Nur77^{GFP} after 3 h stimulation with CpG (**Figure 1B**). Our data further show that the expression in cDCs was highest after CpG and LPS stimulation, whereas the expression was less pronounced in response to R848. pDC and CD103$^+$ DCs revealed highest expression of Nur77^{GFP} after stimulation with CpG, compared with LPS and R848 (**Figure 1C**). These data indicate that in different types of *in vitro* generated DCs, Nur77 expression is quickly induced upon stimulation with inflammatory ligands, and that the expression in response to TLR-specific agonists varies in different DC subsets.

Nur77 Does Not Have a Major Impact on the Development of Murine DCs in Spleen and LNs

To test whether Nur77 expression is required for the development of DCs, we investigated the presence of different DC subsets in spleen and LNs of WT and Nur77$^{-/-}$ mice. We observed a small but significant increase in the percentage of total CD11c^{hi}MHCII^{hi} DCs and in CD11b$^+$ DCs (CD11c^{hi} MHCII^{hi}Sirpα^{pos}CD24^{neg}CD115^{neg}CD4^{pos}) of the spleen of Nur77$^{-/-}$ mice relative to WT mice (**Figure 2A**; Figure S2A in Supplementary Material). The number of CD8α$^+$ spleen DCs (CD11c^{hi}MHCII^{hi}Sirpα^{neg}CD24^{pos}FLT3^{pos}) was similar between WT and Nur77$^{-/-}$ mice. Also in the LNs, the presence of resident

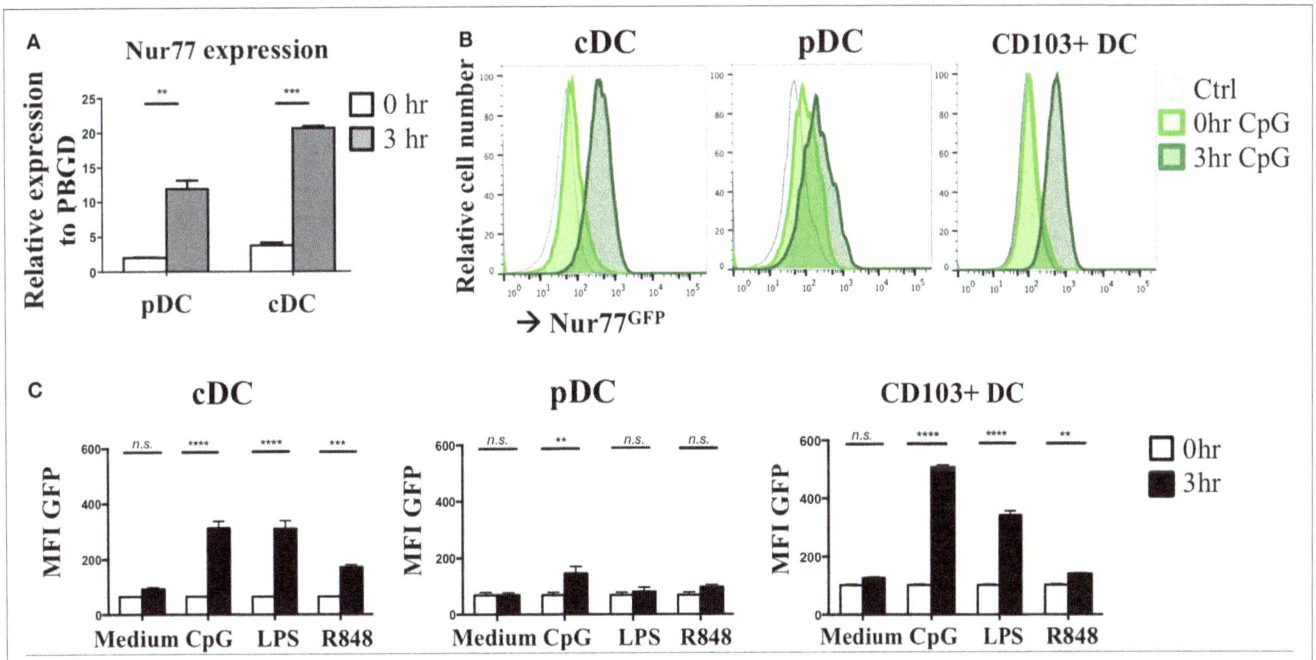

FIGURE 1 | Nur77 expression level in *in vitro* generated murine dendritic cells (DCs). **(A)** Plasmacytoid DCs (pDCs) and conventional DCs (cDCs) were sorted from FLT3L bone marrow cultures pooled from three mice per experiment and immediately lysed for RNA isolation (0 h) or stimulated for 3 h with a combination of R848 and CpG. mRNA expression levels of Nur77 were detected by qPCR analysis. Data shown are the mean of three independent experiments ± SEM, two-tailed unpaired *t*-test: $^*P < 0.05$; $^{**}P < 0.01$; and $^{***}P < 0.001$. **(B)** *In vitro* generated cDCs, pDCs, or CD103$^+$ DCs from Nur77^{GFP} or control mice were stimulated for the indicated times with CpG, and GFP expression was determined by flow cytometry. Shown are the representative data of three mice. **(C)** Quantification of Nur77^{GFP} expression in cDC, pDC, or CD103$^+$ DC stimulated with CpG, LPS, or R848 for 0 or 3 h, presented as the geometric mean (MFI) ± SEM, two-way ANOVA with Sidak's multiple comparisons test ($n = 3$). *n.s.*, not significant; $^*P < 0.05$; $^{**}P < 0.01$; $^{***}P < 0.001$; and $^{****}P < 0.0001$.

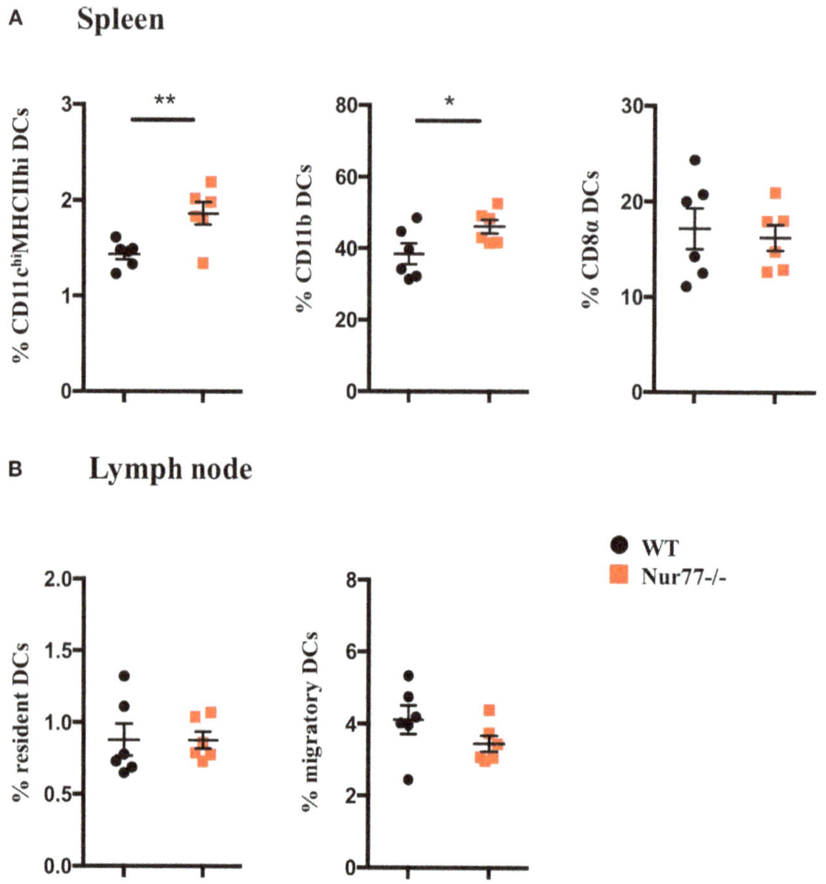

FIGURE 2 | Absence of Nur77 expression does not have a major impact on dendritic cell (DC) development in the spleen and lymph nodes (LNs). % of DCs in **(A)** spleen and **(B)** inguinal LNs of WT or Nur77$^{-/-}$ mice. Shown are the means of pooled data of two independent experiments ± SEM for WT or Nur77$^{-/-}$ mice (n = 3). Two-tailed unpaired t-test: $^{*}P < 0.05$; $^{**}P < 0.01$; and $^{***}P < 0.001$.

(CD11c^{hi}MHCII^{+}) and migratory DCs (CD11c^{+}MHCII^{hi}) was comparable (**Figure 2B**; Figure S2B in Supplementary Material). Also in a transplantable autologous TH-MYCN 9464D mouse model of neuroblastoma (53), we did not observe differences in the presence of the different subsets of DCs in the spleen or (non)draining LN (Figures S3A,B in Supplementary Material). These data indicate that Nur77 is dispensable for DC development. Next, we tested the expression level of Nur77 in different DC subsets by analyzing DCs from the spleen and LNs from transgenic Nur77 reporter mice that express GFP upon activation of the Nur77 promoter. Nur77^{GFP} was clearly expressed in CD11b^{+} spleen DCs. The expression in CD8α^{+} spleen DCs was less well defined and consisted of a population expressing Nur77^{GFP} at a very low level and a population expressing Nur77^{GFP} to a similar level as the CD11b^{+} DCs (**Figures 3A,B**). Resident DCs of inguinal and axillary LN expressed clear levels of Nur77^{GFP}, in contrast to significantly lower expression in migratory DCs of these LN (**Figures 3C,D**). Mice bearing a neuroblastoma tumor showed a similar Nur77^{GFP} expression pattern in DCs (Figures S3C,D in Supplementary Material) as in naïve mice. These data indicate that Nur77 expression does not have a major impact on the development and presence of different DC subsets in the spleen and LNs and that Nur77 is most abundantly expressed in CD11b^{+} spleen DCs and resident DCs of different LNs.

Nur77-Deficient Murine DCs Have Altered Cytokine Production and T Cell Stimulatory Capacity

To assess the functional role of Nur77 in different murine DC subsets, we investigated cytokine production by murine Nur77$^{-/-}$ BMDCs after stimulation with different inflammatory stimuli. We found that Nur77$^{-/-}$ cDCs produced significantly more IL-6, TNFα, and IL-12 upon CpG and R848 stimulation (**Figure 4A**). Nur77$^{-/-}$ pDCs showed increased production of IL-6 and IL-12 upon R848 stimulation, whereas TNFα production was not affected. After stimulation with CpG, type I IFN production was much higher in Nur77$^{-/-}$ pDCs compared with WT pDCs (**Figure 4B**). CD103^{+} DCs showed a stronger response to CpG than to R848, revealing increased production of IL-6, TNFα, and IL-12 (**Figure 4C**). To rule out the possibility that the increase in cytokine production was (partly) mediated by enhanced TLR expression, we profiled TLR7 and TLR9 expression in these cells.

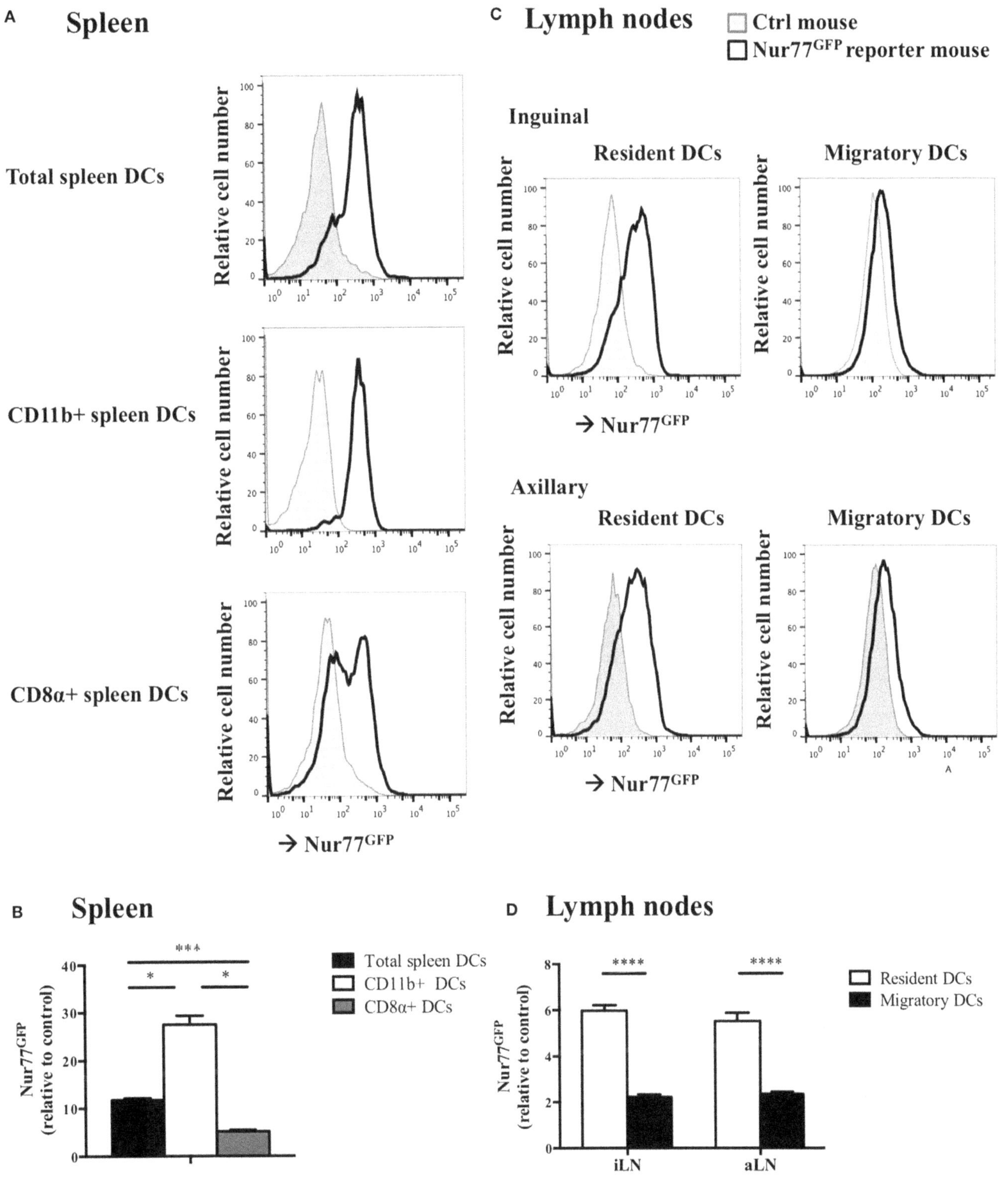

FIGURE 3 | Nur77 expression level in murine dendritic cells (DCs) *ex vivo*. **(A)** *Ex vivo* Nur77^{GFP} expression in the different DC subsets in spleen, shown are the representative data of one out of three transgenic Nur77 reporter mice, where the induction of the Nur77 promoter drives GFP expression (Nur77^{GFP}) mice. **(B)** Quantification of Nur77^{GFP} expression in the different DC subsets in the spleen, presented as the relative Nur77^{GFP} expression to control mice ± SEM, one-way ANOVA with Sidak's multiple comparisons test ($n = 3$). **(C)** *Ex vivo* Nur77^{GFP} expression in the resident and migratory DC subsets of the inguinal and axillary lymph nodes (aLN), shown are the representative data of one out of three transgenic Nur77 reporter mice. **(D)** Quantification of Nur77^{GFP} expression in the resident and migratory DC subsets of the inguinal (iLN) and aLN, presented as the relative Nur77^{GFP} expression to control mice ± SEM, two-way ANOVA with Sidak's multiple comparisons test ($n = 3$): *$P < 0.05$; ***$P < 0.001$; and ****$P < 0.0001$.

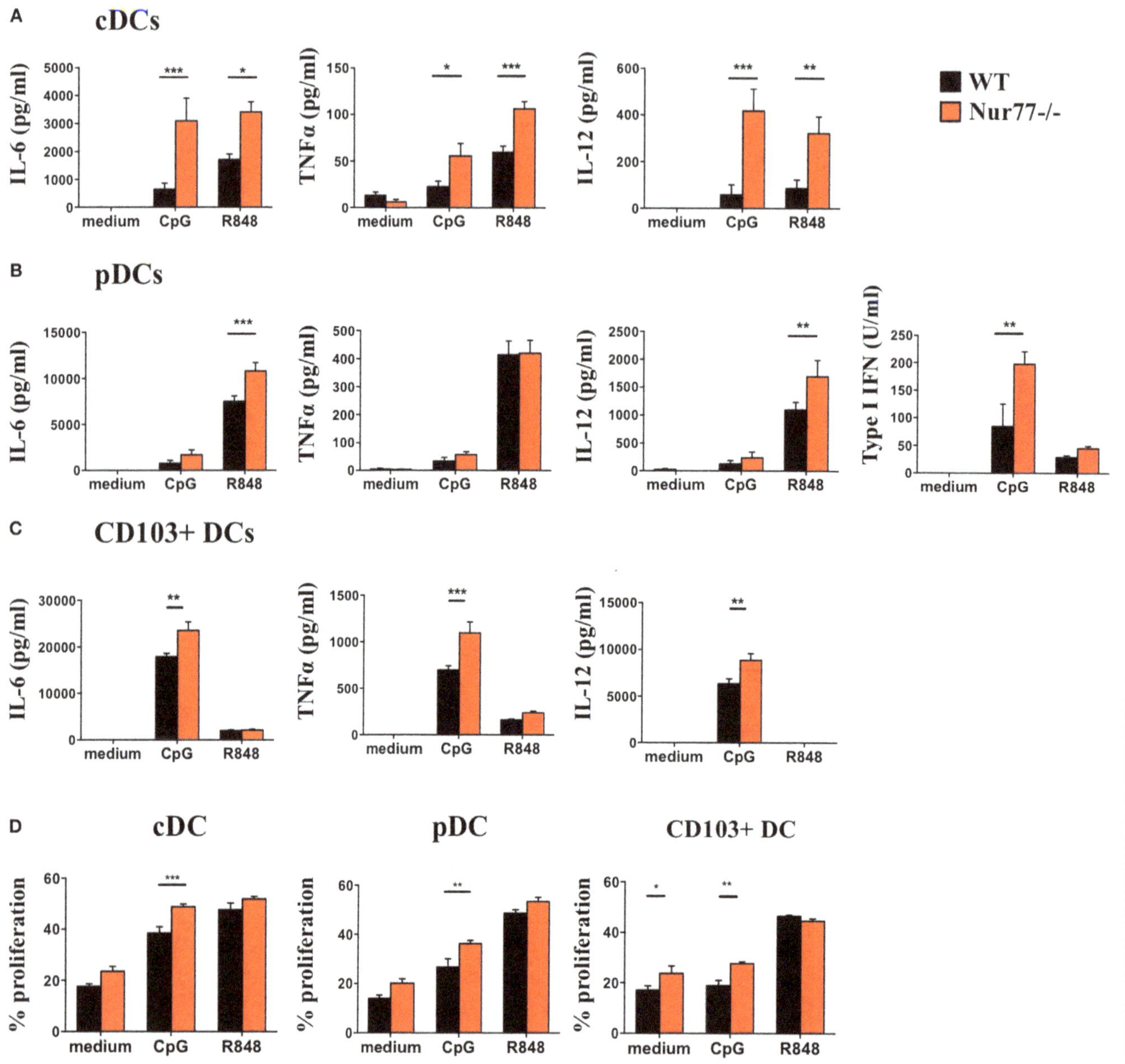

FIGURE 4 | Cytokine production and T cell proliferation by murine Nur77$^{-/-}$ dendritic cells (DCs) are increased compared with WT DCs. Conventional DCs (cDCs) **(A)** and plasmacytoid DCs (pDCs) **(B)** were sorted from FLT3L bone marrow cultures or CD103^{+} DCs **(C)** derived from FLT3L/GM-CSF cultures were stimulated with CpG or R848, cytokine production was measured with ELISA. T cell proliferation **(D)** was measured after coculture of CpG or R848 stimulated cDCs, pDCs, or CD103^{+} DCs with BalB/C T cells and was measured as indicated by CFSE dilution on day 3. Data are shown as the mean ± SEM, two-way ANOVA with Bonferroni posttest (n = 3–6 different mice) (*P < 0.05; **P < 0.01; and ***P < 0.001).

TLR7 and TLR9 expression was similar in WT and Nur77$^{-/-}$ cDCs, whereas TLR7 expression was reduced in Nur77$^{-/-}$ pDCs (Figure S4 in Supplementary Material). In addition to cytokine production, we investigated the T-cell stimulatory capacities for Nur77-deficient DCs. To this end, control, CpG, or R848 stimulated DCs were added to an allogeneic MLR. All Nur77-deficient DC subsets were significantly more potent in inducing T cell proliferation than WT DCs upon stimulation with CpG (**Figure 4D**). These data indicate that Nur77 deficiency in DCs leads to enhanced cytokine production and subsequent increased T cell proliferation.

Nur77 Expression and Function in Human DCs

In addition to defining its expression and function in murine DCs we profiled Nur77 mRNA expression in human moDCs after stimulation with LPS and R848. In accordance with murine DCs, human moDCs quickly upregulated Nur77 mRNA expression and the expression remained stable for 24 h after stimulation with either LPS or R848 (**Figure 5A**). To investigate Nur77 expression in freshly isolated BDCA1+ blood myeloid DCs, purified BDCA1+ DCs were stimulated for different time periods with LPS or R848 (**Figure 5B**). Compared with moDCs, freshly isolated BDCA1+ DCs had much higher expression levels of Nur77 expression under resting conditions. Stimulation with R848 led to a further increase of Nur77 expression, which diminished to lower levels 16 h after stimulation. These data indicate that in different subsets of human DCs Nur77 is expressed with varying expression levels.

Human Nur77-Modified DCs Have Altered Cytokine Production and T Cell Stimulatory Capacity

To test Nur77 function in human DCs, we silenced Nur77 expression in moDCs using a siRNA smartpool. Nur77 expression in moDCs decreased by 60–70% using siNur77 compared with control siRNA (siCTRL) (**Figure 6A**). These siNur77 targeted DCs had increased mRNA and protein expression of IL-6 and TNFα compared with siCTRL-treated DCs (**Figures 6B,C**), especially after R848 stimulation. Nur77-deficient DCs also showed enhanced IL-12 protein production. Profiling of TLR4, TLR7, and TLR8 expression (Figure S5 in Supplementary Material), revealed no change in TLR expression, indicating that the effect on cytokine production is not mediated *via* altered TLR expression. As NR4A family members have been reported to crosstalk with the NF-κB pathway (54), we investigated whether the enhanced cytokine production was dependent on NF-κB signaling. Blocking NF-κB signaling with the NF-κB inhibitor BAY11-7082 inhibited IL-6 and TNFα production in siNur77 DCs and siCTRL DCs to the same level (**Figure 6D**), indicating that the enhanced expression of IL-6 and TNFα was indeed dependent on NF-κB signaling. We next determined the expression of CD40, CD86, and CCR7 in siNur77 DCs. While siNur77 and siCTRL DCs show similar expression of the co-stimulatory markers CD40 and CD86, a significantly lower percentage of CCR7+ DCs were present in siNur77 DCs (**Figure 6E**). To further substantiate these data, we treated DCs with 6-MP, an activator of Nur77 (55–59). Treating DCs with 6-MP before stimulation with R848, led to a dose-dependent decrease of IL-6 and IL-12 production, while TNFα levels were not altered (**Figure 6F**). No effect of 6-MP on cell viability could be detected (Figure S6 in Supplementary Material). In line with decreased IL-6 and IL-12 production, DCs pretreated with 6-MP were less capable of inducing IFNγ production by T cells in an allogeneic MLR (**Figure 6G**). These data show that human Nur77-modified moDCs have altered NF-κB-dependent inflammatory responses that are important in inducing T cell activation.

DISCUSSION

Nuclear receptors have been shown to play a critical role in immune cell function, including members of the NR4A subgroup. However, the expression and function of Nur77 in different DC subsets has not been studied so far. We now show that Nur77 is expressed in different human as well as murine DC subsets. Its expression is rapidly upregulated upon stimulation with different TLR ligands. Deficiency of Nur77 leads to enhanced NF-κB dependent cytokine production and T cell stimulatory capacity of DCs, while stimulation with the Nur77 activator 6-MP limits cytokine production by DCs and its capacity to stimulate allogeneic T cells.

Nur77 expression has been shown to be essential in the differentiation and survival of Ly-6C− monocytes (34, 35), in the polarization of macrophages (37, 38, 60) and in the function and negative selection of T cells (31, 32). This NR is also expressed in infiltrating monocytes and monocyte-derived macrophages of the CNS that are important in experimental autoimmune encephalomyelitis (28) and in patrolling monocytes that control metastasis to the lung (61). We now show, in line with its classification as early response gene, that Nur77 expression is quickly upregulated in different human and murine DC subsets after stimulation with distinct TLR ligands *in vitro*. However, the expression levels in the different DC subsets and level of response toward diverse stimuli vary. We also found Nur77 expression in different subsets of DCs

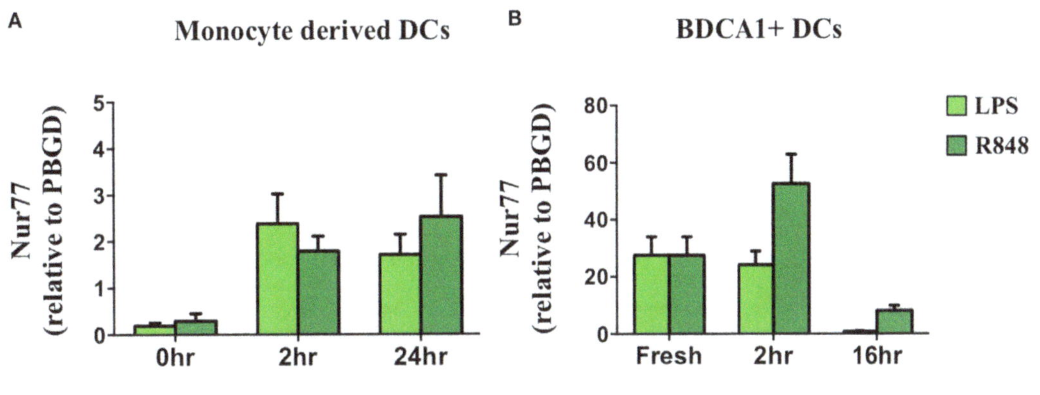

FIGURE 5 | Nur77 mRNA expression in human dendritic cells (DCs). Human day 6 monocyte-derived dendritic cells **(A)** or freshly isolated BDCA1+ DCs **(B)** were stimulated for different time periods with LPS or R848. mRNA expression levels of Nur77 were detected by qPCR analysis. Expression levels shown are related to the housekeeping gene porphobilinogen deaminase (PBGD). Data shown are the mean ± SEM (n = 3–5 different donors).

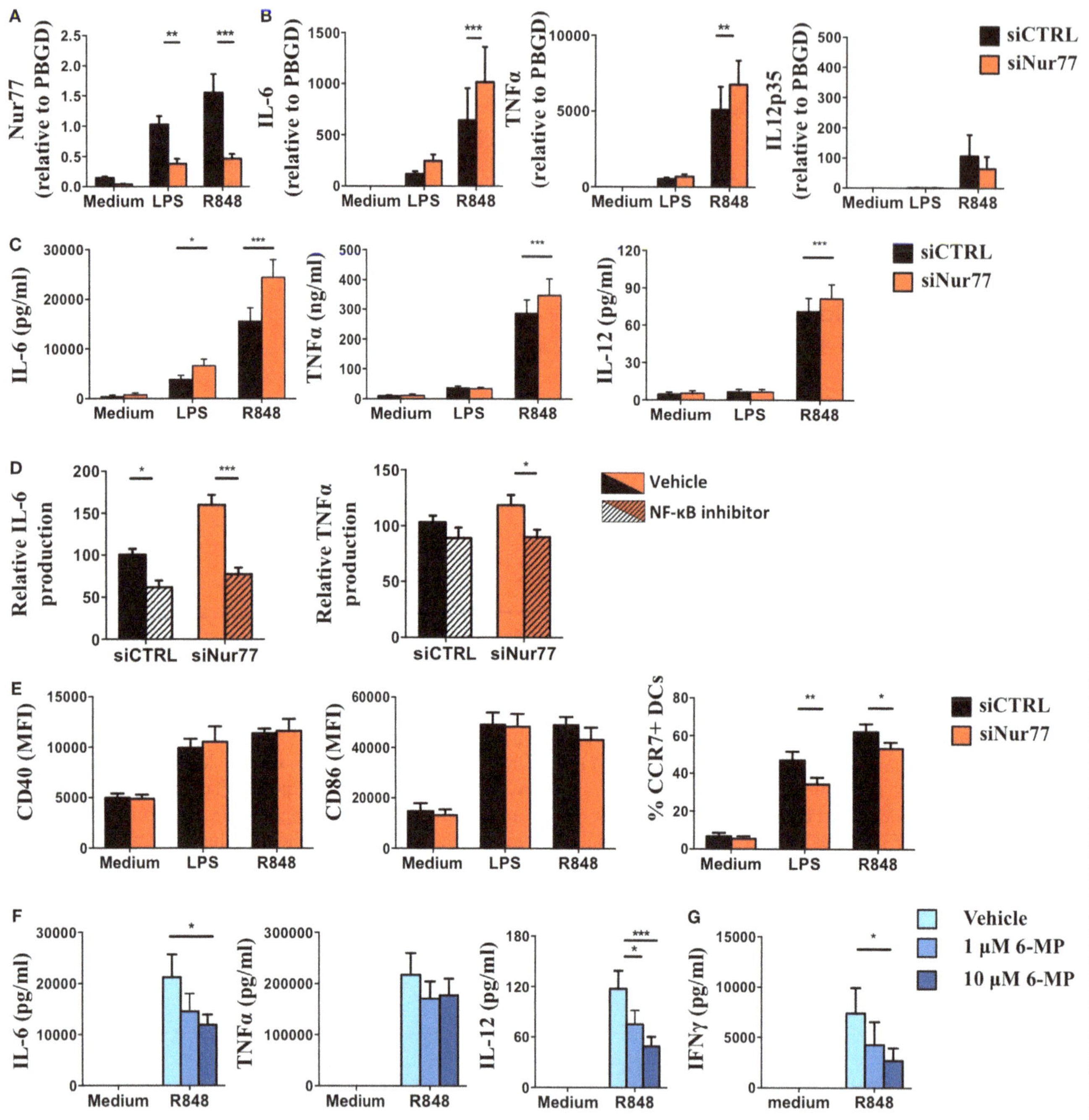

FIGURE 6 | Knockdown or activation of Nur77 in human dendritic cells (DCs) alters DC function and T cell activation. Day 4 monocyte-derived dendritic cells (moDCs) were electroporated with a smartpool siRNA targeting Nur77 (siNur77) or a control siRNA (siCTRL). At day 6, cells were stimulated for 8 h with LPS, and Nur77 mRNA expression was detected by qPCR analysis **(A)**, cytokine mRNA expression after 8 h of stimulation was measured by qPCR analysis **(B)**, and cytokine levels were measured 24 h after stimulation with ELISA. **(C)** Electroporated moDCs were pretreated with Bay11-7082 and then stimulated with R848 for 24 h. Cytokine levels were measured by ELISA. **(D)** CD40, CD86, and CCR7 expression was determined by FACS analysis. **(E)** moDCs were pretreated with 6-mercaptopurine (6-MP) and then stimulated with TLRL for 24 h. Cytokine levels were measured by ELISA. **(F)** moDCs were pretreated with 6-MP and subsequently stimulated with R848, T cell stimulatory capacity was measured in an allogeneic mixed leukocyte reaction by measuring IFNγ production by ELISA **(G)**. Data shown are the mean ± SEM. Two-way ANOVA with Bonferroni posttest (n = 3–12 independent donors): $^{*}P < 0.05$; $^{**}P < 0.01$; and $^{***}P < 0.001$.

in the spleen and LNs directly in naïve and in tumor-bearing mice *ex vivo*. Expression was more pronounced in the CD11b^{+} DCs of the spleen compared with CD8α^{+} DCs and higher in the resident than in the migratory DCs of the LNs. Previously, it has been shown that Nur77 is not required for the differentiation of Ly-6C^{hi} monocytes into moDCs (36). We now also show that Nur77 deficiency does not have a major impact on the presence of different DC subsets in the spleen and LN at steady state conditions as well as mice bearing a neuroblastoma tumor. This confirms that in contrast to its expression in Ly-6C$^-$ monocytes, Nur77 expression is dispensable for the development of spleen and LN DCs.

Although most studies have reported that Nur77 has an anti-inflammatory role in monocytes and macrophages (37, 38, 62), it has been shown that its overexpression in murine macrophages can lead to a pro-inflammatory response (63). Our data point towards an anti-inflammatory role in human and murine DC subsets. Nur77 deficiency in DCs leads to enhanced production of IL-6, TNFα, and IL-12 and subsequent enhanced T cell proliferation, while Nur77 activation leads to reduced IL-6 and IL-12 production and reduced T cell activation. It has been hypothesized that Nur77 acts to resolve inflammation in macrophages (38, 64) and based on our data we now suggest a similar role for Nur77 in DCs.

All NR4A family members, including Nur77, have been shown to modulate immune cell function *via* crosstalk to NF-κB (30, 38, 54, 65). Our data show that also in human DCs, Nur77 affects cytokine production by modulating the NF-κB pathway. It has been shown that Nur77 can affect the NF-κB pathway signaling in numerous ways (38, 63, 65–68). Besides modulating phosphorylation of p65 Ser536 and Ser529 in macrophages (38, 69), Nur77 has also been shown to directly interact with the p65 subunit of NF-κB (65, 66) and block p65 binding to DNA (65). Moreover, Nur77 can regulate TRAF6 auto-ubiquitination (67), important for NF-κB signal transduction (70–72). Future studies should reveal which mechanism underlies Nur77-mediated modulation of NF-κB signaling in DCs and whether different DC subsets or different inflammatory conditions involve specific ways of regulating NF-κB signaling.

While Nur77-deficient DCs show enhanced inflammatory responses, pretreating human DCs with 6-MP led to reduced inflammatory responses and a diminished capacity to induce IFNγ production by T cells in an allogeneic MLR. 6-MP is a nucleic acid analog and has been shown to enhance Nur77 transcriptional activity (55–59). Currently, it is being applied as an immunosuppressive drug for the treatment of several chronic inflammatory diseases such as inflammatory bowel disease, systemic lupus erythematosus, acute lymphoblastic leukemia of childhood, inflammatory myopathies, and rheumatoid arthritis and to prevent acute rejection in organ transplant patients (73–75). It has been shown that besides activating Nur77 (55, 56, 76) 6-MP can also activate the NR4A members Nurr1 (77) and NOR-1 (76) and inhibit the GTPase proteins Rac1 and Rac2 (78, 79). Therefore, the effect observed in moDCs may be a combined effect of 6-MP on the function of either of these proteins. In addition to 6-MP many other pharmacological compounds have been generated to modulate Nur77 function. Among them are different C-DIMs [synthetic 1,1-bis(3′-indolyl)-1-(substituted phenyl)methane analogs] (80), cytosporone B and its structural analogs (81, 82), and TMPA (ethyl 2-[2,3,4-trimethoxy-6-(1-octanoyl)phenyl]acetate) (83). They have been shown to regulate Nur77 function by modulating Nur77-dependent transactivation, influencing its expression levels, inducing nuclear export of Nur77 or affecting binding to other proteins (80–88). Many of these compounds have, as also shown for 6-MP, also Nur77-independent actions (85, 89, 90). In cancer cells, neuronal cells, as well as different immune cells, it has been shown that Nur77 function depends on tissue context, subcellular localization, external stimuli, protein–protein interactions, or post-translational modifications (22–26, 31, 32, 34, 35, 37, 38, 60). How Nur77 function in DCs is exactly regulated upon specific immune stimuli and whether that is different in different DC subsets is currently unknown. Future studies should aim at fully elucidating whether specific stimuli in different subsets of DCs and under specific (pathological) conditions affect Nur77 activation and thereby modulate DC function. More knowledge regarding the exact mechanism(s) of Nur77 activation in DCs will help to choose the best pharmacological compound targeting specific actions of Nur77 in DCs. This will not only be important in optimizing current DC-based immunotherapies but also when more generally targeting Nur77 in different cell types and pathological conditions.

Interestingly, in tumor cells, the natural steroid Dendrogenin A has been shown to stimulate expression of Nur77 *via* binding to LXRβ and induce lethal autophagy (91, 92), opening up new perspectives for cancer treatment (93). Moreover, it has been shown that Dendrogenin A, in addition to inducing growth control and improve overall survival in mice, also induces immune cell infiltration, including DCs, in the tumor (94). As LXR has been shown to affect DC differentiation, maturation and migration (95–101), it is tempting to speculate that part of these effects are mediated *via* regulation of Nur77 expression, especially when DCs are stimulated with Dendrogenin A.

One striking observation is that the percentage of CCR7 expressing human DCs was decreased in siNur77 treated moDCs. Interestingly, another member of the NR4A subfamily, NOR-1, has been shown to affect CCR7-dependent murine CD103$^+$ DC migration from tissues to LNs *in vivo* (42). Nevertheless, we did not observe a similar effect on CCR7 expression in *in vitro* cultured murine CD103$^+$ DCs (data not shown). In agreement with Park et al., we did not find differences in the number of migratory murine DCs present in the LN in Nur77$^{-/-}$ mice compared with WT mice, suggesting a less pronounced role for Nur77 in CCR7-dependent DC migration in mice. However, since NR4A family members are highly homologous proteins and can have redundant functions (102–104), it is also possible that the absence of Nur77 is compensated by NOR-1 in murine DCs.

Given that Nur77 modifies DC function with altered inflammatory responses, Nur77 may be an interesting therapeutic target to either boost or diminish the activation status of DCs in DC-based vaccination strategies in cancer or treatment of autoimmune diseases, respectively.

ETHICS STATEMENT

All animal experiments were approved by the Radboud University's Animal Welfare Body (AWB) (*Instantie voor Dierenwelzijn IvD*) and the Animal Experiment Committee (*DierExperimentenCommissie, RUDEC*) that is recognized by the CCD (Central Authority for Scientific Procedures on Animals). The experiments were performed according to institutional, national, and European guidelines as stipulated in the *Wet op de dierproeven* (WOD) and in the *Dierproevenbesluit*. All experiments involving human material were carried out after obtaining written informed consent from all subjects as per the Declaration of Helsinki. The study was approved by the Institutional Review Board of the Radboud University Nijmegen Medical Center, Commissie Mensgebonden Onderzoek.

AUTHOR CONTRIBUTIONS

NT-K and MA planned and performed experiments. EK-R and ML performed experiments. HI generated and provided mice. NT-K, CV, and MA contributed to the interpretation of the data. MA wrote the manuscript. NT-K, EK-R, ML, HI, and CV contributed to the review of the manuscript. MA designed the study.

ACKNOWLEDGMENTS

We are grateful for the constructive discussions and critically reading of the manuscript to Prof. G. J. Adema. This work is supported by project number 016.156.093 of the Netherlands Organisation for Scientific Research (NWO-Veni) (to MA). NT-K is recipient of a PhD grant from the Radboud University Nijmegen Medical Centre. MA is a recipient of a long-term fellowship (BUIT 2012-5347) from the Dutch Cancer Society.

REFERENCES

1. Granucci F, Foti M, Ricciardi-Castagnoli P. Dendritic cell biology. *Adv Immunol* (2005) 88:193–233. doi:10.1016/S0065-2776(05)88006-X
2. Adema GJ. Dendritic cells from bench to bedside and back. *Immunol Lett* (2009) 122(2):128–30. doi:10.1016/j.imlet.2008.11.017
3. Merad M, Sathe P, Helft J, Miller J, Mortha A. The dendritic cell lineage: ontogeny and function of dendritic cells and their subsets in the steady state and the inflamed setting. *Annu Rev Immunol* (2013) 31:563–604. doi:10.1146/annurev-immunol-020711-074950
4. Granot T, Senda T, Carpenter DJ, Matsuoka N, Weiner J, Gordon CL, et al. Dendritic cells display subset and tissue-specific maturation dynamics over human life. *Immunity* (2017) 46(3):504–15. doi:10.1016/j.immuni.2017.02.019
5. Pakalniskyte D, Schraml BU. Tissue-specific diversity and functions of conventional dendritic cells. *Adv Immunol* (2017) 134:89–135. doi:10.1016/bs.ai.2017.01.003
6. Jacobs JF, Punt CJ, Lesterhuis WJ, Sutmuller RP, Brouwer HM, Scharenborg NM, et al. Dendritic cell vaccination in combination with anti-CD25 monoclonal antibody treatment: a phase I/II study in metastatic melanoma patients. *Clin Cancer Res* (2010) 16(20):5067–78. doi:10.1158/1078-0432.CCR-10-1757
7. Strioga MM, Felzmann T, Powell DJ Jr, Ostapenko V, Dobrovolskiene NT, Matuskova M, et al. Therapeutic dendritic cell-based cancer vaccines: the state of the art. *Crit Rev Immunol* (2013) 33(6):489–547. doi:10.1615/CritRevImmunol.2013008033
8. Aarntzen EH, De Vries IJ, Lesterhuis WJ, Schuurhuis D, Jacobs JF, Bol K, et al. Targeting CD4(+) T-helper cells improves the induction of antitumor responses in dendritic cell-based vaccination. *Cancer Res* (2013) 73(1):19–29. doi:10.1158/0008-5472.CAN-12-1127
9. Aarntzen EH, Schreibelt G, Bol K, Lesterhuis WJ, Croockewit AJ, de Wilt JH, et al. Vaccination with mRNA-electroporated dendritic cells induces robust tumor antigen-specific CD4+ and CD8+ T cells responses in stage III and IV melanoma patients. *Clin Cancer Res* (2012) 18(19):5460–70. doi:10.1158/1078-0432.CCR-11-3368
10. Aarntzen EH, Srinivas M, Schreibelt G, Heerschap A, Punt CJ, Figdor CG, et al. Reducing cell number improves the homing of dendritic cells to lymph nodes upon intradermal vaccination. *Oncoimmunology* (2013) 2(7):e24661. doi:10.4161/onci.24661
11. Lo J, Clare-Salzler MJ. Dendritic cell subsets and type I diabetes: focus upon DC-based therapy. *Autoimmun Rev* (2006) 5(6):419–23. doi:10.1016/j.autrev.2005.12.001
12. Dannull J, Haley NR, Archer G, Nair S, Boczkowski D, Harper M, et al. Melanoma immunotherapy using mature DCs expressing the constitutive proteasome. *J Clin Invest* (2013) 123(7):3135–45. doi:10.1172/JCI67544
13. Sabado RL, Bhardwaj N. Directing dendritic cell immunotherapy towards successful cancer treatment. *Immunotherapy* (2010) 2(1):37–56. doi:10.2217/imt.09.43
14. Hansen M, Met O, Svane IM, Andersen MH. Cellular based cancer vaccines: type 1 polarization of dendritic cells. *Curr Med Chem* (2012) 19(25):4239–46. doi:10.2174/092986712802884213
15. Garg AD, Vara Perez M, Schaaf M, Agostinis P, Zitvogel L, Kroemer G, et al. Trial watch: dendritic cell-based anticancer immunotherapy. *Oncoimmunology* (2017) 6(7):e1328341. doi:10.1080/2162402X.2017.1328341
16. Chow EK, Razani B, Cheng G. Innate immune system regulation of nuclear hormone receptors in metabolic diseases. *J Leukoc Biol* (2007) 82(2):187–95. doi:10.1189/jlb.1206741
17. Ogawa S, Lozach J, Benner C, Pascual G, Tangirala RK, Westin S, et al. Molecular determinants of crosstalk between nuclear receptors and toll-like receptors. *Cell* (2005) 122(5):707–21. doi:10.1016/j.cell.2005.06.029
18. Chute JP, Ross JR, McDonnell DP. Minireview: nuclear receptors, hematopoiesis, and stem cells. *Mol Endocrinol* (2010) 24(1):1–10. doi:10.1210/me.2009-0332
19. Hontelez S, Karthaus N, Looman MW, Ansems M, Adema GJ. DC-SCRIPT regulates glucocorticoid receptor function and expression of its target GILZ in dendritic cells. *J Immunol* (2013) 190(7):3172–9. doi:10.4049/jimmunol.1201776
20. Karthaus N, van Spriel AB, Looman MW, Chen S, Spilgies LM, Lieben L, et al. Vitamin D controls murine and human plasmacytoid dendritic cell function. *J Invest Dermatol* (2014) 134(5):1255–64. doi:10.1038/jid.2013.501
21. Hamers AA, Hanna RN, Nowyhed H, Hedrick CC, de Vries CJ. NR4A nuclear receptors in immunity and atherosclerosis. *Curr Opin Lipidol* (2013) 24(5):381–5. doi:10.1097/MOL.0b013e3283643eac
22. Beard JA, Tenga A, Chen T. The interplay of NR4A receptors and the oncogene-tumor suppressor networks in cancer. *Cell Signal* (2015) 27(2):257–66. doi:10.1016/j.cellsig.2014.11.009
23. Wei X, Gao H, Zou J, Liu X, Chen D, Liao J, et al. Contra-directional coupling of Nur77 and Nurr1 in neurodegeneration: a novel mechanism for memantine-induced anti-inflammation and anti-mitochondrial impairment. *Mol Neurobiol* (2016) 53(9):5876–92. doi:10.1007/s12035-015-9477-7
24. Gao H, Chen Z, Fu Y, Yang X, Weng R, Wang R, et al. Nur77 exacerbates PC12 cellular injury in vitro by aggravating mitochondrial impairment and endoplasmic reticulum stress. *Sci Rep* (2016) 6:34403. doi:10.1038/srep34403
25. Montarolo F, Perga S, Martire S, Navone DN, Marchet A, Leotta D, et al. Altered NR4A subfamily gene expression level in peripheral blood of parkinson's and alzheimer's disease patients. *Neurotox Res* (2016) 30(3):338–44. doi:10.1007/s12640-016-9626-4
26. Zou J, Chen Z, Wei X, Chen Z, Fu Y, Yang X, et al. Cystatin C as a potential therapeutic mediator against Parkinson's disease via VEGF-induced angiogenesis and enhanced neuronal autophagy in neurovascular units. *Cell Death Dis* (2017) 8(6):e2854. doi:10.1038/cddis.2017.240
27. Rothe T, Ipseiz N, Faas M, Lang S, Perez-Branguli F, Metzger D, et al. The nuclear receptor Nr4a1 acts as a microglia rheostat and serves as a therapeutic target in autoimmune-driven central nervous system inflammation. *J Immunol* (2017) 198(10):3878–85. doi:10.4049/jimmunol.1600638

28. Shaked I, Hanna RN, Shaked H, Chodaczek G, Nowyhed HN, Tweet G, et al. Transcription factor Nr4a1 couples sympathetic and inflammatory cues in CNS-recruited macrophages to limit neuroinflammation. *Nat Immunol* (2015) 16(12):1228–34. doi:10.1038/ni.3321
29. Maxwell MA, Muscat GE. The NR4A subgroup: immediate early response genes with pleiotropic physiological roles. *Nucl Recept Signal* (2006) 4:e002. doi:10.1621/nrs.04002
30. McMorrow JP, Murphy EP. Inflammation: a role for NR4A orphan nuclear receptors? *Biochem Soc Trans* (2011) 39(2):688–93. doi:10.1042/BST0390688
31. Fassett MS, Jiang W, D'Alise AM, Mathis D, Benoist C. Nuclear receptor Nr4a1 modulates both regulatory T-cell (Treg) differentiation and clonal deletion. *Proc Natl Acad Sci U S A* (2012) 109(10):3891–6. doi:10.1073/pnas.1200090109
32. Zhou T, Cheng J, Yang P, Wang Z, Liu C, Su X, et al. Inhibition of Nur77/Nurr1 leads to inefficient clonal deletion of self-reactive T cells. *J Exp Med* (1996) 183(4):1879–92. doi:10.1084/jem.183.4.1879
33. Sekiya T, Kashiwagi I, Yoshida R, Fukaya T, Morita R, Kimura A, et al. Nr4a receptors are essential for thymic regulatory T cell development and immune homeostasis. *Nat Immunol* (2013) 14(3):230–7. doi:10.1038/ni.2520
34. Hanna RN, Carlin LM, Hubbeling HG, Nackiewicz D, Green AM, Punt JA, et al. The transcription factor NR4A1 (Nur77) controls bone marrow differentiation and the survival of Ly6C- monocytes. *Nat Immunol* (2011) 12(8): 778–85. doi:10.1038/ni.2063
35. Carlin LM, Stamatiades EG, Auffray C, Hanna RN, Glover L, Vizcay-Barrena G, et al. Nr4a1-dependent Ly6C(low) monocytes monitor endothelial cells and orchestrate their disposal. *Cell* (2013) 153(2):362–75. doi:10.1016/j.cell.2013.03.010
36. Briseno CG, Haldar M, Kretzer NM, Wu X, Theisen DJ, Kc W, et al. Distinct transcriptional programs control cross-priming in classical and monocyte-derived dendritic cells. *Cell Rep* (2016) 15(11):2462–74. doi:10.1016/j.celrep.2016.05.025
37. Bonta PI, van Tiel CM, Vos M, Pols TW, van Thienen JV, Ferreira V, et al. Nuclear receptors Nur77, Nurr1, and NOR-1 expressed in atherosclerotic lesion macrophages reduce lipid loading and inflammatory responses. *Arterioscler Thromb Vasc Biol* (2006) 26(10):2288–94. doi:10.1161/01.ATV.0000238346.84458.5d
38. Hanna RN, Shaked I, Hubbeling HG, Punt JA, Wu R, Herrley E, et al. NR4A1 (Nur77) deletion polarizes macrophages toward an inflammatory phenotype and increases atherosclerosis. *Circ Res* (2012) 110(3):416–27. doi:10.1161/CIRCRESAHA.111.253377
39. Wang T, Jiang Q, Chan C, Gorski KS, McCadden E, Kardian D, et al. Inhibition of activation-induced death of dendritic cells and enhancement of vaccine efficacy via blockade of MINOR. *Blood* (2009) 113(13):2906–13. doi:10.1182/blood-2008-08-176354
40. Karthaus N, Hontelez S, Looman MW, van Spriel AB, Ansems M, Adema GJ. Nuclear receptor expression patterns in murine plasmacytoid and conventional dendritic cells. *Mol Immunol* (2013) 55(3–4):409–17. doi:10.1016/j.molimm.2013.03.020
41. Grajales-Reyes GE, Iwata A, Albring J, Wu X, Tussiwand R, Kc W, et al. Batf3 maintains autoactivation of Irf8 for commitment of a CD8alpha(+) conventional DC clonogenic progenitor. *Nat Immunol* (2015) 16(7):708–17. doi:10.1038/ni.3197
42. Park K, Mikulski Z, Seo GY, Andreyev AY, Marcovecchio P, Blatchley A, et al. The transcription factor NR4A3 controls CD103+ dendritic cell migration. *J Clin Invest* (2016) 126(12):4603–15. doi:10.1172/JCI87081
43. Saini A, Mahajan S, Gupta P. Nuclear receptor expression atlas in BMDCs: Nr4a2 restricts immunogenicity of BMDCs and impedes EAE. *Eur J Immunol* (2016) 46(8):1842–53. doi:10.1002/eji.201546229
44. Nagaoka M, Yashiro T, Uchida Y, Ando T, Hara M, Arai H, et al. The orphan nuclear receptor NR4A3 is involved in the function of dendritic cells. *J Immunol* (2017) 199(8):2958–67. doi:10.4049/jimmunol.1601911
45. Sekiya T, Kashiwagi I, Inoue N, Morita R, Hori S, Waldmann H, et al. The nuclear orphan receptor Nr4a2 induces Foxp3 and regulates differentiation of CD4+ T cells. *Nat Commun* (2011) 2:269. doi:10.1038/ncomms1272
46. Jiang Z, Georgel P, Du X, Shamel L, Sovath S, Mudd S, et al. CD14 is required for MyD88-independent LPS signaling. *Nat Immunol* (2005) 6(6):565–70. doi:10.1038/ni1207
47. Hontelez S, Ansems M, Karthaus N, Zuidscherwoude M, Looman MW, Triantis V, et al. Dendritic cell-specific transcript: dendritic cell marker and regulator of TLR-induced cytokine production. *J Immunol* (2012) 189(1):138–45. doi:10.4049/jimmunol.1103709
48. Sondergaard JN, Poghosyan S, Hontelez S, Louche P, Looman MW, Ansems M, et al. DC-SCRIPT regulates IL-10 production in human dendritic cells by modulating NF-kappaBp65 activation. *J Immunol* (2015) 195(4):1498–505. doi:10.4049/jimmunol.1402924
49. Livak KJ, Schmittgen TD. Analysis of relative gene expression data using real-time quantitative PCR and the 2(-delta delta C(T)) method. *Methods* (2001) 25(4):402–8. doi:10.1006/meth.2001.1262
50. Naik SH, Proietto AI, Wilson NS, Dakic A, Schnorrer P, Fuchsberger M, et al. Cutting edge: generation of splenic CD8+ and CD8- dendritic cell equivalents in Fms-like tyrosine kinase 3 ligand bone marrow cultures. *J Immunol* (2005) 174(11):6592–7. doi:10.4049/jimmunol.174.11.6592
51. Moran AE, Holzapfel KL, Xing Y, Cunningham NR, Maltzman JS, Punt J, et al. T cell receptor signal strength in Treg and iNKT cell development demonstrated by a novel fluorescent reporter mouse. *J Exp Med* (2011) 208(6):1279–89. doi:10.1084/jem.20110308
52. Mayer CT, Ghorbani P, Nandan A, Dudek M, Arnold-Schrauf C, Hesse C, et al. Selective and efficient generation of functional Batf3-dependent CD103+ dendritic cells from mouse bone marrow. *Blood* (2014) 124(20): 3081–91. doi:10.1182/blood-2013-12-545772
53. Kroesen M, Nierkens S, Ansems M, Wassink M, Orentas RJ, Boon L, et al. A transplantable TH-MYCN transgenic tumor model in C57Bl/6 mice for preclinical immunological studies in neuroblastoma. *Int J Cancer* (2014) 134(6):1335–45. doi:10.1002/ijc.28463
54. Murphy EP, Crean D. Molecular interactions between NR4A orphan nuclear receptors and NF-kappaB are required for appropriate inflammatory responses and immune cell homeostasis. *Biomolecules* (2015) 5(3):1302–18. doi:10.3390/biom5031302
55. Yoo YG, Na TY, Yang WK, Kim HJ, Lee IK, Kong G, et al. 6-Mercaptopurine, an activator of Nur77, enhances transcriptional activity of HIF-1alpha resulting in new vessel formation. *Oncogene* (2007) 26(26):3823–34. doi:10.1038/sj.onc.1210149
56. Pires NM, Pols TW, de Vries MR, van Tiel CM, Bonta PI, Vos M, et al. Activation of nuclear receptor Nur77 by 6-mercaptopurine protects against neointima formation. *Circulation* (2007) 115(4):493–500. doi:10.1161/CIRCULATIONAHA.106.626838
57. Huang HY, Chang HF, Tsai MJ, Chen JS, Wang MJ. 6-Mercaptopurine attenuates tumor necrosis factor-alpha production in microglia through Nur77-mediated transrepression and PI3K/Akt/mTOR signaling-mediated translational regulation. *J Neuroinflammation* (2016) 13(1):78. doi:10.1186/s12974-016-0543-5
58. Qin Q, Chen M, Yi B, You X, Yang P, Sun J. Orphan nuclear receptor Nur77 is a novel negative regulator of endothelin-1 expression in vascular endothelial cells. *J Mol Cell Cardiol* (2014) 77:20–8. doi:10.1016/j.yjmcc.2014.09.027
59. Shao Q, Shen LH, Hu LH, Pu J, Qi MY, Li WQ, et al. Nuclear receptor Nur77 suppresses inflammatory response dependent on COX-2 in macrophages induced by oxLDL. *J Mol Cell Cardiol* (2010) 49(2):304–11. doi:10.1016/j.yjmcc.2010.03.023
60. Hamers AA, Argmann C, Moerland PD, Koenis DS, Marinkovic G, Sokolovic M, et al. Nur77-deficiency in bone marrow-derived macrophages modulates inflammatory responses, extracellular matrix homeostasis, phagocytosis and tolerance. *BMC Genomics* (2016) 17:162. doi:10.1186/s12864-016-2469-9
61. Hanna RN, Cekic C, Sag D, Tacke R, Thomas GD, Nowyhed H, et al. Patrolling monocytes control tumor metastasis to the lung. *Science* (2015) 350(6263):985–90. doi:10.1126/science.aac9407
62. Hilgendorf I, Gerhardt LM, Tan TC, Winter C, Holderried TA, Chousterman BG, et al. Ly-6Chigh monocytes depend on Nr4a1 to balance both inflammatory and reparative phases in the infarcted myocardium. *Circ Res* (2014) 114(10):1611–22. doi:10.1161/CIRCRESAHA.114.303204
63. Pei L, Castrillo A, Tontonoz P. Regulation of macrophage inflammatory gene expression by the orphan nuclear receptor Nur77. *Mol Endocrinol* (2006) 20(4):786–94. doi:10.1210/me.2005-0331
64. Pei L, Castrillo A, Chen M, Hoffmann A, Tontonoz P. Induction of NR4A orphan nuclear receptor expression in macrophages in response to inflammatory stimuli. *J Biol Chem* (2005) 280(32):29256–62. doi:10.1074/jbc.M502606200

65. Li L, Liu Y, Chen HZ, Li FW, Wu JF, Zhang HK, et al. Impeding the interaction between Nur77 and p38 reduces LPS-induced inflammation. *Nat Chem Biol* (2015) 11(5):339–46. doi:10.1038/nchembio.1788
66. Hong CY, Park JH, Ahn RS, Im SY, Choi HS, Soh J, et al. Molecular mechanism of suppression of testicular steroidogenesis by proinflammatory cytokine tumor necrosis factor alpha. *Mol Cell Biol* (2004) 24(7):2593–604. doi:10.1128/MCB.24.7.2593-2604.2004
67. Li XM, Zhang S, He XS, Guo PD, Lu XX, Wang JR, et al. Nur77-mediated TRAF6 signalling protects against LPS-induced sepsis in mice. *J Inflamm (Lond)* (2016) 13:4. doi:10.1186/s12950-016-0112-9
68. Hamers AA, van Dam L, Teixeira Duarte JM, Vos M, Marinkovic G, van Tiel CM, et al. Deficiency of nuclear receptor Nur77 aggravates mouse experimental colitis by increased NFkappaB activity in macrophages. *PLoS One* (2015) 10(8):e0133598. doi:10.1371/journal.pone.0133598
69. Ipseiz N, Uderhardt S, Scholtysek C, Steffen M, Schabbauer G, Bozec A, et al. The nuclear receptor Nr4a1 mediates anti-inflammatory effects of apoptotic cells. *J Immunol* (2014) 192(10):4852–8. doi:10.4049/jimmunol.1303377
70. Kobayashi T, Walsh PT, Walsh MC, Speirs KM, Chiffoleau E, King CG, et al. TRAF6 is a critical factor for dendritic cell maturation and development. *Immunity* (2003) 19(3):353–63. doi:10.1016/S1074-7613(03)00230-9
71. Deng L, Wang C, Spencer E, Yang L, Braun A, You J, et al. Activation of the IkappaB kinase complex by TRAF6 requires a dimeric ubiquitin-conjugating enzyme complex and a unique polyubiquitin chain. *Cell* (2000) 103(2):351–61. doi:10.1016/S0092-8674(00)00126-4
72. Wang Y, Tang Y, Teng L, Wu Y, Zhao X, Pei G. Association of beta-arrestin and TRAF6 negatively regulates toll-like receptor-interleukin 1 receptor signaling. *Nat Immunol* (2006) 7(2):139–47. doi:10.1038/ni1294
73. Murray JE, Merrill JP, Harrison JH, Wilson RE, Dammin GJ. Prolonged survival of human-kidney homografts by immunosuppressive drug therapy. *N Engl J Med* (1963) 268:1315–23. doi:10.1056/NEJM196306132682401
74. Kornbluth A, George J, Sachar DB. Immunosuppressive drugs in Crohn's disease. *Gastroenterologist* (1994) 2(3):239–46.
75. Aarbakke J, Janka-Schaub G, Elion GB. Thiopurine biology and pharmacology. *Trends Pharmacol Sci* (1997) 18(1):3–7. doi:10.1016/S0165-6147(96)01007-3
76. Wansa KD, Harris JM, Yan G, Ordentlich P, Muscat GE. The AF-1 domain of the orphan nuclear receptor NOR-1 mediates trans-activation, coactivator recruitment, and activation by the purine anti-metabolite 6-mercaptopurine. *J Biol Chem* (2003) 278(27):24776–90. doi:10.1074/jbc.M300088200
77. Ordentlich P, Yan Y, Zhou S, Heyman RA. Identification of the antineoplastic agent 6-mercaptopurine as an activator of the orphan nuclear hormone receptor Nurr1. *J Biol Chem* (2003) 278(27):24791–9. doi:10.1074/jbc.M302167200
78. Marinkovic G, Hamers AA, de Vries CJ, de Waard V. 6-Mercaptopurine reduces macrophage activation and gut epithelium proliferation through inhibition of GTPase Rac1. *Inflamm Bowel Dis* (2014) 20(9):1487–95. doi:10.1097/MIB.0000000000000122
79. Marinkovic G, Kroon J, Hoogenboezem M, Hoeben KA, Ruiter MS, Kurakula K, et al. Inhibition of GTPase Rac1 in endothelium by 6-mercaptopurine results in immunosuppression in nonimmune cells: new target for an old drug. *J Immunol* (2014) 192(9):4370–8. doi:10.4049/jimmunol.1302527
80. Lee SO, Li X, Hedrick E, Jin UH, Tjalkens RB, Backos DS, et al. Diindolylmethane analogs bind NR4A1 and are NR4A1 antagonists in colon cancer cells. *Mol Endocrinol* (2014) 28(10):1729–39. doi:10.1210/me.2014-1102
81. Zhan Y, Du X, Chen H, Liu J, Zhao B, Huang D, et al. Cytosporone B is an agonist for nuclear orphan receptor Nur77. *Nat Chem Biol* (2008) 4(9):548–56. doi:10.1038/nchembio.106
82. Liu JJ, Zeng HN, Zhang LR, Zhan YY, Chen Y, Wang Y, et al. A unique pharmacophore for activation of the nuclear orphan receptor Nur77 in vivo and in vitro. *Cancer Res* (2010) 70(9):3628–37. doi:10.1158/0008-5472.CAN-09-3160
83. Zhan YY, Chen Y, Zhang Q, Zhuang JJ, Tian M, Chen HZ, et al. The orphan nuclear receptor Nur77 regulates LKB1 localization and activates AMPK. *Nat Chem Biol* (2012) 8(11):897–904. doi:10.1038/nchembio.1069
84. Chintharlapalli S, Burghardt R, Papineni S, Ramaiah S, Yoon K, Safe S. Activation of Nur77 by selected 1,1-Bis(3'-indolyl)-1-(p-substituted phenyl) methanes induces apoptosis through nuclear pathways. *J Biol Chem* (2005) 280(26):24903–14. doi:10.1074/jbc.M500107200
85. Cho SD, Lei P, Abdelrahim M, Yoon K, Liu S, Guo J, et al. 1,1-bis(3'-indolyl)-1-(p-methoxyphenyl)methane activates Nur77-independent proapoptotic responses in colon cancer cells. *Mol Carcinog* (2008) 47(4):252–63. doi:10.1002/mc.20378
86. Safe S, Jin UH, Morpurgo B, Abudayyeh A, Singh M, Tjalkens RB. Nuclear receptor 4A (NR4A) family – orphans no more. *J Steroid Biochem Mol Biol* (2016) 157:48–60. doi:10.1016/j.jsbmb.2015.04.016
87. Yoon K, Lee SO, Cho SD, Kim K, Khan S, Safe S. Activation of nuclear TR3 (NR4A1) by a diindolylmethane analog induces apoptosis and proapoptotic genes in pancreatic cancer cells and tumors. *Carcinogenesis* (2011) 32(6):836–42. doi:10.1093/carcin/bgr040
88. Lee SO, Li X, Khan S, Safe S. Targeting NR4A1 (TR3) in cancer cells and tumors. *Expert Opin Ther Targets* (2011) 15(2):195–206. doi:10.1517/14728222.2011.547481
89. Dawson MI, Ye M, Cao X, Farhana L, Hu QY, Zhao Y, et al. Derivation of a retinoid X receptor scaffold from peroxisome proliferator-activated receptor gamma ligand 1-Di(1H-indol-3-yl)methyl-4-trifluoromethylbenzene. *ChemMedChem* (2009) 4(7):1106–19. doi:10.1002/cmdc.200800447
90. Cho SD, Yoon K, Chintharlapalli S, Abdelrahim M, Lei P, Hamilton S, et al. Nur77 agonists induce proapoptotic genes and responses in colon cancer cells through nuclear receptor-dependent and nuclear receptor-independent pathways. *Cancer Res* (2007) 67(2):674–83. doi:10.1158/0008-5472.CAN-06-2907
91. Segala G, David M, de Medina P, Poirot MC, Serhan N, Vergez F, et al. Dendrogenin A drives LXR to trigger lethal autophagy in cancers. *Nat Commun* (2017) 8(1):1903. doi:10.1038/s41467-017-01948-9
92. Poirot M, Silvente-Poirot S. The tumor-suppressor cholesterol metabolite, dendrogenin A, is a new class of LXR modulator activating lethal autophagy in cancers. *Biochem Pharmacol* (2018) 153:75–81. doi:10.1016/j.bcp.2018.01.046
93. Silvente-Poirot S, Segala G, Poirot MC, Poirot M. Ligand-dependent transcriptional induction of lethal autophagy: a new perspective for cancer treatment. *Autophagy* (2018) 14(3):555–7. doi:10.1080/15548627.2018.1425059
94. de Medina P, Paillasse MR, Segala G, Voisin M, Mhamdi L, Dalenc F, et al. Dendrogenin A arises from cholesterol and histamine metabolism and shows cell differentiation and anti-tumour properties. *Nat Commun* (2013) 4:1840. doi:10.1038/ncomms2835
95. Zhong L, Yang Q, Xie W, Zhou J. Liver X receptor regulates mouse GM-CSF-derived dendritic cell differentiation in vitro. *Mol Immunol* (2014) 60(1):32–43. doi:10.1016/j.molimm.2014.03.006
96. Canavan M, McCarthy C, Larbi NB, Dowling JK, Collins L, O'Sullivan F, et al. Activation of liver X receptor suppresses the production of the IL-12 family of cytokines by blocking nuclear translocation of NF-kappaBp50. *Innate Immun* (2014) 20(7):675–87. doi:10.1177/1753425913501915
97. Geyeregger R, Zeyda M, Bauer W, Kriehuber E, Saemann MD, Zlabinger GJ, et al. Liver X receptors regulate dendritic cell phenotype and function through blocked induction of the actin-bundling protein fascin. *Blood* (2007) 109(10):4288–95. doi:10.1182/blood-2006-08-043422
98. Torocsik D, Barath M, Benko S, Szeles L, Dezso B, Poliska S, et al. Activation of liver X receptor sensitizes human dendritic cells to inflammatory stimuli. *J Immunol* (2010) 184(10):5456–65. doi:10.4049/jimmunol.0902399
99. Villablanca EJ, Raccosta L, Zhou D, Fontana R, Maggioni D, Negro A, et al. Tumor-mediated liver X receptor-alpha activation inhibits CC chemokine receptor-7 expression on dendritic cells and dampens antitumor responses. *Nat Med* (2010) 16(1):98–105. doi:10.1038/nm.2074
100. Beceiro S, Pap A, Czimmerer Z, Sallam T, Guillen JA, Gallardo G, et al. LXR nuclear receptors are transcriptional regulators of dendritic cell chemotaxis. *Mol Cell Biol* (2018) 38(10):e00534-17. doi:10.1128/MCB.00534-17
101. Bruckner M, Dickel D, Singer E, Legler DF. Converse regulation of CCR7-driven human dendritic cell migration by prostaglandin E(2) and liver X receptor activation. *Eur J Immunol* (2012) 42(11):2949–58. doi:10.1002/eji.201242523
102. Cheng LE, Chan FK, Cado D, Winoto A. Functional redundancy of the Nur77 and Nor-1 orphan steroid receptors in T-cell apoptosis. *EMBO J* (1997) 16(8):1865–75. doi:10.1093/emboj/16.8.1865
103. Maira M, Martens C, Philips A, Drouin J. Heterodimerization between members of the Nur subfamily of orphan nuclear receptors as a novel mechanism

for gene activation. *Mol Cell Biol* (1999) 19(11):7549–57. doi:10.1128/MCB.19.11.7549

104. Tontonoz P, Cortez-Toledo O, Wroblewski K, Hong C, Lim L, Carranza R, et al. The orphan nuclear receptor Nur77 is a determinant of myofiber size and muscle mass in mice. *Mol Cell Biol* (2015) 35(7):1125–38. doi:10.1128/MCB.00715-14

8

Langerin$^+$ CD8α^+ Dendritic Cells Drive Early CD8$^+$ T Cell Activation and IL-12 Production During Systemic Bacterial Infection

Kelly A. Prendergast[1,2†], *Naomi J. Daniels*[3], *Troels R. Petersen*[1†], *Ian F. Hermans*[1,2,4] *and Joanna R. Kirman*[3,4*]

[1] *Malaghan Institute of Medical Research, Wellington, New Zealand,* [2] *School of Biological Sciences, Victoria University of Wellington, Wellington, New Zealand,* [3] *Department of Microbiology and Immunology, University of Otago, Dunedin, New Zealand,* [4] *Maurice Wilkins Centre for Molecular Biodiscovery, Auckland, New Zealand*

***Correspondence:**
Joanna R. Kirman
jo.kirman@otago.ac.nz

Bloodstream infections induce considerable morbidity, high mortality, and represent a significant burden of cost in health care; however, our understanding of the immune response to bacteremia is incomplete. Langerin$^+$ CD8α^+ dendritic cells (DCs), residing in the marginal zone of the murine spleen, have the capacity to cross-prime CD8$^+$ T cells and produce IL-12, both of which are important components of antimicrobial immunity. Accordingly, we hypothesized that this DC subset may be a key promoter of adaptive immune responses to blood-borne bacterial infections. Utilizing mice that express the diphtheria toxin receptor under control of the langerin promoter, we investigated the impact of depleting langerin$^+$ CD8α^+ DCs in a murine model of intravenous infection with *Mycobacterium bovis* bacille Calmette–Guerin (BCG). In the absence of langerin$^+$ CD8α^+ DCs, the immune response to blood-borne BCG infection was diminished: bacterial numbers in the spleen increased, serum IL-12p40 decreased, and delayed CD8$^+$ T cell activation, proliferation, and IFN-γ production was evident. Our data revealed that langerin$^+$ CD8α^+ DCs play a pivotal role in initiating CD8$^+$ T cell responses and IL-12 production in response to bacteremia and may influence the early control of systemic bacterial infections.

Keywords: langerin, dendritic cell, diphtheria toxin, bacille Calmette–Guerin, systemic infection

INTRODUCTION

Bloodstream infections are commonly associated with significant morbidity and mortality, with substantial costs to health-care systems (1). Comprehensive knowledge of the essential constituents of an effective immune response to blood-borne bacterial exposure is, therefore, critical for reducing the associated burden to human health. The spleen is an important site for the induction of adaptive immunity. With extensive vasculature and associated lymphoid tissue, blood-borne bacteria or associated particulate components such as immune complexes are efficiently captured by a network of resident antigen-presenting cells (APCs) that include macrophages, B cells, and dendritic cells (DCs) (2). The acquisition of immunogenic elements and subsequent ligation of pathogen recognition receptors, primarily in the marginal zone of the spleen, drives activation of APCs, with some of these cells then moving to the white pulp to initiate adaptive immune responses. The precise roles of different APCs in promoting immune responses to infectious agents, however, have not been fully elucidated.

Splenic DCs can be broadly classified into conventional or plasmacytoid DCs, with conventional DCs further subdivided into three distinct populations: CD4+ DCs, CD8α+ DCs, and double negative DCs (3, 4). The CD8α+ DC population as a whole are reportedly efficient at cross-presenting antigen to CD8+ T cells (5, 6) and are major producers of IL-12, which is known to play a key role in promoting differentiation of IFN-γ-producing T cells (7, 8). However, despite their localization and ability to promote both IL-12 and CD8+ T cell responses, little is known about the importance of CD8α+ DCs in mediating immune responses to systemic bacterial infections.

Confounding the situation, however, it is recognized that there is heterogeneity in function between subpopulations of CD8α+ DCs. A subset of CD8α+ DCs expressing CX_3CR1 has been identified, which lack the ability to produce IL-12 and cross-prime CD8+ T cells and have rearranged immunoglobulin genes—a feature more related to plasmacytoid DCs (9). The CD8α+ DC population can also be subdivided on the basis of expression of the c-type lectin receptor langerin (CD207). The langerin+ CD8α+ DCs in steady state are predominantly localized in the marginal zone (10, 11), a prime location for sampling bloodstream constituents. They have been shown to take up dying cells from the circulation and move to the T cell areas of the spleen to induce tolerance to acquired cell-associated antigens, a process thought to be involved in maintaining self-tolerance (11). However, in response to protein/adjuvant recognition, it was predominantly this langerin-expressing subset of CD8α+ DCs that produced IL-12 in the spleen, and these cells were critical for the priming of potent CD8+ T cell responses to circulating antigens (12). Given these characteristics, we hypothesized that the langerin+ CD8α+ DC subset may be involved in inducing protective responses to systemic infections. To address this hypothesis, we used knock-in mice expressing diphtheria toxin receptor (DTR) under the control of the langerin promoter (*lang*-DTREGFP mice) so that diphtheria toxin (DT) could be used to transiently deplete langerin-expressing DCs during blood-borne bacterial infection.

Bloodstream infections can be caused by a wide range of pathogenic microorganisms. *Escherichia coli*, *Staphylococcus aureus*, and *Streptococcus pneumoniae* are the most common causes of community-acquired bloodstream infection (13); however, mycobacterial species are also an important cause of bloodstream infection, particularly in immune-suppressed individuals (14–16). Since studies in mice depleted of CD11c+ DCs identified a crucial role for splenic DCs in mediating protective adaptive immunity after *Mycobacterium tuberculosis* (*Mtb*) infection (17), we chose to utilize a murine model of intravenous mycobacterial exposure.

To date, there is little information on which subgroups of DCs are important to the antimycobacterial response (18). However, as mice lacking either IFN-γ or IL-12p40 are highly susceptible to infection with *Mtb* (19–23), we considered it likely that the IL-12 producing capabilities of langerin+ CD8α+ DCs would contribute to control of a systemic mycobacterial infection. In addition, the ability of langerin+ CD8α+ DCs to cross-prime CD8+ T cells may be important in the context of mycobacterial infection as studies have shown that antigen-specific CD8+ T cells proliferate rapidly and contribute to immunity in the antimycobacterial response (21–24).

We report herein that during intravenous *Mycobacterium bovis* bacille Calmette–Guerin (BCG) infection, the depletion of langerin+ CD8α+ DCs led to a diminished immune response, with decreased serum IL-12p40 and delayed CD8+ T cell activation, proliferation, and IFN-γ production during infection. An increase in the bacterial burden in the spleen was also evident. These findings suggest that langerin+ CD8α+ DCs may play an important role in the response to blood-borne bacterial infection.

MATERIALS AND METHODS

Mice

Male *lang*-DTREGFP (24), *lang*-EGFP (24), and C57BL/6J mice were bred and housed in the Biomedical Research Unit at the Malaghan Institute of Medical Research. Male *lang*-DTREGFP mice crossed with *lang*-EGFP mice (*lang*-DTREGFP × *lang*-EGFP) were used to better visualize GFP expression on langerin+ cells. OT-I and OT-II mice were crossed with B6.SJL-$Ptprc^a Pep3^b$/BoyJArc congenic mice to enable cell tracking through the congenic marker CD45.1. All mice were housed under specific pathogen-free conditions. All experiments were undertaken within the provisions of the Animal Welfare Act (1999) of New Zealand and approved by the Victoria University of Wellington Animal Ethics Committee.

Mycobacteria

Mycobacterium bovis BCG Pasteur strain 1173P2 was grown at 37°C in Dubos broth (Difco, BD Diagnostics Systems, Sparks, MD, USA), supplemented with 10% Middlebrook oleic acid-albumin-dextrose-catalase (OADC) (Difco), until mid log phase and stored at −80°C in 0.05% PBS Tween80. For recombinant BCG-OVA (25) (a gift from Dr. James Triccas, University of Sydney, NSW, Australia), 50 μg/mL hygromycin (Roche, Manheim, Germany) was added. Before use, defrosted BCG stocks were sonicated briefly prior to dilution in PBS. BCG Pasteur and rBCG-OVA were injected intravenously (i.v.) in the lateral tail vein at 10^5 CFU per mouse.

Depletion of Langerin+ CD8α+ DCs In Vivo

Lang-DTREGFP mice were injected i.p. with 350 ng DT (Sigma-Aldrich, St. Louis, MO, USA) every 2 days for the period of time indicated in each experiment, commencing 2 days before BCG infection.

Determination of Bacterial Burden

Spleens and livers were homogenized in PBS with 0.5% Tween80 (Sigma-Aldrich) and serial dilutions were plated on 7H11 agar (Difco) supplemented with 10% OADC, 25 mg carbenicillin and 100,000 U polymyxin B (Gibco, Invitrogen, Auckland, New Zealand). Plates were incubated at 37°C and bacterial counts performed after 2–3 weeks growth.

Tissue Preparation

Spleens were digested in Liberase TL/DNAse I (Roche) in IMDM (Gibco, Life Technologies) for 30 min at 37°C. Cells were passed through a 70 μm strainer and red blood cells were lysed

(Qiagen, MD, USA) before live cells were counted by Trypan blue exclusion.

Flow Cytometry

Cells were blocked with anti-CD32/16 (clone 2.4G2, produced in-house) and stained with surface antibodies as indicated; CD8-PE (53-6.7), CD62L-APC (MEL-14), IFNγ-PE Cy7 (XMG1.2), CD11b APC CY7 (M1-70), and GR-1 FITC (RB6-8C5) from BD Pharmingen; B220-A647 (RA3-6B2), CD3-PE Cy7 (145-2C11), CD8-A700 (53-6.7), CD11c-eFluor450 (N418), CD44-PE Cy7 (IM7), CD45.1-PE (A20), Vα2-APC (B20.1) from eBioscience, CD11c-PE Cy7 (N418) from BioLegend. A viability dye, live/dead fixable blue (Invitrogen), was included before fixing cells with formalin (Sigma-Aldrich). Samples were collected on an LSRII SORP (BD, San Jose, CA, USA). Data were analyzed using FlowJo version 9.6 (Tree Star, Ashland, OR, USA).

Adoptive Transfer of Carboxyflourescein Diacetate Succinimidyl Ester (CFSE)-Labeled OT-I and OT-II Cells

Spleens and lymph nodes from OT-I × B6 or OT-II × B6 mice were pooled and labeled with 2.5 μM CFSE (Molecular Probes, Eugene, OR, USA) at 37°C for 10 min. On day −1, 5×10^6 cells were transferred intravenously to *lang*-DTREGFP recipient mice. On day 0, mice received 10^5 CFU rBCG-OVA intravenously, and spleens were harvested at indicated time points to assess the CFSE proliferation profile by flow cytometry.

In Vitro Re-Stimulation of OT-I Cells

Seven days after rBCG-OVA infection of OT-I transfer recipients, splenocytes were cultured with 1 μg/mL $OVA_{257-265}$ (SIINFEKL) peptide (GenScript Corporation, Piscataway, NJ, USA) and 2 μg/mL anti-CD28 (clone 37.51, produced in-house) for 6 h at 37°C in complete IMDM (Gibco, Life Technologies), which contained 5% FCS (PAA Laboratories GmbH, Pasching, Austria), 1,000 μg/mL penicillin/streptomycin, 2 mM Glutamax, and 2-Mercaptoethanol (all Gibco, Invitrogen). 2 μM monensin (Sigma-Aldrich) was added for the last 4 h of incubation. Cells were fixed with formalin containing 4% formaldehyde (Sigma-Aldrich) and permeabilized with 0.1% Saponin buffer (Sigma-Aldrich) before being stained for intracellular IFN-γ, which was measured by flow cytometry.

ELISA

Blood was collected at indicated time points from the lateral tail vein and left overnight to clot. The serum was separated by centrifugation and frozen at −20°C. IL-12p40 and IFN-γ ELISAs were performed following the manufacturer's instructions (BD OptEIA) and the plate was read using a Versamax plate reader (Molecular Devices).

Statistics

Bar graphs show mean + SEM error bars. For graphs displaying CFU ($\log_{10}$), the geometric mean + 95% CI is shown. Statistical significance was determined by one-way ANOVA with the Tukey posttest or Kruskal–Wallis test as indicated; significance within groups was determined by two-way ANOVA with the Bonferroni posttest. Graphpad Prism 5 software (Graphpad Software Inc., San Diego, CA, USA) was used for all analyses.

RESULTS

Serum IL-12p40 Is Decreased, and Splenic Bacterial Burden Increased, in the Absence of Langerin⁺ CD8α⁺ DCs in BCG-Infected Mice

To determine if splenic langerin⁺ CD8α⁺ DCs were required for control of systemic BCG infection, we used *lang*-DTREGFP mice (referred to as Lang-DTR mice), which allowed depletion of langerin-expressing cells with DT during the course of infection. Multiple doses of DT were well tolerated and resulted in effective depletion of langerin⁺ CD8α⁺ DCs in the spleen [**Figures 1A,B**; (26)]. Depletion of langerin⁻ CD8α⁺ DCs was not evident (Figure S1 in Supplementary Material). Langerin⁺ CD8α⁺ DCs repopulated the spleen within 2–3 days of the final DT treatment (26).

To determine the effect of early depletion of splenic langerin⁺ CD8α⁺ DC on control of systemic blood-borne infection, the bacterial burden in the spleen was assessed over a 10-week period. BCG-infected, Lang-DTR mice were treated with DT from day −2 until day 6 of infection and spleens were harvested at 1, 3, 4, 6, and 10 weeks and then cultured to determine bacterial counts.

In langerin⁺ CD8α⁺ DC-depleted mice, a significant increase in spleen bacterial burden was evident 1 week after infection, compared to non-depleted mice, and this difference was maintained until 3 weeks after infection when spleen bacterial counts peaked (**Figures 1C,D**). In the later stage of infection, from 4 weeks onward, the difference in splenic bacterial burden between depleted and non-depleted mice was insignificant; by 10 weeks after infection, there was no discernible difference (**Figure 1C**). Extended depletion of langerin⁺ CD8α⁺ DCs (DT-treatment sustained until the 3-week peak of bacterial burden) had no further effect on the bacterial load in the spleen (Figure S2 in Supplementary Material).

Depletion of langerin⁺ CD8α⁺ DCs resulted in a small, but statistically insignificant, increase in the bacterial load of the liver compared to non-depleted mice (**Figure 1D**). DT treatment of C57BL/6 mice did not result in an increase in bacterial load in the liver or spleen (**Figure 1D**), confirming that the depletion of langerin⁺ CD8α⁺ DCs, rather than the DT treatment itself, was the cause of the increased bacterial burden during systemic BCG infection. These data may suggest the role of langerin⁺ CD8α⁺ DCs in the control of blood-borne bacterial infection is particularly important in, and potentially limited to, the spleen.

It has been reported in the CD11c-DTR mouse model that neutrophilia occurred after DT treatment in both naïve and bacterially infected mice, suggesting that neutrophilia was induced by DT itself (27). In the present study, an influx of neutrophils into the spleen was also observed early after BCG infection; however, this was significantly higher in DT-treated BCG-infected mice compared to DT-treated uninfected mice, suggesting that neutrophil influx was a response to BCG infection rather than DT treatment (Figure S3 in Supplementary Material). Indeed, uninfected mice treated with DT did not exhibit splenic neutrophilia.

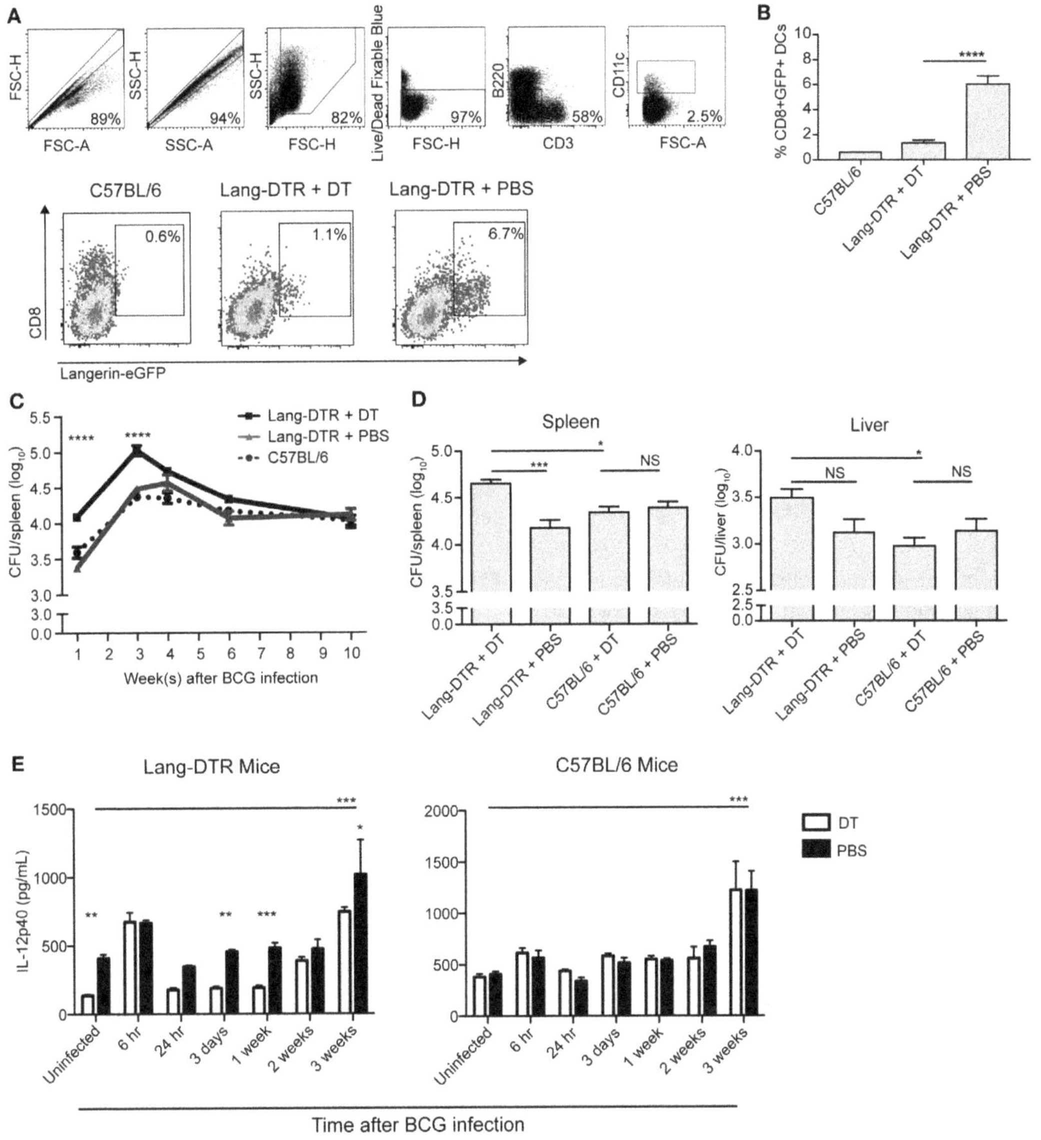

FIGURE 1 | Serum IL-12p40 is decreased, and splenic bacterial burden increased, in the absence of langerin+ CD8α+ dendritic cells in bacille Calmette–Guerin (BCG)-infected mice. Mice were treated with 350 ng diphtheria toxin (DT) i.p. (or PBS as a control) every 2 days from day −2 to day 6 after BCG infection. **(A,B)** Day 7 after BCG infection, GFP expression in the spleens of lang-DTR x lang-EGFP mice and C57BL/6 controls was assessed by flow cytometry after gating on live CD3− B220− CD11c+ cells ($n = 5$ mice per group). $^{****}p < 0.0001$, one-way ANOVA. The results are representative of two pooled experiments. **(C,D)** On day 0, all groups of mice were infected with BCG i.v. At the times indicated, mice were culled and spleens and livers removed, homogenized, and plated on 7H11 agar. Colonies were counted after 2–3 weeks. **(C)** Spleens were then harvested from mice culled at 1, 3, 4, 6, and 10 weeks after BCG infection ($n = 5$–6 mice per group). $^{****}p < 0.0001$, two-way ANOVA between DT and PBS groups. **(D)** In an additional experiment, spleens and livers were harvested from mice culled 3 weeks after BCG infection ($n = 10$ mice per group). The results are representative of two independent experiments. $^{*}p < 0.05$, $^{***}p < 0.001$, NS, not significant. **(E)** Mice were infected with BCG i.v. on day 0. At the times indicated, mice were tail-bled and serum IL-12p40 was measured by ELISA ($n = 4$–8 mice per group). $^{*}p < 0.05$, $^{**}p < 0.01$, $^{***}p < 0.001$, two-way ANOVA between DT and PBS-treated groups, $^{***}p < 0.001$, one-way ANOVA between uninfected and 3-week PBS-treated groups.

IL-12p40 is essential for immune control of mycobacterial infections (19–21), and as such, the concentration in serum was measured during systemic BCG infection in the presence or absence of langerin+ CD8α+ DCs. Interestingly, the concentration of IL-12p40 was significantly lower in the serum of uninfected mice that were depleted of langerin+ CD8α+ DCs (**Figure 1E**), compared to non-depleted mice, suggesting that these DCs contribute to basal IL-12p40 production. After a transient increase in IL-12p40 in both DT-treated and non-depleted mice 6 h after infection, no significant increase in IL-12p40 above basal levels was measured until 3 weeks after infection, at which point the serum concentration was significantly higher in BCG-infected, non-depleted mice compared to uninfected controls; the depletion of langerin+ CD8α+ DCs resulted in reduced IL-12p40 production at this time point. Importantly, in C57BL/6 controls, DT treatment did not affect the serum concentration of IL-12p40, which was significantly increased 3 weeks after BCG infection.

To determine if the decreased IL-12p40 levels in infected langerin$^+$ CD8α^+ DC-depleted mice resulted in reduced IFN-γ production, serum IFN-γ was measured, although typically Th1 IFN-γ responses do not develop until 4 weeks after BCG infection (28). As anticipated, IFN-γ was undetectable in the serum early after BCG infection (weeks 1, 2, and 3; data not shown); however, at 4 weeks post BCG infection, when it was detected, the depletion of langerin$^+$ CD8α^+ DCs had no effect on IFN-γ levels in the serum (Figure S4 in Supplementary Material).

Proliferation of OVA-Specific CD8$^+$ T Cells in Response to Recombinant BCG-OVA Infection Is Delayed, and Activation Diminished, in the Absence of Langerin$^+$ CD8α^+ DCs

CD8α^+ DCs are reportedly the most efficient splenic DC population for cross-presentation of antigen to CD8$^+$ T cells (5, 6). It is also known that mice deficient in CD8$^+$ T cells are impaired in their ability to control mycobacterial infections (29–31). Therefore, the proliferation of CD8$^+$ T cells was assessed in the context of CD8α^+ DC depletion. CFSE-labeled transgenic OVA-specific CD8$^+$ T cells (OT-I cells) were adoptively transferred into Lang-DTR mice, followed by i.v. infection the next day with recombinant BCG that expressed the model antigen ovalbumin (rBCG-OVA). Control animals were infected with non-recombinant BCG, or were left uninfected (OT-I only controls). Animals were then treated with DT every 2 days for the first week of infection, or continuously until the end of the experiment (cont) as indicated, to deplete langerin-expressing cells.

As expected (25), 1 week after rBCG-OVA infection, OT-I cells in the non-depleted recipient mice (rBCG-OVA + PBS) revealed diluted CFSE expression, indicative of proliferation (**Figure 2A**). In contrast, there was little proliferation at this time point in mice depleted of langerin$^+$ CD8α^+ DCs. Two weeks after infection, however, OT-I proliferation was diminished in DT-treated mice, and by 3 weeks after infection, OT-I proliferation occurred regardless of whether langerin$^+$ CD8α^+ DCs had been depleted (data not shown). Mice treated continuously with DT for the duration of the experiment did not have significantly different OT-I proliferation than mice depleted for just the first week of infection. These data suggest that depletion of langerin$^+$ CD8α^+ DCs delayed rather than prevented OT-I activation.

Infection with wild-type BCG did not induce significant OT-I proliferation compared to uninfected controls (OT-I only) at any time point assessed, confirming that the T cell activation was antigen-specific. The overall number of OT-I cells, and the percentage of proliferating cells, was significantly lower in the spleen of langerin$^+$ CD8α^+ DC-depleted mice 1 week after rBCG-OVA infection, as well as at 2 weeks after infection in terms of OT-I number, compared to non-depleted mice (**Figure 2B**). Three weeks after infection, however, OT-I cells in the spleen had increased significantly in response to rBCG-OVA infection in both depleted and non-depleted mice, compared to uninfected controls.

The apparently diminished CD8$^+$ T cell response in the absence of langerin$^+$ CD8α^+ DCs was also reflected in the activation status and IFN-γ production of OT-I cells. One week after rBCG-OVA infection, OT-I cells in langerin$^+$ CD8α^+ DC-depleted mice displayed higher CD62L and lower CD44 compared to OT-I cells in non-depleted mice (**Figure 2C**), indicative of reduced activation. In addition, in OT-I cells isolated from mice depleted of langerin$^+$ CD8α^+ DC during infection, the proportion of IFN-γ^+ OT-I cells in response to *in vitro* stimulation with OVA$_{257-265}$ peptide was diminished compared to non-depleted mice (**Figure 2D**). Together, these data suggest that langerin$^+$ CD8α^+ DCs are important for early CD8$^+$ T cell activation and function after BCG infection.

In analogous experiments, using adoptively transferred CFSE-labeled transgenic OVA-specific CD4$^+$ T cells (OT-II cells), we did not observe any effect of langerin$^+$ CD8α^+ DC depletion on OT-II cell proliferation or the total number of OT-II cells in the spleen (**Figure 3**). As such, additional effects of depletion on these cells were not investigated further in this study.

DISCUSSION

Langerin$^+$ CD8α^+ DCs, resident in the marginal zone of the spleen, are localized for effective sampling of the blood; however, to the best of our knowledge, the role of these DCs in protection against systemic bacterial infection is yet to be reported. Here, we show that *in vivo* depletion of langerin$^+$ CD8α^+ DCs during intravenous BCG infection resulted in decreased IL-12p40 in the serum and a delay in antigen-specific CD8$^+$ T cell proliferation, with reduced activation and IFN-γ production associated. An increased bacterial burden in the spleen was also evident. Together, these results suggest that langerin$^+$ CD8α^+ DCs may play an important role in the immune response against blood-borne bacterial infection.

In similar experimental contexts, several *in vivo* DC-depletion studies have demonstrated protective antimicrobial DC-mediated responses. Depletion of CD11c$^+$ DCs during *S. aureus* bloodstream infection resulted in decreased serum IL-12, concomitant with an increased bacterial load (32). Similarly, bacterial numbers were increased after depletion of CD11c$^+$ DCs during intravenous *Mtb* infection (17). Depletion of dermal langerin$^+$ DCs in the context of *Leishmania major* infection resulted in a significant reduction in CD8$^+$ T cell proliferation, with no effect on CD4$^+$ T cell responses; however, no impact on parasite clearance was demonstrated (33).

By contrast, a number of reports have shown that depletion of DCs enhances, rather than impairs, host defense to the infective organism. A study of *Listeria monocytogenes* infection revealed a direct role for CD8α^+ DCs in promoting bacterial disease. In the absence of CD8α^+ DCs, bacteria were unable to traffic into the periarteriolar sheath and remained trapped in the marginal zone of the spleen, suggesting that the DCs facilitated entry of these microorganisms into the spleen. Not surprisingly, the absence of CD8α^+ DCs during *L. monocytogenes* infection resulted in a reduced bacterial load compared to wild-type animals (34). Depletion of CD11c$^+$ DCs prior to *Yersinia enterocolitica* infection also led to the surprising finding that animal survival increased; this was discovered to be due to neutrophil accumulation in the spleen following DC depletion, rather than a direct effect of the

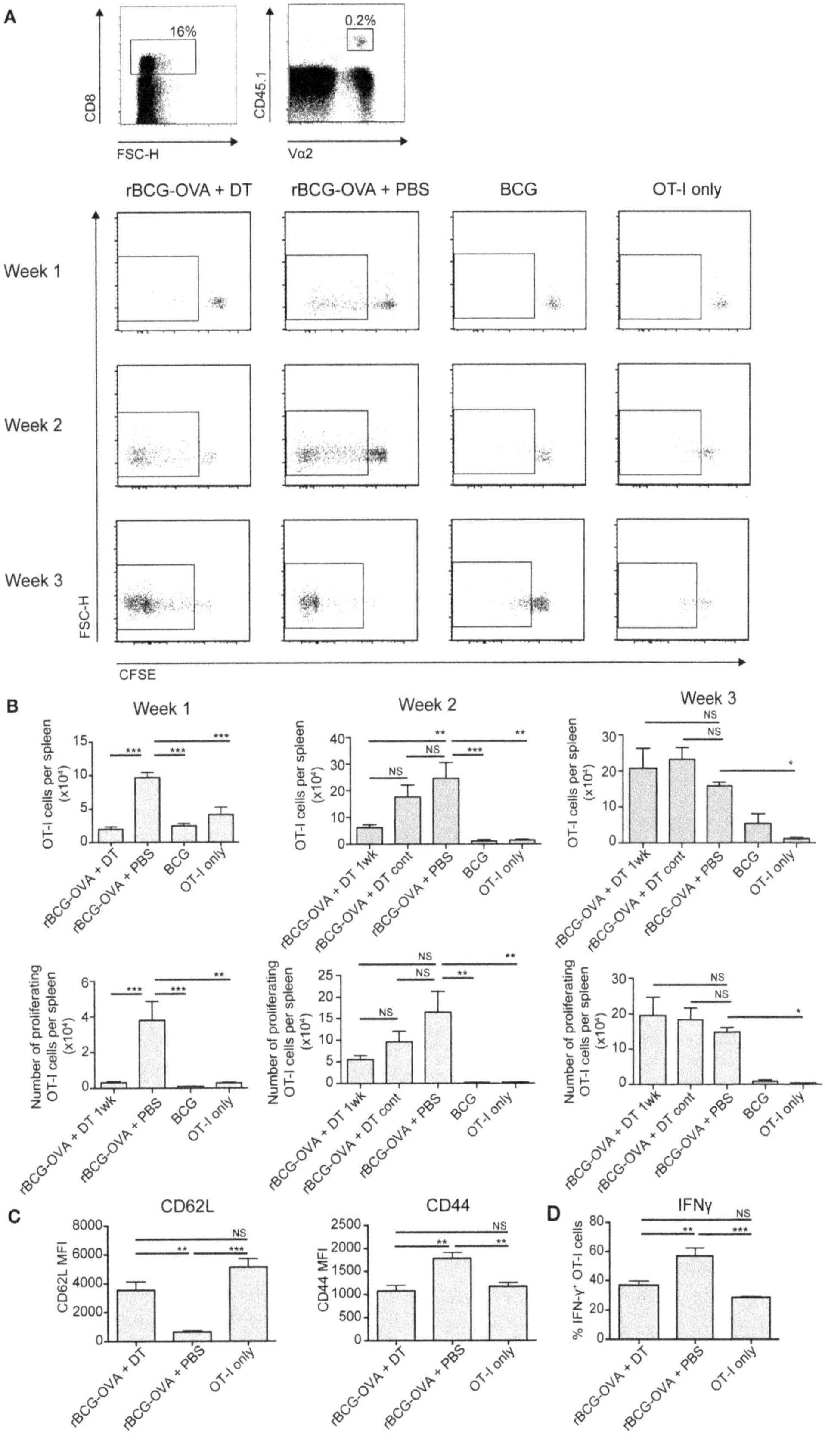

FIGURE 2 | Continued

FIGURE 2 | OT-I T cell proliferation in response to rBCG-OVA infection is delayed, and activation diminished, in the absence of langerin+ CD8α+ dendritic cells (DCs). Lang-diphtheria toxin receptor mice received 5 × 10^6 carboxyflourescein diacetate succinimidyl ester (CFSE)-labeled splenocytes from OT-I × B6 donor mice 1 day before i.v. infection with rBCG-OVA or BCG. One group of mice were not infected (OT-I only group). Mice infected with rBCG-OVA were treated with 350 ng diphtheria toxin (DT) i.p. (or PBS as a control) starting on day −2, every 2 days for the first week of infection, or until the end of the experiment as denoted. At the indicated time points, mice were culled and spleens removed. The CFSE profile of splenic OT-I cells was assessed by flow cytometry. **(A)** Representative flow cytometry plots of the CFSE profile after gating on CD8+ CD45.1+ Vα2+ OT-I cells; flow plots show the proliferating cells in mice depleted with DT for 1 week. **(B)** The number of OT-I cells, and the number of proliferating OT-I cells within the spleen are shown, for mice receiving 1 week or continuous DT treatment (cont). **(C)** One week after rBCG-OVA infection, the median fluorescent intensity (MFI) of CD62L and CD44 expressed on OT-I cells was measured by flow cytometry. **(D)** One week after rBCG-OVA infection, splenocytes were cultured with 1 μg/mL $OVA_{257-265}$ peptide for 6 h. Intracellular IFN-γ production by OT-I cells was measured by flow cytometry (n = 3–6 mice per group). *$p < 0.05$, **$p < 0.01$, ***$p < 0.001$, NS, not significant, one-way ANOVA. The results are representative of two independent experiments.

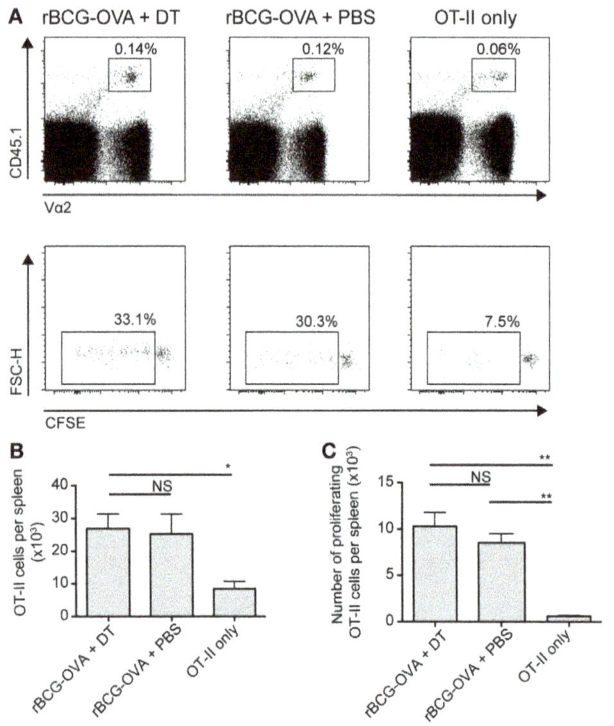

FIGURE 3 | OT-II proliferation is unaffected by depletion of langerin+ CD8α+ dendritic cells. Lang-diphtheria toxin receptor mice received 5 × 10^6 carboxyflourescein diacetate succinimidyl ester (CFSE)-labeled splenocytes from OT-II × B6 donor mice 1 day before i.v. infection with 10^5 CFU rBCG-OVA. One group of mice was not infected (OT-II only group). Mice infected with rBCG-OVA were treated with 350 ng DT i.p. (or PBS as a control) starting on day −2, every 2 days until day 6. On day 9 after infection, mice were culled and spleens were removed. The CFSE profile of splenic OT-II cells was assessed by flow cytometry. **(A)** Representative plots of CD4+ CD45.1+ Vα2+ OT-II cells and their CFSE profiles, gated on proliferating (CFSE intermediate and negative) OT-II cells. **(B)** The number of OT-II cells and **(C)** the number of proliferating OT-II cells per spleen are shown (n = 3 mice per group). NS, not significant, *$p < 0.05$, **$p < 0.01$, one-way ANOVA. The results are representative of two independent experiments.

DCs (35). It appears, therefore, that while DCs are key players in the antibacterial response to blood-borne bacteria, specific DC subsets may be protective or detrimental to the immune response, depending on the infecting bacterial species.

The effect of depletion of CD8α+ DCs during systemic mycobacterial infection has not been reported, to date. In terms of the langerin+ CD8α+ DC subset, we have previously shown the functional specialization of these DCs *in vitro* (12), and *in vivo* (36) in protein/adjuvant models, particularly, with respect to enhanced IL-12 production. CD8α+ DCs, as a whole population, were superior to CD8α− DCs in their ability to induce protective responses against BCG infection in an adoptive transfer setting (37), and have also been implicated as transient producers of IL-12p40 5 h after i.v. BCG exposure (38). In light of these findings, it could be expected that langerin+ CD8α+ DCs would be important for IL-12p40 production in the context of BCG infection; however, as our data show a transient increase of IL-12p40 6 h after infection in both DT-treated and non-depleted mice, it suggests that perhaps langerin− CD8α+ DCs may be the early producers of IL-12p40, before langerin+ CD8α+ DCs are implicated by 3 weeks after infection.

The role of CD8α+ DCs has also been examined in *Batf3*−/− mice. These mice lack the Batf3 transcription factor and, reportedly, as a consequence are deficient in CD8α+ DCs (39). However, as we and others have recently discovered, CD8α+ DCs do develop in these mice when bred on a C57BL/6 background under certain, as yet undefined, conditions (36, 40). We suggest that langerin− CX3CR1− CD8α+ cells that remain in *Batf3*−/− mice are in fact precursors for the mature langerin+ population. Moreover, others have shown that infection with *Mtb*, *Toxoplasma gondii* or *L. monocytogenes* causes restoration of fully functional CD8α+ cDCs in *Batf3*−/− mice, attributed to compensatory pathways involving the related transcription factors Batf and Batf2 (41). Therefore, the findings reported in this depletion study provide important novel insights into the role of langerin+ CD8α+ DCs in the immune response to blood-borne mycobacteria.

While we acknowledge that DT treatment also depletes Langerhans cells and langerin+ dermal DCs (24, 42), these cells do not have access to the spleen. Therefore, they likely play no role in the protection observed in non-depleted, BCG-infected mice. Furthermore, when comparing DT-treated Lang-DTR mice and splenectomized mice, CD8+ T cell activation in response to antigen and synthetic NKT cell ligand exposure is severely compromised in both models (43), indicating that the presence of the splenic langerin-expressing cells are crucial for promoting effective CD8+ T cell responses to circulating antigens. However, we cannot entirely discount the possibility that DT treatment led to a decrease in early killing efficiency by macrophages or DCs due to the uptake of apoptotic cells. It is also possible that the observed impact of depleting langerin-expressing cells in the context of BCG infection could have resulted from a reduction in a functional activity that can be attributed to the CD8α+ DC population as a whole. In this situation, it is possible the effect of depleting langerin-expressing cells could, therefore, simply reflect a large reduction [up to 60% (26)] of total $CD8\alpha^+$ DCs in spleens of these mice.

Interestingly, our work revealed that the depletion of langerin $CD8\alpha^+$ DCs lead to reduced $CD8^+$ T cell activation and proliferation during the first week of BCG infection; however, 2 and 3 weeks after infection, $CD8^+$ T cells proliferated in both depleted and non-depleted mice. As this effect was similarly apparent in mice treated with DT for either the first week or the full duration of the experiment, this suggested that $langerin^+$ $CD8\alpha^+$ DCs primarily drive $CD8^+$ T cell proliferation early after BCG infection, and may be redundant after this time. It is possible that other subsets of cross-presenting DCs, such as $langerin^-$ $XCR1^+$ DCs, were responsible for stimulating $CD8^+$ T cells during these later time points, as these cells would not have been depleted in the langerin-DTR mice. In contrast, an increase in the spleen bacterial load was detected whether DT treatment was continued throughout the experiment or only administered for the first week after infection (in the latter case, DCs would have reconstituted during the second week). This suggests the role of $langerin^+$ $CD8\alpha^+$ DCs in antimycobacterial control may be of particular significance in the first week after infection, and the importance of this early effect on the ensuing immune response is maintained throughout the bacterial proliferation phase.

Although significant insights into the beneficial role of $langerin^+$ $CD8\alpha^+$ DCs in blood-borne bacterial infection are presented in this study, the mechanism of protection was not fully elucidated in this work. Interestingly, numerous reports have shown that *Mtb*-infected mice deficient in IL-12 or $CD8^+$ T cells have increased bacterial burdens after 3–4 or 4–6 weeks of infection, respectively (20, 29, 31, 44). Therefore, in concordance with our findings, the IL-12 production and $CD8^+$ T cell stimulation of $langerin^+$ $CD8\alpha^+$ DCs may represent important aspects of the antibacterial response.

In this study, we report a previously unobserved role for $langerin^+$ $CD8\alpha^+$ DCs during the initiation of the immune response against systemic mycobacterial infection. The functional heterogeneity of $CD8\alpha^+$ DCs has been underappreciated in the literature to date; thus, the data presented herein provide important insights specifically related to the $langerin^+$ DC subset. These significant findings provide a platform for further investigations to more conclusively determine the mechanism of protective influence of $langerin^+$ $CD8\alpha^+$ DCs, and whether this extends to other blood-borne bacterial infections.

AUTHOR CONTRIBUTIONS

KP planned and performed all experimental work, analyzed and prepared figures, and assisted with writing of the manuscript; ND assisted with figure preparation and wrote the manuscript in consultation with KP and JK; TP assisted with experimental conception and analysis; IH assisted with experimental conception and planning; JK was in charge of overall direction and planning of the project, as well as experimental conception and manuscript preparation.

ACKNOWLEDGMENTS

We would like to thank Dr. Lindsay Ancelet, Ms. Fenella Rich, and Ms. Clare Burn for technical assistance, the Malaghan Institute Biomedical Research Unit for animal husbandry, and the Cell Technology Suit for flow cytometry support. This work was supported by the Marsden Fund, New Zealand.

SUPPLEMENTARY MATERIAL

FIGURE S1 | Diphtheria toxin (DT) treatment mediates specific depletion of $langerin^+$ $CD8\alpha^+$ DCs. Mice were treated with 350 ng DT i.p. (or PBS as a control) every 2 days from day −2 to day 6 after bacille Calmette–Guerin (BCG) infection. On day 7 after BCG infection, GFP expression in the spleens of lang-diphtheria toxin receptor × lang-EGFP mice was assessed by flow cytometry after gating on live $CD3^-$ $B220^-$ $CD11c^+$ cells ($n = 5$ mice per group), as per **Figure 1A**. **(A)** Gating strategy for $langerin^+$ $CD8\alpha^+$ and $langerin^-$ $CD8\alpha^+$ DC populations. **(B)** Bar graphs show the mean + SEM percentage of $langerin^+$ $CD8\alpha^+$ and $langerin^-$ $CD8\alpha^+$ DCs in mice treated with DT or PBS. NS, not significant, $^{****}p < 0.0001$, one-way ANOVA. The results are representative of two pooled experiments.

FIGURE S2 | Extended depletion of $langerin^+$ $CD8\alpha^+$ DCs had no further effect on the bacterial load in the spleen. Mice were treated with 350 ng diphtheria toxin (DT) i.p. (or PBS as a control) every 2 days from day −2 to day 6 after bacille Calmette–Guerin (BCG) infection, or until 3 weeks after BCG infection. On day 0, all groups of mice were infected with BCG i.v. At 3 weeks after BCG infection, mice were culled and spleens removed, homogenized, and plated on 7H11 agar ($n = 10$–11 mice per group). Colonies were counted after 2–3 weeks. Graph shows the geometric mean of spleen bacterial CFU + 95% CI for mice treated with DT for 1 or 3 weeks, or PBS control. NS, not significant, $^{**}p < 0.01$, one-way ANOVA. The results are representative of two independent experiments.

FIGURE S3 | Diphtheria toxin (DT) treatment itself did not induce neutrophilia Lang-diphtheria toxin receptor mice were treated with 350 ng DT i.p. (or PBS as a control) on day −1. Bacille Calmette–Guerin (BCG) infection was carried out on day 0, and mice were culled and spleens removed 2 or 24 h after infection; uninfected mice were culled at the 24 h time point. **(A)** Representative flow cytometry plots of neutrophil proportions in BCG infected and uninfected mice, treated with DT or PBS. **(B)** The percentage of neutrophils ($CD11b^+$ $GR1^{high}$) in the spleens of BCG infected or uninfected mice, treated with DT or PBS is shown ($n = 3$–4 mice per group). NS, not significant, $^{*}p < 0.05$, $^{**}p < 0.01$, $^{***}p < 0.001$, one-way ANOVA.

FIGURE S4 | Depletion of $langerin^+$ $CD8\alpha^+$ DCs had no effect on IFN-γ levels in the serum 4 weeks after bacille Calmette–Guerin (BCG) infection Lang-diphtheria toxin receptor or C57BL/6 mice were infected with 10^5 CFU BCG i.v. on day 0 and treated with 350 ng diphtheria toxin i.p. (or PBS as a control) starting on day −2 and continuing every 2 days for 1 week. Four weeks after BCG infection, mice were tail-bled and serum IFN-γ levels were measured by ELISA ($n = 10$ mice per group). NS, not significant, Kruskal–Wallis test. This result is representative of two independent experiments.

REFERENCES

1. Kollef MH, Zilberberg MD, Shorr AF, Vo L, Schein J, Micek ST, et al. Epidemiology, microbiology and outcomes of healthcare-associated and community-acquired bacteremia: a multicenter cohort study. *J Infect* (2011) 62(2):130–5. doi:10.1016/j.jinf.2010.12.009
2. Mebius RE, Kraal G. Structure and function of the spleen. *Nat Rev Immunol* (2005) 5(8):606–16. doi:10.1038/nri1669
3. Vremec D, Pooley J, Hochrein H, Wu L, Shortman K. CD4 and CD8 expression by dendritic cell subtypes in mouse thymus and spleen. *J Immunol* (2000) 164(6):2978–86. doi:10.4049/jimmunol.164.6.2978
4. Moore AJ, Anderson MK. Dendritic cell development: a choose-your-own-adventure story. *Adv Hematol* (2013) 2013:949513. doi:10.1155/2013/949513
5. den Haan JM, Lehar SM, Bevan MJ. CD8+ but not CD8− dendritic cells cross-prime cytotoxic T cells in vivo. *J Exp Med* (2000) 192(12):1685–96. doi:10.1084/jem.192.12.1685
6. Pooley JL, Heath WR, Shortman K. Cutting edge: intravenous soluble antigen is presented to CD4 T cells by CD8− dendritic cells, but cross-presented to CD8 T cells by CD8+ dendritic cells. *J Immunol* (2001) 166(9):5327–30. doi:10.4049/jimmunol.166.9.5327
7. Manetti R, Parronchi P, Giudizi MG, Piccinni MP, Maggi E, Trinchieri G, et al. Natural killer cell stimulatory factor (interleukin 12 [IL-12]) induces T helper type 1 (Th1)-specific immune responses and inhibits the development of IL-4-producing Th cells. *J Exp Med* (1993) 177(4):1199–204. doi:10.1084/jem.177.4.1199
8. Macatonia SE, Hosken NA, Litton M, Vieira P, Hsieh CS, Culpepper JA, et al. Dendritic cells produce IL-12 and direct the development of Th1 cells from naive CD4+ T cells. *J Immunol* (1995) 154(10):5071–9.
9. Bar-On L, Birnberg T, Lewis KL, Edelson BT, Bruder D, Hildner K, et al. CX3CR1+ CD8alpha+ dendritic cells are a steady-state population related to plasmacytoid dendritic cells. *Proc Natl Acad Sci U S A* (2010) 107(33):14745–50. doi:10.1073/pnas.1001562107
10. Idoyaga J, Suda N, Suda K, Park CG, Steinman RM. Antibody to langerin/CD207 localizes large numbers of CD8alpha+ dendritic cells to the marginal zone of mouse spleen. *Proc Natl Acad Sci U S A* (2009) 106(5):1524–9. doi:10.1073/pnas.0812247106
11. Qiu C-H, Miyake Y, Kaise H, Kitamura H, Ohara O, Tanaka M. Novel subset of CD8alpha+ dendritic cells localized in the marginal zone is responsible for tolerance to cell-associated antigens. *J Immunol* (2009) 182(7):4127–36. doi:10.4049/jimmunol.0803364
12. Farrand KJ, Dickgreber N, Stoitzner P, Ronchese F, Petersen TR, Hermans IF. Langerin+CD8 alpha+ dendritic cells are critical for cross-priming and IL-12 production in response to systemic antigens. *J Immunol* (2009) 183(12):7732–42. doi:10.4049/jimmunol.0902707
13. Laupland KB, Church DL. Population-based epidemiology and microbiology of community-onset bloodstream infections. *Clin Microbiol Rev* (2014) 27(4):647–64. doi:10.1128/CMR.00002-14
14. El Helou G, Hachem R, Viola GM, El Zakhem A, Chaftari AM, Jiang Y, et al. Management of rapidly growing mycobacterial bacteremia in cancer patients. *Clin Infect Dis* (2013) 56(6):843–6. doi:10.1093/cid/cis1032
15. El Helou G, Viola GM, Hachem R, Han XY, Raad II. Rapidly growing mycobacterial bloodstream infections. *Lancet Infect Dis* (2013) 13(2):166–74. doi:10.1016/S1473-3099(12)70316-X
16. Jacob ST, Pavlinac PB, Nakiyingi L, Banura P, Baeten JM, Morgan K, et al. *Mycobacterium tuberculosis* bacteremia in a cohort of HIV-infected patients hospitalized with severe sepsis in Uganda-high frequency, low clinical suspicion [corrected] and derivation of a clinical prediction score. *PLoS One* (2013) 8(8):e70305. doi:10.1371/journal.pone.0070305
17. Tian T, Woodworth J, Sköld M, Behar SM. In vivo depletion of CD11c+ cells delays the CD4+ T cell response to *Mycobacterium tuberculosis* and exacerbates the outcome of infection. *J Immunol* (2005) 175(5):3268–72. doi:10.4049/jimmunol.175.5.3268
18. Prendergast KA, Kirman JR. Dendritic cell subsets in mycobacterial infection: control of bacterial growth and T cell responses. *Tuberculosis* (2013) 93(2):115–22. doi:10.1016/j.tube.2012.10.008
19. Khader SA, Pearl JE, Sakamoto K, Gilmartin L, Bell GK, Jelley-Gibbs DM, et al. IL-23 compensates for the absence of IL-12p70 and is essential for the IL-17 response during tuberculosis but is dispensable for protection and antigen-specific IFN-gamma responses if IL-12p70 is available. *J Immunol* (2005) 175(2):788–95. doi:10.4049/jimmunol.175.2.788
20. Cooper AM, Kipnis A, Turner J, Magram J, Ferrante J, Orme IM. Mice lacking bioactive IL-12 can generate protective, antigen-specific cellular responses to mycobacterial infection only if the IL-12 p40 subunit is present. *J Immunol* (2002) 168(3):1322–7. doi:10.4049/jimmunol.168.3.1322
21. Feng CG, Jankovic D, Kullberg M, Cheever A, Scanga CA, Hieny S, et al. Maintenance of pulmonary Th1 effector function in chronic tuberculosis requires persistent IL-12 production. *J Immunol* (2005) 174(7):4185–92. doi:10.4049/jimmunol.174.7.4185
22. Flynn JL, Chan J, Triebold KJ, Dalton DK, Stewart TA, Bloom BR. An essential role for interferon gamma in resistance to *Mycobacterium tuberculosis* infection. *J Exp Med* (1993) 178(6):2249–54. doi:10.1084/jem.178.6.2249
23. Cooper AM, Dalton DK, Stewart TA, Griffin JP, Russell DG, Orme IM. Disseminated tuberculosis in interferon gamma gene-disrupted mice. *J Exp Med* (1993) 178(6):2243–7. doi:10.1084/jem.178.6.2243
24. Kissenpfennig A, Henri S, Dubois B, Laplace-Builhé C, Perrin P, Romani N, et al. Dynamics and function of Langerhans cells in vivo: dermal dendritic cells colonize lymph node areas distinct from slower migrating Langerhans cells. *Immunity* (2005) 22(5):643–54. doi:10.1016/j.immuni.2005.04.004
25. Ryan AA, Nambiar JK, Wozniak TM, Roediger B, Shklovskaya E, Britton WJ, et al. Antigen load governs the differential priming of CD8 T cells in response to the bacille Calmette Guerin vaccine or *Mycobacterium tuberculosis* infection. *J Immunol* (2009) 182(11):7172–7. doi:10.4049/jimmunol.0801694
26. Prendergast KA, Osmond TL, Ochiai S, Hermans IF, Kirman JR. Sustained in vivo depletion of splenic langerin+ CD8α+ dendritic cells is well-tolerated by lang-DTREGFP mice. *J Immunol Methods* (2014) 406:104–9. doi:10.1016/j.jim.2014.02.005
27. Tittel AP, Heuser C, Ohliger C, Llanto C, Yona S, Hammerling GJ, et al. Functionally relevant neutrophilia in CD11c diphtheria toxin receptor transgenic mice. *Nat Methods* (2012) 9(4):385–90. doi:10.1038/nmeth.1905
28. Kamath AT, Groat NL, Bean AG, Britton WJ. Protective effect of DNA immunization against mycobacterial infection is associated with the early emergence of interferon-gamma (IFN-gamma)-secreting lymphocytes. *Clin Exp Immunol* (2000) 120:476–82. doi:10.1046/j.1365-2249.2000.01240.x
29. Behar SM, Dascher CC, Grusby MJ, Wang CR, Brenner MB. Susceptibility of mice deficient in CD1D or TAP1 to infection with *Mycobacterium tuberculosis*. *J Exp Med* (1999) 189(12):1973–80. doi:10.1084/jem.189.12.1973
30. Flynn JL, Goldstein MM, Triebold KJ, Koller B, Bloom BR. Major histocompatibility complex class I-restricted T cells are required for resistance to *Mycobacterium tuberculosis* infection. *Proc Natl Acad Sci U S A* (1992) 89(24):12013–7. doi:10.1073/pnas.89.24.12013
31. Sousa AO, Mazzaccaro RJ, Russell RG, Lee FK, Turner OC, Hong S, et al. Relative contributions of distinct MHC class I-dependent cell populations in protection to tuberculosis infection in mice. *Proc Natl Acad Sci U S A* (2000) 97(8):4204–8. doi:10.1073/pnas.97.8.4204
32. Schindler D, Gutierrez MG, Beineke A, Rauter Y, Rohde M, Foster S, et al. Dendritic cells are central coordinators of the host immune response to *Staphylococcus aureus* bloodstream infection. *Am J Pathol* (2012) 181(4):1327–37. doi:10.1016/j.ajpath.2012.06.039
33. Brewig N, Kissenpfennig A, Malissen B, Veit A, Bickert T, Fleischer B, et al. Priming of CD8+ and CD4+ T cells in experimental leishmaniasis is initiated by different dendritic cell subtypes. *J Immunol* (2009) 182(2):774–83. doi:10.4049/jimmunol.182.2.774
34. Edelson BT, Bradstreet TR, Hildner K, Carrero JA, Frederick KE, KC W, et al. CD8α+ dendritic cells are an obligate cellular entry point for productive infection by *Listeria monocytogenes*. *Immunity* (2011) 35(2):236–48. doi:10.1016/j.immuni.2011.06.012
35. Autenrieth SE, Warnke P, Wabnitz GH, Lucero Estrada C, Pasquevich KA, Drechsler D, et al. Depletion of dendritic cells enhances innate anti-bacterial host defense through modulation of phagocyte homeostasis. *PLoS Pathog* (2012) 8(2):e1002552. doi:10.1371/journal.ppat.1002552
36. Petersen TR, Knight DA, Tang CW, Osmond TL, Hermans IF. Batf3-independent langerin− CX3CR1− CD8alpha+ splenic DCs represent a precursor for classical cross-presenting CD8alpha+ DCs. *J Leukoc Biol* (2014) 96:1001–10. doi:10.1189/jlb.1A0314-130R
37. Gao X, Wang S, Fan Y, Bai H, Yang J, Yang X. CD8+ DC, but not CD8− DC, isolated from BCG-infected mice reduces pathological reactions induced by

mycobacterial challenge infection. *PLoS One* (2010) 5(2):e9281. doi:10.1371/journal.pone.0009281

38. Rothfuchs AG, Egen JG, Feng CG, Antonelli LRV, Bafica A, Winter N, et al. In situ IL-12/23p40 production during mycobacterial infection is sustained by CD11bhigh dendritic cells localized in tissue sites distinct from those harboring bacilli. *J Immunol* (2009) 182(11):6915–25. doi:10.4049/jimmunol.0900074
39. Hildner K, Edelson BT, Purtha WE, Diamond M, Matsushita H, Kohyama M, et al. *Batf3* deficiency reveals a critical role for CD8alpha+ dendritic cells in cytotoxic T cell immunity. *Science* (2008) 322:1097–100. doi:10.1126/science.1164206
40. Mott KR, Maazi H, Allen SJ, Zandian M, Matundan H, Ghiasi YN, et al. Batf3 deficiency is not critical for the generation of CD8alpha dendritic cells. *Immunobiology* (2014) 220(4):518–24. doi:10.1016/j.imbio.2014.10.019
41. Tussiwand R, Lee WL, Murphy TL, Mashayekhi M, Kc W, Albring JC, et al. Compensatory dendritic cell development mediated by BATF-IRF interactions. *Nature* (2012) 490(7421):502–7. doi:10.1038/nature11531
42. Poulin LF, Henri S, de Bovis B, Devilard E, Kissenpfennig A, Malissen B. The dermis contains langerin+ dendritic cells that develop and function independently of epidermal Langerhans cells. *J Exp Med* (2007) 204(13):3119–31. doi:10.1084/jem.20071724
43. Osmond TL, Farrand KJ, Painter GF, Ruedl C, Petersen TR, Hermans IF. Activated NKT cells can condition different splenic dendritic cell subsets to respond more effectively to TLR engagement and enhance cross-priming. *J Immunol* (2015) 195(3):821–31. doi:10.4049/jimmunol.1401751
44. Cooper AM, Magram J, Ferrante J, Orme IM. Interleukin 12 (IL-12) is crucial to the development of protective immunity in mice intravenously infected with *Mycobacterium tuberculosis*. *J Exp Med* (1997) 186(1):39–45. doi:10.1084/jem.186.1.39

9

Novel Cre-Expressing Mouse Strains Permitting to Selectively Track and Edit Type 1 Conventional Dendritic Cells Facilitate Disentangling their Complexity *in vivo*

Raphaël Mattiuz[1], Christian Wohn[1], Sonia Ghilas[1], Marc Ambrosini[1], Yannick O. Alexandre[1], Cindy Sanchez[1], Anissa Fries[1], Thien-Phong Vu Manh[1], Bernard Malissen[1,2], Marc Dalod[1] and Karine Crozat[1*]*

[1] Centre d'Immunologie de Marseille-Luminy, Turing Center for Living Systems, CNRS, INSERM, Aix Marseille Univ, Marseille, France, [2] Centre d'Immunophénomique, Aix Marseille Univ, CNRS, INSERM, Marseille, France

***Correspondence:**
Marc Dalod
dalod@ciml.univ-mrs.fr
Karine Crozat
crozat@ciml.univ-mrs.fr

Type 1 conventional DCs (cDC1) excel in the cross-priming of $CD8^+$ T cells, which is crucial for orchestrating efficient immune responses against viruses or tumors. However, our understanding of their physiological functions and molecular regulation has been limited by the lack of proper mutant mouse models allowing their conditional genetic targeting. Because the *Xcr1* and *A530099j19rik* (*Karma/Gpr141b)* genes belong to the core transcriptomic fingerprint of mouse cDC1, we used them to engineer two novel Cre-driver lines, the *Xcr1*^{Cre} and *Karma*^{Cre} mice, by knocking in an IRES-Cre expression cassette into their 3′-UTR. We used genetic tracing to characterize the specificity and efficiency of these new models in several lymphoid and non-lymphoid tissues, and compared them to the *Clec9a*^{Cre} mouse model, which targets the immediate precursors of cDCs. Amongst the three Cre-driver mouse models examined, the *Xcr1*^{Cre} model was the most efficient and specific for the fate mapping of all cDC1, regardless of the tissues examined. The *Karma*^{Cre} model was rather specific for cDC1 when compared with the *Clec9a*^{Cre} mouse, but less efficient than the *Xcr1*^{Cre} model. Unexpectedly, the *Xcr1*^{Cre} model targeted a small fraction of $CD4^+$ T cells, and the *Karma*^{Cre} model a significant proportion of mast cells in the skin. Importantly, the targeting specificity of these two mouse models was not changed upon inflammation. A high frequency of germline recombination was observed solely in the *Xcr1*^{Cre} mouse model when both the *Cre* and the *floxed* alleles were brought by the same gamete irrespective of its gender. *Xcr1*, *Karma*, and *Clec9a* being differentially expressed within the cDC1 population, the three CRE-driver lines examined showed distinct recombination patterns in cDC1 phenotypic subsets. This advances our understanding of cDC1 subset heterogeneity and the differentiation trajectory of these cells. Therefore, to the best of our knowledge, upon informed use, the *Xcr1*^{Cre} and *Karma*^{Cre} mouse models represent the best tools currently reported to specifically and faithfully target cDC1 *in vivo*, both at steady state and upon inflammation. Future use of these mutant mouse models will undoubtedly boost our understanding of the biology of cDC1.

Keywords: dendritic cells, cDC1, XCR1, Gp141b, Karma, Clec9a, Cre, fate mapping

INTRODUCTION

Dendritic cells (DCs) constitute a heterogeneous population of antigen presenting cells (APCs) which are instrumental for the orchestration of innate and adaptive immune responses. In mice and in humans, three distinct types of DCs differing in their phenotype, localization and functions populate all lymphoid and most non-lymphoid tissues at steady state. Plasmacytoid DCs (pDCs) are the major source of type I interferon (IFN) upon many viral infections. Conventional DCs (cDCs) consist of two populations, coined as type 1 and type 2 cDCs and which excel in the cross-priming of CD8$^+$ T cells or in the promotion of CD4$^+$ T cell and humoral immunity, respectively. The functions of cDCs and their molecular regulation have been studied *in vivo* by using a wealth of mouse models that enable their depletion or genetic manipulation, namely *Cd11c (Itgax)*^{hDTR} (1) or *Cd11c (Itgax)*^{Cre} (2, 3) and more recently the *Zbtb46*^{hDTR} (4) or *Zbtb46*^{Cre} (5). However, interpretation of the results obtained using those mice can be difficult due to the expression of *Cd11c* by many other cell types than cDCs and of *Zbtb46* by committed erythroid progenitors and endothelial cell populations (6). Moreover, these mutant mouse models are not suited to study the respective functions of each of the two cDC types. This goal requires the use of refined mutant mouse models enabling specific targeting of either cDC1 or cDC2.

Constitutive (*Batf3*-KO mice) or conditional (*Itgax*^{Cre}; *Irf8*$^{fl/fl}$ mice) genetic inactivation of transcription factors required for the differentiation of cDC1 allowed to study their specific functions *in vivo* (7, 8). However, interpretation of the results obtained with these models can be difficult because they are not targeting solely cDC1 (7, 9–11). Moreover, cDC1 are replenished in *Batf3*-KO mice under inflammatory conditions, due to expression of other Batf transcription factors that compensate for Batf3 loss (12). Finally, these models do not allow the editing of cDC1 genome, which would be a powerful method to decipher the molecular regulation of their functions. Hence, novel mutant mouse models are needed to reach this goal.

In all tissues with the exception of the intestine, cDC1 can be defined as CD24$^+$ SIRPα/CD172a$^-$ cDCs (13–15). In addition, lymphoid-tissue resident cDC1 express CD8α, whereas the cDC1 residing in the parenchyma of non-lymphoid tissues and their counterparts that have migrated in secondary lymphoid organs express CD103. CLEC9A, a C type lectin receptor that allows efficient cross-presentation by cDC1 of dying cell-associated antigens (16) has been identified as a good candidate to generate mice enabling selective targeting of cDC1 *in vivo* due to its selective expression in these cells and to a lesser extent in pDCs (17–20). However, a thorough analysis of mice expressing a Cre recombinase under the *Clec9a* promoter showed that Cre-driven recombination occurred not only in cDC1 and to some extent in pDCs, but also in cDC2, leading to the discovery that *Clec9a* is expressed in a progenitor cell common to both cDC types (21). Hence, the *Clec9a*^{Cre} mouse is not suitable for specific targeting of cDC1.

A major breakthrough in the field of cDC1 was the identification of XCR1 as a universal marker of all cDC1 regardless of their tissues of residency, and present in all the warm-blooded vertebrate species studied to date (22–27). *Xcr1* encodes the chemokine receptor XCR1, which ligand XCL1 is strongly upregulated in natural killer (NK) cells, CD8$^+$ T cells and memory T cells upon activation in mice (24, 26, 28–31). Recently, a mouse model based on the expression of the Cre recombinase under the control of the *Xcr1* promoter has been generated to specifically manipulate gene expression in cDC1. This mutant mouse model was engineered by replacing the single coding exon of *Xcr1* by the *Cre* gene (32). This strategy assumes that the *Xcr1* gene is haplosufficient. However, this hypothesis has to be tested considering that XCR1 promotes the cross-talk between cDC1 and NK cells or CD8$^+$ T lymphocytes, by facilitating their reciprocal recruitment and/or activation (24, 26, 29). Regardless of its potential limitation, this *Xcr1*$^{tm4(cre)Ksho}$ mouse model has been useful to decipher the role of cDC1 in intraepithelial T cell homeostasis in the intestine (32). However, to the best of our knowledge, it has not been used yet for conditional gene targeting of the cDC1 lineage. Besides *Xcr1*, the *A530099j19rik* gene (named *Karma* hereafter) has also been identified as selectively expressed in cDC1 by bulk transcriptomic analysis on immune cell subsets and organs (10, 33). The *Karma* gene encodes a protein with 7 transmembrane domains, likely corresponding to a G protein-coupled receptor, leading to its recent denomination as *Gpr141b* by the Mouse Genome Informatics. Recently, we generated the *Karma* knock-in reporter/deleter mouse model, which expresses in the *Karma* locus a construct encoding both the fluorescent tandem dimer Tomato (tdTomato) and the human diphtheria toxin receptor (hDTR), allowing specific tracking and conditional depletion of cDC1 *in vivo*. Results obtained with this reporter mouse validated the *Karma* locus as highly reliable to functionally target cDC1 *in vivo* (33).

To match the unmet need of a mouse model allowing specific and efficient *in vivo* genetic manipulation of cDC1, we generated two novel Cre-driver lines, the *Xcr1*^{Cre} and *Karma*^{Cre} mice, by knocking in an IRES-Cre expression cassette in the 3′-UTR of the *Xcr1* or *Karma* locus, respectively. In this study, we used genetic tracing to characterize the specificity and efficiency of the Cre-mediated recombination in these new models at steady state and upon infection, and compared them with the *Clec9a*^{Cre} model. This study also advanced our understanding of the phenotypic heterogeneity of cDC1 with regard to their differentiation trajectory.

MATERIALS AND METHODS

Generation of cDC1 Targeting Cre Constructs and Mice

Xcr1^{Cre} (*B6-Xcr1*^{tm1Ciphe}) and *Karma*^{Cre} (*B6-Gpr141b*^{tm2Ciphe}) mice were made according to a standard gene targeting approach in C57BL/6N-derived ES cells. They were constructed by inserting, through ET homologous recombination, a cassette containing the internal ribosome entry site (IRES) followed by a gene encoding the codon-improved version of Cre recombinase (34), into the 3′-UTR of the *Xcr1* or *A530099j19rik/Gpr141b* genes, 34 and 98 bp after the stop codon, respectively. These mice were outcrossed for three generations with wild type (*Wt*) C57BL/6J mice purchased from Charles River Laboratories. All experiments were performed with sex-matched littermate mice at 6–12 weeks of age. *Clec9a*^{Cre} (*Clec9a*$^{tm2.1(icre)Crs}$) (21) knock-in mice [kindly provided by Caetano Reis e Sousa (The Francis Crick Institute, UK)], *Karma-tdTomato-hDTR* (*Gp141b*^{tm1Ciphe}) (33) were maintained on the C57BL/6J background. *Rosa26*$^{lox-stop-lox-tdRFP}$ (*Gt(ROSA)26Sor*^{tm1Hjf}) mice in which expression of the tandem dimer Red Fluorescent Protein (tdRFP) is driven through the deletion of a "lox-stop-lox" sequence (35) were purchased from the Jackson Laboratory and maintained on the C57BL/6J background. *Rosa26*$^{lox-stop-lox-DTA}$ (*Gt(ROSA)26Sor*$^{tm1(DTA)Lky}$) mice in which expression of active domain of the diphtheria toxin (DTA) is driven through the deletion of a "lox-stop-lox" sequence (36) were obtained from Prs. David Voehringer and Richard M. Locksley, and maintained on the C57BL/6J background. Mice were bred and maintained in our specific pathogen—free animal facility. This study was carried out in accordance with institutional guidelines and with protocols approved by the Comité National de Réflexion Ethique sur l'Expérimentation Animale #14.

Preparation of Cell Suspension From Blood and Tissues, and Analysis by Flow Cytometry

Splenocytes were prepared by infusing spleens with an enzymatic cocktail made of Collagenase D (1 mg/ml) and DNase I (70 µg/ml, both Roche) in plain RPMI 1640, and further incubation for 25 min at 37°C. Ice cold EDTA (2 mM) was added for additional 5 min. Cells were filtered through a 70-µm nylon sieve, and exposed to 0.155 M NH_4Cl, 10 mM $KHCO_3$, 0.127 M EDTA to lyse red blood cells. Liver and lungs were minced in an enzymatic cocktail (1 mg/ml of Collagenase D and 70 µg/ml of DNase I), incubated for 25 min at 37°C. Ice-cold EDTA (2 mM) was added for additional 5 min, then digested tissues were filtered through a 70 µm nylon sieve (BD Falcon). Low-density cells were further enriched by centrifugation over a 1.069 g/ml density gradient (OptiPrep, Axis-Shield), washed and resuspended in PBS, EDTA 2 mM, 2% BSA, and red blood cells were lysed as detailed above. Cutaneous LNs (inguinal and axillar LNs) were cut into small pieces and digested for 25 min at 37°C with a mixture of type II collagenase (Worthington Biochemical) and DNase I (Sigma-Aldrich) in plain RPMI 1640. The resulting cell suspension was treated with 5 mM EDTA and filtered through a 70 µm nylon sieve (BD Falcon). For the skin, ears were split into a ventral and dorsal parts and incubated for 105 min at 37°C in RPMI containing 0.25 mg/ml Liberase TL (Roche Diagnostic Corp.) and 0.5 mg/ml DNase I (Sigma Aldrich). Digested tissue was homogenized using Medicons and Medimachine (Becton Dickinson) to obtain homogenous cell suspensions. For skin mast cells, we used a protocol recently described (37). To test the germline recombination in blood cells, peripheral blood mononuclear cells (PBMCs) were enriched by centrifugation over a 1.077 g/ml density gradient (Ficoll-Paque Plus, GE Healthcare), washed and resuspended in PBS, EDTA 2 mM, 2% BSA before staining. Staining of cells for flow cytometry started with a pre-incubation with 2.4G2 mAb to block unspecific binding to Fc-receptors. Staining with mAb (**Supplementay Table S1**) was then performed in PBS, 2% BSA, 2 mM EDTA for 25 min on ice. For exclusion of dead cells 4′,6-diamidino-2-phenylindole (DAPI, Thermo Fisher Scientific) was added 5 min before acquisition. Data were acquired on a LSRFortessa X-20 flow cytometer (BD Biosciences), and analyzed using FlowJo (Tree Star, Inc.).

Bone Marrow-Derived DC Differentiation

FLT3-L-BMDCs were generated as described (38) with some modifications. BM cell suspensions were prepared and red blood cells were lysed as detailed in the previous section. After washing in complete RPMI 1640 medium, cells were cultured at 3×10^6 cells/ml in 24 well plates, with 10% FBS, RPMI 1640 medium containing murine FLT3-L (in house supernatant from B16-*Flt3l* cells, used at 1/20 final) at 37°C in 5% CO2. Four days after, half of the culture medium was replaced by fresh FLT3-L. Cells were harvested at indicated times for flow cytometry analysis after staining for CD11c, SiglecH, CD24, SIRPα, XCR1, and CD11b (**Supplementay Table S1**).

Microarray Data Generation and Analysis

DCs were generated *in vitro* from mouse BM FLT3-L cultures and sorting by flow cytometry to over 98% purity, as live, singlet, CD11c$^+$ cells that were SiglecH$^+$ for eq-pDCs, SIRPα$^-$CD24^{high} for eq-cDC1 and SIRPα$^+$CD24$^{-/low}$ for eq-cDC2. Total RNA (50 ng) was used as starting material for each sample to synthesize biotinylated probes, using the NuGen protocol as described previously (39). Affymetrix Mouse Gene 1.0 ST raw. CEL files were analyzed in the R statistical environment (version 3.4.1). Data were RMA normalized using the oligo package and processed as described previously (40). Heatmaps of Log2-normalized expression values of selected genes were performed using the Morpheus website from the Broad Institute (https://software.broadinstitute.org/morpheus/). Hierarchical clusterings were performed using the One-Pearson correlation as a metric and the average linkage as a clustering method for samples and genes, except for **Figure 5B** where the complete linkage method was used for the genes. The microarray data have been deposited in the GEO database under the series accession number GSE121859.

Mouse Cytomegalovirus Infection

Animals were infected intraperitoneally with 2×10^5 PFU of salivary gland-extracted MCMV Smith strain (3rd *in vivo* passage). Forty-Eight hours later, spleen and liver were harvested and prepared for flow cytometry analysis as described above.

Analysis of Germline Recombination

Four females and 2 males of each *Xcr1*$^{Cre/wt}$; *Rosa26*$^{tdRFP/wt}$ and *Karma*$^{Cre/wt}$; *Rosa26*$^{tdRFP/wt}$ genotype were backcrossed to C57BL/6J mice. Their progeny was genotyped and bled to analyse tdRFP expression in circulating T and B cells as a sign of germline recombination.

RESULTS

Generation of New cDC1-Targeting Cre-Driver Lines

By comparative gene expression profiling, we and other have previously identified *Xcr1* and *a530099j19rik* (*Gpr141b*/*Karma*) genes as specifically expressed by mouse cDC1 in different tissues throughout the body (10, 22–26, 31, 33). We used such unique gene expression profile to genetically target cDC1 *in vivo* by generating $Xcr1^{Cre}$ (**Figure 1A**) and $Karma^{Cre}$ (**Figure 1B**) knock-in mouse models. The insertion of an IRES-Cre cassette after the STOP codon of *Xcr1* and *Karma* genes allows the translation of two separate proteins resulting in the expression of the Cre recombinase. Expression of endogenous XCR1 was not significantly altered in the $Xcr1^{Cre}$ mouse model (**Supplementary Figure S1A**, top).

The $XCR1^{Cre}$ Mouse Model Allows Selective and Efficient Recombination of loxP Sequences in Migratory and Resident cDC1 in All Tissues Examined

To determine the specificity of the Cre-induced recombination in $Xcr1^{Cre}$ (**Figure 1A**) and $Karma^{Cre}$ (**Figure 1B**) mice, we bred them with the Cre-reporter line $Rosa26^{lox-stop-lox-tdRFP}$ (named hereafter $Rosa26^{tdRFP}$) (35), and analyzed the tdRFP expression pattern in immune cells of lymphoid organs [spleen and cutaneous lymph-nodes (CLNs)] (**Supplementary Figures S1A,B**) and non-lymphoid tissues (lungs, liver, and skin) (**Supplementary Figures S1C–E**). To define DC cell populations, we applied gating strategies adapted from (41). As a control Cre-driver line, we used the $Clec9a^{Cre}$ mice (21) bred to $Rosa26^{tdRFP}$. Regardless of the tissues examined, we found that all three mouse models achieved effective targeting of the cDC1-lineage, with $Xcr1^{Cre}$, and $Clec9a^{Cre}$ being the most efficient (**Figure 2**). In contrary to $Clec9a^{Cre}$, the $Xcr1^{Cre}$ and $Karma^{Cre}$ mouse models did not show any significant Cre activity, neither in pDCs nor in macrophages (**Figure 2**). However, Cre recombination (tdRFP signal) was detected in a fraction of other cell types. In $Xcr1^{Cre/wt}$; $Rosa26^{tdRFP/wt}$ mice, a minute proportion (<1%) of $CD4^+$ T cells expressed tdRFP in the spleen, CLNs, lung and liver, which increased to a much higher fraction of $CD4^+$ T cells in the skin (8.4 ± 6.4%). The $CD4^+$ T cells harboring *Xcr1*-driven Cre recombination lacked detectable level of XCR1 (**Supplementary Figure S1E**, bottom). Hence, they likely derived from progenitors cells that transiently expressed *Xcr1*. In the skin, lungs and CLNs of $Karma^{Cre/wt}$; $Rosa26^{tdRFP/wt}$ mice, a fraction of cDC2 had undergone recombination, although to a lesser extent than in $Clec9a^{Cre/wt}$; $Rosa26^{tdRFP/wt}$ mice where cDC2 were targeted in all tissues (**Figure 2**). Surprisingly, in the skin of $Karma^{Cre/wt}$; $Rosa26^{tdRFP/wt}$ mice, a large proportion of mast cells (61.1 ± 12.8%) also expressed the tdRFP (**Figure 2**).

To further assess cDC1-targeting specificity in the three Cre-driver mouse strains, we analyzed the proportion of different immune cell types within the $tdRFP^+$ cells (**Figure 3**, **Supplementary Figure S2**). As expected on the basis of previous report (21), other cells than cDC1, in particular cDC2 and to some extent pDCs, represented the major fraction of the cells targeted in $Clec9a^{Cre}$ mice (**Figure 3**). In contrast, in all examined organs, except for the CLNs, cDC1 represented the major fraction of the cells targeted in $Xcr1^{Cre}$ mice, $CD4^+$ T cells constituting the second most frequent cell types expressing tdRFP in these organs, and the most frequent in the CLNs. This reflects the higher numbers of $CD4^+$ T cells as compared to cDC1s in all these organs. Finally, cDC1 represented the major fraction of targeted cells in $Karma^{Cre}$ mice in all examined organs, except for the skin where 64.4 ± 5.8% of the $tdRFP^+$ cells were mast cells (**Figure 3**). We assessed the expression pattern of the *Karma* gene in mast cells and compared it to a variety of other immune cell types, using the database from the Immgen consortium. These results revealed that mast cells express similar levels of the *Karma* gene as cDC1 in all organs examined, trachea, tongue, esophagus, skin, and peritoneal cavity (**Supplementary Figure S3**), consistent with the efficient genetic tracing of mast cells in the skin of $Karma^{Cre}$ mice. Altogether, these results show that our novel $Xcr1^{Cre}$ and $Karma^{Cre}$ mouse models constitute the most reliable Cre-driver lines reported to date for selective and efficient *in vivo* targeting of cDC1, with the $Xcr1^{Cre}$ model performing the best. However, it should be noted that a small fraction of $CD4^+$ T cells is targeted in $Xcr1^{Cre}$ mice and that mast cells are largely targeted in $Karma^{Cre}$ animals.

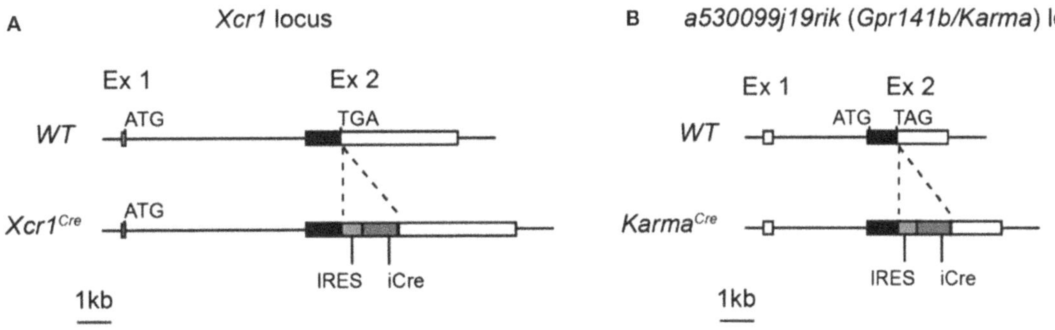

FIGURE 1 | Schematic representations of $Xcr1^{Cre}$ and $Karma^{Cre}$ genetic constructions. A cassette containing an IRES sequence upstream of a gene encoding a codon-improved CRE recombinase was inserted by homologous ET recombination downstream of the stop codon of *Xcr1* exon 2 **(A)** and of *a530099j19rik/Karma/Gpr141b* exon 2 **(B)** genes, to produce $Xcr1^{Cre}$ and $Karma^{Cre}$ mouse mutants, respectively, on a C57BL/6J background.

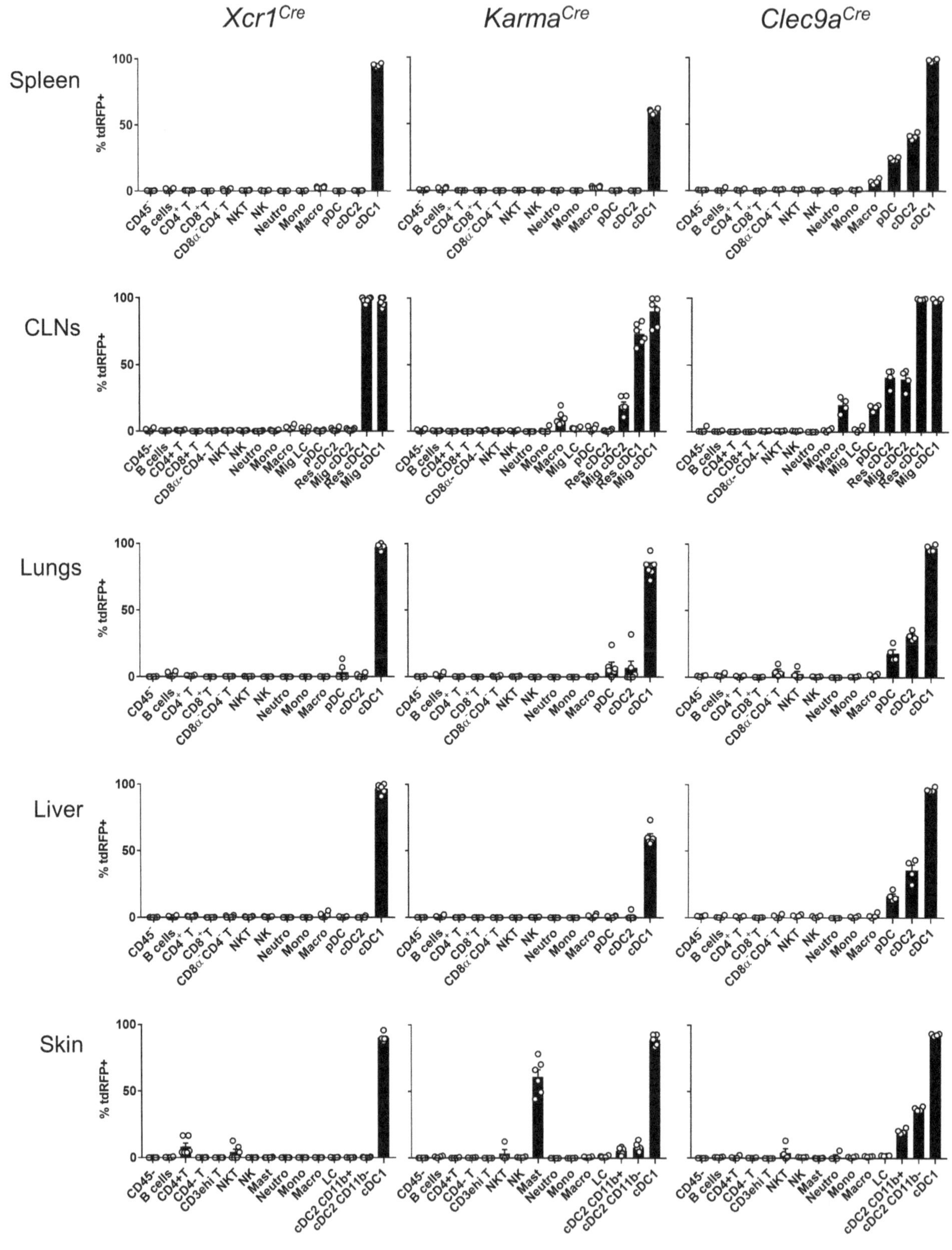

FIGURE 2 | *Xcr1*^{Cre} and *Karma*^{Cre} mouse models target with high specificity cDC1 in lymphoid and non-lymphoid tissues. Flow cytometry analysis of the tdRFP expression by different immune cell populations (as defined in **Supplementary Figure S1**), from spleen, CLNs, lungs, liver, and skin of *Xcr1*$^{Cre/wt}$; *Rosa26*$^{tdRFP/wt}$, *Karma*$^{Cre/wt}$; *Rosa26*$^{tdRFP/wt}$ and *Clec9a*$^{Cre/wt}$; *Rosa26*$^{tdRFP/wt}$ mice. Gating strategies are detailed in **Supplementary Figure S1**. Data show one dot per individual value, mean +/− SEM per group, and are from two pooled experiments with at least two mice per group.

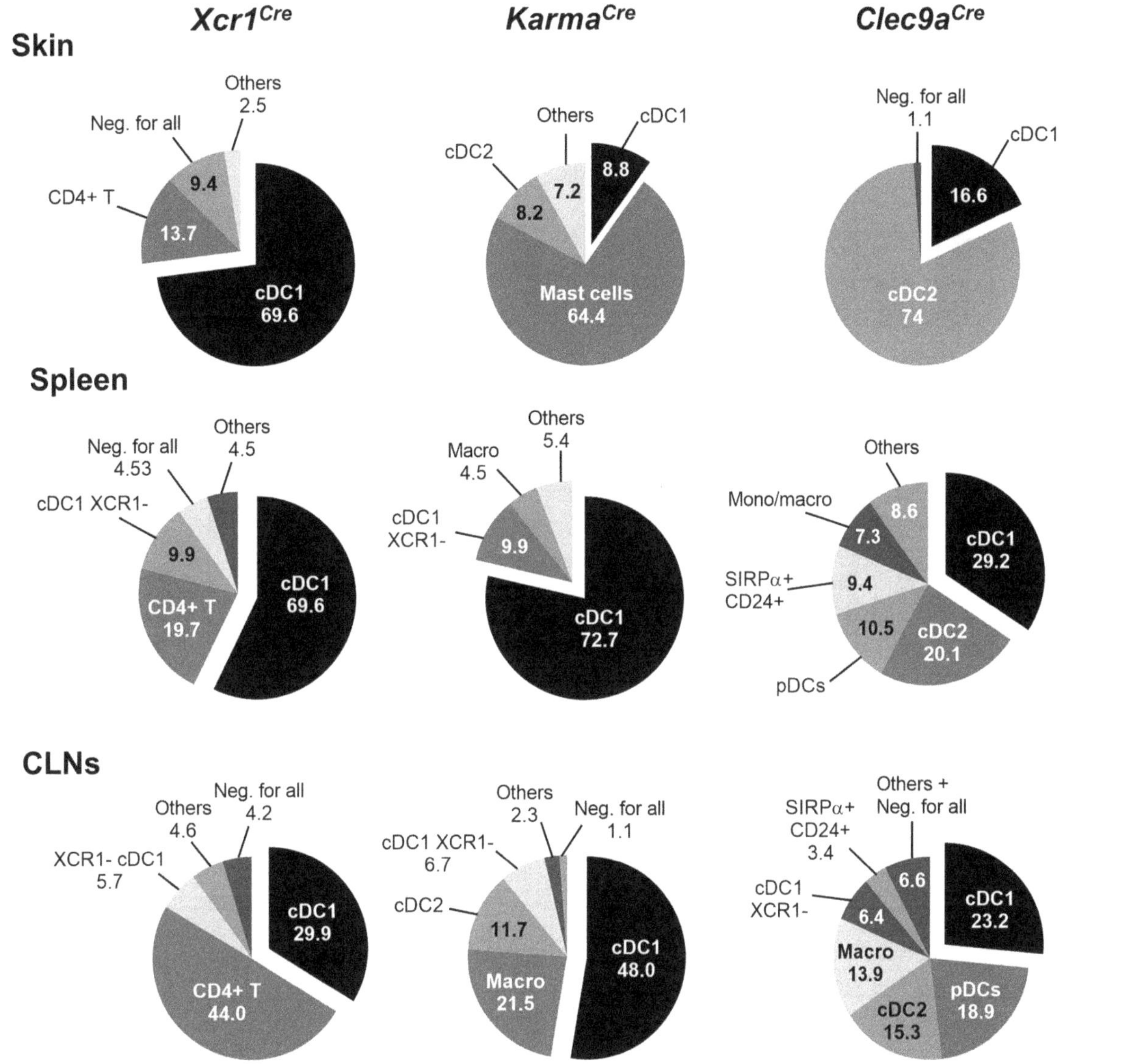

FIGURE 3 | Proportion of cell types within tdRFP$^+$ cells in the skin, spleen, and CLNs of each genotype. The back gating strategy used to define the relative proportions of cell types among tdRFP$^+$ cells was performed by using the antibody staining detailed in the upper side of **Supplementary Figure S1**. Exceptions were made as follow for *Xcr1*$^{Cre/wt}$; *Rosa26*$^{tdRFP/wt}$ mice: to define further the tdRFP$^+$ cells that fell within the Lin$^+$ (CD19/CD3ε/NKp46/Ly6G) gate, the antibody staining detailed in the bottom side of **Supplementary Figure S1** was used. The proportion of CD4$^+$ T lymphocytes within tdRFP$^+$ cells when using the latter ("lymphoid") antibody panel was matching the proportion of Lin$^+$ cells within tdRFP$^+$ cells when using the former antibody ("myeloid") panel. For *Karma*$^{Cre/wt}$; *Rosa26*$^{tdRFP/wt}$ mice, mast cells were defined as Lin$^-$ CD11b$^-$ CD11c$^-$ XCR1$^-$ MHC-II$^-$ CD64$^-$ F4/80$^-$ FcεRIα$^+$ CD117$^+$. Others: sum of all the other cell subsets not detailed in the pie charts. Neg. for all, negative for all: cells that did not stain positive for the markers used in the upper antibody panel. Data are shown for one experiment representative of three with three mice per group.

The Use of Different cDC1-Specific Promoters for Driving Cre Expression Reveals Heterogeneity in the cDC1 Population Defined as CD24$^+$ SIRPα$^-$ cDCs

To try understanding the lower efficiency of the *Karma*^{Cre} model for cDC1 targeting, as compared to the *Xcr1*^{Cre} or *Clec9a*^{Cre} mice, we examined the expression pattern of the tdRFP reporter within the splenic cDC1 defined as CD24$^+$SIRPα$^-$ cDCs (gated in the CD45$^+$Lin$^-$SiglecH$^-$MerTK$^-$CD64$^-$CD11c$^+$MHC-II$^+$CD26$^+$ cells) (13). CD24$^+$SIRPα$^-$ cDC1 can be split into 4 subsets according to their heterogeneous expression of CD8α and XCR1 (**Figure 4**). XCR1 expression was reported to correlate with a better crosspresentation by cDC1 (23, 42). The CD8α$^+$XCR1$^+$ cDC1 subset was reported to be phenotypically and functionally homogenous (23, 42), and likely corresponds to full-fledged differentiated cDC1 endowed with a high

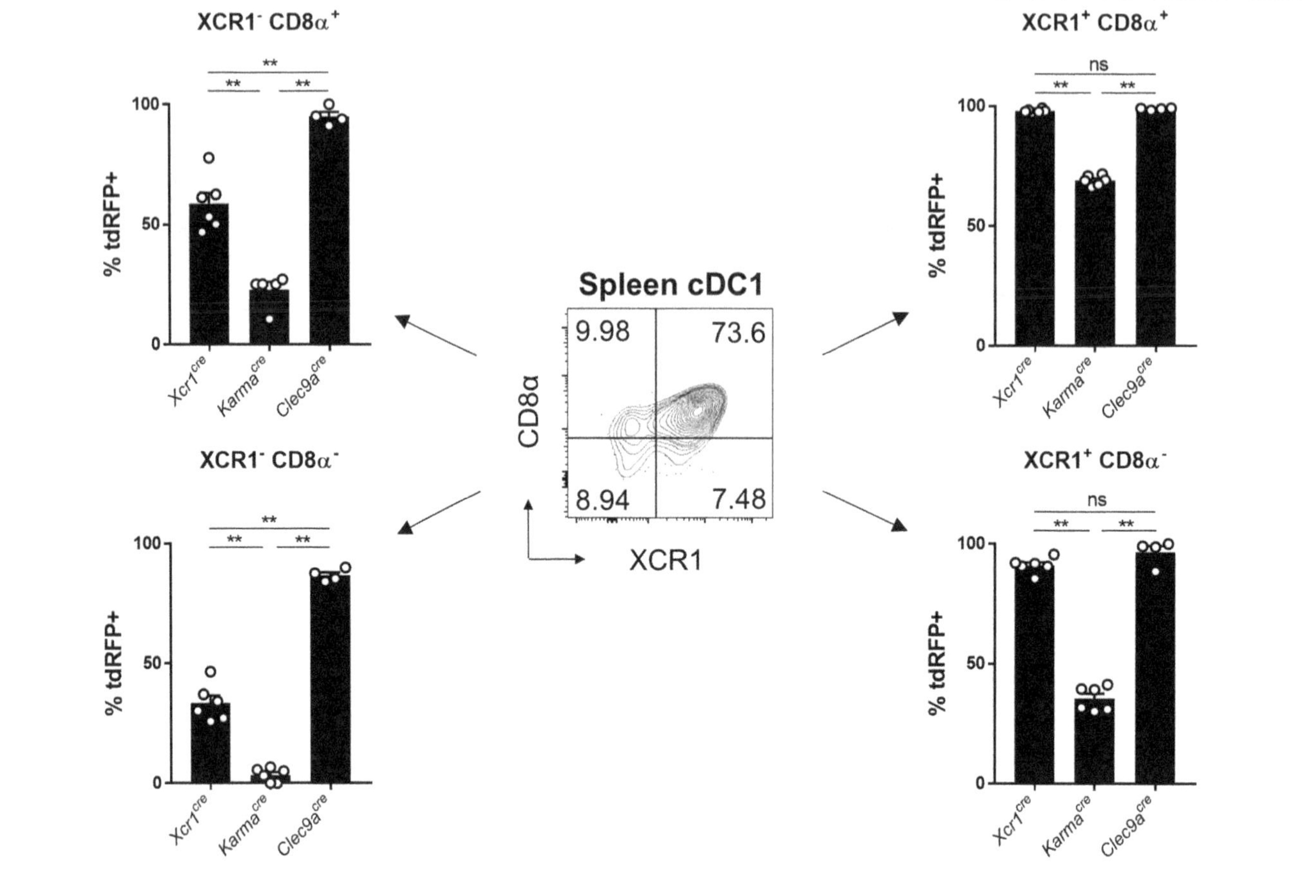

FIGURE 4 | Tracing of *Xcr1* and *Karma* expression in the cDC1 population in spleen. Flow cytometry analysis of the tdRFP expression in the 4 CD24$^+$ cDC1 subsets defined as CD8α$^+$XCR1$^-$, CD8α$^+$XCR1$^+$, CD8α$^-$XCR1$^+$, and CD8α$^-$XCR1$^-$, in the spleen of $Xcr1^{Cre/wt}$; $Rosa26^{tdRFP/wt}$, $Karma^{Cre/wt}$; $Rosa26^{tdRFP/wt}$, and $Clec9a^{Cre/wt}$; $Rosa26^{tdRFP/wt}$ mice. Data show one dot per individual value, mean +/- SEM per group, and are from two pooled experiments with at least two mice per group. Statistical analyses were performed using nonparametric Mann-Whitney tests in all experiments (**, $p < 0.01$; n.s, non-significant).

crosspresentation activity (43). However, the three other cDC1 subsets, CD8α$^+$XCR1$^-$, CD8α$^-$XCR1$^+$, and CD8α$^-$XCR1$^-$, have not been extensively characterized. The CD8α$^-$XCR1$^-$ cells may encompass pre-cDC1 (13, 44). The CD8α$^-$XCR1$^+$ cells likely correspond to pre-terminally differentiated cDC1. The CD8α$^+$XCR1$^-$ cells could correspond to the small fraction of homeostatically matured splenic cDC1 that have downregulated XCR1 expression, similarly to what occurs at steady state in the skin, the intestine or the thymus (25, 32, 39). It could also be possible that XCR1$^-$ cells encompass other cell types contaminating the SIRPα$^-$CD24$^+$ cDC1 gate. However, the exclusion of CD3ε$^+$ and SiglecH$^+$ cells in our gating strategy ensured that the CD8α$^+$XCR1$^-$ cDC1 subset was not contaminated by CD8$^+$ T cells nor CD8α$^+$ pDCs (45–47). Consistent with the early expression of *Clec9a* starting at the pre-DC stage (21), $Clec9a^{Cre}$ model targeted efficiently all 4 subsets, regardless of XCR1 and CD8α acquisition, with more than 85% of the cells in each subset expressing tdRFP (**Figure 4**). Although the $Xcr1^{Cre}$ model was more efficient in targeting XCR1$^+$ cDC1 as initially expected, a significant Cre activity was also detected both in XCR1$^-$CD8α$^-$ and XCR1$^-$CD8α$^+$ cDC1 subsets, with 37% and 53% of tdRFP expression, respectively (**Figure 4**). This indicated that a significant proportion of these cells from these two subsets derived from XCR1-expressing precursors, consistent with the hypothesis that they respectively encompass pre-cDC1 and terminally matured cDC1. The $Karma^{Cre}$ model was effective in targeting the XCR1$^+$CD8α$^+$ cDC1 subset, contrasting with no recombination detected in the XCR1$^-$CD8α$^-$ subset and with only a weak Cre activity in the XCR1$^+$CD8α$^-$ subset (**Figure 4**). The fraction of XCR1$^-$CD8α$^+$ cDC1 targeted in $Karma^{Cre}$ mice (22.8 ± 6.1%) was lower than that of XCR1$^+$CD8α$^+$ cDC1 (69.0 ± 2.1%). This suggest that most of XCR1$^-$CD8α$^+$ cDC1 do not derive from XCR1$^+$CD8α$^+$ cDC1 contrary to our expectation that the majority of the former cells correspond to an advanced maturation state of the latter ones. Altogether, the combined use of our fate mapping mouse models suggests consecutive expression of the corresponding genes along the differentiation of the cDC1 lineage in the spleen, with *Clec9a* expressed from the common cDC progenitor stage, *Xcr1* likely starting at the pre-cDC1 stage and *Karma* turned on only at a later stage similarly to CD8α.

Comparison of the Three Fate Mapping Mouse Strains Advances Our Understanding of the Differentiation Trajectory of cDC1

We further investigated to which extent our fate mapping mutant mouse models could help refining the differentiation trajectory of cDC1, using as a simple model bone marrow (BM) cells cultured with Fms-like tyrosine kinase 3 ligand (FLT3-L) (38). This model allows *in vitro* generation of three subsets of DCs, which are phenotypically and functionally equivalent to *in vivo* cDC1 (eq-cDC1), cDC2 (eq-cDC2) and pDCs (eq-pDCs) (38, 48–50). To refine the differentiation trajectory of cDC1, we followed the acquisition of the tdRFP signal over time in FLT3-L-differentiated DCs generated from BM of our fate mapping mutant mice (**Supplementary Figure S4**, **Figure 5A**). *Xcr1*^{Cre} and *Clec9a*^{Cre} models allowed efficient recombination in eq-cDC1 (56 vs. 90%) (**Figure 5A**). Interestingly, *Karma*^{Cre} did not present any recombinase activity in any of the DC populations (**Figure 5A**). Consistently, whereas gene expression profiling of the eq-DC subsets generated in standard BM FLT3-L cultures confirmed their close homology to their *in vivo* counterparts isolated from the spleen (**Figure 5B**), it also showed that eq-cDC1 lacked expression of the *Karma*, *Cd8a* and *Ly75* (*Cd205*) genes (**Figure 5B**, black arrows). This was confirmed using our previously published *Karma* reporter mouse model knocked-in for tdTomato in the 3′UTR of the *Karma* gene (33) (**Supplementary Figure S5A**). However, these eq-cDC1 acquired *Karma* and CD8α expression upon *in vivo* transfer (**Supplementary Figures S5B,C**). *Karma* was also expressed in eq-cDC1 differentiated from BM cells cultured with FLT3-L on feeder cells expressing the Notch ligand Delta-like 1 (**Figure 5C**, black arrows), similarly to what has been recently reported for CD8α and CD205 expression (43). Altogether, these results demonstrate a sequential expression of *Clec9a*, *Xcr1* and *Karma* during cDC1 ontogeny, with *Clec9a* being induced early starting at the common cDC progenitor stage (21), then followed by *Xcr1* which induction might be initiated already at the pre-cDC1 stage. Likewise to CD8α, *Karma* is acquired at a more advanced differentiation stage that is not reached under classical conditions of DC differentiation from BM in FLT3-L *in vitro* cultures but can be promoted by Notch signaling. This work thus significantly extends two recent studies showing that cDC1 derived *in vitro* from mouse or human hematopoietic precursors with a combination of cytokines and growth factors need additional signals to reach a terminal state of differentiation including acquisition of CD8α expression for mouse cDC1 (43, 51).

The Cre Expression Under *Xcr1* or *Karma* Promoters Remains cDC1-Specific Upon Infection-Induced Inflammation

The expression of many membrane proteins or transcription factors changes upon inflammation (12, 52). An important incentive for generating *Xcr1*^{Cre} and *Karma*^{Cre} models, was that the expression of the *Xcr1* and *Karma* genes was specific for cDC1 both at steady state and under inflammatory conditions (53). To confirm this observation based on transcriptomic studies, we examined cDC1-targeting specificity of the *Karma*^{Cre} and *Xcr1*^{Cre} mouse models in an inflammatory context, namely systemic mouse cytomegalovirus (MCMV) infection, using the *Rosa26*^{tdRFP} reporter as a read out. We adapted a gating strategy adapted from (52) to identify inflammatory DCs (InflDCs) in spleen and liver (**Supplementary Figure S6**). Although we could observe the appearance of InflDCs upon MCMV infection, tdRFP expression remained unchanged in infected animals as compared to control mice, being still essentially confined to the cDC1 population, both in *Xcr1*$^{Cre/wt}$; *Rosa26*$^{tdRFP/wt}$ and *Karma*$^{Cre/wt}$; *Rosa26*$^{tdRFP/wt}$ mice (**Supplementary Figure 6**). This demonstrated that both cDC1-targeting models are stable and allow excision of a floxed genomic sequence efficiently and largely selectively in cDC1 at steady state and upon inflammation.

Germline Recombination of loxP Sequences Is Frequent in the Offspring of *Xcr1*^{Cre} but Not *Karma*^{Cre} Mice

Recombination of loxP-flanked genomic sequences in germ cells have been described in many Cre mouse models (54–56). To test whether germline recombination occurs in our cDC1-targeting Cre-driver lines, we backcrossed *Xcr1*$^{Cre/wt}$; *Rosa26*$^{tdRFP/wt}$ and *Karma*$^{Cre/wt}$; *Rosa26*$^{tdRFP/wt}$ mice to C57BL/6J mice, and analyzed their offspring for ubiquitous tdRFP expression, using blood T and B cells as a readout (**Figure 7A**). Total or partial germline recombination of the *Rosa26*^{tdRFP} locus occurred in 95% of the offspring who had inherited one loxP-flanked allele from *Xcr1*$^{Cre/wt}$; *Rosa26*$^{tdRFP/wt}$ male mice (**Figure 7B**). Germline recombination occurred with the same frequency irrespective of the segregation of the paternal *Cre* and loxP-flanked alleles in the offspring, demonstrating that this process occurred during meiosis rather than in the embryo. No germline recombination was observed when both alleles were from maternal germ cells (**Figure 7B**). In ongoing crosses using the *Xcr1*^{Cre} mouse model with different loxP-flanked mouse strains, we could also observe germline recombination in the progeny even when the floxed alleles were brought together with the *Xcr1*^{Cre} allele by the maternal gamete (data not shown). This indicates that, contrary to what the results of the *Rosa26*$^{tdRFP/wt}$ backcross appears to suggest, off-target activity of the Cre recombinase in germline is not a gender effect. Additionally, the incidence of germline recombination depended on the loxP-flanked allele (data not shown). No occurrence of germline recombination was detected so far for the *Karma*^{Cre} model (**Figure 7B**). Therefore, the *Karma*^{Cre} model might be more appropriate than the *Xcr1*^{Cre} model to obtain rapidly mice in which cDC1 are inactivated for candidate genes, through conventional breeding strategies. Germline recombination in the offspring should however always be assessed for any novel loxP-flanked allele.

DISCUSSION

Xcr1 and *A530099j19rik* (*Karma/Gpr141b)* genes code for the chemokine receptor XCR1 and for the putative G protein-coupled receptor Gpr141b, respectively, and are among the core

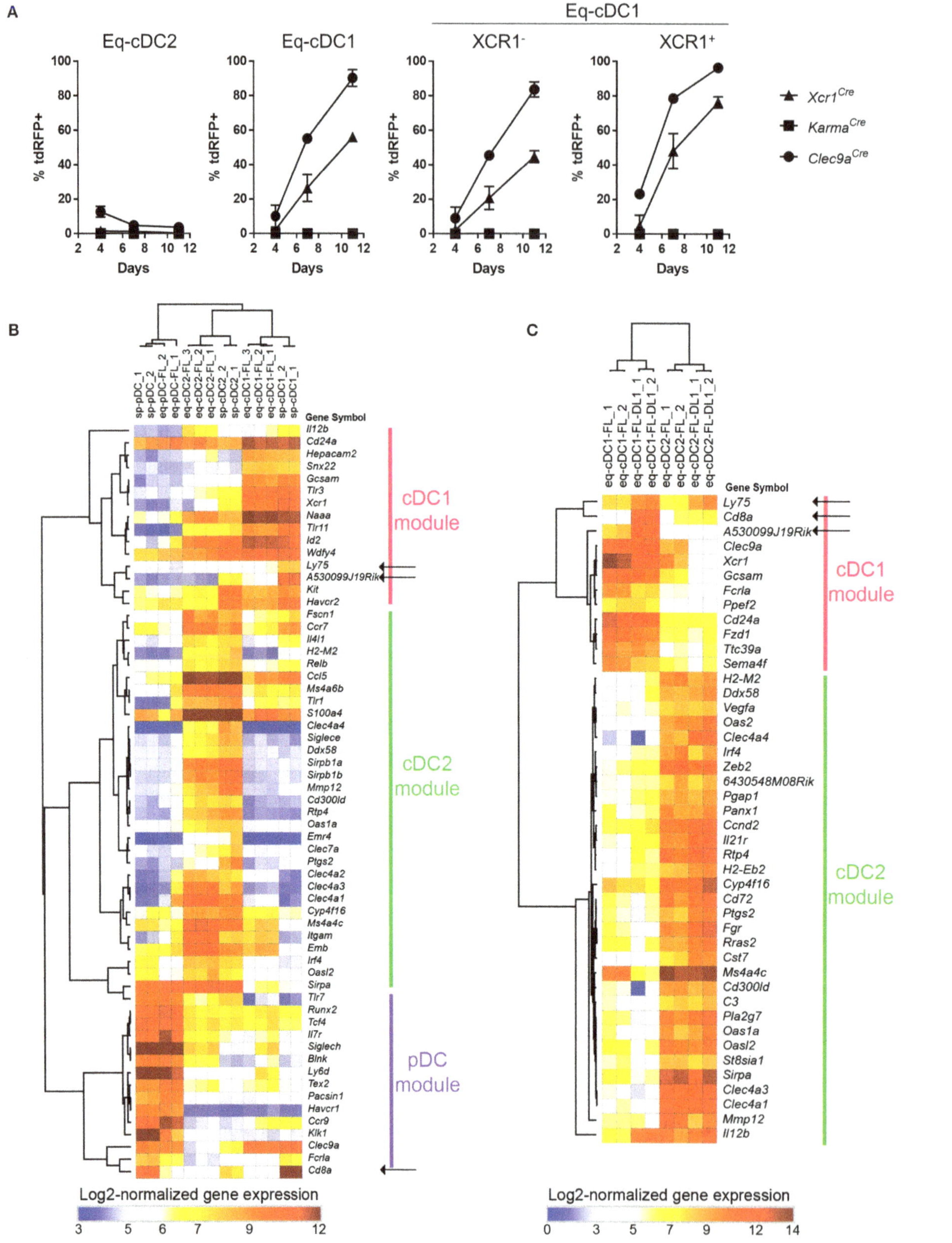

FIGURE 5 | Sequential regulation of *Clec9a*, *Xcr1* and *Karma* expression during cDC1 differentiation. **(A)** Kinetic analysis of the tdRFP expression in DCs differentiated *in vitro* from $Xcr1^{Cre/wt}$; $Rosa26^{tdRFP/wt}$, $Karma^{Cre/wt}$; $Rosa26^{tdRFP/wt}$ and $Clec9a^{Cre/wt}$; $Rosa26^{tdRFP/wt}$ BM cells cultured with FLT3-L. Eq-cDC2 were gated as *(Continued)*

FIGURE 5 | CD11c$^+$MHC-II$^+$CD24$^-$SIRPα$^+$ cells, and eq-cDC1 as CD11c+ MHC-II$^+$CD24$^+$SIRPα$^-$ cells (**Supplementay Figure S4**). Data are shown for one experiment representative of two, with three mice per group. **(B,C)** Heatmaps display the expression profiles of archetypical genes previously shown to be selectively expressed in cDC1, cDC2, or pDC. **(B)** Gene expression across DC types either isolated from murine spleens (sp-pDC, sp-cDC1, and sp-cDC2), or derived *in vitro* in standard FLT3-L BM cultures (eq-pDC-FL, eq-cDC1-FL, and eq-cDC2-FL), as assessed with microarrays. **(C)** Gene expression patterns across cDC types derived *in vitro* from FLT3-L BM cultures under standard conditions (-FL) or on DL1-expression OP9 feeder cells (-FL-DL1), as assessed from public RNA-seq data (GEO accession number GSE110577).

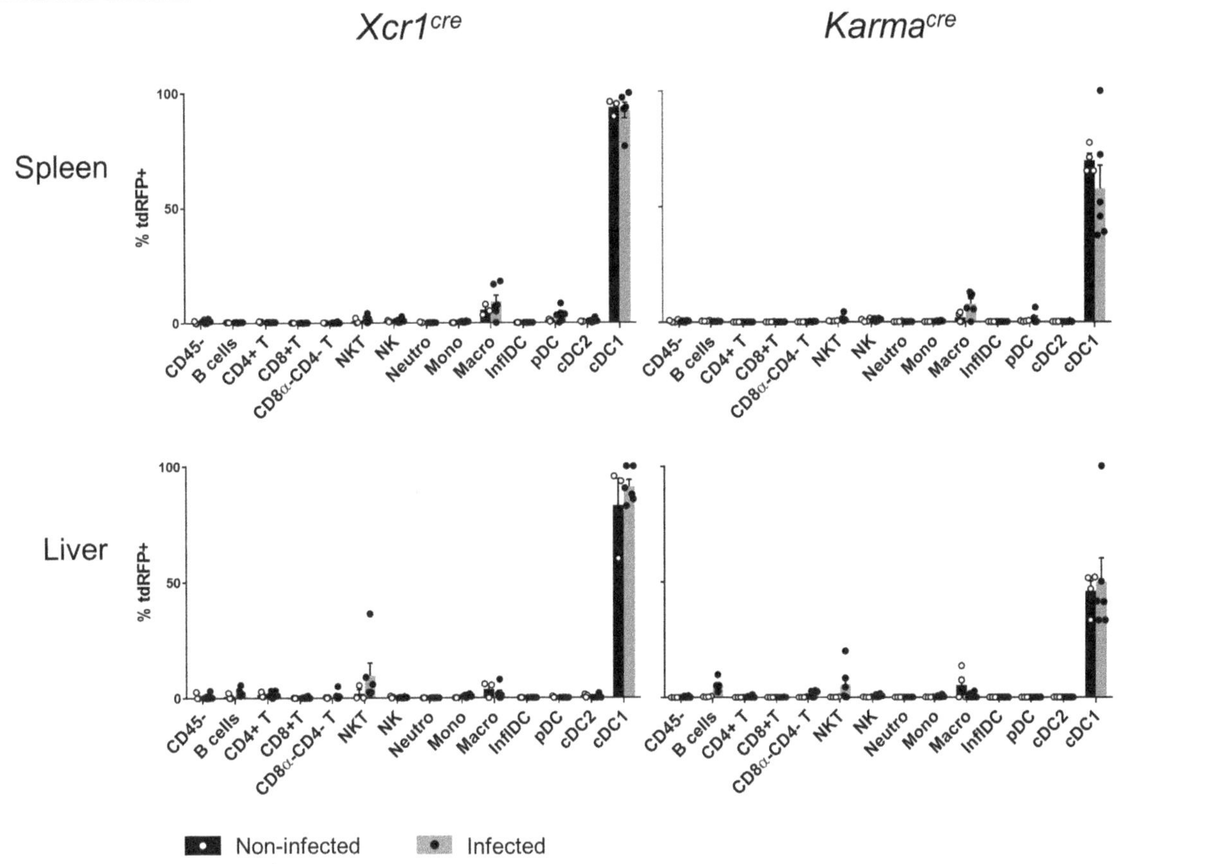

FIGURE 6 | *Xcr1* and *Karma* expressions remain confined to cDC1 upon virus-induced inflammatory responses. Flow cytometry analysis of the tdRFP expression by different immune cell populations as in **Figure 2A**, from spleen, CLNs, and liver of *Xcr1*$^{Cre/wt}$; *Rosa26*$^{tdRFP/wt}$, and *Karma*$^{Cre/wt}$; *Rosa26*$^{tdRFP/wt}$ mice 2 days after MCMV infection. Cell population gating strategy detailed in **Supplementay Figure S3**. Data show one dot per individual value, mean +/- SEM per group, and are from two pooled experiments with at least three individuals per group of infected mice. Statistical analyses were performed using nonparametric Mann-Whitney tests when possible, and the difference between non infected and infected was non-significant in each cell population. NI, non-infected; InflDCs, inflammatory DCs.

gene signature specifically identifying mouse cDC1 throughout the organism (10, 22–25, 33). We have inserted an IRES-Cre cassette into the 3′ UTR of the *Xcr1* and *Karma* coding exon to generate *Xcr1*^{Cre} and *Karma*^{Cre} mouse models, respectively. In this study, we have characterized the efficiency and specificity of Cre-mediated recombination in these novel mouse models at steady state and upon viral infection, comparing them to the *Clec9a*^{Cre} model. To the best of our knowledge, this study demonstrated that our novel *Xcr1*^{Cre} and *Karma*^{Cre} mouse models are the most trustful and robust for the genetic tracking and manipulation of cDC1 *in vivo*.

Amongst the three Cre-driver mouse models examined, *Xcr1*^{Cre} model is the most efficient and specific for fate mapping all cDC1 regardless of the tissues examined. The *Karma*^{Cre} model is rather specific for cDC1 when compared with *Clec9a*^{Cre} mouse, but much less efficient than the *Xcr1*^{Cre} model. Unexpectedly, a fraction of CD4$^+$ T cells is labeled with tdRFP in the *Xcr1*^{Cre};*Rosa26*$^{tdRFP/wt}$ mouse (**Figure 2**) without expressing any detectable XCR1 at their cell surface (**Supplementary Figure S1E**). Further analysis need to be conducted to determine whether XCR1 was transiently turned on in the distant progenitors of these cells or on the contrary during their terminal differentiation. Interestingly, the proportion of *Xcr1*^{cre} fate-mapped CD4$^+$ T cells was much higher in the skin than in the other organs examined, suggesting that these cells may be polarized toward specific functions and/or develop under instructive signals encountered preferentially in barrier organs. Further studies will be needed to test these hypotheses. In the

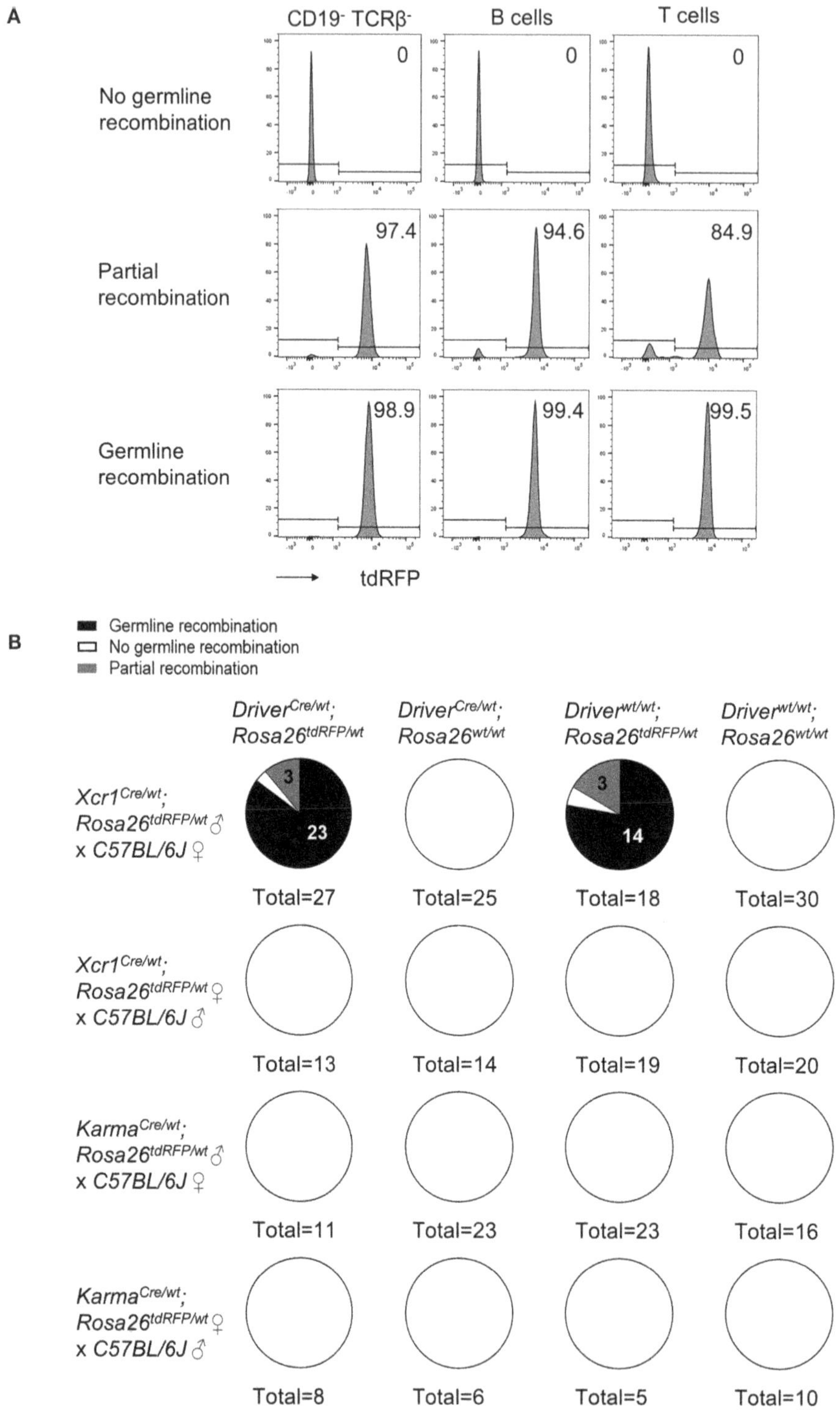

FIGURE 7 | The Cre expression under *Xcr1* but not *Karma* promoter efficiently recombines Lox-sequences in germ cells. **(A)** Representative flow cytometry analysis of tdRFP expression in CD19$^-$ TCRβ$^-$, B and T cells in blood of mice with no germline recombination, partial recombination, and germline recombination. One sample representative of each is shown. **(B)** Analysis of germline recombination in offspring from backcrosses of *Xcr1*$^{Cre/wt}$; *Rosa26*$^{tdRFP/wt}$ and *Karma*$^{Cre/wt}$; *Rosa26*$^{tdRFP/wt}$ mice of both sexes with wild-type (*WT*; C57BL/6J) mice. Germline recombination shown here occurred when both *Cre* and *floxed* alleles were of paternal origin. However, with other type of flox constructs, we regularly observed occurrences of germline recombination when both alleles were brought together, either by the father or by the mother.

skin of the *Karma*^{Cre}; *Rosa26*$^{tdRFP/wt}$ mouse model, the vast majority of the tdRFP^{+} cells were of mast cell origin (**Figure 3B**). Microarray data released recently by the Immgen consortium (https://www.immgen.org) show that mast cells from the skin, peritoneal cavity, trachea and esophagus express high level of the *Karma* gene (**Supplementary Figure S3**), confirming our observation. To the best of our knowledge, this is the first report of a gene that is selectively shared by both cDC1 and mast cells. The *Karma*^{Cre} mice will therefore be of special interest to researchers aiming at genetically manipulating mast cells in tissues. In all tissues and in all mouse models examined, no tdRFP expression was detected in the CD45-negative cells present in cell suspensions (**Figure 2**). Although, we did not examine tdRFP expression in other non-hematopoietic cells, it is unlikely that some of these cell types would be targeted in *Xcr1*^{Cre} or *Karma*^{Cre} mice considering that the *Xcr1* and *Gp141b* genes were not expressed outside of the hematopoietic system in all of the transcriptomic databases we queried.

To inactivate specifically a candidate gene in cDC1, both alleles of this candidate gene should be excised. This requires a breeding strategy in which one *Cre* allele and one floxed allele of the gene to be inactivated are brought by the same germ cells, where unexpected recombination could occur. We have tested the frequency of germline recombination for both the *Xcr1*^{Cre} and *Karma*^{Cre} models. Only the *Xcr1*^{Cre} model showed adventitious Cre activity in germ cells resulting in progeny with recombined *Rosa26*^{tdRFP} locus in all their cells. Interestingly, this was paternal inherited in this specific experimental setting. However, this may depend on the loxP-flanked construct, as we had events of germline recombination transmitted by females for other floxed genes than the *Rosa26*^{tdRFP} reporter. Therefore, to reach specific recombination in cDC1 using the *Xcr1*^{Cre} model, the *Cre* allele and the loxP-flanked allele should be inherited from different parents. We recommend breeding one parent homozygous for both the *Cre* allele and a null allele of the target gene, to another parent homozygous for the floxed allele of the target gene. Each investigator using the *Xcr1*^{Cre} model should always test their progeny for unexpected off-target recombination. A recent publication strongly suggested to include, in each experimental procedure of publication using Cre mouse models, detailed procedures about the breeding strategies used and the method the investigators applied to detect any unexpected and unspecific recombination (56).

Our genetic tracing of cDC1 *in vivo* in the spleen (**Figure 4**), or *in vitro* in FLT3-L-differentiated BM-DC cultures (**Figure 5A**) revealed heterogeneity in the cDC1 population. The differential expression of *Xcr1* and *Karma* genes within the cDC1 population qualifies *Xcr1*^{Cre} and *Karma*^{Cre} mouse models as powerful tools to describe further these cDC1 subsets *in vivo*. *In vitro*, BM-DCs derived from *Karma*^{Cre} mice did not show any sign of Cre activity (**Figure 5A**), confirming that the *Karma* gene is not transcriptionally active in these cells as directly assessed through their gene expression profiling (**Figure 5B**), akin to *Cd8a* or *Ly75* (*Dec205*) (43). We show here that expression of the *Karma* gene on cDC1 requires accessory signals, which can be provided upon *in vivo* transfer, or *in vitro* by Notch signaling likewise to what has been recently reported for *Cd8a* and *Ly75* (43). Of note, in FLT3-L *in vitro* BM-DC culture, detection in eq-cDC1 of the activity of the Cre recombinase as readout by tdRFP expression seemed to be delayed over time as compared to cell surface acquisition of XCR1 (**Figure 5**), although the *Cre* and *Xcr1* genes were expressed under the same promoter from one bi-cistronic mRNA. This might be explained by a delayed translation of the *Cre* gene as compared to *Xcr1*, or because efficient recombination of DNA by the Cre requires time. This latter case might especially apply to the *Rosa26*^{tdRFP} reporter mouse line used in this study, because it was engineered as requiring two consecutive rounds of Cre-excision to generate detectable tdRFP signal, in order to limit any leaky transcription of the fluorescent reporter gene across the stopper at steady state (35). This contrasts to most reporter lines which require only one sequence of recombination to emit signal (57, 58) and must therefore require lower and/or less sustained Cre activity to allow recombination. Breeding the *Xcr1*^{Cre} model with a Cre-reporter mouse which is easily recombined (57) might allow a better synchronization of XCR1 surface expression with Cre activity.

Our results advanced our understanding of the differentiation trajectory of cDC1, and validated the *Xcr1*^{Cre} mouse model as a robust tool to inactivate genes selectively in cDC1 either *in vivo* or *in vitro* using BM-derived DC cultures. Future use of these mutant mouse models will undoubtedly boost the advancing of our understanding of the biology of cDC1.

AUTHOR CONTRIBUTIONS

MD and KC: Conceptualization. RM, CW, BM, MD, and KC: Methodology, Validation, Formal Analysis. RM, CW, SG, MA, YA, CS, and AF: Investigation. T-PV, MD: bioinformatics analyses. BM: Mouse model construction supervision. RM, KC: Visualization. RM, KC, and MD: Writing. All authors: Editing. BM, MD, and KC: Project Supervision and Administration.

FUNDING

This work was in part carried out in the frame of the Innate Immunocytes in Health and Disease (I2HD) collaborative project between CIML, AVIESAN, and SANOFI. It was supported by grants from the European Research Council under the European Community's Seventh Framework Program [FP7/2007–2013 grant agreement number 281225 to M. Dalod; FP7/2007-2013 grant no. 322465 (Integrate) to BM], from the Agence Nationale de la Recherche (ANR; XCR1-DirectingCells to KC), from the Fondation pour la Recherche Médicale (label Equipe FRM 2011, project number DEQ20110421284 to MD), which supported the *Karma*^{Cre} mouse generation, from the Program Hubert Curien (PHC) Maïmonide-Israel 2017 project number 38155SJ (to MD) supported by the French Ministries of Foreign Affairs (MAEDI) and of Research and Higher Education (MENESR) and from the Fondation ARC pour la recherche sur le cancer (to KC). CIPHE is supported by the French Ministry of Research via PHENOMIN (French National Infrastructure for mouse Phenogenomics; ANR10-INBS-07 to BM). This work also benefited from institutional funding from CNRS and INSERM. RM was supported by doctoral fellowships from the Biotrail PhD program (Fondation A*MIDEX). RM, CW, SG, and YA were supported by fellowships from Fondation ARC pour la recherche sur le cancer.

ACKNOWLEDGMENTS

We thank Frédéric Fiore and members of the Centre d'Immunophénomique (CIPHE) (Aix Marseille Univ, INSERM US012, CNRS UMS3367, Marseille, France) for generating the *Xcr1*^{Cre} and *Karma*^{Cre} mice, and for taking care of mouse breeding; Marilyn Boyron, the cytometry core, and animal house facilities (CIML, UMR7280, France) for critical technical assistance. The authors also thank Rebecca Gentek (Aix Marseille Univ, CNRS, INSERM, CIML, France) for helpful discussion and protocol sharing. This work benefited from data assembled by the ImmGen consortium.

REFERENCES

1. Jung S, Unutmaz D, Wong P, Sano G-I, De los Santos K, Sparwasser T, et al. *In vivo* depletion of CD11c+ dendritic cells abrogates priming of CD8+ T cells by exogenous cell-associated antigens. *Immunity* (2002) 17:211–20. doi: 10.1016/S1074-7613(02)00365-5
2. Caton ML, Smith-Raska MR, Reizis B. Notch–RBP-J signaling controls the homeostasis of CD8 $^-$ dendritic cells in the spleen. *J Exp Med.* (2007) 204:1653–64. doi: 10.1084/jem.20062648
3. Stranges PB, Watson J, Cooper CJ, Choisy-Rossi C-M, Stonebraker AC, Beighton RA, et al. Elimination of antigen-presenting cells and autoreactive T cells by fas contributes to prevention of autoimmunity. *Immunity* (2007) 26:629–41. doi: 10.1016/j.immuni.2007.03.016
4. Meredith MM, Liu K, Darrasse-Jeze G, Kamphorst AO, Schreiber HA, Guermonprez P, et al. Expression of the zinc finger transcription factor zDC (Zbtb46, Btbd4) defines the classical dendritic cell lineage. *J Exp Med.* (2012) 209:1153–65. doi: 10.1084/jem.20112675
5. Loschko J, Schreiber HA, Rieke GJ, Esterházy D, Meredith MM, Pedicord VA, et al. Absence of MHC class II on cDCs results in microbial-dependent intestinal inflammation. *J Exp Med.* (2016) 213:517–34. doi: 10.1084/jem.20160062
6. Satpathy AT, Kc W, Albring JC, Edelson BT, Kretzer NM, Bhattacharya D, et al. Zbtb46 expression distinguishes classical dendritic cells and their committed progenitors from other immune lineages. *J Exp Med.* (2012) 209:1135–152. doi: 10.1084/jem.20120030
7. Hildner K, Edelson BT, Purtha WE, Diamond M, Matsushita H, Kohyama M, et al. Batf3 deficiency reveals a critical role for CD8α+ dendritic cells in cytotoxic T cell immunity. *Science* (2008) 322:1097–100. doi: 10.1126/science.1164206
8. Luda KM, Joeris T, Persson EK, Rivollier A, Demiri M, Sitnik KM, et al. IRF8 transcription-factor-dependent classical dendritic cells are essential for intestinal T cell homeostasis. *Immunity* (2016) 44:860–74. doi: 10.1016/j.immuni.2016.02.008
9. Lee W, Kim HS, Hwang SS, Lee GR. The transcription factor Batf3 inhibits the differentiation of regulatory T cells in the periphery. *Exp Mol Med.* (2017) 49:e393. doi: 10.1038/emm.2017.157
10. Robbins SH, Walzer T, Dembélé D, Thibault C, Defays A, Bessou G, et al. Novel insights into the relationships between dendritic cell subsets in human and mouse revealed by genome-wide expression profiling. *Genome Biol.* (2008) 9:R17. doi: 10.1186/gb-2008-9-1-r17
11. Sichien D, Scott CL, Martens L, Vanderkerken M, Van Gassen S, Plantinga M, et al. IRF8 transcription factor controls survival and function of terminally differentiated conventional and plasmacytoid dendritic cells, respectively. *Immunity* (2016) 45:626–40. doi: 10.1016/j.immuni.2016.08.013
12. Tussiwand R, Lee W-L, Murphy TL, Mashayekhi M, Kc W, Albring JC, et al. Compensatory dendritic cell development mediated by BATF–IRF interactions. *Nature* (2012) 490:502–7. doi: 10.1038/nature 11531
13. Grajales-Reyes GE, Iwata A, Albring J, Wu X, Tussiwand R, Kc W, et al. Batf3 maintains autoactivation of Irf8 for commitment of a CD8α(+) conventional DC clonogenic progenitor. *Nat Immunol.* (2015) 16:708–17. doi: 10.1038/ni.3197
14. Lahoud MH, Proietto AI, Gartlan KH, Kitsoulis S, Curtis J, Wettenhall J, et al. Signal regulatory protein molecules are differentially expressed by CD8– dendritic cells. *J Immunol.* (2006) 177:372–82. doi: 10.4049/jimmunol.177.1.372
15. Merad M, Sathe P, Helft J, Miller J, Mortha A. The dendritic cell lineage: ontogeny and function of dendritic cells and their subsets in the steady state and the inflamed setting. *Annu Rev Immunol.* (2013) 31:563–604. doi: 10.1146/annurev-immunol-020711-074950
16. Sancho D, Joffre OP, Keller AM, Rogers NC, Martínez D, Hernanz-Falcón P, et al. Identification of a dendritic cell receptor that couples sensing of necrosis to immunity. *Nature* (2009) 458:899–903. doi: 10.1038/nature07750
17. Caminschi I, Proietto AI, Ahmet F, Kitsoulis S, Shin Teh J, Lo JCY, et al. The dendritic cell subtype-restricted C-type lectin Clec9A is a target for vaccine enhancement. *Blood* (2008) 112:3264–73. doi: 10.1182/blood-2008-05-155176
18. Huysamen C, Willment JA, Dennehy KM, Brown GD. CLEC9A is a novel activation C-type lectin-like receptor expressed on BDCA3+ dendritic cells and a subset of monocytes. *J Biol Chem.* (2008) 283:16693–701. doi: 10.1074/jbc.M709923200
19. Poulin LF, Reyal Y, Uronen-Hansson H, Schraml BU, Sancho D, Murphy KM, et al. DNGR-1 is a specific and universal marker of mouse and human Batf3-dependent dendritic cells in lymphoid and nonlymphoid tissues. *Blood* (2012) 119:6052–62. doi: 10.1182/blood-2012-01-406967
20. Sancho D, Mourão-Sá D, Joffre OP, Schulz O, Rogers NC, Pennington DJ, et al. Tumor therapy in mice via antigen targeting to a novel, DC-restricted C-type lectin. *J Clin Invest.* (2008) 2098–110. doi: 10.1172/JCI34584
21. Schraml BU, van Blijswijk J, Zelenay S, Whitney PG, Filby A, Acton SE, et al. Genetic tracing via DNGR-1 expression history defines dendritic cells as a hematopoietic lineage. *Cell* (2013) 154:843–58. doi: 10.1016/j.cell.2013.07.014
22. Bachem A, Güttler S, Hartung E, Ebstein F, Schaefer M, Tannert A, et al. Superior antigen cross-presentation and XCR1 expression define human CD11c $^+$ CD141 $^+$ cells as homologues of mouse CD8 $^+$ dendritic cells. *J Exp Med.* (2010) 207:1273–81. doi: 10.1084/jem.20100348
23. Bachem A, Hartung E, Güttler S, Mora A, Zhou X, Hegemann A, et al. Expression of XCR1 characterizes the Batf3-dependent lineage of dendritic cells capable of antigen cross-presentation. *Front Immunol.* (2012) 3:214. doi: 10.3389/fimmu.2012.00214
24. Crozat K, Guiton R, Contreras V, Feuillet V, Dutertre C-A, Ventre E, et al. The XC chemokine receptor 1 is a conserved selective marker of mammalian cells homologous to mouse CD8α $^+$ dendritic cells. *J Exp Med.* (2010) 207:1283–92. doi: 10.1084/jem.20100223
25. Crozat K, Tamoutounour S, Vu Manh T-P, Fossum E, Luche H, Ardouin L, et al. Cutting edge: expression of XCR1 defines mouse lymphoid-tissue resident and migratory dendritic cells of the CD8 + Type. *J Immunol.* (2011) 187:4411–5. doi: 10.4049/jimmunol.1101717

26. Dorner BG, Dorner MB, Zhou X, Opitz C, Mora A, Güttler S, et al. Selective expression of the chemokine receptor XCR1 on cross-presenting dendritic cells determines cooperation with CD8+ T Cells. *Immunity* (2009) 31:823–33. doi: 10.1016/j.immuni.2009.08.027
27. Vu Manh T-P, Elhmouzi-Younes J, Urien C, Ruscanu S, Jouneau L, Bourge M, et al. Defining mononuclear phagocyte subset homology across several distant warm-blooded vertebrates through comparative transcriptomics. *Front Immunol.* (2015) 6:299. doi: 10.3389/fimmu.2015.00299
28. Bottcher JP, Bonavita E, Chakravarty P, Blees H, Cabeza-Cabrerizo M, Sammicheli S, et al. NK cells stimulate recruitment of cDC1 into the tumor microenvironment promoting cancer immune control. *Cell* (2018) 172:1022–37 e14. doi: 10.1016/j.cell.2018.01.004
29. Brewitz A, Eickhoff S, Dahling S, Quast T, Bedoui S, Kroczek RA, et al. CD8+ T cells orchestrate pDC-XCR1+ dendritic cell spatial and functional cooperativity to optimize priming. *Immunity* (2017) 46:205–19. doi: 10.1016/j.immuni.2017.01.003
30. Dorner BG, Smith HRC, French AR, Kim S, Poursine-Laurent J, Beckman DL, et al. Coordinate expression of cytokines and chemokines by NK cells during murine cytomegalovirus infection. *J Immunol.* (2004) 172:3119–31. doi: 10.4049/jimmunol.172.5.3119
31. Yamazaki C, Miyamoto R, Hoshino K, Fukuda Y, Sasaki I, Saito M, et al. Conservation of a chemokine system, XCR1 and its ligand, XCL1, between human and mice. *Biochem Biophys Res Commun.* (2010) 397:756–61. doi: 10.1016/j.bbrc.2010.06.029
32. Ohta T, Sugiyama M, Hemmi H, Yamazaki C, Okura S, Sasaki I, et al. Crucial roles of XCR1-expressing dendritic cells and the XCR1-XCL1 chemokine axis in intestinal immune homeostasis. *Sci Rep.* (2016) 6:23505. doi: 10.1038/srep23505
33. Alexandre YO, Ghilas S, Sanchez C, Le Bon A, Crozat K, Dalod M. XCR1 + dendritic cells promote memory CD8 + T cell recall upon secondary infections with *Listeria monocytogenes* or certain viruses. *J Exp Med.* (2016) 213:75–92. doi: 10.1084/jem.20142350
34. Shimshek DR, Kim J, Hübner MR, Spergel DJ, Buchholz F, Casanova E, et al. Codon-improved Cre recombinase (iCre) expression in the mouse. *Genes* (2002) 32:19–26. doi: 10.1002/gene.10023
35. Luche H, Weber O, Nageswara Rao T, Blum C, Fehling HJ. Faithful activation of an extra-bright red fluorescent protein in "knock-in" Cre-reporter mice ideally suited for lineage tracing studies. *Eur J Immunol.* (2007) 37:43–53. doi: 10.1002/eji.200636745
36. Voehringer D, Liang H-E, Locksley RM. Homeostasis and effector function of lymphopenia-induced "Memory-Like" T cells in constitutively T cell-depleted mice. *J Immunol.* (2008) 180:4742–53. doi: 10.4049/jimmunol.180.7.4742
37. Gentek R, Ghigo C, Hoeffel G, Bulle MJ, Msallam R, Gautier G, et al. Hemogenic endothelial fate mapping reveals dual developmental origin of mast cells. *Immunity* (2018) 48:1160–171.e5. doi: 10.1016/j.immuni.2018.04.025
38. Naik SH, Proietto AI, Wilson NS, Dakic A, Schnorrer P, Fuchsberger M, et al. Cutting edge: generation of splenic CD8+ and CD8- dendritic cell equivalents in Fms-like tyrosine kinase 3 ligand bone marrow cultures. *J Immunol.* (2005) 174:6592–7. doi: 10.4049/jimmunol.174.11.6592
39. Ardouin L, Luche H, Chelbi R, Carpentier S, Shawket A, Montanana Sanchis F, et al. Broad and largely concordant molecular changes characterize tolerogenic and immunogenic dendritic cell maturation in thymus and periphery. *Immunity* (2016) 45:305–18. doi: 10.1016/j.immuni.2016.07.019
40. Baranek T, Manh T-PV, Alexandre Y, Maqbool MA, Cabeza JZ, Tomasello E, et al. Differential responses of immune cells to type I interferon contribute to host resistance to viral infection. *Cell Host Microbe* (2012) 12:571–84. doi: 10.1016/j.chom.2012.09.002
41. Guilliams M, Dutertre C-A, Scott CL, McGovern N, Sichien D, Chakarov S, et al. Unsupervised high-dimensional analysis aligns dendritic cells across tissues and species. *Immunity* (2016) 45:669–84. doi: 10.1016/j.immuni.2016.08.015
42. Kroczek RA, Henn V. The Role of XCR1 and its ligand XCL1 in antigen cross-presentation by murine and human dendritic cells. *Front Immunol.* (2012) 3:14. doi: 10.3389/fimmu.2012.00014
43. Kirkling ME, Cytlak U, Lau CM, Lewis KL, Resteu A, Khodadadi-Jamayran A, et al. Notch signaling facilitates *in vitro* generation of cross-presenting classical dendritic cells. *Cell Rep.* (2018) 23:3658–72.e6. doi: 10.1016/j.celrep.2018.05.068
44. Schlitzer A, Sivakamasundari V, Chen J, Sumatoh HRB, Schreuder J, Lum J, et al. Identification of cDC1- and cDC2-committed DC progenitors reveals early lineage priming at the common DC progenitor stage in the bone marrow. *Nat Immunol.* (2015) 16:718–28. doi: 10.1038/ni.3200
45. Bar-On L, Birnberg T, Lewis KL, Edelson BT, Bruder D, Hildner K, et al. CX3CR1+ CD8alpha+ dendritic cells are a steady-state population related to plasmacytoid dendritic cells. *Proc Natl Acad Sci USA.* (2010) 107:14745–50. doi: 10.1073/pnas.1001562107
46. Dalod M, Salazar-Mather TP, Malmgaard L, Lewis C, Asselin-Paturel C, Brière F, et al. Interferon alpha/beta and interleukin 12 responses to viral infections: pathways regulating dendritic cell cytokine expression *in vivo*. *J Exp Med.* (2002) 195:517–28. doi: 10.1084/jem.20011672
47. O'Keeffe M, Hochrein H, Vremec D, Caminschi I, Miller JL, Anders EM, et al. Mouse plasmacytoid cells: long-lived cells, heterogeneous in surface phenotype and function, that differentiate into CD8(+) dendritic cells only after microbial stimulus. *J Exp Med.* (2002) 196:1307–19. doi: 10.1084/jem.20021031
48. Brasel K, De Smedt TD, Smith JL, Maliszewski CR. Generation of murine dendritic cells from flt3-ligand–supplemented bone marrow cultures. *Blood* (2000) 96:3029–39.
49. Brawand P, Fitzpatrick DR, Greenfield BW, Brasel K, Maliszewski CR, De Smedt T. Murine plasmacytoid pre-dendritic cells generated from Flt3 ligand-supplemented bone marrow cultures are immature APCs. *J Immunol.* (2002) 169:6711–6719. doi: 10.4049/jimmunol.169.12.6711
50. Gilliet M, Boonstra A, Paturel C, Antonenko S, Xu X-L, Trinchieri G, et al. The development of murine plasmacytoid dendritic cell precursors is differentially regulated by FLT3-ligand and granulocyte/macrophage colony-stimulating factor. *J Exp Med.* (2002) 195:953–8. doi: 10.1084/jem.20020045
51. Balan S, Arnold-Schrauf C, Abbas A, Couespel N, Savoret J, Imperatore F, et al. Large-scale human dendritic cell differentiation revealing notch-dependent lineage bifurcation and heterogeneity. *Cell Rep.* (2018) 24:1902–15.e6. doi: 10.1016/j.celrep.2018.07.033
52. Greter M, Helft J, Chow A, Hashimoto D, Mortha A, Agudo-Cantero J, et al. GM-CSF controls nonlymphoid tissue dendritic cell homeostasis but is dispensable for the differentiation of inflammatory dendritic cells. *Immunity* (2012) 36:1031–1046. doi: 10.1016/j.immuni.2012.03.027
53. Manh T-PV, Alexandre Y, Baranek T, Crozat K, Dalod M. Plasmacytoid, conventional, and monocyte-derived dendritic cells undergo a profound and convergent genetic reprogramming during their maturation. *Eur J Immunol.* (2013) 43:1706–15. doi: 10.1002/eji.201243106
54. Becher B, Waisman A, Lu L-F. Conditional gene-targeting in mice: problems and solutions. *Immunity* (2018) 48:835–6. doi: 10.1016/j.immuni.2018.05.002
55. Schmidt-Supprian M, Rajewsky K. Vagaries of conditional gene targeting. *Nat Immunol.* (2007) 8:665–68. doi: 10.1038/ni0707-665
56. Song AJ, Palmiter RD. Detecting and avoiding problems when using the Cre–lox system. *Trends Genet.* (2018) 34:333–40. doi: 10.1016/j.tig.2017.12.008
57. Liu J, Willet SG, Bankaitis ED, Xu Y, Wright CVE, Gu G. Non-parallel recombination limits cre-loxP-based reporters as precise indicators of conditional genetic manipulation: Cre-Recombinations are Non-Parallel Events. *Genesis* (2013) 51:436–42. doi: 10.1002/dvg.22384
58. Srinivas S, Watanabe T, Lin C-S, William CM, Tanabe Y, Jessell TM, et al. Cre reporter strains produced by targeted insertion of EYFP and ECFP into the ROSA26 locus. *BMC Dev Biol.* (2001) 1:4. doi: 10.1186/1471-213X-1-4

10

Staphylococcus aureus PSM Peptides Modulate Human Monocyte-Derived Dendritic Cells to Prime Regulatory T Cells

*Jennifer R. Richardson, Nicole S. Armbruster, Manina Günter, Jörg Henes and Stella E. Autenrieth**

Department of Internal Medicine II, University of Tübingen, Tübingen, Germany

***Correspondence:**
Stella E. Autenrieth
stella.autenrieth@med.uni-tuebingen.de

Staphylococcus aureus (Sa), as one of the major human pathogens, has very effective strategies to subvert the human immune system. Virulence of the emerging community-associated methicillin-resistant Sa (CA-MRSA) depends on the secretion of phenol-soluble modulin (PSM) peptide toxins e.g., by binding to and modulation of innate immune cells. Previously, by using mouse bone marrow-derived dendritic cells we demonstrated that PSMs in combination with various Toll-like receptor (TLR) ligands induce a tolerogenic DC phenotype (tDC) characterized by the production of IL-10 and impaired secretion of pro-inflammatory cytokines. Consequently, PSM-induced tDCs favored priming of $CD4^+CD25^+FoxP3^+$ T_{regs} with suppressor function while impairing the Th1 response. However, the relevance of these findings for the human system remained elusive. Here, we analyzed the impact of PSMα3 on the maturation, cytokine production, antigen uptake, and T cell stimulatory capacity of human monocyte-derived DCs (moDCs) treated simultaneously with either LPS (TLR4 ligand) or Sa cell lysate (TLR2 ligand). Herein, we demonstrate that PSMs indeed modulate human moDCs upon treatment with TLR2/4 ligands via multiple mechanisms, such as transient pore formation, impaired DC maturation, inhibited pro- and anti-inflammatory cytokine secretion, as well as reduced antigen uptake. As a result, the adaptive immune response was altered shown by an increased differentiation of naïve and even $CD4^+$ T cells from patients with Th1/Th17-induced diseases (spondyloarthritis and rheumatoid arthritis) into $CD4^+CD127^-CD25^{hi}CD45RA^-FoxP3^{hi}$ regulatory T cells (T_{regs}) with suppressor function. This T_{reg} induction was mediated most predominantly by direct DC-T-cell interaction. Thus, PSMs from highly virulent Sa strains affect DC functions not only in the mouse, but also in the human system, thereby modulating the adaptive immune response and probably increasing the tolerance toward the bacteria. Moreover, PSMα3 might be a novel peptide for tolerogenic DC induction that may be used for DC vaccination strategies.

Keywords: monocyte-derived dendritic cells, *Staphylococcus aureus*, phenol-soluble modulins, immune tolerance, immunity, regulatory T cells

INTRODUCTION

Dendritic cells (DCs) are specialized antigen presenting cells (APCs) able to prime naïve T cells thereby inducing a primary immune response and maintaining self-tolerance (1). Initially DCs occur in an immature state, specialized for antigen uptake with a high endocytic capability (2). The recognition of pathogens via germ-line encoded pattern-recognition receptors, like Toll-like Receptors (TLRs), leads to DC maturation (3). This event is characterized by the loss of their endocytic capacities and the upregulation of CCR7, co-stimulatory molecules, and HLA-DR, necessary for homing into the draining lymph node and T-cell priming (4). Furthermore, DCs secrete pro-inflammatory cytokines, such as TNF-α, IL-6 or IL-12, which recruit other immune cells for pathogen clearance and contribute to T helper cell (Th) differentiation (5). Apart from inducing an efficient immune response, DCs are also crucial for maintaining immune tolerance in the steady-state. Although the specific phenotype of so-called tolerogenic DCs (tDCs) and the molecular mechanism involved in tolerance induction by these cells are not entirely defined (6–9) they are characterized by an immature phenotype and produce high amounts of anti-inflammatory cytokines, e.g., IL-10 and TGF-ß, which possess critical immunoregulatory functions like controlling/regulating the production of pro-inflammatory cytokines. They have the potential to induce regulatory T cell (T_{reg}) expansion thereby impairing effector T cell responses (8, 10–12).

Various pathogens and tumors can induce tDCs and subsequent T_{reg} differentiation as immune escape strategy to impair clearance. This process is mediated by pathogenic products from e.g., *C. albicans*, *S. mansoni* and *V. cholerae*, which are partially used for the production of immunosuppressive drugs. These are widely used for therapy of autoimmune diseases or transplant rejections even though they have severe side effects by suppressing the entire host immune system (11, 13). Therefore, DC vaccination strategies by applying tDCs are an attractive alternative (8, 9, 13). Several clinical trials started to analyze the effect of tDCs as treatment option for patients with autoimmune disorders (8).

Phenol-soluble modulins (PSMs) are short amphipathic α-helical peptides, which are produced by highly virulent Staphylococci, such as community-associated Methicillin-resistant *Staphylococcus aureus* (Sa) promoting, e.g., cell lysis thereby evading clearance by immune cells (14, 15). Two types of PSMs are distinguished according to their length: α-type PSMs (~20–25 AA) and β-type PSMs (~44 AA) (16). The PSMα peptides are the most potent PSMs regarding cytolysis and highly contribute to the virulence of Sa (16, 17). Own previous studies with mouse bone-marrow derived DCs (BM-DCs) showed that PSMα3 prime tDCs when co-incubated with various TLR ligands (TLRL), regardless which TLR was activated. Molecularly, this event is characterized by the increased activation of the p38-CREB pathway, which in consequence leads to diminished pro-inflammatory cytokine production but increased IL-10 secretion. These PSM-induced tDCs favored priming of $CD4^+CD25^+FoxP3^+$ T_{regs} with suppressor function (10, 12, 18). Thus, we hypothesized that PSMs of Sa likewise induce tDCs in the human system.

Herein, we show that PSMα3 penetrates and modulates human monocyte-derived DCs (moDCs) by altering the TLR2- or TLR4-induced maturation, inhibiting pro- and anti-inflammatory cytokine production and reducing antigen uptake, but producing indolamin-2,3-dioxygenase (IDO). As a result, the frequency of $CD4^+CD127^-CD25^{hi}CD45RA^-Foxp3^{hi}$ T_{regs} is increased, while Th1 responses are diminished. Moreover, PSMα3-induced tDCs from healthy donors even enhanced differentiation of $CD4^+$ T cells from patients with Th17-associated autoimmune diseases to T_{regs}. Thus, PSMα3 might be a novel peptide for manipulating DCs to become tolerogenic for DC vaccination strategies.

Abbreviations: APC, antigen presenting cell; BM-DCs, bone-marrow derived DCs; CA-MRSA, community-associated methicillin-resistant Sa; DCs, dendritic cells; IDO, indolamin-2,3-dioxygenase; iT_{regs}, induced regulatory T cells; LDH, L-lactate dehydrogenase; moDCs, monocyte-derived DCs; PBMCs, peripheral blood mononuclear cells; PSM, phenol-soluble modulin peptides; Sa, *Staphylococcus aureus*; Sa lysate, *Staphylococcus aureus* cell lysate; tDCs, tolerogenic DCs; Th, T helper cell; TLR, Toll-like receptor; TLRL, Toll-like receptor ligand; T_{regs}, regulatory T cells.

MATERIALS AND METHODS

Research Subjects

Buffy coats from healthy volunteers were obtained from the ZKT Tübingen GmbH. Fresh blood was obtained from healthy volunteers with informed consent. This was approved by the ethical review committee of the medical faculty of the Eberhard-Karls-University of Tübingen with the project number 633/2012BO2. Blood from patients with TH17-associated autoimmune diseases were obtained from the division of Rheumatology, Department of Internal Medicine II, University Hospital Tübingen. This was approved by the ethical review committee of the medical faculty of the Eberhard-Karls-University of Tübingen with the project number 046/2015BO2.

Reagents

Formylated PSM peptides (PSMα3, δ-Toxin) were synthesized at the Interfaculty Institute of Cell Biology, Department of Immunology, University of Tübingen. FITC-labeled PSMα2 was synthesized at the Group of Hubert Kalbacher, Interfaculty Institute of Biochemistry, University of Tübingen. Sa cell lysate (Sa lysate) containing lipopeptides and specifically activating TLR2 was prepared from a protein A-deficient Sa mutant strain (SA113) and provided by Andreas Peschel, Interfaculty Institute of Microbiology and Infection Medicine, University of Tübingen.

Isolation of Peripheral Blood Mononuclear Cells

Buffy coats or fresh blood was diluted with Dulbecco's PBS (Life Technologies) (Buffy Coats 1:7 blood: PBS; Fresh blood 1:1 blood: PBS). Peripheral blood mononuclear cells (PBMCs) were obtained by density gradient centrifugation at 2000 rpm for 20 min at room temperature with 35 mL cell suspension stacked on 15 mL Biocoll separation solution (Biochrom). The interphase containing the PBMCs was abstracted and washed twice with

PBS. PBMCs were further used to generate human moDCs and for the isolation of naïve CD4+ T cells and CD4+ T cells.

Generation of Human Monocyte-Derived DCs

PBMCs were plated in a tissue-treated 6-well plate (6 × 10^6 cells per well) in DC medium [RPMI1640 (Merck), 10% FBS (Sigma), 2 mM L-Glutamine (Life Technologies), 100 U/mL Penicillin-Streptomycin (Life Technologies), 1 × non-essential amino acids (Merck), 1 mM sodium pyruvate (Merck) and 50 μM 2-mercaptoethanol (Roth)] and incubated for 1 h at 37°C, 5% CO_2. After that, wells were washed with medium and PBS discarding the non-adherent cells. 3 mL/well DC medium containing 50 ng IL-4 and 100 ng GM-CSF (both from Miltenyi) was added to the remaining cells. Cells were incubated for 6 d at 37°C, 5% CO_2. Cytokines were again added on day 2 and day 4. At day 6 the cells were used for the following experiments. The purity of the moDC culture was always >90% of leukocytes (**Figure S1**).

Cytokine/Indolamin-2,3-Dioxygenase Production by moDCs

MoDCs (2.5 × 10^5) were seeded in a 96-well plate and treated with 3 μg/mL Sa lysate or 100 ng/mL LPS in combination with or without PSMα3 (10 μM). For some experiments moDCs were treated with different concentrations of PSMα3 or additionally stimulated with 100 ng/mL Pam2CSK4 (for TLR2/TLR6; InvivoGen), 1 μg/mL Pam3CSK4 (for TLR1/TLR2; InvivoGen), 1 μg/mL CpG ODN 2395 (for TLR9; InvivoGen), 5 μg/mL Imiquimod (for TLR7; InvivoGen), 2 μg/mL Flagellin (for TLR5; InvivoGen) or 10 μg/mL LTA (for TLR2/TLR4; InvivoGen) in combination with or without PSMα3 (10 μM). Supernatants were collected after 6 h, 24 h or 48 h and analyzed for TNF, IL-10, IL-12 and IDO production, respectively. Cytokines and IDO in the supernatants were determined by sandwich ELISA [eBioscience (TNF, IL-10, IL-12), R&D Systems (IDO)] according to the manufacturer's instructions.

Flow Cytometry

For moDC surface marker analysis of the costimulatory and inhibitory molecules, moDCs (2 × 10^5) were seeded in a 96-well plate and stimulated with 3 μg/mL Sa lysate or 100 ng/mL LPS with or without PSMα3 (10 μM) or PSMα3 alone for 6 h or 24 h. Cells were removed from the plate using Accutase (Sigma-Aldrich) and treated with IgG from human serum (1 μg of human IgG per 100,000 cells; Sigma-Aldrich) for 20 min at room temperature to avoid unspecific binding via Fc receptors. Cells were stained with ZombieAqua (BioLegend) to exclude dead cells and fluorochrome conjugated extracellular antibodies: HLA-DR BV650 (L243, BioLegend), CD11b BV510 (ICRF44, BioLegend), CD11c APC (MJ4-27G121, Miltenyi), CD11c PE-Cy7 (Bu15, BioLegend), CD40 FITC (5C3, eBioscience), CD80 PE-Cy7 (2D10, BioLegend), CD83 PE-Dazzle 594 (HB15e, BioLegend), CD86 BV605 (IT2.2, BioLegend), PD-L1 PE (29E.2A3, BioLegend), PD-L2 PE (MIH18), ILT3 PE (ZM4.1, BioLegend) for 20 min at 4°C. FACS buffer [PBS containing 1% FBS, 2 mM EDTA (Merck) and 0.09% NaN_3 (Sigma-Aldrich)] was used for all incubations and washing steps. At least 50,000 cells were acquired using a LSR Fortessa flow cytometer (BD Biosciences) with the DIVA software (BD Biosciences) and were further analyzed using FlowJo 10.4.2 software (Tree Star).

Phosphoflow

For the experiments analyzing phosphorylation of signaling cascades, moDCs (2 × 10^5) were seeded in a 96-well plate and treated for 1 h with 100 ng/mL LPS with or without PSMα3 (10 μM) or PSMα3 alone. Cells were removed from the plate using Accutase and treated with IgG from human serum (1 μg of human IgG per 100,000 cells) for 20 min at room temperature to avoid unspecific binding via Fc receptors. Cells were stained with ZombieAqua (BioLegend) to exclude dead cells and fluorochrome conjugated extracellular antibodies: HLA-DR PE (L243; BD Biosciences) and CD11c APC/Cy7 (Bu15; BioLegend) for 20 min at 4°C. To detect intracellular p-p38 and p-NF-κB cells were fixed with 2% paraformaldehyde (VWR) in PBS, permeabilized with 90% freezing methanol (Applichem) overnight and stained with the primary Abs to phospho-p38 MAPK (Thr180/Tyr182; clone 12F8) or phospho-NF-κB p65 (Ser536; clone: 93H1) (both from Cell Signaling) for 1 h in the dark at room temperature followed by DyLight649-conjugated AffiniPure Goat At-Rabbit IgG (Jackson ImmunoResearch) for 15 min at 4°C. PBS with 0.5% BSA (Biomol) was used for incubation and washing steps of intracellular antibody stainings. At least 50,000 cells were acquired using a Canto-II (BD Biosciences) with DIVA software (BD Biosciences) and were further analyzed using the FlowJo 10.4.2 software (Tree Star).

Measurement of Antigen Uptake by Flow Cytometry or Multispectral Imaging Flow Cytometry

MoDCs (5 × 10^5) were seeded in a 48-well plate and stimulated for 24 h with 3 μg/mL Sa lysate or 100 ng/mL LPS with or without PSMα3 (10 μM) or PSMα3 alone prior to the incubation with Ovalbumin (OVA)-AlexaFluor647 (5 μg/mL, Invitrogen) together with PSMα2 FITC (0.5 μM) for 30 min at 37°C, 5% CO_2. Unspecific binding of OVA/PSMα2 was assessed by incubating the cells on ice. Cells were washed twice with ice-cold PBS containing 2% FBS. Subsequently, cells were blocked and stained with ZombieAqua (BioLegend), HLA-DR BV650 (L243, BioLegend), HLA-DR APC-Cy7 (L243, BioLegend) and CD11c PE-Cy7 (Bu15, BioLegend) as described above and analyzed by flow cytometry or by multispectral imaging flow cytometry. For the latter, images of 10,000 living moDCs were acquired using the Image-Stream mkII (Amnis) with the INSPIRE instrument controller software. The data were analyzed using the IDEAS analysis software (Merck Millipore).

Lactate Dehydrogenase Release

MoDCs (2 × 10^5) were seeded in a 96-well plate and treated with Triton X100 (1%; Sigma-Aldrich), DMSO (2%, Fluka), PSMα2 (10 μM), PSMα3 (2.5, 5, 7.5, and 10 μM), δ-Toxin (10 μM) or OVA (10 μg, Sigma-Aldrich) for 10 min at 37°C, 5% CO_2. Cell death was determined using 7-aminoactinomycin D (7-AAD, Biomol) staining and acquisition on a Canto II flow cytometer.

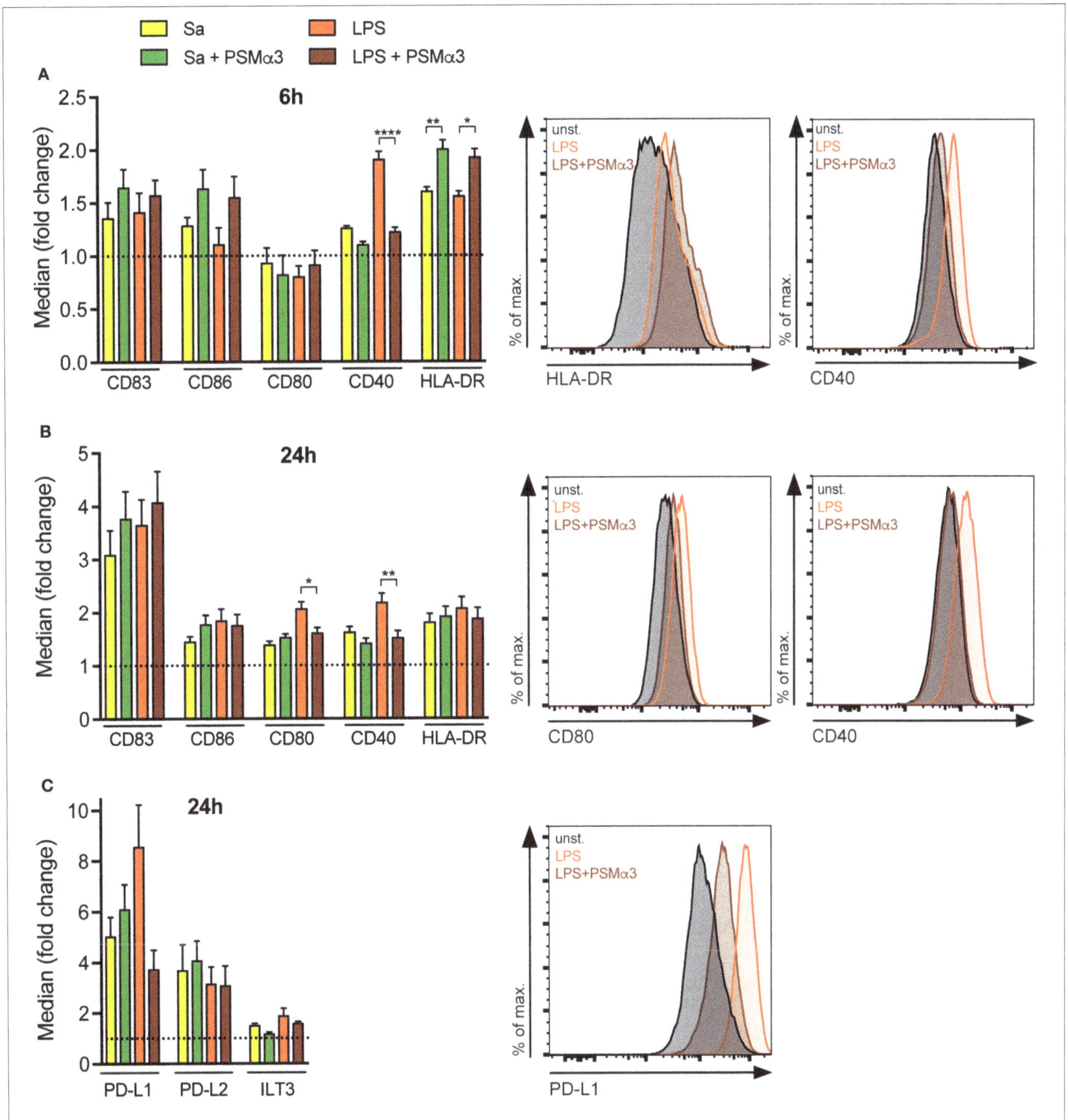

FIGURE 1 | PSMs modulate surface molecule expression of TLR-treated moDCs. MoDCs were treated with Sa lysate or LPS with or without PSMα3 for 6 h **(A)** or 24 h **(B,C)** and analyzed by flow cytometry. MoDCs were characterized as living $CD11c^{+}HLA\text{-}DR^{+}$ cells and the expression of the indicated costimulatory **(A,B)** and inhibitory molecules **(C)** was determined. The graphs show the mean fluorescence intensity of the respective marker expression as fold change of untreated cells. The graphs show $n \geq 3$ independent experiments (mean ± SEM) performed in triplicates. Representative histogram overlays of HLA-DR and CD40 after 6 h **(A)**, CD80, CD40 **(B)**, and PD-L1 **(C)** after 24 h. $^{*}p < 0.05$, $^{**}p < 0.005$ or $^{****}p < 0.0001$, one-way ANOVA with Turkey's posttest or Kruskal-Wallis with Dunn's posttest.

Supernatants were used for the analysis of lactate dehydrogenase (LDH) release using the Cytotoxicity Detection Kit (Roche) according to the manufacturer's instructions. Absorbance was measured at 492 nm and 620 nm over a period of 1 h with an interval of 5 min using the Spark 10 M microplate reader (Tecan).

T-Cell Assay

MoDCs (5×10^4) were seeded in a 96-well plate and stimulated with 3 µg/mL Sa lysate or 100 ng/mL LPS with or without PSMα3 (10 µM) or PSMα3 alone for 24 h. For some experiments moDCs were pre-treated with 200 µM 1-Methyl-D-tryptophan (1-DMT) for 1 h prior to the stimulation. Human naïve $CD4^+$ T cells were isolated from PBMCs using the MojoSort™ Human CD4 Naïve T Cell Isolation Kit (BioLegend) according to the manufacturer's instructions. For the magnetic cell separation, a LS column (Miltenyi Biotech) was placed into the QuadroMACS Separator (Miltenyi Biotech) and rinsed with MACS buffer (PBS containing 0,5% BSA (Biomol) and 2 mM EDTA). The cell suspension was applied to the column, and the column was washed three times with 3 mL MACS buffer. The untouched naïve $CD4^+$ T cells were collected in the flow through. The purity of isolated (naïve) $CD4^+$ T cells was always ≈85% (**Figure S4**). The naïve $CD4^+$ T cells were labeled with CFSE (5 μM, BioLegend) according to the manufacturer's instructions. 2×10^5 T cells diluted in 100 μL T cell medium [RPMI1640 (Merck), 10% FBS (Sigma), 2 mM L-Glutamine (Life Technologies), 100 U/mL penicillin-streptomycin (Life Technologies), 1 × non-essential amino acids (Merck), 1 mM sodium pyruvate (Merck), 10 mM HEPES (Biochrom) and 50 μM 2-mercaptoethanol (Roth)] were added to the moDCs. To investigate whether secreted factors from DCs upon PSM-treatment mediate T_{reg} priming, T cells were co-cultured with untreated moDCs adding conditioned medium from LPS or LPS + PSMα3 stimulated DCs. In a second assay moDCs treated as described above were splitted using Accutase (Sigma-Aldrich) for 5 min at room temperature and again sowed with either fresh or conditioned DC medium (TLRL or TLRL + PSMα3). In some conditions, DC were fixed with 1% paraformaldehyde for 10 min at 4°C to address the impact of newly secreted factors on T_{reg} priming by DCs. 3–4 d after co-culture T cells were blocked with IgG from human serum for 15 min at room temperature and subsequently stained with ZombieAqua, CD4 APC-Vio770 (REA623, Miltenyi), CD3 Pacific Blue (SK7, BioLegend), CD25 PE-Cy7 (BC96, eBiosciences), CD127 PE (eBioRDR5, eBiosciences) and CD45RA BV605 (HI100, BioLegend) for 20 min at 4°C. For intracellular staining, cells were fixed and permeabilized with the Foxp3/ Transcription Factor Staining Buffer Set (eBiosciences), blocked and stained with CD4 APC-Vio770, CD3 Pacific Blue, FoxP3 AlexaFluor647 (259D, BioLegend), T-bet PE-Dazzle 594 (4B10, BioLegend), GATA3 PerCP-Cy5.5 (16E10A23, BioLegend) and RORγt BV650 (Q21-559, BD Biosciences) for 45 min at 4°C. FACS buffer was used for all incubations and washing steps for the extracellular staining, and 1 × permeabilization buffer (Foxp3/Transcription Factor Staining Buffer Set (eBiosciences) was used for all incubations and washing steps for the intracellular staining. At least 70,000 cells were acquired using an LSR Fortessa flow cytometer (BD Biosciences) with the DIVA software (BD Biosciences) and were further analyzed using FlowJo 10.4.2 software (Tree Star).

Autologous T-Cell Assay

$CD14^+$ cells from PBMCs of patients with TH17-associated autoimmune diseases were isolated by MACS using CD14 MicroBeads (Miltenyi Biotech) and plated in a tissue-treated 6-well plate (1.3×10^6 cells per well) in DC medium containing 50 ng IL-4 and 100 ng GM-CSF for 6 d to generate moDCs. The remaining $CD14^-$ cells were frozen at −80°C in RPMI1640 supplemented with 20 % FBS and 10% DMSO. After 6 d moDCs (5×10^4) were seeded in a 96-well plate and stimulated with 100 ng/mL LPS with or without PSMα3 (10 μM) for 24 h. The $CD14^-$ cells were thawed and used to isolate $CD4^+$ T cells by MACS with CD4 MicroBeads (Miltenyi Biotech). The $CD4^+$ T cells were labeled with CFSE (5 μM, BioLegend) according to the manufacturer's instructions and 2×10^5 T cells diluted in 100 μL T cell medium were added to the moDCs. 3–4 days after co-culture T cells were stained as above and iT_{regs} were analyzed by flow cytometry using an LSR Fortessa flow cytometer (BD Biosciences) with the DIVA software (BD Biosciences) and were further analyzed using FlowJo 10.4.2 software (Tree Star).

Cytokine Production in the moDC T Cell Co-culture

Fifty microliter cell culture supernatants from the T cell assay were taken on day 1, 2 and 3 and cytokine production from 15 μL was analyzed by performing bead-based immunoassays in a 96-well plate [LEGENDplex human B cell Panel (13-Plex) and LEGENDplex Free Active/Total TGF-β1 (BioLegend)] according to the manufacturer's instructions, using the Lyric flow cytometer with autosampler (BD Bioscience).

T Cell Suppression Assay

MoDCs (2×10^5) were seeded in a 48-well plate and stimulated with 100ng/mL LPS and 10 μM PSMα3 for 24 h. Human $CD4^+$ T cells were isolated from PBMCs using the human CD4 MicroBeads Kit (Miltenyi) according to the manufacturer's instructions using LS columns. 8×10^5 T cells were added to the stimulated moDCs and cultured for 4 d at 37°C, 5% CO_2. T cells were stained with CD4 APC-Vio770, CD25 PE-Cy7, CD127 PE and CD45RA PerCP (HI100, BioLegend) as described above and dead cells were excluded using DAPI (Sigma-Aldrich,16,7 ng/mL). T_{regs} were purified by FACS sorting using an ARIA IIu cell sorter (BD Bioscience), according to the surface molecule expression ($CD4^+CD127^-CD25^{hi}CD45RA^-$, see **Figure S7**). $CD4^+$ T cells isolated from PBMCs from a different donor were used as T effector (T_{eff}) cells purified with CD4 MicroBeads Kit (Miltenyi). The T_{effs} were labeled with CFSE (5 μM), and 8×10^4 cells were seeded in a 96- well plate in T cell medium together with the indicated numbers of sorted T_{regs}. For T cell activation of the T_{effs} Dynabeads (Human T-Activator CD3/CD28Proliferation; Gibco) were added according to the manufacturer's instructions. The proliferation of T_{effs} was assessed after 3 d by flow cytometry. Dead cells were excluded by staining the cells with ZombieAqua. 20,000 cells were acquired at the Canto II with the DIVA software (BD Biosciences) and were further analyzed using the proliferation tool in FlowJo 10.4.2 software (Tree Star).

Statistical Analysis

Statistical analysis was performed using GraphPad Prism 7.0a software (GraphPad, San Diego, CA). Statistical differences were determined using one-way ANOVA with Turkey's posttest in case data were normally distributed (Shapiro-Wilk normality test). Otherwise, data were analyzed using the Kruskal-Wallis nonparametric test. The differences were considered as

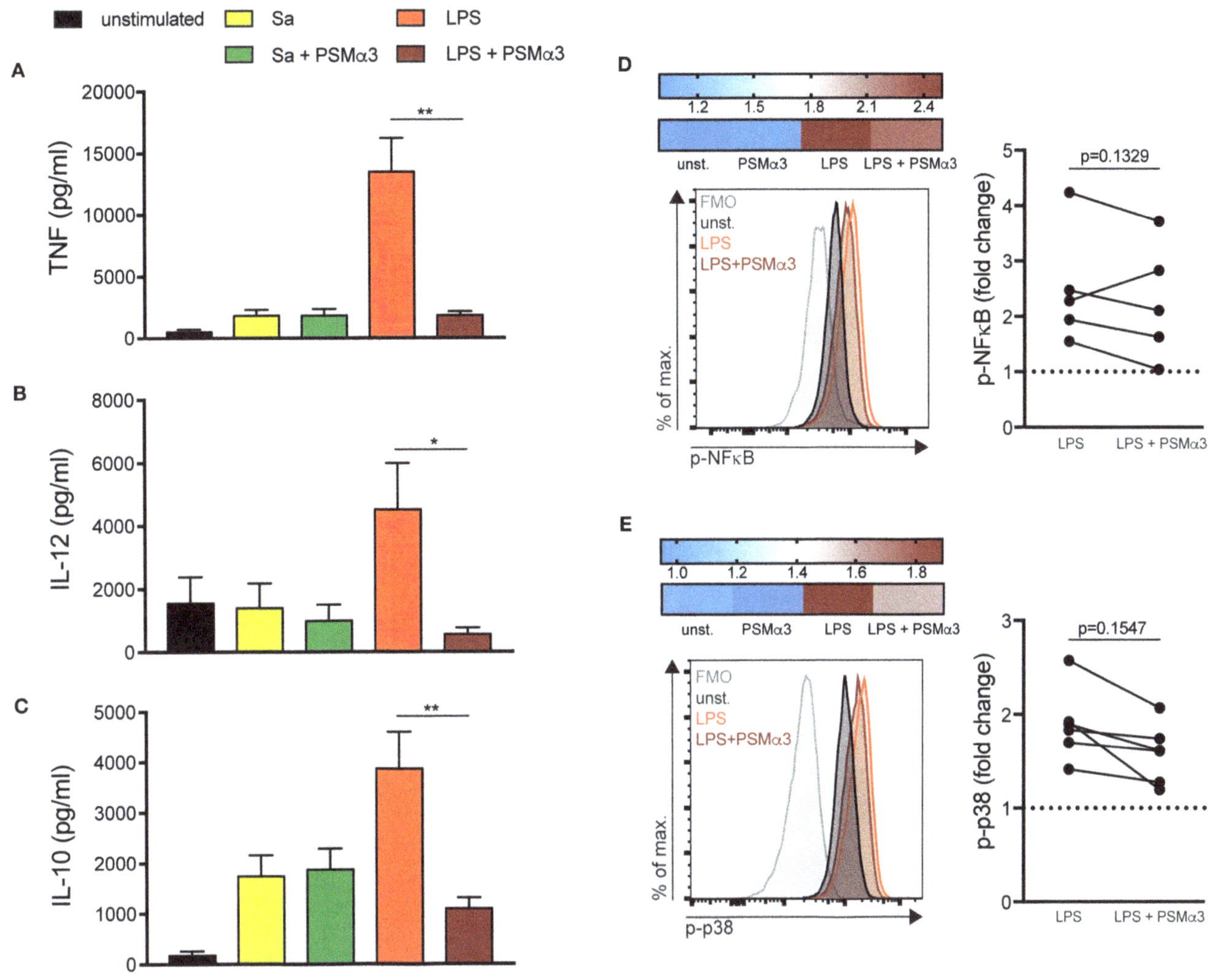

FIGURE 2 | PSMs impair pro- and anti-inflammatory cytokine secretion by moDCs. **(A–C)** MoDCs were treated with Sa lysate or LPS with or without PSMα3 for 6 h **(A)** or 24 h **(B,C)**. The cell culture supernatants were collected and analyzed for TNF **(A)**, IL-12 **(B)** and IL-10 **(C)** production by sandwich ELISA. The graphs show $n \geq 10$ independent experiments (mean ± SD/SEM) performed in triplicates. **(D,E)** MoDCs were treated with LPS with or without PSMα3 or PSMα3 alone for 60 min. Thereafter, the cells were stained extracellularly with anti-CD11c and anti-HLA-DR antibodies, followed by fixation, permeabilization and subsequent intracellular staining using anti-phospho-NF-κB **(D)** and anti-phospho-p38 antibodies **(E)**. Representative histogram overlays of p-NF-κB **(D)** and p-p38 **(E)** in DCs (gated on $CD11c^{+}HLA\text{-}DR^{+}$ cells). The heat map shows fold-change of p-NF-κB **(D)** and p-p38 **(E)** normalized to untreated DCs (unst.). The graphs show the statistical analysis of p-NF-κB **(D)** and p-p38 **(E)** from $n = 5$ different donors. $^{*}p < 0.05$ or $^{**}p < 0.005$, Kruskal-Wallis with Dunn's posttest or one-way ANOVA with Turkey's posttest.

statistically significant if $p < 0.05$ (*), $p < 0.005$ (**), $p < 0.001$ (***), or $p < 0.0001$ (****).

RESULTS

PSMs Modulate Surface Molecule Expression of TLR-Treated moDCs

The maturation of DCs is an essential event for successful T-cell activation comprising the upregulation of maturation markers (e.g., CD83 and HLA-DR), co-stimulatory (e.g., CD80, CD86, CD40) and co-inhibitory molecules (e.g., PD-L1, PD-L2 or ILT3). To investigate if the Sa-derived toxin PSMα3 has an impact on DC maturation, moDCs were treated with either the TLR2 ligand Sa lysate (12) or the TLR4 ligand LPS with or without PSMα3. Surface marker expression was analyzed by flow cytometry after 6 or 24 h (Gating see **Figure S1**). All surface molecules analyzed were increased upon TLRL treatment compared to untreated moDCs at 6 and 24 h with the exception of CD80 after 6 h (**Figure 1**) confirming DC maturation (mDCs - mature DCs). Simultaneous treatment of moDCs with TLRLs and PSMα3 for 6h revealed a tendency, but no significant increase of the maturation marker CD83 and CD86 compared to treatment with TLRLs alone (**Figure 1A**). In contrast, HLA-DR was significantly increased 6h (Sa $p = 0.0081$; LPS $p = 0.0226$) after TLRL treatment in combination with PSMα3 whereas CD40 was less expressed on mDCs treated with LPS in combination with PSMα3 compared to LPS treated cells after 6 h (LPS $p < 0.0001$) and 24 h (LPS $p < 0.0049$) (**Figures 1A,B**). Similarly, CD80

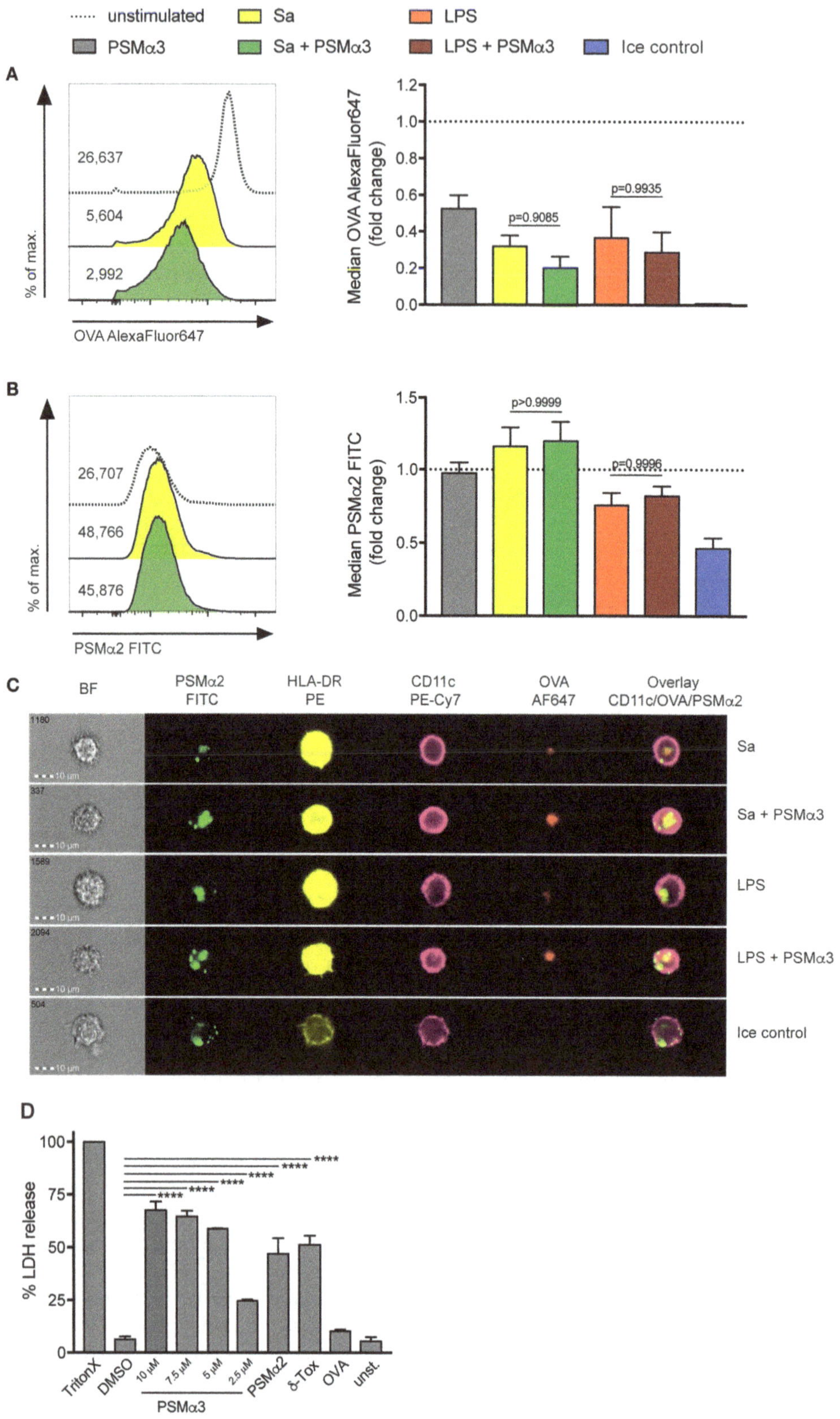

FIGURE 3 | PSMs inhibit antigen uptake by moDCs and penetrate the membrane via transient pore formation. **(A–C)** MoDCs treated for 24 h with Sa lysate or LPS with or without PSMα3 or PSMα3 alone were incubated with AlexaFluor647-labeled OVA and FITC-labeled PSMα2 at 37°C or on ice for 30 min. **(A,B)** The uptake of *(Continued)*

FIGURE 3 | OVA and PSMα2 by living CD11c$^+$HLA-DR$^+$ moDCs was assessed by flow cytometry. The histogram overlays (left) and the bar graphs (right, collected data) show the mean fluorescence intensity of OVA-AlexaFluor647 **(A)** or PSMα2-FITC **(B)**, in case of the collected data as fold change of unstimulated cells ($n \geq 5$, performed in triplicates, mean ± SEM). **(C)** The localization of OVA-AlexaFluor647 and PSMα2-FITC in CD11c$^+$HLA-DR$^+$ moDCs was analyzed by multispectral imaging flow cytometry (one representative experiment of $n = 3$ independent experiments; mean ± SEM). Representative bright field (BF) and fluorescence images of moDCs are shown for the different treatments. **(D)** MoDCs were either not treated (unst.) or incubated with 1% Triton X-100, 2% DMSO, PSMα3 (2.5 μM, 5 μM, 7.5 μM or 10 μM), 10 μM PSMα2, 10 μM δ-Toxin or 5 μg/mL OVA for 10 min. The LDH release was determined in the cell culture supernatants (one representative experiment of $n = 3$ independent experiments; mean ± SEM). ****$p < 0.0001$, one-way ANOVA with Turkey's posttest or Kruskal-Wallis with Dunn's posttest.

up-regulation on TLR4-stimulated mDCs was impaired when the cells were treated with PSMα3 for 24 h (LPS $p = 0.0135$) (**Figure 1B**). The analysis of co-inhibitory molecule expression revealed no significant differences after 24 h; however, PSMα3 showed a tendency to prevent the upregulation of the co-inhibitory molecule PD-L1 in TLR4-stimulated moDCs (LPS $p = 0.0615$) (**Figure 1C**). In summary, PSMα3 enhanced the early upregulation of HLA-DR on DCs but prevented that of the co-stimulatory molecules CD40 and CD80 especially upon TLR4 stimulation.

PSMs Impair Pro- and Anti-inflammatory Cytokine Secretion by TLR4-Treated moDCs

Stimulation of TLRs not only leads to DC maturation but also to the expression of cytokines to initiate an immune response. Previously, we showed that PSMα3 impaired the pro-inflammatory cytokine production triggered by various TLRLs in mouse BM-DCs, whereas it induced the expression of the anti-inflammatory cytokine IL-10 (12, 18). Therefore, cell culture supernatants from moDCs treated with Sa lysate or LPS with or without PSMα3 were analyzed after 6 h for TNF (**Figure 2A**) and after 24 h for IL-12 (**Figure 2B**), IL-10 (**Figure 2C**) or TNF production (**Figure S2A**). TLRL treatment led to an overall induction of cytokine secretion with the exception of IL-12 (**Figure 2B**) in TLR2-ligand treated mDCs (**Figure 2**). The production of TNF, IL-12 and IL-10 was impaired by PSMα3 in LPS treated mDCs (TNF 1.800 vs. 13.500 pg/ml, $p = 0.0082$; IL-12 550 vs. 4.500 pg/ml, $p = 0.021$; IL-10 1090 vs. 3850 pg/ml, $p = 0.0080$) (**Figure 2**) the latter in a concentration dependent manner (**Figure S2B**), but not in Sa lysate treated mDCs. The treatment of DCs with PSMα3 in combination with other TLR-ligands like Pam2CSK4, Pam3CSK4, LTA, Flagellin, CpG, and Imiquimod showed no significant differences in the production of TNF and IL-10 compared to TLR-L treatment alone (**Figure 2** and **Figure S2C**). In summary, PSMα3 inhibited pro- as well as anti-inflammatory cytokine production by LPS-treated mDCs.

PSMs Impair NF-κB and p38 Phosphorylation in LPS-Treated moDCs

To investigate the signaling pathways involved in the cytokine modulation by PSMs, DCs were treated with LPS in the presence or absence of PSMα3 for 60 min and phosphorylation of NF-κB p65 (p-NF-κB) (**Figure 2D**) and p38 MAPK (p-p38) (**Figure 2E**) was analyzed by flow cytometry. Treatment of DCs with PSMα3 did not affect p- NF-κB or p-p38 compared to untreated DCs (**Figures 2D,E** heatmap), whereas after LPS treatment a 2.5-fold and 2-fold increase of p- NF-κB and p-p38, respectively, was observed compared to untreated DCs (**Figures 2D,E**). DCs incubated with LPS combined with PSMα3 revealed a 2.0-fold and 1.5-fold increase of NF-κB or p38 phosphorylation (**Figures 2D,E**). Analyzing signaling pathways in moDCs from 5 donors revealed by trend a reduced, but not significant, NF-κB or p38 phosphorylation upon PSMα3 treatment. These data indicate that impaired phosphorylation of both NF-κB and p38 pathways by PSMα3 may account for impaired cytokine production as well as co-stimulatory molecule expression by moDCs upon LPS treatment.

PSMs Inhibit Antigen Uptake by moDCs

Antigen uptake is a pivotal task of DCs and necessary for T-cell activation. To elucidate possible effects of PSMs on this event, moDCs were treated with or without either Sa lysate or LPS in the presence or absence of PSMα3 for 24 h. Subsequently cells were incubated with the fluorescently-labeled (AlexaFluor647) model antigen OVA in combination with FITC-labeled PSMα2 for 30 min. Immature DCs (iDCs - immature DCs) take up OVA mainly by clathrin-mediated endocytosis and macropinocytosis, whereas mature DCs retain antigen uptake by receptor-mediated endocytosis (12, 19–21). This effect was observed when moDCs matured after treatment with either Sa lysate or LPS by ~68 or ~63%, respectively (**Figure 3A**). OVA uptake was reduced by ~48% after solely treatment with PSMα3 ($p < 0.0001$) (**Figure 3A**), showing that iDCs are affected in their task to take up antigen by PSMs. A trend to further impaired antigen uptake by TLRL and PSMα3 treated moDCs was observed (Sa $p = 0.6603$, LSP $p = 0.9054$) (**Figure 3A**). Incubation of iDCs with OVA on ice was used to exclude unspecific binding (**Figure 3A**) thereby preventing remodeling of the actin cytoskeleton, which is required for clathrin-mediated endocytosis and micropinocytosis (22). In conclusion, PSMα3 affects moDCs in their antigen uptake capacity.

PSMs Penetrate the Membrane of moDCs Via Transient Pore Formation

Previously, we and others showed that PSMs form transient pores into the cell membrane thereby entering the cytosol (10, 15). To address whether PSMs are internalized by human moDCs via mechanisms of antigen uptake or by pore formation iDCs were incubated with fluorescently-labeled PSMα2 as described above and analyzed by flow cytometry and multispectral imaging flow cytometry. Despite the uptake of OVA-AlexaFluor647, PSMα2-FITC was observed in moDCs regardless of their maturation

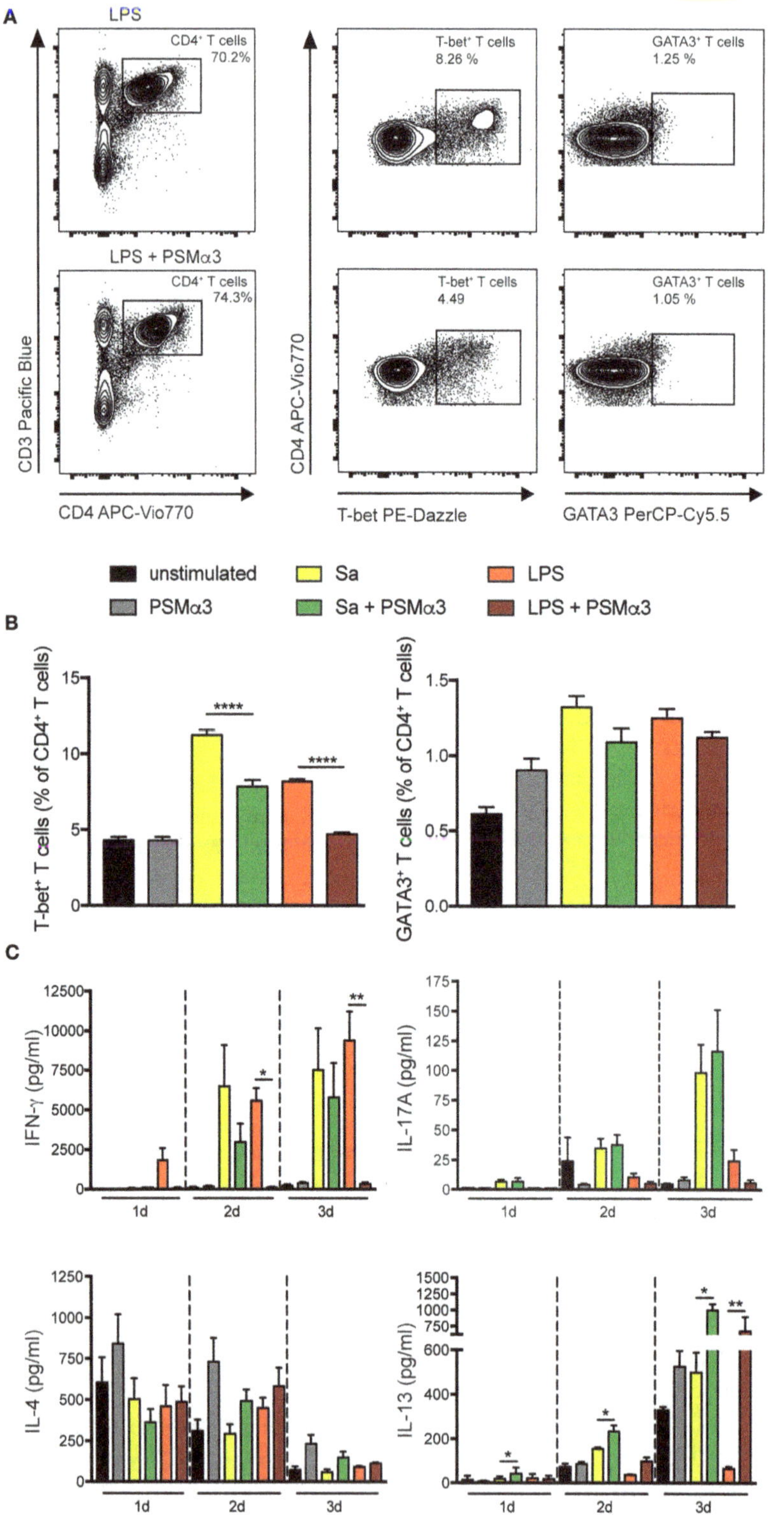

FIGURE 4 | Polarization of Th1 is impaired by PSMs. MoDCs treated for 24 h with Sa lysate or LPS with or without PSMα3 or PSMα3 alone were co-cultured with CFSE-labeled naïve $CD4^+$ T cells for 3 d. The different Th subsets were analyzed by flow cytometry; Th1 cells were characterized as $CD3^+CD4^+$T-bet^+ T cells, Th2 cells were characterized as $CD3^+CD4^+GATA3^+$ T cells **(A)**. **(B)** The bar graphs show the frequency of T-bet^+ Th1 and $GATA3^+$ Th2 cells from $CD4^+$ T cells (one representative of $n = 4$ independent experiments performed in triplicates, mean ± SEM). **(C)** Cell culture supernatants from the DC T cell co-culture were collected after 1 d, 2 d or 3 d and analyzed for Th-associated cytokine production ($n \geq 3$ performed in triplicates; mean ± SEM). $^*p < 0.05$, $^{**}p < 0.005$, or $^{****}p < 0.0001$, one-way ANOVA with Turkey's posttest or Kruskal-Wallis with Dunn's posttest.

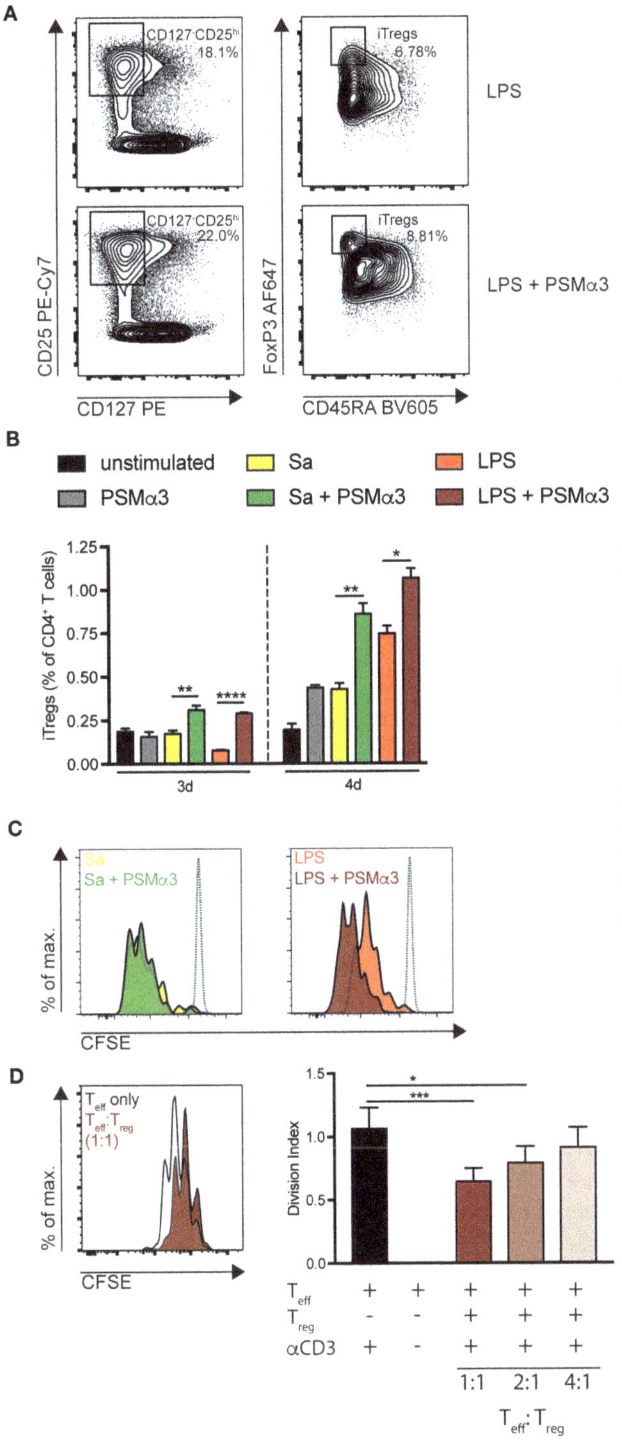

FIGURE 5 | PSMα3-treated moDCs increase the proliferation and frequency of iT_{regs}. **(A–C)** MoDCs treated for 24 h with Sa lysate or LPS with or without PSMα3 or PSMα3 alone were co-cultured with CFSE-labeled naïve $CD4^+$ T cells for 3 d or 4 d. iT_{regs} were analyzed by flow cytometry and characterized as $CD4^+CD127^-CD25^{hi}CD45RA^-Foxp3^{hi}$ cells **(A)**. The frequency of iT_{regs} from $CD4^+$ T cells **(B)** and the proliferation of iT_{regs} **(C)** co-cultured with TLRL-only or in combination with PSMα3-treated mDCs was analyzed ($n \geq 5$ performed in triplicates, mean ± SEM). Proliferation was compared to T cells *(Continued)*

FIGURE 5 | cultured without DCs (gray dotted line). **(D)** Allogenic suppression assay of CFSE-labeled T_{effs} cultured in different ratios with or without sorted T_{regs} ($CD4^+CD127^-CD25^{hi}CD45RA^-$, **Figure S7**) from DC T cell co-culture described in **(A)**. Proliferation of the CFSE-labeled T_{effs} with or without activation via αCD3-beads was assessed after 3 d ($n = 2$ performed in triplicates; mean ± SEM). *$p < 0.05$, **$p < 0.005$, ***$p < 0.001$, or ****$p < 0.0001$, one-way ANOVA with Turkey's posttest or Kruskal-Wallis with Dunn's posttest.

status (**Figure 3B**). Moreover, PSMα2-FITC was also detected in moDCs incubated on ice but reduced by ~54% ($p = 0.0003$), indicating that the uptake was not an active process requiring actin remodeling (**Figure 3B**). These observations were confirmed by multispectral imaging flow cytometry, showing PSMα2-FITC located at the membrane when actin-cytoskeleton rearrangement is blocked (ice control) as well as co-localized with OVA most likely in the phagosome when moDCs were incubated at 37°C regardless of the treatment (**Figure 3C**).

Transient pore formation in the membrane of moDCs mediated by PSMα3 was demonstrated by measuring L-lactate dehydrogenase (LDH) in the supernatant of moDCs treated with PSMα2 various concentrations of PSMα3 (**Figure 3D**). Triton-X, which disrupts the membrane completely as well as δ-Toxin, which is known to form transient pores (23) were used as positive controls (**Figure 3D**). Neither treatment of moDCs with OVA, the peptide-dissolvent DMSO or medium alone had any effects on LDH release (**Figure 3D**), whereas PSMα3 significantly induced LDH release in a concentration-dependent manner. Further, flow cytometric analysis of the moDCs showed that apart from treatment with Triton-X, none of the reagents affected their viability (**Figure S3**). Together the data show that PSMs enter moDCs via transient pore formation without cytolytic effects.

Polarization of T Helper1 Cells Is Impaired by PSMs

DCs play a crucial role in the activation and polarization of T cells. Not only the direct interaction, but also the local cytokine milieu is important for the outcome and distinct transcription factors control the differentiation of the T cell subsets (24, 25). To assess the impact of PSMα3-treated moDCs on the polarization of T helper (Th) cell subsets, moDCs were treated with or without Sa lysate or LPS in combination with PSMα3 for 24 h. Subsequently, the cells were co-cultured with naive $CD4^+$ T cells for 3–4 d. Flow cytometry analysis of the Th subsets showed that TLRL-treated mDCs primed significantly more $T\text{-}bet^+$ Th1 cells whereas mDCs co-treated with PSMα3 prevented Th1 priming (Sa 11.2 vs. 7.8%, $p < 0.0001$; LPS 8.2 vs. 4.7%, $p < 0.0001$) (**Figures 4A,B**). In contrast, stimulation of iDCs with PSMα3 alone did not show any difference compared to untreated cells (**Figure 4B**), indicating that PSMα3 without TLRL has no influence on the priming capacity of moDCs. Analyzing Th2 cells by GATA3 expression after co-culture with moDCs treated with TLRL alone or in combination with PSMα3 revealed the same tendency as T-bet expression, but no significant differences (Sa 1.32 vs. 1.1%, $p = 0.27$; LPS 1.25 vs. 1.1%, $p = 0.8$) (**Figures 4A,B** and **Figure S6B**). However, no difference in the frequency of RORγt$^+$CD4$^+$ T cells was observed (data not shown).

Cytokine secretion analysis of the major Th1, Th2, and Th17 cytokines in co-culture after 1–3 days showed that IFN-γ secretion was completely prevented when TLR4 ligand-treated mDCs were co-treated with PSMα3 (LPS day 1 1.800 vs. 80 pg/ml, $p = 0.5617$; day 2 5.600 vs. 120 pg/ml, $p = 0.0146$, day 3 9.400 vs. 330 pg/ml, $p < 0.0001$), which in part, but not significant, was also seen for TLR2-stimulated mDCs (Sa day 1 60 vs. 40 pg/ml, $p>0.999$; day 2 6.500 vs. 3.000 pg/ml, $p = 0.2534$, day 3 7.500 vs. 5,800 pg/ml, $p = 0.9105$) (**Figure 4C**). Comparable results, but without significance, were observed for IL-17A secretion at day 2 and 3 by TLR4 ligand-treated mDCs together with PSMα3 (LPS day 2 10.8 vs. 5.1 pg/ml, $p = 0.9658$, day3 24.4 vs. 5.7 pg/ml, $p = 0.4336$). Similarly, no significant effects of PSMα3 were observed for IL-17A secretion after co-culture of CD4$^+$ T cells with mDCs treated with Sa lysate. Further, IL-4 secretion showed no difference after treatment with either Sa lysate or LPS, respectively (**Figure 4C**). However, the expression of the closely related cytokine IL-13 significantly increased 3 days after coculture of CD4$^+$ T cells with moDCs treated with TLRLs and PSMα3 (Sa 500 vs. 1.000 pg/ml, $p = 0.0327$; LPS 65 vs. 680 pg/ml, $p = 0.0057$) (**Figure 4C**). This Th cytokine expression is connected with the impaired production of pro-inflammatory cytokines in co-cultures of CD4$^+$ T cells with moDCs treated with TLRLs and PSMα3 (**Figures S5A–C**).

Thus, PSMα3-treated TLR2- and TLR4- stimulated mDCs decreased the frequency of T-bet$^+$ Th1 cells, as well as IFN-γ secretion.

PSMα3-Treated moDCs Induce T_{reg} Priming Via Direct Cell Interaction and IDO Production

Previously, our group showed that PSMα3 primes mouse tDCs thereby enhancing the frequency and proliferation of T_{regs} (10, 12). Further, as PSMα3 treatment of moDCs attenuated the priming of Th1 cells, we investigated whether PSMα3-treated moDCs also increased T_{reg} priming. Therefore, moDCs were treated with or without Sa lysate or LPS in combination with PSMα3 for 24 h. Next, the cells were co-cultured with naïve CFSE-labeled CD4$^+$ T cells for 3–4 d and analyzed by flow cytometry. Newly primed T_{regs} were characterized as CD4$^+$CD127$^-$CD25^{hi}CD45RA$^-$FoxP3^{hi} induced T_{regs} [iT_{regs}; (26)]. PSMα3 increased the frequency of iT_{regs} upon co-culture with moDCs after TLR2 or TLR4 ligand treatment (Sa day 3 0.17 vs. 0.31%, $p < 0.0033$; Sa day 4 0.43 vs. 0.86%, $p = 0.0054$; LPS day 3 0.08 vs. 0.29%, $p < 0.0001$; LPS day 4 0.75 vs. 1.07%, $p = 0.0204$) (**Figures 5A,B**). Treating CD4$^+$ T cells with PSMα3 in combination with TLRLs without moDCs did not result in CD4$^+$ T cell activation or priming of iT_{regs} (**Figure S6**).

Further, these iT_{regs} showed a greater proliferation potential than the iT_{regs} primed without PSMα3 (**Figure 5C**). To test the functionality of these iT_{regs}, we sorted iT_{regs} (CD4$^+$CD127$^-$CD25^{hi}CD45RA$^-$) after 4 d of co-culture with LPS + PSMα3-treated moDCs (**Figure S7**). Sorted iT_{regs} were again cultured with CFSE-labeled CD4$^+$ T cells (T_{eff}) in the presence of anti-CD3/CD28 coated beads to induce T_{eff} proliferation for 4 d. T_{regs} significantly decreased T_{eff} proliferation analyzed by CFSE-dilution in a concentration-dependent manner (1:1 reduction ~38%, $p = 0.0004$; 1:2 reduction ~25%, $p = 0.0176$; 1:4 reduction ~12%, $p = 0.2603$) (**Figure 5D**), demonstrating that PSMα3-induced iT_{regs} suppress T_{eff} proliferation.

To investigate whether secreted factors from DCs upon PSM-treatment mediate iT_{reg} priming, T cells were co-cultured with iDCs simultaneously adding medium from LPS or LPS with PSMα3-treated moDCs (conditioned medium) (**Figure 6A** condition 2). As described above, PSMα3 increased the frequency of iT_{regs} upon co-culture of naïve CD4$^+$ T cells with moDCs (**Figure 6A** condition 1 and **Figure 6B**). A similar increase of iT_{regs} was mediated by iDCs incubated with conditioned medium from LPS + PSMα3, whereas LPS conditioned medium had no effect (0.31% compared to 0.09%, respectively, $p = 0.0757$) **Figure 6A** condition 2 and **Figure 6B**). These observations show that PSM-induced secretion of soluble factors by mDCs modulate iDCs to prime iT_{regs}.

In another assay DCs were washed 24 h after treatment with LPS or LPS + PSMα3 (mDCs) and further cultured for 3–4 days with CD4$^+$ T cells in fresh medium. These conditions revealed an even higher frequency of iT_{regs} (0.52 or 1.32%, respectively; $p < 0.0001$) compared to mDCs without medium change (**Figure 6A** condition 3 and **Figure 6B**) and suggest that the interaction of mDCs with CD4$^+$ T cells as well as secreted factors produced by mDCs after interaction with T cells are important for iT_{reg} priming.

To further address the impact of direct DC-T-cell interaction on T_{reg} priming, mDCs were fixed and either cultured with naïve CD4$^+$ T cells in fresh or conditioned medium. Fixation of mDCs treated with or without PSMα3 led to low frequencies of iT_{regs} after co-culture with naïve CD4$^+$ T cells in fresh medium (0.08% vs. 0.2%, $p = 0.6038$) (**Figure 6A** condition 4 and **Figure 6B**). Similar results were obtained by the addition of conditioned medium to this co-culture showing that mainly direct interaction of mDCs with naïve CD4$^+$ T cells is essential for iT_{reg} induction. However, in this experimental setting we cannot exclude that soluble factors produced by mDCs after DC-T cell interaction are involved in iT_{reg} priming. To address this issue, culture supernatants of mDCs with naïve CD4$^+$T cells were analyzed over time for soluble factors, which were shown to be responsible for iT_{reg} priming and proliferation, like TGF-β, IL-10, IL-2, CD40L and IDO. Neither, IL-10 (**Figure 6C**), TGF-ß (**Figure 6D**), CD40L nor IL-2 (**Figure S5** were increased in the co-culture of PSMα3-treated mDCs with naïve CD4$^+$ T cells compared to mDCs independently of the TLRL used. Moreover, T helper cell priming cytokines like IL-4, IL-6, IL-12p70, IL17A and IFN-γ were hardly detectable in the co-culture supernatants of LPS + PSMα3 treated mDCs with CD4$^+$ T cells (**Figure 4C** and **Figure S5**) as described above.

In contrast, secretion of the enzyme IDO, which is important for T_{reg} differentiation from naïve T cells (8), was significantly increased by mDCs in response to PSMα3 treatment after 1 (11.000 vs. 1.440 pg/ml, $p < 0.0001$) and 2 days (42.000 vs. 33.800 pg/ml, $p = 0.0006$) compared to mDCs alone (**Figure 6E**).

As previously described, LPS treatment alone also led to IDO secretion by moDCs (27). We addressed the impact of IDO on iT_{reg} priming by mDCs using the specific IDO inhibitor 1-Methyl-D-Tryptophan (1-DMT) prior to treatment of iDCs with LPS or LPS + PSMα3. These mDCs were then co-cultured with $CD4^+$ T cells and the frequency of iT_{regs} determined as described above. Surprisingly, IDO inhibition revealed increased frequencies of iT_{regs} by 2 fold independently whether cells were treated with LPS + PSMα3 or the inhibitor alone (see **Figure S8**). No difference in the proliferation of $CD4^+$ T cells was observed upon IDO inhibition. Moreover, IDO inhibition had hardly any effect on the frequency of Th1, Th2 and Th17 cells in the culture (data not shown). Thus, the increased IDO production by PSM-treated DCs seems not to be essential for iT_{reg} induction.

Together, these data indicate that PSMα3 modulates moDCs to prime predominantly T_{regs} via mechanisms involving mainly direct DC-T cell interaction in combination with DC-secreted yet unknown factors.

PSMα3-Treated moDCs Induce T_{regs} From $CD4^+$ T Cells of Patients With Autoimmune Diseases

In order to address whether PSMα3 can be used for therapeutic approaches by modulating moDCs for iT_{reg} priming in a setting of T cell associated autoimmune diseases, moDCs from healthy donors were co-cultured after treatment with LPS or LPS + PSMα3 with $CD4^+$ T cells from patients with spondyloarthritis (**Figure 7A**) and rheumatoid arthritis (RA) (data not shown). These patients suffer from spondylitis/enthesitis of the spine or peripheral arthritis with pain, morning stiffness and consecutive ankylosing of the spine and/or joint destruction. These diseases display a high frequency of pro-inflammatory Th1 and Th17 cells. As shown for T cells from healthy donors, PSMα3 increased the frequency of iT_{regs} upon co-culture with LPS-treated mDCs by > 10-fold compared to LPS treatment alone ($p = 0.024$), whereas no effects were observed for Th1, Th2, and Th17 priming of T cells from patients with spondylitis (**Figure 7A**). Moreover, similar, but not significant results ($p = 0.0919$) could be observed in an autologous setting using mDCs and $CD4^+$ T cells from patients with spondyloarthritis (**Figure 7B** and **Figure S9**). This shows that PSMα3 indeed modulates moDCs to prime iT_{regs} even in allogenic and autologous disease settings, indicating its potential for DC therapy in chronic inflammatory diseases.

DISCUSSION

There is a need for particular therapeutic approaches preventing or inhibiting immune activation in autoimmune diseases, allograft rejection, allergies, asthma and various forms of hyper-sensitivity. Current therapies, which mainly use nonspecific systemic immunosuppressants, are associated with severe side effects. Thus, *ex vivo* generated tDCs are an attractive alternative to enhance, maintain or restore immunological tolerance.

Here, we addressed the possibility of PSMα3, which is secreted by highly virulent CA-MRSA strains, to induce human tDCs as potential therapeutic for DC vaccination strategies. PSMs form transient pores into the membrane of neutrophils (15), and DCs thereby getting access to the cytosol, in the case of DCs without cell lysis (**Figure 3**) (10). Molecularly, PSMα3 enhanced the activation of the p38-CREB pathway upon TLR ligation, which in consequence diminished pro-inflammatory cytokine production but induced IL-10 secretion by mouse bone marrow-derived DCs (10). Here, we show that PSMα2 enters human moDCs via endocytosis and transient pore formation and is located in the cytosol as well as close to the membrane. Indeed, NF-κB as well as p38 activation are necessary for DC maturation including upregulation of CD80, CD86, and CD40, but also cytokine production (28–30). We believe that PSMα3 prevents TLR-activation either extracellularly and/or intracellularly thereby inducing tDCs. Direct extracellular interaction of PSMα1-3 with TLR4 was shown to prevent binding of HMGB1 to TLR4 and thus downstream activation of NF-κB (31). Similarly, we here show that PSMα3 prevents activation of NF-κB as well as p38 MAPK signaling. Whether PSMα3 also blocks binding of LPS to TLR4 remains to be shown. Moreover, our findings are in agreement with several studies showing that NF-κB inhibition favors an immature or tolerogenic DC phenotype, which stimulates the expansion of Foxp3 expressing regulatory T cells (32–35).

A hallmark of tDCs is their immature phenotype characterized by low surface levels of MHC class II and costimulatory molecules, such as CD86, CD40, CD54, and PD-L2, but increased expression of TLRs, chemokine receptors and PD-L1. *In vivo* studies showed that the tissue or even tumor microenvironment is important for regulating the development and function of tDCs (36). Although PSMα3 had little influence on TLR-induced up-regulation of HLA-DR, CD83, CD86, and PD-L2, up-regulation of costimulatory molecules CD80, PD-L1, and CD40 was inhibited, preventing full DC-maturation. Likewise, cholera toxin in combination with LPS induced CD80 and CD86 but reduced CD40 and CD54 expression by DCs (37). Mechanistically, the inhibition of TNFα production, which among others regulates CD40 expression, upon synergistic treatment with TLRLs and PSMα3 could explain the impaired up-regulation of CD40 (38). This fits to the fact that the lack of CD40 expression on DCs was shown to be important for the generation of T_{regs} while suppressing primary immune responses (39). Moreover, some studies have shown that phenotypically mature DCs are also able to promote T_{regs} and act superior in activating their suppressor function (40, 41).

In addition, PSMα3 dramatically changed the cytokine secretion pattern of moDCs upon TLRL treatment by preventing the secretion of the pro-inflammatory cytokines TNF, IL-12, but also of anti-inflammatory IL-10, which is produced by DCs in response to TLR-stimulation. This is in contrast to the data observed by mouse bone-marrow derived DC, where IL-10 secretion is even increased upon PSM and TLRL treatment compared to TLRL treatment alone (12). However, PSM-treated moDCs still impair Th1 but promote T_{reg} priming. Tolerogenic DCs are defined by their capacity to induce T_{regs} via production of anti-inflammatory molecules that may be secreted, membrane bound, or both. A variety of studies demonstrated the necessity of IL-10 secretion by tDCs for T_{reg} induction (42–45) and for the maintenance of suppressive T_{regs} upon strong inflammatory

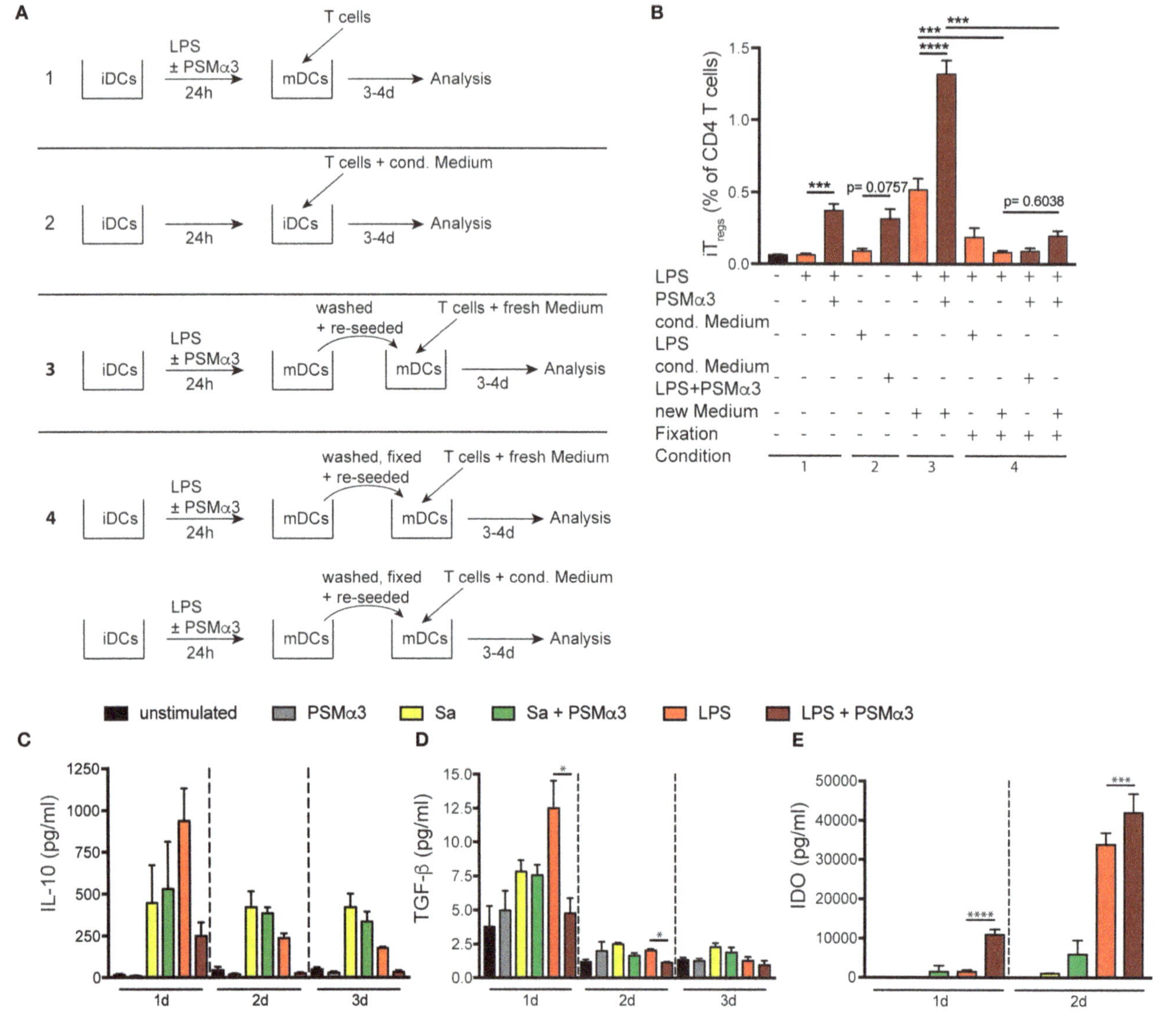

FIGURE 6 | PSMα3-treated moDCs increase the proliferation and frequency of iT$_{regs}$ by direct interaction and IDO production. **(A)** Schematic overview of the experimental setting: T cells were co-cultured for 3–4 d (1) with mDCs (LPS or LPS + PSMα3 for 24 h), with (2) untreated moDCs (iDCs) in the presence of conditioned medium from LPS or LPS + PSMα3 treated DCs, with (3) washed and re-seeded mDCs together with new medium or (4) with fixed moDCs together with either new medium or conditioned medium. **(B)** The bar graphs show the frequency of iT$_{regs}$ from CD4$^+$ T cells analyzed by flow cytometry from the experiments described in **(A)** (one representative of $n \geq 3$ independent experiments performed in triplicates). **(C,D)** Cell culture supernatants from the DC T cell co-culture ($n \geq 3$ performed in triplicates; mean ± SEM) were analyzed for IL-10 **(C)** and TGF-β production **(D)** after 1 d, 2 d or 3 d by a bead-based immunoassay. **(E)** Cell culture supernatants ($n = 2$ performed in triplicates; mean ± SEM) from moDCs treated with Sa lysate or LPS with or without PSMα3 were analyzed for IDO production by sandwich ELISA. $^*p < 0.05$, $^{***}p < 0.001$ or $^{****}p < 0.0001$, one-way ANOVA with Turkey's posttest or Kruskal-Wallis with Dunn's posttest.

signals (12, 44, 46, 47). The data described herein raise the question whether IL-10 secretion is a hallmark of tDCs.

As T-cell differentiation is mainly controlled by cytokines mediating polarizing signals (48) we addressed other factors as mediators for T$_{reg}$ induction. IDO, an immune-regulatory enzyme, which is mainly expressed in DCs, was shown to modulate adaptive immune responses by promoting immune-suppression and tolerance (49–51). IDO expression in DCs is induced either by IFN-γ or by TLR activation via the non-canonical NF- κB pathway. IDO acts through tryptophan (TRP) depletion and production of TRP metabolites thereby inducing differentiation of new T$_{regs}$ from naïve T cells (27, 51–55). PSM treatment of moDCs resulted in an even enhanced IDO expression as compared to Sa lysate or LPS treatment alone. The latter was recently shown to induce IDO together with the transcription factor aryl-hydrocarbon receptor (AhR) (27). However, our results obtained with IDO inhibition by 1-DMT argue against a mechanistically role of IDO in PSM-mediated T$_{reg}$ induction. Thus, it is tempting to speculate that PSMα3 modulated moDCs prime T$_{regs}$ via mechanisms involving

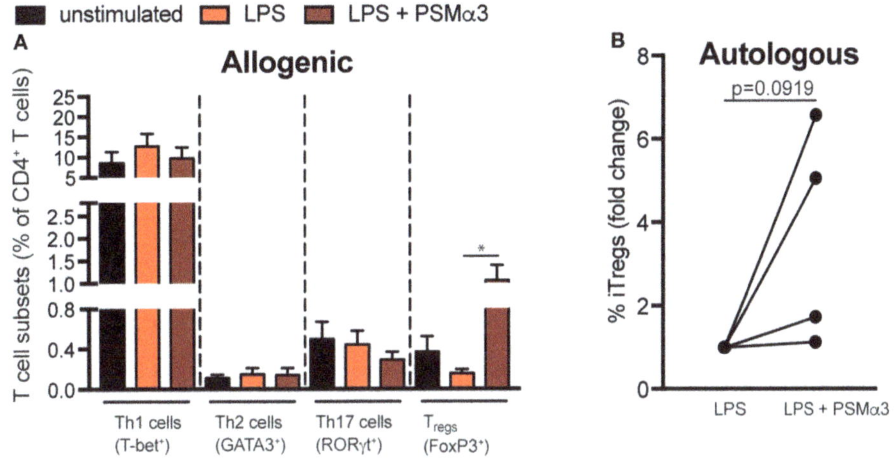

FIGURE 7 | PSMα3-treated moDCs induce T_{regs} from $CD4^+$ T cells of patients with autoimmune diseases. **(A)** Allogenic T-cell assay: MoDCs from healthy donors were treated for 24 h with LPS with or without PSMα3 and co-cultured with CFSE-labeled $CD4^+$ T cells from patients with Th17-associated spondyloarthritis for 3 d or 4 d. The different T cell subsets were analyzed by flow cytometry. The graph shows the frequency of the T-bet$^+$ Th1, GATA3$^+$ Th2, RORγt$^+$ Th17 cells and $CD127^-CD25^{hi}CD45RA^-Foxp3^{hi}$ iT_{regs} from $CD4^+$ T cells ($n = 6$ patients; mean ± SEM). $^*p < 0.05$, one-way ANOVA with Turkey's posttest or Kruskal-Wallis with Dunn's posttest. **(B)** Autologous T-cell assay: MoDCs from spondyloarthritis patients were treated as described in **(A)** and co-cultured with CFSE-labeled $CD4^+$ T cells from the same patient. $CD127^-CD25^{hi}CD45RA^-Foxp3^{hi}$ iT_{regs} were analyzed by flow cytometry. The graph shows the frequency of iT_{regs} as fold change from LPS-treated cells of 4 different spondyloarthritis patients. Data were analyzed by unpaired student's *T*-test.

predominantly direct DC-T cell interaction in combination with the absence of Th-priming cytokines and probably yet unknown DC-secreted factors.

The data from this study are a proof of concept of the potential use of Sa-derived PSMα3 to induce tolerogenic human DCs with the ability to prime iT_{regs}. Especially, when using PSMα3-induced tDCs to prime iT_{regs} in allogenic and autologous settings of $CD4^+$ T cells from spondylitis patients. It is believed that tolerogenic DCs may induce tolerance to the pathologic immune responses in a patient without affecting the immune defense against pathogens or tumors. There are two strategies to restore tolerance in autoimmunity: improve the induction and function of tolerogenic DC or generating tolerogenic DC *in vitro* for subsequent administration *in vivo* as cell therapy (13, 56, 57). Different immune-modulatory agents such as dexamethasone, vitamin D3, TNF or IL-10, but also pathogen-derived products have been used in order to modify the phenotype, cytokine profiles and activity of DCs (58–65). Pre-clinical models of arthritis (65), EAE (66), and type 1 diabetes [T1D; (67)] have demonstrated the efficacy of *in vitro* induced tolerogenic DC-based cell therapy.

There is a need for the complete understanding of the mechanisms that control tolerance and immunity in the context of the complexity and heterogeneity of autoimmune diseases, in which multiple cell types are affected and various genetic backgrounds are involved.

AUTHOR CONTRIBUTIONS

SA, JR, and NA contributed to the conception and design of the study. JR and MG performed the experiments and statistical analysis. SA and JR wrote the first draft of the manuscript. SA, JR, NA, MG, and JH wrote sections of the manuscript. All authors read and approved the submitted version of the manuscript.

ACKNOWLEDGMENTS

We thank Johannes Morschl for technical assistance and Peter Richardson for critical reading of the manuscript. Cell sorting and flow cytometry sample acquisition was done on shared instruments of the Flow Cytometry Core Facility Tübingen. Imaging flow cytometry sample acquisition, and data analysis was done on shared instruments of the Imaging Flow Cytometry Core Facility Tübingen. The Imaging Flow Cytometry Core Facility was supported by a grant from the Ministry of Science, Research and Arts of Baden Württemberg (Az.: SI-BW 01222-91) and the Deutsche Forschungsgemeinschaft DFG (German Research Foundation) (Az.: INST 2388/33-1).

REFERENCES

1. Merad M, Sathe P, Helft J, Miller J, Mortha A. The dendritic cell lineage: ontogeny and function of dendritic cells and their subsets in the steady state and the inflamed setting. *Annu Rev Immunol.* (2013) 31:563–604. doi: 10.1146/annurev-immunol-020711-074950
2. Villadangos JA, Schnorrer P. Intrinsic and cooperative antigen-presenting functions of dendritic-cell subsets *in vivo*. *Nat Rev Immunol.* (2007) 7:543–55. doi: 10.1038/nri2103
3. Banchereau J, Steinman RM. Dendritic cells and the control of immunity. *Nature* (1998) 392:245–52. doi: 10.1038/32588
4. Banchereau J, Briere F, Caux C, Davoust J, Lebecque S, Liu Y-J, et al. Immunobiology of dendritic cells. *Annu Rev Immunol.* (2000) 18:767–811. doi: 10.1146/annurev.immunol.18.1.767
5. Coquet JM, Rausch L, Borst J. The importance of co-stimulation in the orchestration of T helper cell differentiation. *Immunol Cell Biol.* (2015) 93:780–8. doi: 10.1038/icb.2015.45
6. Gordon JR, Ma Y, Churchman L, Gordon SA, Dawicki W. Regulatory dendritic cells for immunotherapy in immunologic diseases. *Front Immunol.* (2014) 5:7. doi: 10.3389/fimmu.2014.00007
7. Kushwah R, Hu J. Role of dendritic cells in the induction of regulatory T cells. *Cell Biosci.* (2011) 1:20. doi: 10.1186/2045-3701-1-20
8. Raker VK, Domogalla MP, Steinbrink K. Tolerogenic dendritic cells for regulatory T cell induction in man. *Front Immunol.* (2015) 6:569. doi: 10.3389/fimmu.2015.00569
9. Yoo S, Ha S-J. Generation of tolerogenic dendritic cells and their therapeutic applications. *Immune Netw.* (2016) 16:52–9. doi: 10.4110/in.2016.16.1.52
10. Armbruster NS, Richardson JR, Schreiner J, Klenk J, Günter M, Kretschmer D, et al. PSM peptides of *Staphylococcus aureus* activate the p38-CREB pathway in dendritic cells, thereby modulating cytokine production and T cell priming. *J Immunol.* (2016) 196:1284–92. doi: 10.4049/jimmunol.1502232
11. Ouyang W, Rutz S, Crellin NK, Valdez PA, Hymowitz SG. Regulation and functions of the IL-10 family of cytokines in inflammation and disease. *Annu Rev Immunol.* (2011) 29:71–109 doi: 10.1146/annurev-immunol-031210-101312
12. Schreiner J, Kretschmer D, Klenk J, Otto M, Bühring H-J, Stevanovic S, et al. *Staphylococcus aureus* phenol-soluble modulin peptides modulate dendritic cell functions and increase *in vitro* priming of regulatory T cells. *J Immunol.* (2013) 190:3417–26. doi: 10.4049/jimmunol.1202563
13. Maldonado RA, Andrian von UH. How tolerogenic dendritic cells induce regulatory T cells. *Adv Immunol.* (2010) 108:111–65. doi: 10.1016/B978-0-12-380995-7.00004-5
14. Otto M. Phenol-soluble modulins. *Int J Med Microbiol.* (2014) 304:164–9. doi: 10.1016/j.ijmm.2013.11.019
15. Wang R, Braughton KR, Kretschmer D, Bach T-HL, Queck SY, Li M, et al. Identification of novel cytolytic peptides as key virulence determinants for community-associated MRSA. *Nat Med.* (2007) 13:1510–4. doi: 10.1038/nm1656
16. Peschel A, Otto M. Phenol-soluble modulins and staphylococcal infection. *Nat Rev Microbiol.* (2013) 11:667–73. doi: 10.1038/nrmicro3110
17. Cheung GYC, Kretschmer D, Duong AC, Yeh AJ, Ho TV, Chen Y, et al. Production of an attenuated phenol-soluble modulin variant unique to the MRSA clonal complex 30 increases severity of bloodstream infection. *PLoS Pathog.* (2014) 10:e1004298. doi: 10.1371/journal.ppat.1004298.s002
18. Armbruster NS, Richardson JR, Schreiner J, Klenk J, Günter M, Autenrieth SE. *Staphylococcus aureus* PSM peptides induce tolerogenic dendritic cells upon treatment with ligands of extracellular and intracellular TLRs. *Int J Med Microbiol.* (2016) 306:666–74. doi: 10.1016/j.ijmm.2016.09.002
19. Autenrieth SE, Soldanova I, Rösemann R, Gunst D, Zahir N, Kracht M, et al. Yersinia enterocolitica YopP inhibits MAP kinase-mediated antigen uptake in dendritic cells. *Cell Microbiol.* (2007) 9:425–37. doi: 10.1111/j.1462-5822.2006.00800.x
20. Burgdorf S, Kautz A, Böhnert V, Knolle PA, Kurts C. Distinct pathways of antigen uptake and intracellular routing in CD4 and CD8 T cell activation. *Science* (2007) 316:612–6. doi: 10.1126/science.1137971
21. Platt CD, Ma JK, Chalouni C, Ebersold M, Bou-Reslan H, Carano RAD, et al. Mature dendritic cells use endocytic receptors to capture and present antigens. *Proc Natl Acad Sci USA.* (2010) 107:4287–92. doi: 10.1073/pnas.0910609107
22. West MA, Wallin RPA, Matthews SP, Svensson HG, Zaru R, Ljunggren H-G, et al. Enhanced dendritic cell antigen capture via toll-like receptor-induced actin remodeling. *Science* (2004) 305:1153–7. doi: 10.1126/science.1099153
23. Pokorny A, Yandek LE, Elegbede AI, Hinderliter A, Almeida PFF. Temperature and composition dependence of the interaction of δ-lysin with ternary mixtures of sphingomyelin/cholesterol/POPC. *Biophys J.* (2006) 91:2184–97. doi: 10.1529/biophysj.106.085027
24. Li P, Spolski R, Liao W, Leonard WJ. Complex interactions of transcription factors in mediating cytokine biology in T cells. *Immunol Rev.* (2014) 261:141–56. doi: 10.1111/imr.12199
25. Zou W, Restifo NP. TH17 cells in tumour immunity and immunotherapy. *Nat Rev Immunol.* (2010) 10:248–56. doi: 10.1038/nri2742
26. Santegoets SJAM, Dijkgraaf EM, Battaglia A, Beckhove P, Britten CM, Gallimore A, et al. Monitoring regulatory T cells in clinical samples: consensus on an essential marker set and gating strategy for regulatory T cell analysis by flow cytometry. *Cancer Immunol Immunother.* (2015) 64:1271–86. doi: 10.1007/s00262-015-1729-x
27. Salazar F, Awuah D, Negm OH, Shakib F, Ghaemmaghami AM. The role of indoleamine 2,3-dioxygenase-aryl hydrocarbon receptor pathway in the TLR4-induced tolerogenic phenotype in human DCs. *Sci Rep.* (2017) 7:43337. doi: 10.1038/srep43337
28. Ardeshna KM, Pizzey AR, Devereux S, Khwaja A. The PI3 kinase, p38 SAP kinase, and NF-kappaB signal transduction pathways are involved in the survival and maturation of lipopolysaccharide-stimulated human monocyte-derived dendritic cells. *Blood* (2000) 96:1039–46.
29. Dalod M, Chelbi R, Malissen B, Lawrence T. Dendritic cell maturation: functional specialization through signaling specificity and transcriptional programming. *EMBO J.* (2014) 33:1104–16. doi: 10.1002/embj.201488027
30. Kaisho T, Akira S. Dendritic-cell function in toll-like receptor- and MyD88- knockout mice. *Trends Immunol.* (2001) 22:78–83. doi: 10.1016/S1471-4906(00)01811-1
31. Chu M, Zhou M, Jiang C, Chen X, Guo L, Zhang M, et al. *Staphylococcus aureus* phenol-soluble modulins $\alpha 1$–$\alpha 3$ act as novel toll-like receptor (TLR) 4 antagonists to inhibit HMGB1/TLR4/NF-κB signaling pathway. *Front Immunol.* (2018) 9:862. doi: 10.3389/fimmu.2018.00862
32. Iruretagoyena MI. Inhibition of nuclear factor- B enhances the capacity of immature dendritic cells to induce antigen-specific tolerance in experimental autoimmune encephalomyelitis. *J Pharmacol Exp Therapeut.* (2006) 318:59–67. doi: 10.1124/jpet.106.103259
33. Li M, Zhang X, Zheng X, Lian D, Zhang ZX, Ge W, et al. Immune modulation and tolerance induction by RelB-silenced dendritic cells through RNA interference. *J Immunol.* (2007) 178:5480–7. doi: 10.4049/jimmunol.178.9.5480
34. Martin E, Capini C, Duggan E, Lutzky VP, Stumbles P, Pettit AR, et al. Antigen-specific suppression of established arthritis in mice by dendritic cells deficient in NF-kappaB. *Arthritis Rheum.* (2007) 56:2255–66. doi: 10.1002/art.22655
35. Thompson AG, O'Sullivan BJ, Beamish H, Thomas R. T cells signaled by NF-kappa B- dendritic cells are sensitized not anergic to subsequent activation. *J Immunol.* (2004) 173:1671–80. doi: 10.4049/jimmunol.173.3.1671
36. Li H, Shi B. Tolerogenic dendritic cells and their applications in transplantation. *Cell Mol Immunol.* (2015) 12:24–30. doi: 10.1038/cmi.2014.52
37. Lavelle EC, McNeela E, Armstrong ME, Leavy O, Higgins SC, Mills KHG. Cholera toxin promotes the induction of regulatory T cells specific for bystander antigens by modulating dendritic cell activation. *J Immunol.* (2003) 171:2384–92. doi: 10.4049/jimmunol.171.5.2384
38. Danese S, Sans M, Scaldaferri F, Sgambato A, Rutella S, Cittadini A, et al. TNF- blockade down-regulates the CD40/CD40L pathway in the mucosal microcirculation: a novel anti-inflammatory mechanism of infliximab in Crohn's disease. *J Immunol.* (2006) 176:2617–24. doi: 10.4049/jimmunol.176.4.2617
39. Quezada SA, Jarvinen LZ, Lind EF, Noelle RJ. CD40/CD154 interactions at the interface of tolerance and immunity. *Annu Rev Immunol.* (2004) 22:307–28. doi: 10.1146/annurev.immunol.22.012703.104533
40. Pletinckx K, Döhler A, Pavlovic V, Lutz MB. Role of dendritic cell maturity/costimulation for generation, homeostasis, and suppressive activity of regulatory T cells. *Front Immun.* (2011) 2:39. doi: 10.3389/fimmu.2011.00039

41. Spörri R, Reis e Sousa C. Inflammatory mediators are insufficient for full dendritic cell activation and promote expansion of $CD4^+$ T cell populations lacking helper function. *Nat Immunol.* (2005) 6:163–70. doi: 10.1038/ni1162
42. Akbari O, DeKruyff RH, Umetsu DT. Pulmonary dendritic cells producing IL-10 mediate tolerance induced by respiratory exposure to antigen. *Nat Immunol.* (2001) 2:725–31. doi: 10.1038/90667
43. McGuirk P, McCann C, Mills KHG. Pathogen-specific T regulatory 1 cells induced in the respiratory tract by a bacterial molecule that stimulates interleukin 10 production by dendritic cells: a novel strategy for evasion of protective T helper type 1 responses by *Bordetella pertussis. J Exp Med.* (2002) 195:221–31. doi: 10.1084/jem.20011288
44. Murai M, Turovskaya O, Kim G, Madan R, Karp CL, Cheroutre H, et al. Interleukin 10 acts on regulatory T cells to maintain expression of the transcription factor Foxp3 and suppressive function in mice with colitis. *Nat Immunol.* (2009) 10:1178–84. doi: 10.1038/ni.1791
45. Wakkach A, Fournier N, Brun V, Breittmayer J-P, Cottrez F, Groux H. Characterization of dendritic cells that induce tolerance and T regulatory 1 cell differentiation *in vivo. Immunity* (2003) 18:605–17. doi: 10.1016/S1074-7613(03)00113-4
46. Bonifazi P, Zelante T, D'Angelo C, De Luca A, Moretti S, Bozza S, et al. Balancing inflammation and tolerance *in vivo* through dendritic cells by the commensal *Candida albicans. Mucosal Immunol.* (2009) 2:362–74. doi: 10.1038/mi.2009.17
47. Falcón C, Carranza F, Martínez FF, Knubel CP, Masih DT, Motrán CC, et al. Excretory-secretory products (ESP) from Fasciola hepatica induce tolerogenic properties in myeloid dendritic cells. *Vet Immunol Immunopathol.* (2010) 137:36–46. doi: 10.1016/j.vetimm.2010.04.007
48. Campbell DJ, Koch MA. Phenotypical and functional specialization of $FOXP3^+$ regulatory T cells. *Nat Rev Immunol.* (2011) 11:119–30. doi: 10.1038/nri2916
49. Bubnoff Von D, Scheler M, Wilms H, Fimmers R, Bieber T. Identification of IDO-positive and IDO-negative human dendritic cells after activation by various proinflammatory stimuli. *J Immunol.* (2011) 186:6701–9. doi: 10.4049/jimmunol.1003151
50. Harden JL, Egilmez NK. Indoleamine 2,3-dioxygenase and dendritic cell tolerogenicity. *Immunol Invest.* (2012) 41:738–64. doi: 10.3109/08820139.2012.676122
51. Munn DH, Mellor AL. Indoleamine 2,3 dioxygenase and metabolic control of immune responses. *Trends Immunol.* (2013) 34:137–43. doi: 10.1016/j.it.2012.10.001
52. Baban B, Chandler PR, Sharma MD, Pihkala J, Koni PA, Munn DH, et al. IDO activates regulatory T cells and blocks their conversion into Th17-like T cells. *J Immunol.* (2009) 183:2475–83. doi: 10.4049/jimmunol.0900986
53. Chen W, Liang X, Peterson AJ, Munn DH, Blazar BR. The indoleamine 2,3-dioxygenase pathway is essential for human plasmacytoid dendritic cell-induced adaptive T regulatory cell generation. *J Immunol.* (2008) 181:5396–404. doi: 10.4049/jimmunol.181.8.5396
54. Hwu P, Du MX, Lapointe R, Do M, Taylor MW, Young HA. Indoleamine 2,3-dioxygenase production by human dendritic cells results in the inhibition of T cell proliferation. *J Immunol.* (2000) 164:3596–9. doi: 10.4049/jimmunol.164.7.3596
55. Salazar F, Hall L, Negm OH, Awuah D, Tighe PJ, Shakib F, et al. The mannose receptor negatively modulates the toll-like receptor 4-aryl hydrocarbon receptor-indoleamine 2,3-dioxygenase axis in dendritic cells affecting T helper cell polarization. *J Allergy Clin Immunol.* (2016) 137:1841–51.e2. doi: 10.1016/j.jaci.2015.10.033
56. Amodio G, Gregori S. Dendritic cells a double-edge sword in autoimmune responses. *Front Immunol.* (2012) 3:233. doi: 10.3389/fimmu.2012.00233
57. Lutz MB. Therapeutic potential of semi-mature dendritic cells for tolerance induction. *Front Immunol.* (2012) 3:123. doi: 10.3389/fimmu.2012.00123
58. Gregori S, Tomasoni D, Pacciani V, Scirpoli M, Battaglia M, Magnani CF, et al. Differentiation of type 1 T regulatory cells (Tr1) by tolerogenic DC-10 requires the IL-10-dependent ILT4/HLA-G pathway. *Blood* (2010) 116:935–44. doi: 10.1182/blood-2009-07-234872
59. Penna G, Adorini L. 1 Alpha,25-dihydroxyvitamin D3 inhibits differentiation, maturation, activation, and survival of dendritic cells leading to impaired alloreactive T cell activation. *J Immunol.* (2000) 164:2405–11. doi: 10.4049/jimmunol.164.5.2405
60. Piemonti L, Monti P, Allavena P, Sironi M, Soldini L, Leone BE, et al. Glucocorticoids affect human dendritic cell differentiation and maturation. *J Immunol.* (1999) 162:6473–81.
61. Sato M, Takayama T, Tanaka H, Konishi J, Suzuki T, Kaiga T, et al. Generation of mature dendritic cells fully capable of T helper type 1 polarization using OK-432 combined with prostaglandin E(2). *Cancer Sci.* (2003) 94:1091–8. doi: 10.1111/j.1349-7006.2003.tb01405.x
62. Steinbrink K, Graulich E, Kubsch S, Knop J, Enk AH. $CD4^+$ and $CD8^+$ anergic T cells induced by interleukin-10-treated human dendritic cells display antigen-specific suppressor activity. *Blood* (2002) 99:2468–76. doi: 10.1182/blood.V99.7.2468
63. Steinbrink K, Wölfl M, Jonuleit H, Knop J, Enk AH. Induction of tolerance by IL-10-treated dendritic cells. *J Immunol.* (1997) 159:4772–80.
64. Van Brussel I, Lee WP, Rombouts M, Nuyts AH, Heylen M, De Winter BY, et al. Tolerogenic dendritic cell vaccines to treat autoimmune diseases: can the unattainable dream turn into reality? *Autoimmun Rev.* (2014) 13:138–50. doi: 10.1016/j.autrev.2013.09.008
65. van Duivenvoorde LM, Han WGH, Bakker AM, Louis-Plence P, Charbonnier L-M, Apparailly F, et al. Immunomodulatory dendritic cells inhibit Th1 responses and arthritis via different mechanisms. *J Immunol.* (2007) 179:1506–15. doi: 10.4049/jimmunol.179.3.1506
66. Menges M, Rößner S, Voigtländer C, Schindler H, Kukutsch NA, Bogdan C, et al. Repetitive injections of dendritic cells matured with tumor necrosis factor alpha induce antigen-specific protection of mice from autoimmunity. *J Exp Med.* (2002) 195:15–21. doi: 10.1084/jem.20011341
67. Feili-Hariri M, Falkner DH, Morel PA. Regulatory Th2 response induced following adoptive transfer of dendritic cells in prediabetic NOD mice. *Eur J Immunol.* (2002) 32:2021–30. doi: 10.1002/1521-4141(200207)32:7<2021::AID-IMMU2021>3.0.CO;2-J

11

Intestinal CD103$^+$CD11b$^+$ cDC2 Conventional Dendritic Cells are Required for Primary CD4$^+$ T and B Cell Responses to Soluble Flagellin

Adriana Flores-Langarica[1], Charlotte Cook[2], Katarzyna Müller Luda[3], Emma K. Persson[4], Jennifer L. Marshall[5], Nonantzin Beristain-Covarrubias[1], Juan Carlos Yam-Puc[1], Madelene Dahlgren[3], Jenny J. Persson[3], Satoshi Uematsu[6,7], Shizuo Akira[8], Ian R. Henderson[2], Bengt Johansson Lindbom[3,9], William Agace[3,9] and Adam F. Cunningham[1]*

[1] Institute of Immunology and Immunotherapy, College of Medical and Dental Sciences, University of Birmingham, Birmingham, United Kingdom, [2] Institute of Microbiology and Infection, College of Medical and Dental Sciences, University of Birmingham, Birmingham, United Kingdom, [3] Immunology Section, Department of Experimental Medical Science, Lund University, Lund, Sweden, [4] VIB-Ugent Center for Inflammation Research, Ghent, Belgium, [5] Institute of Inflammation and Ageing, College of Medical and Dental Sciences, University of Birmingham, Birmingham, United Kingdom, [6] International Research and Development Centre for Mucosal Vaccine, Institute for Medical Science, The University of Tokyo, Tokyo, Japan, [7] Department of Immunology and Genomics, Osaka City University Graduate School of Medicine, Osaka, Japan, [8] World Premier International Immunology Frontier Research Centre, Osaka University, Suita, Japan, [9] Section of Biology and Chemistry, Department for Micro- and Nanotechnology, Technical University of Denmark, Kongens Lyngby, Denmark

Correspondence:
Adriana Flores-Langarica
a.floreslangarica@bham.ac.uk

Systemic immunization with soluble flagellin (sFliC) from *Salmonella* Typhimurium induces mucosal responses, offering potential as an adjuvant platform for vaccines. Moreover, this engagement of mucosal immunity is necessary for optimal systemic immunity, demonstrating an interaction between these two semi-autonomous immune systems. Although TLR5 and CD103$^+$CD11b$^+$ cDC2 contribute to this process, the relationship between these is unclear in the early activation of CD4$^+$ T cells and the development of antigen-specific B cell responses. In this work, we use TLR5-deficient mice and *CD11c-cre.Irf4*$^{fl/fl}$ mice (which have reduced numbers of cDC2, particularly intestinal CD103$^+$CD11b$^+$ cDCs), to address these points by studying the responses concurrently in the spleen and the mesenteric lymph nodes (MLN). We show that CD103$^+$CD11b$^+$ cDC2 respond rapidly and accumulate in the MLN after immunization with sFliC in a TLR5-dependent manner. Furthermore, we identify that whilst CD103$^+$CD11b$^+$ cDC2 are essential for the induction of primary T and B cell responses in the mucosa, they do not play such a central role for the induction of these responses in the spleen. Additionally, we show the involvement of CD103$^+$CD11b$^+$ cDC2 in the induction of Th2-associated responses. *CD11c-cre.Irf4*$^{fl/fl}$ mice showed a reduced primary FliC-specific Th2-associated IgG1 responses, but enhanced Th1-associated IgG2c responses. These data expand our current understanding of the mucosal immune responses promoted by sFliC and highlights the potential of this adjuvant for vaccine usage by taking advantage of the functionality of mucosal CD103$^+$CD11b$^+$ cDC2.

Keywords: flagellin, mucosa, immune response, dendritic cells, cDC2

INTRODUCTION

The systemic and mucosal immune systems are semi-autonomous and engaging systemic immunity does not necessarily induce immunity in mucosal sites. Engaging the two immune systems concurrently could potentially enhance the benefits of vaccination, as most vaccines are administered through subcutaneous (s.c.) or intra-muscular injection. One antigen that can induce both mucosal and systemic immunity concurrently after intraperitoneal (i.p.) or s.c. immunization is purified, soluble flagellin (sFliC) from *Salmonella* Typhimurium (1–3). This 51 kDa bacterial motility protein is the only known ligand for TLR5 (4). Moreover, flagellin is an immunodominant antigen that can induce robust innate and adaptive immune responses, which can also be protective (5–7). These properties, alongside its potential as an adjuvant, mean flagellin is the focus of multiple vaccine strategies in livestock and in humans (8–12). The antigenic environment in which flagellin is encountered influences the type of immune response induced to this protein. When surface-localized on the bacterium, the antigen-specific response is Th1-reflecting, whereas to purified flagellin the response is significantly more Th2-like, including the induction of FliC-specific IgG1 (13, 14).

Conventional dendritic cells (cDC) are key initiators and modulators of adaptive immune responses and as such targeting cDC directly is an approach to enhance responses to vaccines (15, 16). cDCs can be classified into two major subsets; cDC1 that are require the transcription factors IRF8, BATF3, and ID2, and cDC2 that development is independent of these transcription factors, importantly some them require the transcription factor IRF4 for their survival and function. This classification is particularly important since it allows the identification of cDCs equivalents across tissues and even across species (17, 18). In the intestinal mucosa several sub populations of cDC can be found, $CD103^{+}CD11b^{-}$, $CD103^{+}CD11b^{+}$, and $CD103^{-}CD11b^{+}$ cDC. The first corresponds to cDC1 and the latter two to cDC2. Each of these subsets plays key, non-redundant roles in controlling immune homeostasis in the intestinal mucosa (19–21).

In vivo studies have shown that by 24 h after i.p. or s.c. immunization with sFliC, T cell priming is established in multiple sites concurrently, including the mesenteric lymph node (MLN), spleen and peripheral lymph nodes (1). Analysis of cDCs shows that exclusively in the MLN, there is a rapid TLR5-dependent accumulation of $CD103^{+}$ cDC post sFliC-immunization (1). Moreover, using *Cd11c-cre.Irf4*$^{fl/fl}$ mice, which have diminished numbers of $CD103^{+}CD11b^{+}$ cDCs in the small intestine lamina propria and a 90% reduction of this population in the MLN, we showed that this subset was essential for the induction of adaptive immune responses in the MLN, while splenic cDC2 play only a partial role. For clarity, $CD103^{+}CD11b^{+}$ cDCs will be referred to throughout as $CD103^{+}$cDC2 (3). This indicates that i.p., immunization with sFliC can bridge both systemic and mucosal immune systems through the targeting of a single mucosal cDC subset.

Our previous work examining the role of $CD103^{+}$cDC2 in regulating the response to sFliC focused on the long-term antibody response *in vivo* using the *Cd11c-cre.Irf4*$^{fl/fl}$ mice. This necessitated the use of a prime-boost system and did not focus on the primary T and B cell responses. Whilst all elements of the response were lost in the MLN when mucosal $CD103^{+}$cDC2 were reduced, some features of the anti-FliC response were retained in the spleen. This could be because some T and B cell responses were generated in the MLN shortly after immunization, which could lead to the generation of memory T and B cell responses that contribute to the responses observed after secondary immunization. Alternatively, it could be that cDC2 and cDC1 contributed differentially to the anti-sFliC response in the MLN and spleen. Therefore, we examine here the development of the anti-sFliC response in the first days after immunization to characterize the relationship between cDC2 and TLR5 and the early induction of IgG switching.

MATERIAL AND METHODS

Mice

Cd11c-cre.Irf4$^{fl/f}$ (19) and $NAIP5^{-/-}$ mice were maintained at the Biomedical Center at Lund University. Specific pathogen-free 8 week C57BL/6 mice were purchased from Harlan Sprague-Dawley. $TLR5^{-/-}$ mice were maintained in-house at the Biomedical Service Unit at the University of Birmingham. Littermates or age matched mice were used for all experiments. All animal procedures were carried out in strict accordance with the Lund/Malmö Animal Ethics Committee, the University of Birmingham Ethics Committee and were covered under the UK Home Office Project license 30/2850.

Antigen Preparation and Immunization

sFliC was generated as described (22), a his-tagged recombinant protein and purified by nickel affinity chromatography and immunoprecipitation with a FliC-specific monoclonal. Mice were immunized i.p. with 20 μg recombinant sFliC for 24 h or 7 days as indicated.

Cell Isolation and Flow Cytometry

Single cell suspensions from spleens and MLNs were generated by mechanical disruption. When evaluating cDCs, enzymatic digestion was performed using collagenase VIII digestion (400 U/ml; 25 min; 37°C). Cells were processed for flow cytometry using previously described procedures (1). Data acquisition was performed on a LSRII (BD Bioscience) or a CyAn ADP (Beckman Coulter) and analyzed using FlowJo software 9.8.2. (Tree Star). The following FITC-conjugated antibodies were used, CD3 (145-2C11), B220 (RA3-6B2), and NK1,1 (PK136; all from eBioscience). The following PE-conjugated antibodies were used; CD103 (M290) and CD62L (MEL-14; both from eBioscience). CD11c (N418), CD44 (IM7), and CD95 (MFL3; all from eBioscience) were PE-Cy7-conjugated. CD11b (M1/70), CD4 (RM4-5, both BD Biosciences), TCRβ (H57-597, Biolegend), GL7 (eBioscience) were PB-conjugated. MHC-II (M5/114.15.2) and

Abbreviations: Ab, antibody; cDCs, conventional dendritic cells; GC, germinal center; i. p., intraperitoneal; MLN, mesenteric lymph node; s.c., subcutaneous; sFliC, soluble flagellin.

Streptavidin (eBioscience) APC-conjugated where used. B220 (RA3-6B2), CD11b (MI-70), CD11c (N418) and NK1.1 (PK136; all from eBioscience) were Alexa700-conjugated. TCRβ (H57-597, Biolegend) was APC Cy7-conjugated. CD8α (5H10) from Invitrogen was used PO-conjugated.

cDCs were gated as Lin^-[CD3,B220,NK1.1,GR1]$CD11c^+MHC^{hi}$ cells, splenic cDC1 were defined as $CD8\alpha^+$ and cDC2 as $CD11b^+CD4^+$ cells, mucosal cDC1 were defined as $CD103^+CD11b^-$ and cDC2 as $CD103^+CD11b^+$ cells. Activated $CD4^+$ T cells were gated as $CD3^+CD4^+CD44^+CD62L^-$. Germinal center (GC) B cells were defined as $TCR\beta^-CD19^+GL7^+CD95^+$ cells.

Immunohistochemistry and Confocal Microscopy

Immunohistochemistry was performed as described previously (13). Cryosections (6 μm) were incubated with primary unlabelled Abs for 45 min at RT before addition of either HRP-conjugated or biotin-conjugated secondary antibodies. FliC-binding cells were identified as described (1) using soluble biotinylated FliC. Subsequently streptavidin ABComplex alkaline phosphatase (Dako) was used. Signal was detected using diaminobenzidine for HRP activity and naphthol AS-MX phosphate with Fast Blue salt and levamisole for alkaline phosphatase activity. Images were acquired using a Leica microscope DM6000 using 10x and 20x objectives. Quantification of $sFliC^+IgG1^+$ and $sFliC^+IgG2c^+$ was performed in two independent experiments, each with 4 mice per group. A total of 10 random fields were evaluated per slide.

Immunofluorescence was performed on frozen sections. Staining was performed in PBS containing 10% FCS, 0.1% sodium azide and sections were mounted in 2.5% 1,4-Diazabicyclo(2,2,2)octane (pH 8.6) in 90% glycerol in PBS. After incubation with primary Abs (1 h, room temperature), secondary Abs were added (30 min; room temperature). Images were acquired using the Fluorescence Zeiss Axio Scan.Z1, image analysis was performed with Zen, 2012 blue edition.

The following Abs were used for immunofluorescence: CD11c, Dec205, CD103. DCIR2 was used biotinylated. CD11b (eBioscience) and streptavidin (Jackson Immunoresearch) were used A488 conjugated. And AMCA-conjugated anti-IgM (Jackson Immunoresearch) was used. The following Abs were used for immunohistochemistry: IgD, IgG1, and IgG2c. sFliC and PNA (Vector) biotinylated were used.

In vitro Restimulation for the Detection of Antigen-Specific $CD4^+$ T Cells

Antigen-specific $CD4^+$ T cells were detected by their expression of CD154 post-restimulation as previously described (23). In brief, 6×10^6 cells (from spleen or MLN) were cultured in the presence of sFliC (5 μg/ml), anti-CD40 (1C10 2 μg/ml), biotinylated anti-CD154 (MR1 5 μg/ml) and anti-Fcγ receptor (2.4G2 50 μg/ml) for 48 h. Control wells included cells cultured without antigen. The expression of CD154 was evaluated by staining the cells with Streptavidin-APC and gating was done on Lin^-(CD19/CD11b/NK1.1/CD11c)$TCR\beta^+CD4^+CD62L^-$.

Sflic-Specific ELISA

ELISA plates were coated with 5 μg/ml of sFliC (24 h at 4°C) and blocked with 1% BSA overnight at 4°C. Serum was diluted 1:100 in PBS–0.05% Tween, and was further diluted stepwise. Plates were incubated for 1 h at 37°C. Bound antibodies were detected using alkaline phosphatase conjugated, goat anti-mouse IgG, IgG1, and IgG2c Abs (Southern Biotech). Alkaline phosphatase activity was detected using Sigma-Fast p-nitrophenylphosphate (Sigma Aldrich). Relative reciprocal titers were calculated by measuring the dilution at which the serum reached a defined OD_{405}.

Statistics

For statistics we used the non-parametric Mann-Whitney sum of ranks test or two-way ANOVA as appropriate using the GraphPad Prism software (GraphPad).

RESULTS

The Accumulation of $CD103^+$cDC2 in the MLN After sFliC Immunization Is TLR5-Dependent

Intraperitoneal immunization of sFliC induces a rapid MyD88-dependent accumulation of intestinal-derived $CD103^+$cDC2 in the MLN (1, 3). To analyse the role of TLR5 in this response, WT and $TLR5^{-/-}$ mice were immunized with sFliC and the cDC response analyzed by flow cytometry and *in situ* by immunofluorescence 24 h post-immunization. In the MLN of WT mice, immunization with sFliC resulted in an increase in the frequency and absolute numbers of $CD103^+$cDC2, which was abrogated in $TLR5^{-/-}$ mice, no significant change in absolute numbers or frequency was observed for cDC1 or $CD103^-$cDC2 (**Figure 1A**). Immunofluorescence microscopy showed that $CD103^+$cDC2 were mainly located in the T zone, before and after immunization, although they were less abundant in the absence of immunization. The high zoom-insets confirmed that $CD103^+$cDC2 in the T zone express CD11c, CD103, and CD11b. TLR5 is the extracellular receptor for sFliC, however there is an intracellular pathway for flagellin detection controlled by NAIP5 (24). To evaluate the contribution of this alternative pathway we evaluated the $CD103^+$cDC2 in $NAIP5^{-/-}$ mice, we observed a similar accumulation of those cells in comparison with the WT after sFliC immunization, strongly suggesting that TLR5 exclusively controls the response to sFliC by $CD103^+$cDC2 in the MLN (**Figure 1B**).

In contrast to the MLN, in the spleen there was no change in the frequency and absolute numbers of cDC2 (identified as $CD11b^+$ cDC) of WT mice after immunization with sFliC (**Figure 1C**). Furthermore, no difference was observed in the location of cDC2 ($DCIR2^+$) which remain primarily localized in the bridging channels between the red and white pulps (25). Loss of TLR5 did not alter the numbers of cDC2 before or after immunization, nor the distribution of these cells within the spleen (**Figure 1B**). Therefore, immunization with sFliC results

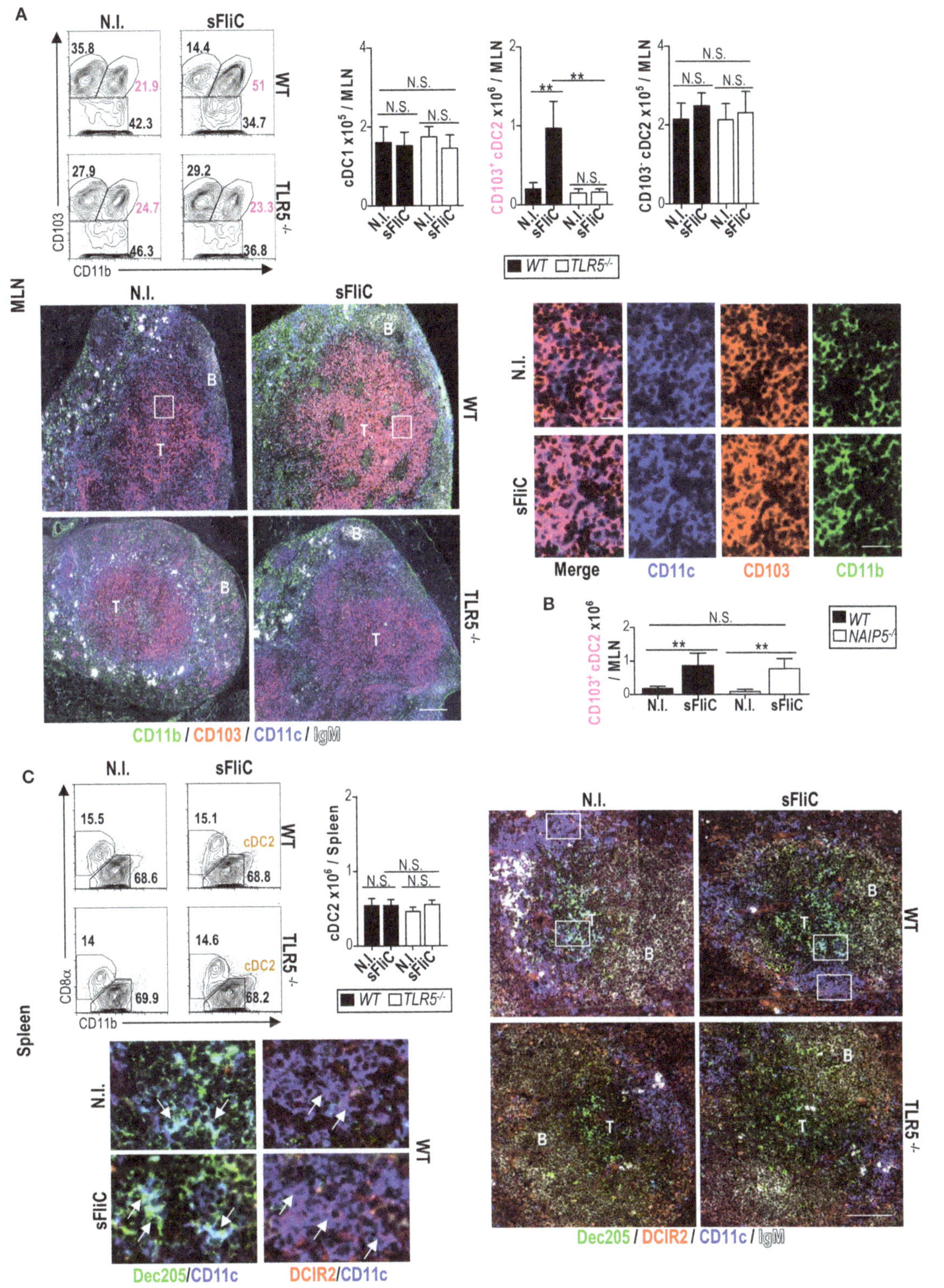

FIGURE 1 | Mucosal CD103$^+$cDC2 respond to sFliC immunization in a TLR5-dependent manner. Wild-type (WT) or TLR5$^{-/-}$ mice were immunized i.p. with sFliC and cDCs (Lin$^-$MHC-II^{hi}CD11c^{hi}) were evaluated 24 h later, alongside non-immunized (N.I.) mice. **(A)** MLN representative flow cytometry plots (including percentages) of cDC1 (Lin$^-$MHC-II^{hi}CD11c^{hi}CD11b$^-$CD103$^+$), CD103$^+$cDC2s (Lin$^-$MHC-II^{hi}CD11c^{hi}CD11b$^+$CD103$^+$) and CD103$^-$cDC2 (Lin$^-$MHC-II^{hi}CD11c^{hi}CD103$^-$) are shown with adjacent graphs of absolute numbers. Representative photomicrographs of MLN sections stained for CD11c; blue, CD103; red, CD11b; green, and IgM; white (scale bar = 200 μm) are shown (top right). Zoom-in insets (white boxes) show single staining and a merge of CD11c, CD103, and CD11b (scale bar = 20 μm).

(Continued)

FIGURE 1 | T, T zone; B, B zone. **(B)** WT or NAIP5$^{-/-}$ mice were immunized i.p., with sFliC and absolute numbers of MLN CD103^{+}cDC2s were evaluated 24 h later, alongside non-immunized (N.I.) mice. **(C)** Wild-type (WT) or TLR5$^{-/-}$ mice were immunized i.p. with sFliC and splenic cDCs (Lin^{-}MHC-II^{hi}CD11c^{hi}) were evaluated 24 h later, alongside non-immunized (N.I.) mice. Representative flow cytometry plots (including percentages) of cDC2s (Lin^{-}MHC-II^{hi}CD11c^{hi}CD11b^{+}) are shown with adjacent graphs of absolute numbers. Representative photomicrographs of spleen sections stained for CD11c; blue, Dec205; green, DCIR2; red, and IgM; white (scale bar = 100 μm). Zoom-in insets (white boxes) show the differential location of cDC1s (Dec205^{+}) in the T zone and cDC2s (DCIR2^{+}) in the bridging channels. Data shown as mean+s.d. of 4 mice and are representative of 3 independent experiments. $^{**}P < 0.001$, by two-way analysis of variance (ANOVA) N.S., not significant.

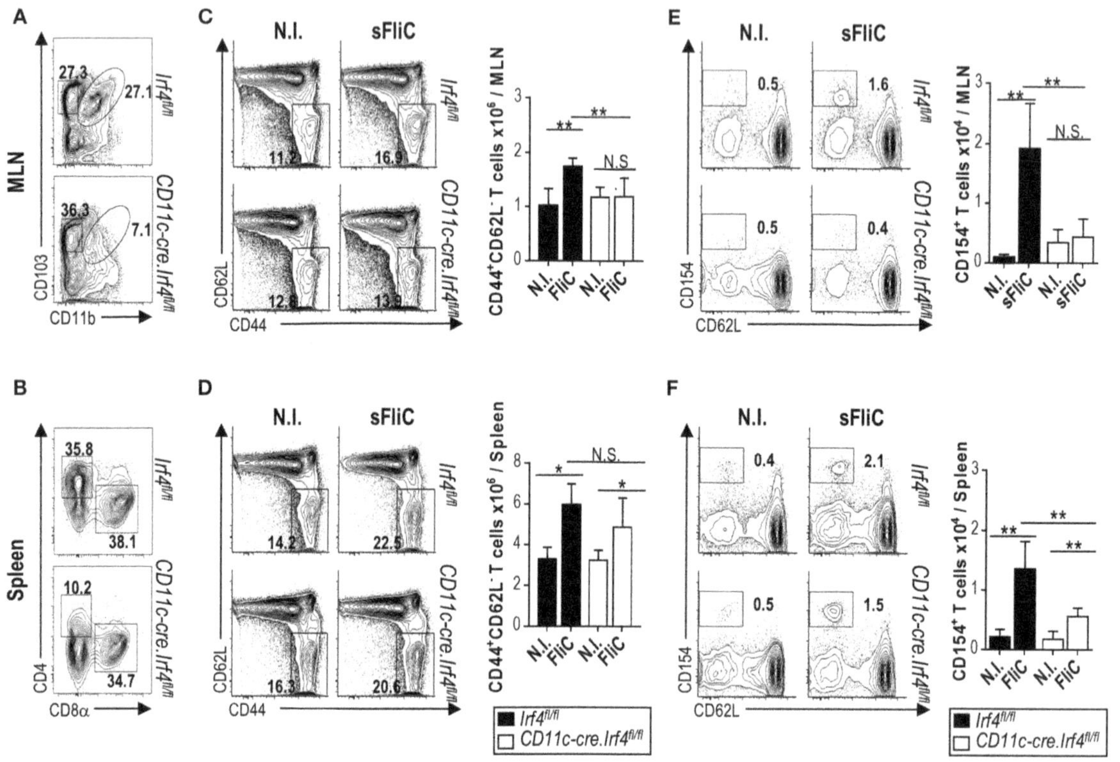

FIGURE 2 | The primary T cell response to sFliC is dependent upon CD103^{+}cDC2 in the mucosa but not in the spleen. cDC populations in *Irf4$^{fl/fl}$* or *Cd11c-cre.Irf4$^{fl/fl}$* mice were evaluated in **(A)** MLN and **(B)** spleen. *Irf4$^{fl/fl}$* or *Cd11c-cre.Irf4$^{fl/fl}$* mice were either non-immunized (N.I.) or immunized with sFliC and T cell responses were evaluated 7 days later. Representative flow cytometry plots (percentages) and absolute numbers (graphs) of activated CD4^{+} T cells (CD3^{+}CD4^{+}CD44^{+}CD62L^{-}) in the **(C)** MLN and **(D)** spleen. *Ex vivo* sFliC-specific restimulations, single cell suspensions were restimulated with 5 μg/ml of sFliC in the presence of anti-CD40 (2 μg/ml), biotinylated anti-CD154 (5 μg/ml) for 48 h. Antigen-specific CD4^{+} T cells were identified by detection of the anti-CD154 by streptavidin. **(E)** MLN and **(F)** spleen representative flow cytometry plots (percentages) and absolute numbers (graphs) of CD154^{+} CD4^{+} T cells. Data shown as mean + s.d. (n = 4 mice/group) representative experiment of 3 performed. $^{**}P < 0.001$; $^{*}P < 0.05$, by two-way analysis of variance (ANOVA), N.S., not significant.

in the selective accumulation of CD103^{+}cDC2 in the MLN, but not in the spleen in a TLR5 dependent manner.

CD103^{+}cDC2 Are Essential for T Cell Priming in the MLN After Immunization With sFliC

To assess the contribution of cDC2 to T cell priming after immunization with sFliC, we assessed responses in *Cd11c-cre.Irf4$^{fl/fl}$* mice. These mice lack IRF4 in cells that express CD11c, resulting in a 50% reduction of CD103^{+}CD11b^{+} cDCs in the small intestine lamina propria and a 90% reduction in the MLN (19). **Figure 2A** shows the significant reduction of MLN CD103^{+}CD11b^{+} cDCs in *Cd11c-cre.Irf4$^{fl/fl}$* mice in comparison with the *Irf4$^{fl/fl}$* mice. Furthermore, we also show the expected reduction of splenic cDC2 in these mice (**Figure 2B**). The frequency and number of activated CD4^{+} T cells in the MLN of *Cd11c-cre.Irf4$^{fl/fl}$* mice 7 days after FliC immunization, was lower compared to *Irf4$^{fl/fl}$* mice and similar to non-immunized mice (**Figure 2C**). In contrast, absolute numbers of activated CD4^{+} T cells in the spleen were similar between *Cd11c-cre.Irf4$^{fl/fl}$* and *Irf4$^{fl/fl}$* mice (**Figure 2D**). To examine the endogenous antigen-specific T cell response we performed an *in vitro* re-stimulation essay that uses the transient expression of CD154 to identify antigen-specific CD4^{+} T cells (23). In the MLN from immunized *Cd11c-cre.Irf4$^{fl/fl}$* mice, the frequency and number of CD154^{+} sFliC-specific CD4^{+} T cells was significantly lower than those in immunized *Irf4$^{fl/fl}$* mice and similar to levels observed in from non-immunized mice (**Figure 2E**). In contrast, in the spleen an increase of CD154^{+} sFliC-specific CD4^{+} T cells was observed

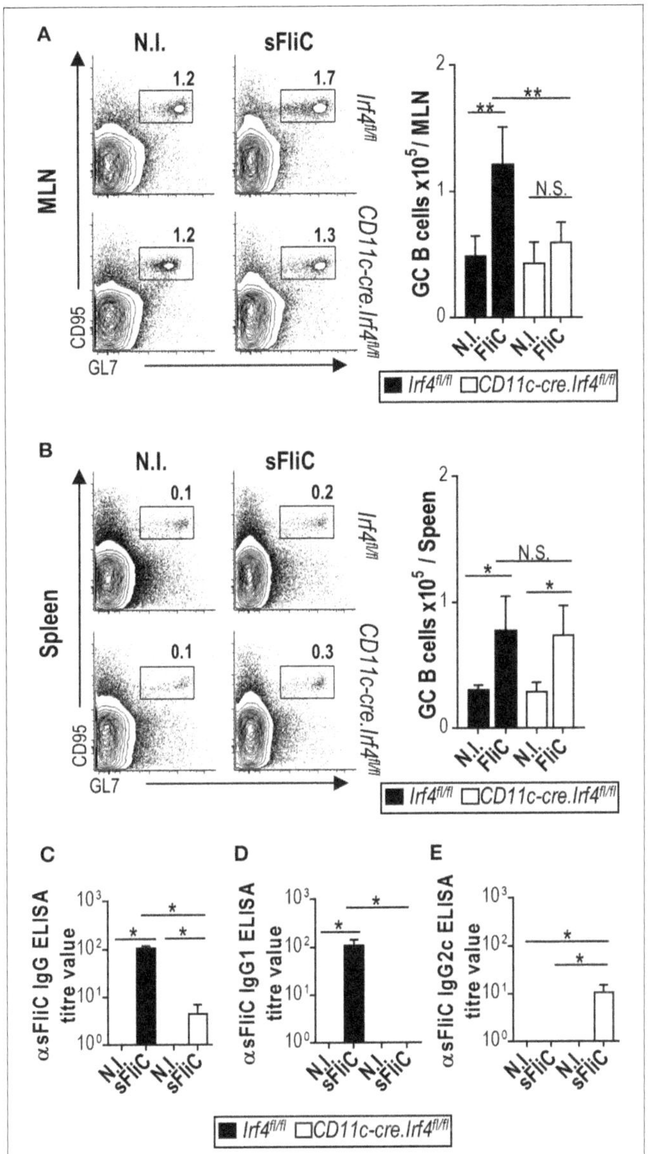

FIGURE 3 | The generation of primary B cell responses to sFliC in the MLN, but not the spleen, are dependent upon CD103$^+$cDC2. *Irf4$^{fl/fl}$* or *Cd11c-cre.Irf4$^{fl/fl}$* mice were either non-immunized (N.I.) sFliC-immunized and GC B cells (TCRβ$^-$CD19$^+$GL7$^+$CD95$^+$) were evaluated 7 days later. **(A)** MLN and **(B)** spleen representative flow cytometry plots (percentages) and absolute numbers (graphs) of GC B cells. Data are mean+s.d. ($n = 4$ mice/group) representative experiment of 3 performed. $^{**}P < 0.001$; $^{*}P < 0.05$, by two-way analysis of variance (ANOVA), NS, not significant. **(C)** Serum anti-sFliC IgG, IgG1, and IgG2c evaluated by enzyme-linked immunosorbent assay (ELISA). Data shown as mean + s.d. ($n = 12$ mice/group) and shows three independent experiments pooled together. $^{*}P < 0.05$, two-way analysis of variance (ANOVA), N.S., not significant.

in the *Cd11c-cre.Irf4$^{fl/fl}$* mice compared to the non-immunized mice but it was significantly lower compared to *Irf4$^{fl/fl}$* mice (**Figure 2F**). Collectively, these results demonstrate that the early T cell response induced to sFliC is dependent on mucosal CD103$^+$cDC2s, however in the spleen IRF4 expression by cDCs only impacts partially on T cell priming.

cDC2 Influence the Extent and Direction of IgG Switching

In order to address how the B cell response to sFliC is affected in the *Cd11c-cre.Irf4$^{fl/fl}$* mice we analyzed GC B cells by flow cytometry 7-days post-immunization. In the MLN, *Cd11c-cre.Irf4$^{fl/fl}$* mice showed no increase in the number of GC B cells in comparison to non-immunized and *Irf4$^{fl/fl}$* sFliC-immunized mice (**Figure 3A**). In contrast, in the spleen, immunized *Cd11c-cre.Irf4$^{fl/fl}$* and *Irf4$^{fl/fl}$* mice displayed a similar increase in GC B cell numbers (**Figure 3B**). To analyse the FliC-specific Ab response in more detail, serum Ab titres were evaluated by ELISA. Total sFliC-specific IgG titers were reduced in *Cd11c-cre.Irf4$^{fl/fl}$* mice in comparison with *Irf4$^{fl/fl}$* mice (**Figure 3C**). In mice, sFliC induces some Th2-associated features including antigen-specific IgG1 (13, 14). FliC-specific IgG1 was detected in sFliC-immunized *Irf4$^{fl/fl}$* mice, but was absent in *Cd11c-cre.Irf4$^{fl/fl}$* mice (**Figure 3D**). This was unexpected since some sFliC-specific IgG was detected in *Cd11c-cre.Irf4$^{fl/fl}$* mice and so titers of Th1-associated IgG2c were assessed. This isotype was detected exclusively in sFliC-immunized *Cd11c-cre.Irf4$^{fl/fl}$* mice (**Figure 3E**), suggesting that cDC2 contribute to IgG1 switching.

We hypothesized that the serum IgG2c derived from spleen. To analyze this possibility *in situ*, we performed immunohistochemistry on serial sections from the MLN and spleen of sFliC-immunized *Irf4$^{fl/fl}$* and *Cd11c-cre.Irf4$^{fl/fl}$* mice. GCs were identified as follicular areas that bind PNA and sFliC-specific cells were identified by using biotinylated sFliC in conjunction with either anti-IgG1 or anti-IgG2c Abs. In the MLN, sFliC-specific cells were exclusively observed in *Irf4$^{fl/fl}$* mice and were IgG1$^+$ (**Figure 4A**). In contrast, sFliC-binding cells were found in the spleens of both *Irf4$^{fl/fl}$* and *Cd11c-cre.Irf4$^{fl/fl}$* mice whilst in the *Irf4$^{fl/fl}$* mice, the sFliC-specific cells were IgG1$^+$ and IgG2c$^-$. In contrast, in *Cd11c-cre.Irf4$^{fl/fl}$* mice the sFliC-specific cells were exclusively IgG2c$^+$ (**Figure 4B**). Collectively, these results show that cDC2s play a role in the polarization of the Ab response *in vivo*.

DISCUSSION

We have previously shown that sFliC can drive a long-term mucosal adaptive response after i.p. immunization (1, 3). Furthermore, we also have shown that s.c. and i.p. immunization both induce similar cDC and IgA responses in the MLN, suggesting that our observations are not dependent of the route of immunization, but due to the intrinsic properties of sFliC. When addressing the prime-boost immune response in *Cd11c-cre.Irf4$^{fl/fl}$* mice the immune response to sFliC in the spleen was reduced, but not abrogated, suggesting the possibility that memory cells could contribute to the response. To address this possibility we studied the primary immune response to sFliC and show that the primary T and B cell responses to sFliC in the MLN are completely dependent on CD103$^+$cDC2, while that in the spleen is only partially dependent on cDC2.

Mucosal CD103$^+$cDC2s are probably more efficient at driving responses after sFliC immunization because of their high

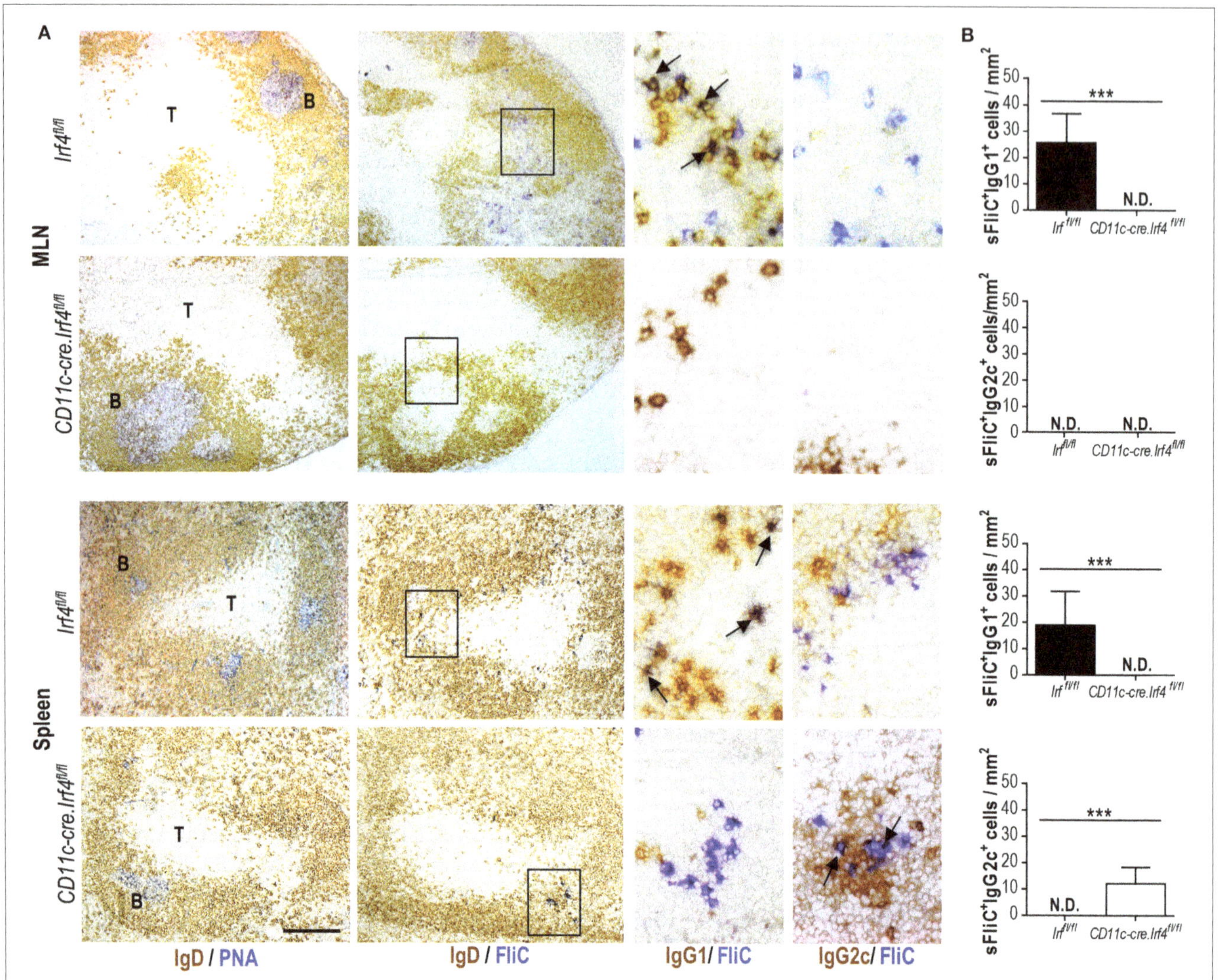

FIGURE 4 | Switching to IgG1 is abrogated in the *CD11c-cre.Irf4*$^{fl/fl}$ mice. *Irf4*$^{fl/fl}$ or *Cd11c-cre.Irf4*$^{fl/fl}$ mice were sFliC-immunized for 7 days. **(A)** Representative photomicrographs of serial sections from MLN and spleen stained for: PNA-binding cells (blue) and IgD-expressing cells (brown) (first column) or sFliC-binding cells (blue) and IgD-expressing cells (brown) (second column), scale bar = 200 μm. The third and fourth columns show zoom-in insets (black-boxed areas) stained to detect sFliC-binding cells and IgG1 and IgG2c respectively (scale bar = 50 μm). T, T zone; B, B zone. **(B)** Quantification of sFliC$^+$IgG1$^+$ cells and sFliC$^+$IgG2c$^+$ cells in the MLN and spleen. A total of 10 random fields were evaluated per slide. Data shown as mean + s.d. (n = 8 mice pooled from two independent experiments). ***P < 0.0001, by Mann-Whitney. N.D. non-detected.

expression levels of TLR5 in comparison to splenic cDCs (26, 27). TLR5 can play an additional role in enhancing antigen capture and presentation through MHC-II and this is not MyD88-dependent (28). Moreover, ligation of TLR5 itself will lead to an upregulation of co-stimulatory molecules and cytokine expression, in a MyD88-dependent manner (4, 14). This is likely to be the mechanism that mediates the accumulation of CD103$^+$cDC2 into the MLN after immunization with sFliC (1, 3). Furthermore, splenic cDCs are able to respond rapidly after sFliC immunization, possibly through activation by a bystander effect (22, 29). Therefore, in the spleen there may be less of a selective advantage for one subset to capture sFliC over another, meaning that both cDC1 and cDC2 are potentially able to present antigen to CD4$^+$ T cells and initiate priming. In support of this idea *ex vivo* data using sorted, *in vivo* loaded, cDCs showed that both splenic cDC1 and cDC2 are able to mediate to T cell priming. Additionally, when flagellin is used as an adjuvant in studies using DEC205 and 33D1 to target splenic cDC1 and cDC2 cells, it shows that the presence of flagellin enhances the capacity of both cDC subsets to mediate T cell proliferation (30). This demonstrates that flagellin can promote responses in both cDC subsets, which indirectly supports our findings. In contrast to this, in the intestinal mucosa only CD103$^+$cDC2 mediate T cell priming (3). Therefore, despite having a similar ontogeny, mucosal CD103$^+$cDC2 and splenic cDC2 show differences in their capacity to capture sFliC and this difference may account for why cDC2 play such a dominant role in driving T cell responses to FliC in the MLN but not the spleen.

After primary immunization of WT mice with sFliC, there is a robust GC response in the spleen, but a limited extrafollicular plasma cell response (13, 22). The predominant antigen-specific IgG isotype detected after immunization with sFliC in the serum is IgG1, associated to a Th2-like response (13, 14). Importantly, in the *Cd11c-cre.Irf4*$^{fl/fl}$ mice there was no significant increase in numbers of GC B cells in the MLN. In contrast, in the spleen, there was a normal GC response, which suggested that a B cell response developed in the spleen but not in the MLN when CD103^{+}cDC2 were reduced. Nevertheless, there were lower serum total IgG titers in the *CD11-cre.Irf4*$^{fl/fl}$ mice and an abrogated IgG response in the BM (3). One interpretation of this is that in the primary response to sFliC, the antibody response generated in the MLN is a significant, if not predominant, contributor, to the serum total FliC-specific IgG pool.

A more detailed analysis of the IgG response showed that there was a difference in the predominant IgG isotype induced between immunized *Cd11c-cre.Irf4*$^{fl/fl}$ and *Irf4*$^{fl/fl}$ mice. Inducing the appropriate IgG isotype is important as the distinct IgG isotypes can influence the level of protection afforded by vaccination (31) or against different pathogens (32). Surprisingly, the residual FliC-specific IgG response observed in *Cd11c-cre.Irf4*$^{fl/fl}$ mice was not of the IgG1 isotype, but instead was of the IgG2c isotype. Immunohistochemistry showed that the FliC-specific IgG2c was being produced locally in the spleen by cells proximal to GC (**Figure 3**). This suggests that although a B cell response is maintained in the spleens of the *Cd11c-cre.Irf4*$^{fl/fl}$ mice, this B cell response is substantially different qualitatively. Further work is needed to identify what B cell associated factors, such as BAFF or APRIL, cDC1 and cDC2 produce that may contribute to this and whether these differ between cDCs from different anatomical sites. In mice, there is a partial association between the direction of the T helper response and IgG isotype switching and so these findings may suggest that cDC2 contribute to Th2-associated responses. An association between cDC2 and Th2 polarization has been described previously in the context of infection or in atopic asthma models (21, 33–35). Moreover, we are working toward developing strategies to conjugate sFliC to different antigens and evaluate if these features that sFliC is able to promote as an adjuvant can be transferred to clinically relevant antigens. Our data helps inform on the relative merits of targeting specific DC populations in vaccination strategies.

AUTHOR CONTRIBUTIONS

Conceptualization: AF-L, AC, and WA. Methodology: AF-L, CC, NB-C, JY-P, IH, MD, and BL. Investigation: AF-L, KM, EP, JM, NB-C, and JY-P. Resources: JP, SU, and SA. Writing—original draft: AF-L. Writing, review, and editing: AF-L, AC, and WA. Funding acquisition: AF-L, AC, and WA.

ACKNOWLEDGMENTS

The authors would like to thank Dr. K. Kotarsky and A. Selberg for animal typing and husbandry (Lund University) and Ian Ricketts at the Biomedical Service Unit at the University of Birmingham.

REFERENCES

1. Flores-Langarica A, Marshall JL, Hitchcock J, Cook C, Jobanputra J, Bobat S, et al. Systemic flagellin immunization stimulates mucosal CD103^{+} dendritic cells and drives Foxp3+ regulatory T cell and IgA responses in the mesenteric lymph node. *J Immunol.* (2012) 189:5745–54. doi: 10.4049/jimmunol.1202283
2. Lopez-Yglesias AH, Zhao X, Quarles EK, Lai MA, VandenBos T, Strong RK, et al. Flagellin induces antibody responses through a TLR5- and inflammasome-independent pathway. *J Immunol.* (2014) 192:1587–96. doi: 10.4049/jimmunol.1301893
3. Flores-Langarica A, Muller Luda K, Persson EK, Cook CN, Bobat S, Marshall JL, et al. CD103(+)CD11b(+) mucosal classical dendritic cells initiate long-term switched antibody responses to flagellin. *Mucosal Immunol.* (2018) 11:681–92. doi: 10.1038/mi.2017.105
4. Hayashi F, Smith KD, Ozinsky A, Hawn TR, Yi EC, Goodlett DR, et al. The innate immune response to bacterial flagellin is mediated by Toll-like receptor 5. *Nature* (2001). 410:1099–103. doi: 10.1038/35074106
5. McSorley SJ, Ehst BD, Yu Y, Gewirtz AT. Bacterial flagellin is an effective adjuvant for CD4+ T cells *in vivo*. *J Immunol.* (2002) 169:3914–9. doi: 10.4049/jimmunol.169.7.3914
6. Bobat S, Flores-Langarica A, Hitchcock J, Marshall JL, Kingsley RA, Goodall M, et al. Soluble flagellin, FliC, induces an Ag-specific Th2 response, yet promotes T-bet-regulated Th1 clearance of *Salmonella typhimurium* infection. *Eur J Immunol.* (2011) 41:1606–18. doi: 10.1002/eji.201041089
7. Vijayan A, Rumbo M, Carnoy C, Sirard JC. Compartmentalized antimicrobial defenses in response to flagellin. *Trends Microbiol.* (2018) 26:423–35. doi: 10.1016/j.tim.2017.10.008
8. McNeilly TN, Naylor SW, Mahajan A, Mitchell MC, McAteer S, Deane D, et al. *Escherichia coli* O157:H7 colonization in cattle following systemic and mucosal immunization with purified H7 flagellin. *Infect Immun.* (2008) 76:2594–602. doi: 10.1128/IAI.01452-07
9. Liu G, Tarbet B, Song L, Reiserova L, Weaver B, Chen Y, et al. Immunogenicity and efficacy of flagellin-fused vaccine candidates targeting 2009 pandemic H1N1 influenza in mice. *PLoS ONE* (2011) 6:e20928. doi: 10.1371/journal.pone.0020928
10. Taylor DN, Treanor JJ, Strout C, Johnson C, Fitzgerald T, Kavita U, et al. Induction of a potent immune response in the elderly using the TLR-5 agonist, flagellin, with a recombinant hemagglutinin influenza-flagellin fusion vaccine (VAX125, STF2.HA1 SI). *Vaccine* (2011). 29:4897–902. doi: 10.1016/j.vaccine.2011.05.001
11. Kajikawa A, Zhang L, Long J, Nordone S, Stoeker L, LaVoy A, et al. Construction and immunological evaluation of dual cell surface display of HIV-1 gag and *Salmonella enterica* serovar Typhimurium FliC in *Lactobacillus acidophilus* for vaccine delivery. *Clin Vaccine Immunol.* (2012) 19:1374–81. doi: 10.1128/CVI.00049-12
12. Sun Y, Shi W, Yang JY, Zhou DH, Chen YQ, Zhang Y, et al. Flagellin-PAc fusion protein is a high-efficacy anti-caries mucosal vaccine. *J Dent Res.* (2012) 91:941–7. doi: 10.1177/0022034512457684

13. Cunningham AF, Khan M, Ball J, Toellner KM, Serre K, Mohr E, et al. Responses to the soluble flagellar protein FliC are Th2, while those to FliC on Salmonella are Th1. *Eur J Immunol.* (2004) 34:2986–95. doi: 10.1002/eji.200425403
14. Didierlaurent A, Ferrero I, Otten LA, Dubois B, Reinhardt M, Carlsen H, et al. Flagellin promotes myeloid differentiation factor 88-dependent development of Th2-type response. *J Immunol.* (2004) 172:6922–30. doi: 10.4049/jimmunol.172.11.6922
15. Trumpfheller C, Longhi MP, Caskey M, Idoyaga J, Bozzacco L, Keler T, et al. Dendritic cell-targeted protein vaccines: a novel approach to induce T-cell immunity. *J Intern Med.* (2012) 271:183–92. doi: 10.1111/j.1365-2796.2011.02496.x
16. Sehgal, K., Dhodapkar, K. M., and Dhodapkar, M. V. (2014). Targeting human dendritic cells *in situ* to improve vaccines. *Immunol Lett.* 162(1 Pt A):59–67. doi: 10.1016/j.imlet.2014.07.004
17. Guilliams M, Ginhoux F, Jakubzick C, Naik SH, Onai N, Schraml BU, et al. Dendritic cells, monocytes and macrophages: a unified nomenclature based on ontogeny. *Nat Rev Immunol.* (2014) 14:571–8. doi: 10.1038/nri3712
18. Guilliams, M., Dutertre, C. A., Scott, C. L., McGovern, N., Sichien, D., Chakarov, S., et al. (2016). Unsupervised high-dimensional analysis aligns dendritic cells across tissues and species. *Immunity* 45, 669–84. doi: 10.1016/j.immuni.2016.08.015
19. Persson EK, Uronen-Hansson H, Semmrich M, Rivollier A, Hagerbrand K, Marsal J, et al. IRF4 transcription-factor-dependent $CD103^+CD11b^+$ dendritic cells drive mucosal T helper 17 cell differentiation. *Immunity* (2013) 38:958–69. doi: 10.1016/j.immuni.2013.03.009
20. Joeris T, Muller-Luda K, Agace WW, Mowat AM. Diversity and functions of intestinal mononuclear phagocytes. *Mucosal Immunol.* (2017) 10:845–64. doi: 10.1038/mi.2017.22
21. Mayer JU, Demiri M, Agace WW, MacDonald AS, Svensson-Frej M, Milling SW. Different populations of CD11b(+) dendritic cells drive Th2 responses in the small intestine and colon. *Nat Commun.* (2017) 8:15820. doi: 10.1038/ncomms15820
22. Flores-Langarica A, Bobat S, Marshall JL, Yam-Puc JC, Cook CN, Serre K, et al. Soluble flagellin coimmunization attenuates Th1 priming to Salmonella and clearance by modulating dendritic cell activation and cytokine production. *Eur J Immunol.* (2015) 45:2299–311. doi: 10.1002/eji.201545564
23. Kirchhoff D, Frentsch M, Leclerk P, Bumann D, Rausch S, Hartmann S, et al. Identification and isolation of murine antigen-reactive T cells according to CD154 expression. *Eur J Immunol.* (2007) 37:2370–7. doi: 10.1002/eji.200737322
24. Lightfield KL, Persson J, Brubaker SW, Witte CE, von Moltke J, Dunipace EA, et al. Critical function for Naip5 in inflammasome activation by a conserved carboxy-terminal domain of flagellin. *Nat Immunol.* (2008) 9:1171–8. doi: 10.1038/ni.1646
25. Dudziak D, Kamphorst AO, Heidkamp GF, Buchholz VR, Trumpfheller C, Yamazaki S, et al. Differential antigen processing by dendritic cell subsets *in vivo*. *Science* (2007) 315:107–11. doi: 10.1126/science.1136080
26. Uematsu S, Jang MH, Chevrier N, Guo Z, Kumagai Y, Yamamoto M, et al. Detection of pathogenic intestinal bacteria by Toll-like receptor 5 on intestinal CD11c+ lamina propria cells. *Nat Immunol.* (2006) 7:868–74. doi: 10.1038/ni1362
27. Feng T, Cong Y, Alexander K, Elson CO. Regulation of Toll-like receptor 5 gene expression and function on mucosal dendritic cells. *PLoS ONE* (2012) 7:e35918. doi: 10.1371/journal.pone.0035918
28. Letran SE, Lee SJ, Atif SM, Uematsu S, Akira S, McSorley SJ. TLR5 functions as an endocytic receptor to enhance flagellin-specific adaptive immunity. *Eur J Immunol.* (2011) 41:29–38. doi: 10.1002/eji.201040717
29. Salazar-Gonzalez RM, Srinivasan A, Griffin A, Muralimohan G, Ertelt JM, Ravindran R, et al. Salmonella flagellin induces bystander activation of splenic dendritic cells and hinders bacterial replication *in vivo*. *J Immunol.* (2007) 179:6169–75. doi: 10.4049/jimmunol.179.9.6169
30. Antonialli R, Sulczewski FB, Amorim K, Almeida BDS, Ferreira NS, Yamamoto MM, et al. CpG oligodeoxinucleotides and flagellin modulate the immune response to antigens targeted to $CD8\alpha^+$ and $CD8\alpha^-$ conventional dendritic cell subsets. *Front Immunol.* (2017) 8:1727. doi: 10.3389/fimmu.2017.01727
31. Zhang Y, Dominguez-Medina C, Cumley NJ, Heath JN, Essex SJ, Bobat S, et al. IgG1 is required for optimal protection after immunization with the purified porin OmpD from Salmonella Typhimurium. *J Immunol.* (2017) 199:4103–9. doi: 10.4049/jimmunol.1700952
32. Lane PJ, MacLennan IC. Impaired IgG2 anti-pneumococcal antibody responses in patients with recurrent infection and normal IgG2 levels but no IgA. *Clin Exp Immunol.* (1986) 65:427–33.
33. Gao, Y., Nish, S. A., Jiang, R., Hou, L., Licona-Limon, P., Weinstein, J. S., et al.. (2013). Control of T helper 2 responses by transcription factor IRF4-dependent dendritic cells. *Immunity* 39, 722–732. doi: 10.1016/j.immuni.2013.08.028
34. Williams JW, Tjota MY, Clay BS, Vander Lugt B, Bandukwala HS, Hrusch CL, et al. Transcription factor IRF4 drives dendritic cells to promote Th2 differentiation. *Nat Commun.* (2013) 4:2990. doi: 10.1038/ncomms3990
35. Demiri M, Muller-Luda K, Agace WW, Svensson-Frej M. Distinct DC subsets regulate adaptive Th1 and 2 responses during *Trichuris muris* infection. *Parasite Immunol.* (2017) 39, 1–10. doi: 10.1111/pim.12458

12

Fas Signaling in Dendritic Cells Mediates Th2 Polarization in HDM-Induced Allergic Pulmonary Inflammation

Miaomiao Han[1,2,3†], *Ran Hu*[2†], *Jingyu Ma*[2], *Baohua Zhang*[2], *Ce Chen*[4], *Huabin Li*[1*], *Jun Yang*[3*] and *Gonghua Huang*[2,4*]

[1] Department of Otolaryngology-Head and Neck Surgery, Center for Allergic and Inflammatory Diseases, Affiliated Eye and ENT Hospital, Fudan University, Shanghai, China, [2] Shanghai Institute of Immunology, Shanghai Jiao Tong University School of Medicine, Shanghai, China, [3] Xin Hua Hospital Affiliated to Shanghai Jiao Tong University School of Medicine, Shanghai, China, [4] Guangdong Provincial Key Laboratory of Medical Molecular Diagnostics, Guangdong Medical University, Dongguan, China

***Correspondence:**
Huabin Li
allergyli@163.com
Jun Yang
yangjun@xinhuamed.com.cn
Gonghua Huang
gonghua.huang@shsmu.edu.cn

These authors have contributed equally to this work

†

Fas–Fas ligand (FasL) signaling plays an important role in the development of allergic inflammation, but the cellular and molecular mechanisms are still not well known. By using the bone marrow-derived dendritic cell (BMDC) transfer-induced pulmonary inflammation model, we found that house dust mite (HDM)-stimulated FAS-deficient BMDCs induced higher Th2-mediated allergic inflammation, associated with increased mucus production and eosinophilic inflammation. Moreover, FAS-deficient BMDCs promoted Th2 cell differentiation upon HDM stimulation *in vitro*. Compared to wild-type BMDCs, the Fas-deficient BMDCs had increased ERK activity and decreased IL-12 production upon HDM stimulation. Inhibition of ERK activity could largely increase IL-12 production, consequently restored the increased Th2 cytokine expression of OT-II CD4$^+$ T cells activated by Fas-deficient BMDCs. Thus, our results uncover an important role of DC-specific Fas signaling in Th2 differentiation and allergic inflammation, and modulation of Fas signaling in DCs may offer a useful strategy for the treatment of allergic inflammatory diseases.

Keywords: allergic inflammation, dendritic cells, Fas, house dust mite, Th2

INTRODUCTION

Allergic inflammation has been generally considered as a T helper (Th) 2-mediated chronic immune response (1). Th2 cells produce effector cytokines such as IL-4, IL-5, and IL-13 to mediate the respiratory symptoms. Among these effector cytokines, IL-4 is involved in IgE synthesis and IL-5 can drive eosinophilia in lung tissue, while IL-13 contributes to mucus overproduction, airway hyper-responsiveness (AHR), goblet cell metaplasia and airway remodeling (1–3). House dust mite (HDM) has been reported to cause 50–85% of allergic asthmatic inflammation (4). The polarization of a Th2-mediated immune response to inhaled allergens (such as HDM) is determined by the status of dendritic cells (DCs). DCs promote Th2 differentiation through upregulation of the expression of several costimulatory molecules such as CD86, OX40L and polarization cytokines including IL-6, IL-10, and IL-33 (5–8), as well as Th2-cell-attracting chemokines, such as CCL17 and CCL22 (9). Although accumulating evidence suggests that DCs are sufficient and necessary to initiate Th2 responses, the underlying signaling mechanism for DCs to direct Th2 differentiation and function is still not well-understood.

Fas (CD95, also named APO-1) signaling is widely considered to mediate apoptosis upon binding to its ligand (FasL, also called "CD95L or APO-1L") or its agonist antibody (10). In an ovalbumin (OVA)-induced mouse asthma model, Fas-deficient mice have delayed resolution of airway hyperresponsiveness (AHR) compared to wild-type mice (11). Further study indicates that Fas deficiency in T cells contributes to the prolonged resolution of airway inflammation (12). Recent studies have shown that Fas–FasL interaction could also activate non-apoptotic pathways, such as Fas signaling leading to T cell activation, proliferation and differentiation (13) and promoting Th17 polarization and Th17-mediated autoimmunity (14). Fas-deficient mice sensitized with OVA increase the expression of IL-4, IL-5, and IL-13 compared to wild-type mice (15). Although DCs are pivotal in regulating T cell activation, proliferation, differentiation and allergic inflammation, the role of Fas signaling in DCs in driving Th2 differentiation and Th2-mediated allergic inflammation still need to be elucidated.

In the present study, we used the well-established model by adoptively transferring HDM-pulsed BMDCs to recipient mice to explore the role of FAS signaling in DCs in pulmonary inflammation. We found that Fas deficiency in DCs led to increased mucus production, eosinophilic inflammation and Th2 response *in vivo*. Fas-deficient BMDCs promoted the production of Th2-related cytokines such as IL-4 and IL-13. Further mechanistic study showed that DCs directed Th2 differentiation by modulating the Fas–ERK–IL-12 axis. Collectively, our results identify an important signaling mechanism of DC-mediated Th2 responses and modulation of Fas signaling in DCs might offer a useful strategy for the treatment of eosinophilic lung inflammatory diseases.

MATERIALS AND METHODS

Mice

B6.MRL-*Tnfrsf6*^{lpr} mice were from The Jackson Laboratory. C57BL/6 mice were from Shanghai SLAC Laboratory Animal Center (Shanghai, China). All mice were kept in a specific pathogen-free (SPF) barrier facility maintained by Shanghai Jiao Tong University School of Medicine. All the experimental mice were used at 6–10 weeks. Animal protocols were approved by Institutional Animal Care and Use Committee of Shanghai Jiao Tong University School of Medicine.

BMDC Culture

BMDCs were cultured as previously described (16). Briefly, bone marrow cells were collected by perfusing mouse femur and tibia. After red blood cell lysis, cells were cultured in RPMI 1640 (Invitrogen Corp.) supplemented with 10% fetal calf serum (FCS, Gibco), penicillin and streptomycin (Invitrogen), 2-mercaptoethanol (Sigma-Aldrich), supernatant from J5 cells (provided by Dr. Qibin Leng, Institut Pasteur of Shanghai, China) expressing GM-CSF (1:50) and 10 ng/ml IL-4 (R&D). On day 3, the entire medium was removed and replaced with fresh differentiation medium. On day 7, the cells were harvested for analyses. The purity of CD11c^{+} BMDCs was >80%.

BMDC Adoptive Transfer Experiment

In BMDC adoptive transfer experiment, wild-type or Fas-deficient BMDCs were pulsed with 50 μg/ml HDM (Greer Laboratories, Lenoir, NC) for 12 h, washed, and then 1×10^6 HDM-pulsed BMDCs were administered intravenously into naïve C57BL/6 recipients. Recipients transferred with un-pulsed wild-type or Fas-deficient BMDCs as control. On day 10–12, all the recipients were lightly anesthetized and challenged intranasally with 10 μg HDM in 40 μl PBS and the mice were sacrificed for analysis on day 13.

Antibodies and Flow Cytometry

Anti-mouse CD11c (N418), MHC-II (M5/114.15.2), CD11b (M1/70), Ly6G (RB6-8C5), siglec F (E50-2440), CD4 (RM4-5), TCRβ (H57-597), IL-4 (11B11), IL-13 (eBio13A), IL-17A (eBio17B7), CD25 (PC61.5), CD44 (IM7), CD62L (MEL-14), CD69 (H1.2F3), Ki-67 (SolA15), IL-12p40 (C17.8), CD45 (30-F11), CD178 (MFL3) antibodies were obtained from eBioscience. Anti-mouse IL-5 (TRFK5) was obtained from BD Biosciences. Anti-mouse CCR3 (J073E5) was obtained from Biolegend. For surface staining, cells were stained with antibodies in PBS containing 1% FCS (Hyclone) on ice for 30 min. For intracellular staining, cells were stimulated with PMA (Sigma-Aldrich) and ionomycin (Sigma-Aldrich) for 5 h in the presence of Golgistop (BD Biosciences) before being stained according to the manufacturer's instructions (eBioscience). CD4^{+}T cell proliferation was detected by anti-Ki-67 staining according to the manufacturer's instructions (eBioscience) 3 days after co-culture. Labeling OTII CD4^{+} T cells with CFSE (carboxyfluorescein diacetate succinimidyl diester; Invitrogen), cell proliferation was detected by flow cytometry 4 days after co-culture. For cell apoptosis analysis, cells were stained with CaspACE™ FITC-VAD-FMK *in situ* Marker (Promega). The samples were acquired on a FACSCantoII (BD) or LSRFortessa™ X-20 (BD) and analyzed with FlowJo software (Treestar).

Bronchoalveolar Lavage Fluid (BALF) Collection and Lung Mononuclear Cell Isolation

For BALF collection, lung tissues were lavaged with 1 ml cold PBS for 3 times and the supernatant was collected. Lung mononuclear cells were prepared as previously described (17). Briefly, lung tissues were removed, minced and digested with 1 mg/ml Collagenase IV (Life Technologies) in RPMI-1640 (Hyclone) with 5% FCS (Hyclone) for 45 min at 37°C. Cells were enriched by using 38% Percoll gradient (GE Healthcare Life Sciences). Red blood cells were lyzed with ACK lysis buffer (R&D Systems). Cells were harvested for analyses.

Histology

Left lobe of lung tissues were removed from mice after BALF collection, fixed with 4% paraformaldehyde (PFA) at room temperature for 24 h and embedded in paraffin, cut into 5-μm sections for hematoxylin and eosin (HE) or periodic acid-Schiff

(PAS) staining. The lung inflammation was blindly quantified using HE-stained sections according to the criteria previously published (18). The quantification of the goblet cell hyperplasia in the airway was done as previously described (19).

RNA Isolation and Quantitative PCR (qPCR)

Total RNAs of lung tissues were isolated using Trizol regent (Invitrogen). Total RNAs of cells were isolated using RNeasy mini Kit (QIAGEN) according to the manufacturer's instructions. 1 μg total RNA was used for reverse transcription with PrimeScript RT Master Mix (TAKARA) according to the manufacturer's instructions in a total volume of 20 μl. qPCR was carried out with SYBR Green PCR Master Mix (Applied Biosystems) in a Vii7 Real-Time PCR system (Applied Biosystems). mRNA expression of genes was normalized to *Hprt*. The primers shown below were from Primerbank: *Hprt*, forward primer: TCAGTCAACGGGGGACATAAA, reverse primer: GGGGCT GTACTGCTTAACCAG; *Il4*, forward primer: GGTCTCAAC CC CCAGCTAGT, reverse primer: GCCGATGATCTCTCT CAAGTGAT; *Il17a*, forward primer: TCAGCGTGTCCAAAC ACTGAG, reverse primer: CGCCAAGGGAG TTAAAGACTT; *Ifng*, forward primer: GCCACGGCACAGTCATTGA, reverse primer: TGCTGATGGCCTGATTGTCTT; *Il6*, forward primer: CTGCAAGAGACTTCCATCCAG, reverse primer: AGTGGT ATAGACAGGTATGTTGG; *Il12p35*, forward primer: CAATCA CGC TACCTCCTCTTT, reverse primer: CAGCAGTGCAGG AATAATGTTTC; *Il12p40*, forward primer: GTCCTCAGAAGC TAACCATCTC, reverse primer: CCAGAGC CTATGACTCCA TGTC; *Il10*, forward primer: CTTACTGACTGGCATGAGGAT CA, reverse prime: GCAGCTCTAGGAGCATGTGG. The other primers were used as described, such as *Il5*, *Il13* (20), *Gata3* (21), *Il9* (22), *Tnfsf4* (8), *Cd86* (23), *Tslp* (24).

Cell Stimulation and Culture

BMDCs were stimulated with HDM in the presence or absence of Fas agonistic antibody Jo2 (1 μg/ml, BD) or Fas antagonistic antibody kp7-6 (1 mM, Merk) for 5 h for RNA analysis. For drug inhibitor treatments, cells were incubated with vehicle (DMSO) or U0126 (10 μM) (from Calbiochem) for 0.5–1 h before adding other stimuli. For BMDC–T cell co-culture, BMDCs and flow cytometry-sorted naïve OT-II $CD4^+$ T cells ($CD4^+25^-CD44^-CD62L^+$, purity >99%) were mixed at a ratio of 1:10 in the presence of $OVA_{323-339}$ peptide and HDM, and then the $CD4^+$ T cells were harvested at 48 h for mRNA analysis or supernatant was harvested at 72 h for ELISA. For cytokine treatment, cultures were supplemented with 1 ng/ml IL-12p70 (R&D).

Protein Analysis

Concentrations of IL-4 and IL-13 were measured by ELISA according to the manufacturer's instructions (R&D; eBioscience). Read the OD values at 450 nm on the MultiSKAN GO microplate reader (Thermo). Immunoblot analysis was performed as described (25) with antibody to ERK phosphorylated at Thr202 and Tyr204, antibody to p38 phosphorylated at Thr180 and Tyr182, antibody to JNK phosphorylated at Thr183 and Tyr185 and antibody to ERK (all from Cell Signaling Technology), antibody to alpha tubulin (Proteintech).

Statistical Analysis

All statistical analyses were performed by unpaired Student's *t*-tests or ANOVA using GraphPad Prism software (version 5.0). $P < 0.05$ was considered significant. Results represent means ± SEM.

RESULTS

Fas-Deficient BMDCs Enhance HDM-Induced Pulmonary Inflammation

To explore the role of Fas signaling in DCs in the regulation of HDM-induced allergic inflammation in mice, we used a BMDC adoptive transfer protocol to induce lung inflammation (**Figure 1A**). We transferred HDM-pulsed or un-pulsed wild-type or Fas-deficient BMDCs into naïve wild-type recipient mice. After HDM re-challenged, mice received HDM-pulsed BMDCs showed higher total cell number in the bronchoalveolar lavage (BAL) compared to mice received un-pulsed BMDCs (**Figure 1B**). A significantly increased total cell number was also observed in the BAL of recipients transferred with HDM-pulsed Fas-deficient BMDCs (**Figure 1B**). We also observed higher inflammatory cell infiltration and mucus production in lung tissues of recipients transferred with HDM-pulsed Fas-deficient BMDCs than those transferred with HDM-pulsed wild-type BMDCs (**Figures 1C,D**). Flow cytometry showed that a dramatically increased eosinophil infiltration both in the BAL and lung tissues of recipients transferred with HDM-pulsed Fas-deficient BMDCs compared to those transferred with HDM-pulsed wild-type BMDCs (**Supplementary Figures 1A,B**). We also analyzed the inflammatory eosinophils (iEos) ($CD45^+$Siglec $F^{int}CCR3^+CD62L^-$) and resident eosinophils (rEos) ($CD45^+$Siglec $F^{int}CCR3^+CD62L^+$) in lung tissues (26). The cell number of iEos was increased in recipients transferred with HDM-pulsed Fas-deficient BMDCs compared to those transferred with HDM-pulsed wild-type BMDCs, but rEos was comparable between recipients transferred with HDM-pulsed wild-type BMDCs and those transferred with Fas-deficient BMDCs (**Figure 1E**). However, the neutrophil infiltration had no difference between the two groups (**Supplementary Figures 1C,D**). Together, these data indicate that HDM-pulsed Fas-deficient BMDCs can induce more severe allergic airway inflammation than HDM-pulsed wild-type BMDCs.

Fas Signaling in BMDCs Does Not Affect $CD4^+$ T Cell Proliferation, Apoptosis, and Activation *in vivo*

In addition to a role of innate immune cells in the development of allergic inflammation, the adaptive immune system also play an important role in driving and sustaining this inflammation (27). A comparable $CD4^+$ T cell activation was observed in lung tissues of the recipients transferred with HDM-pulsed wild-type or Fas-deficient BMDCs (**Figure 2A**). We also

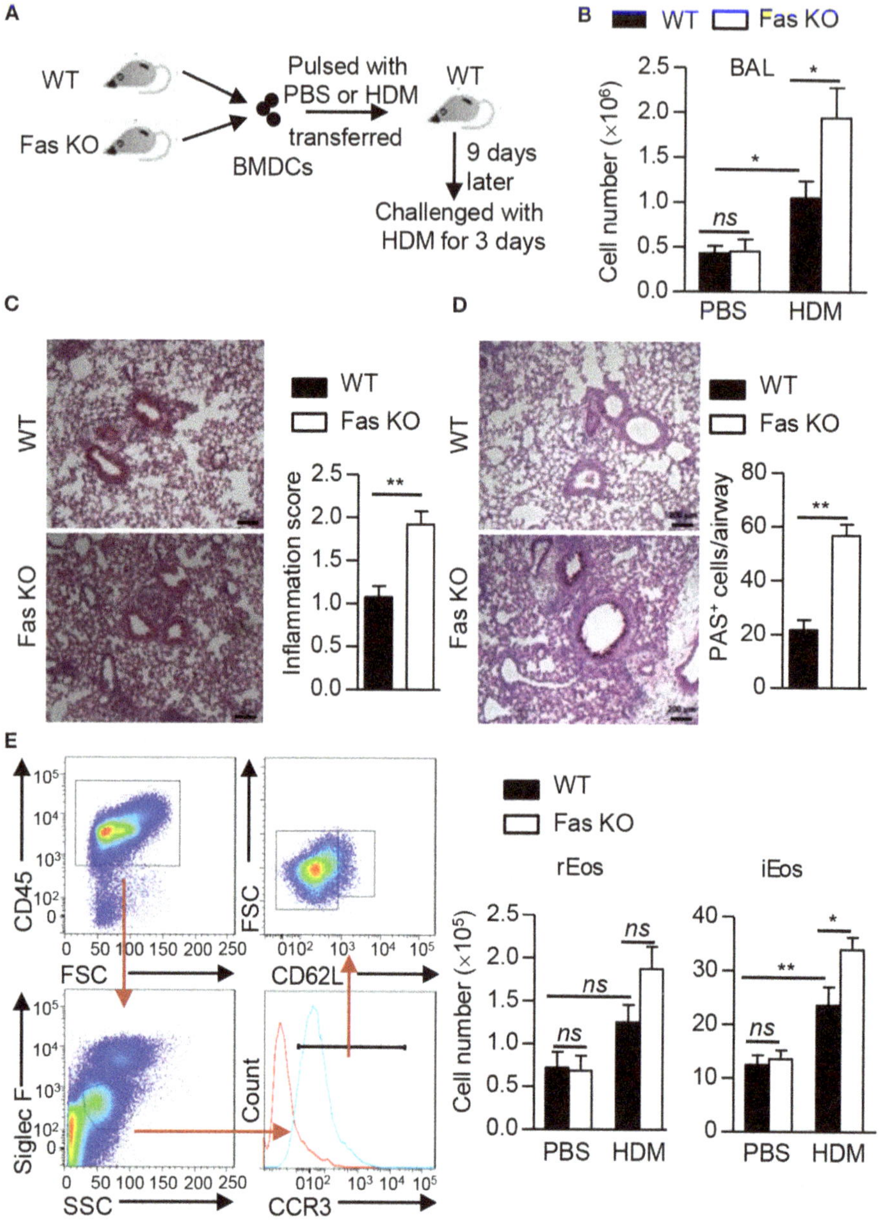

FIGURE 1 | Fas-deficient BMDCs enhance HDM-induced pulmonary inflammation. **(A)** Protocol for HDM-induced allergic airway inflammation using BMDC transfer experiment. **(B)** Total cell number in the BAL. **(C)** HE staining of lung sections from recipients transferred with HDM-pulsed wild-type or Fas-deficient BMDCs and quantitative analysis. Scale Bars represent 200 μm. **(D)** PAS staining of lung sections from recipients transferred with HDM-pulsed wild-type or Fas-deficient BMDCs and quantification of PAS$^+$ cells in airways. Scale Bars represent 200 μm. **(E)** Gating strategy and cell number of inflammatory eosinophils (iEos) ($CD45^+SiglecF^{int}CCR3^+CD62L^-$) and resident eosinophils (rEos) ($CD45^+SiglecF^{int}CCR3^+CD62L^+$) in lung tissues of recipients transferred with wild-type or Fas-deficient BMDCs pulsed or un-pulsed with HDM. $^*P < 0.05$, $^{**}P < 0.01$, *ns*, not significant. Data are representative of two independent experiments with 5–8 mice per group **(B–E)**. Student's *t*-tests **(C,D)** or two-way ANOVA **(B,E)** were performed and data were presented as mean ± SEM.

examined whether Fas-deficient in BMDCs could affect CD4$^+$ T cell proliferation or apoptosis *in vivo*, we performed Ki-67 and VAD staining assay, respectively. Our results showed that the proportion of Ki-67$^+$CD4$^+$ T cells and the median fluorescence intensity (MFI) value of VAD$^+$CD4$^+$ T cell in lung tissues and mediastinal lymph nodes (mLN) had no differences between the recipients transferred with HDM-pulsed wild-type BMDCs and those transferred with Fas-deficient BMDCs (**Figures 2B–E**). Taken together, these results show that Fas signaling in BMDCs is not required for CD4$^+$ T cell activation, proliferation and apoptosis upon HDM treatment.

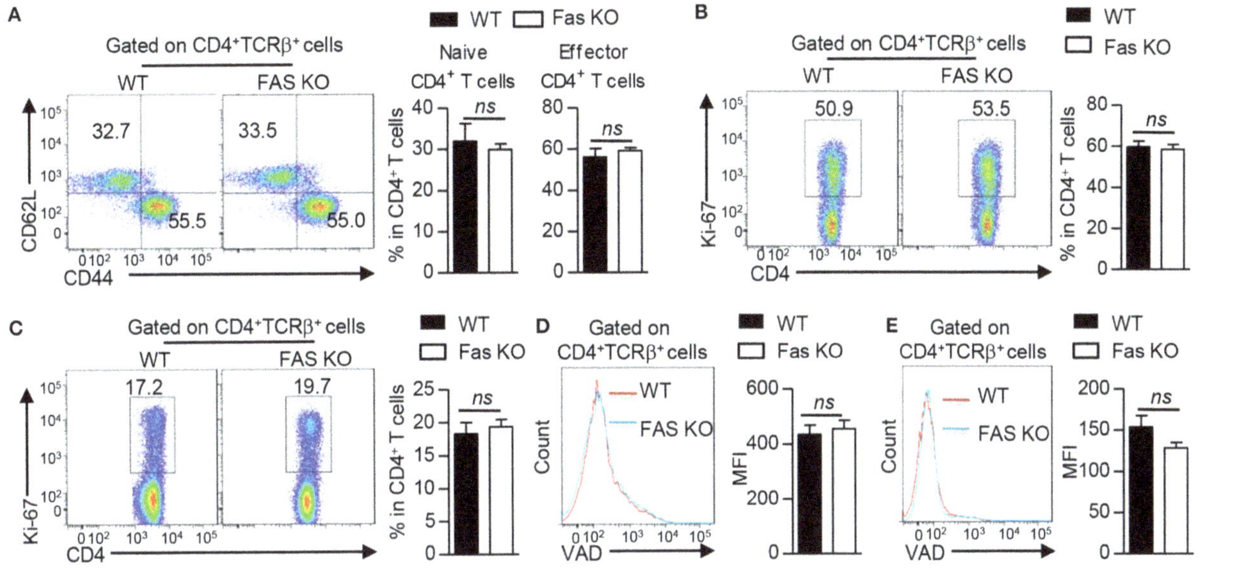

FIGURE 2 | Fas signaling in BMDCs does not affect CD4$^+$ T cell proliferation, apoptosis and activation *in vivo*. Mice were treated as **Figure 1A** described. **(A)** Flow cytometry (left) and proportions (right) of naïve CD4$^+$ T cells (CD4$^+$TCRβ$^+$ CD62L$^+$CD44$^-$) and effector CD4$^+$ T cells (CD4$^+$TCRβ$^+$CD62L$^-$CD44$^+$) in lung tissues. **(B,C)** Flow cytometry (left) and proportion (right) of Ki-67 expression in CD4$^+$ T cells of lung tissues **(B)** and mLN **(C)**. **(D,E)** Flow cytometry (left) and Median Fluorescence Intensity (MFI) of VAD (right) staining in CD4$^+$ T cells of lung tissues **(D)** and mLN **(E)**. *ns*, not significant. Data are representative of two independent experiments with 4–6 mice per group **(A–E)**. Student's *t*-tests **(A–E)** were performed and data were presented as mean ± SEM.

Fas-Deficient BMDCs Promote Th2 Responses Upon HDM Treatment

Given that there was no difference in the proliferation and apoptosis of CD4$^+$ T cells in the recipients transferred with HDM-pulsed wild-type or Fas-deficient BMDCs, we reasoned that the difference in inflammatory response might be due to the potential of these cells to produce inflammatory cytokines. Thus, we first measured cytokine expression in lung tissues of these two group mice. The qPCR results showed that the recipients transferred with HDM-pulsed Fas-deficient BMDCs had higher mRNA expression of *Il4* (encoding IL-4), *Il5* (encoding IL-5), and *Il13* (encoding IL-13), but comparable expression of *Ifng* (encoding IFNγ) and *Il17a* (encoding IL-17A) in lung tissues than those transferred with HDM-pulsed wild-type BMDCs (**Figure 3A**). Although a comparable percentage and cell number of CD4$^+$ T cells was observed in lung tissues of the two HDM-pulsed groups (**Figure 3B**), intracellular staining showed that recipients transferred with HDM-pulsed Fas-deficient BMDCs had higher percentage of IL-4$^+$, IL-5$^+$, and IL-13$^+$CD4$^+$ T cells in lung tissues than those transferred with wild-type BMDCs, along with higher cell number of IL-4$^+$, IL-5$^+$, and IL-13$^+$CD4$^+$ T cells (**Figures 3C,D**), whereas the percentage and cell number of IL-17$^+$CD4$^+$ T cells were similar in the two groups (**Supplementary Figures 2A,B**). However, the percentage and cell number of IL-4$^+$, IL-5$^+$, and IL-13$^+$CD4$^+$ T cells had no difference between the recipients transferred with un-pulsed wild-type and Fas-deficient BMDCs (**Supplementary Figures 2C,D**). Taken together, these results demonstrate that HDM-pulsed Fas-deficient BMDCs promote Th2 responses *in vivo*.

Fas Signaling in BMDCs Instructs Th2 Cell Differentiation *in vitro*

To determine whether the increased Th2 response *in vivo* is due to the direct interaction between DCs and T cells, we co-cultured wild-type or Fas-deficient BMDCs with naïve OT-II CD4$^+$ T cells in the presence of $OVA_{323-339}$ peptide with or without HDM. The polarization of CD4$^+$ T cells was determined by qPCR or ELISA, respectively. OT-II CD4$^+$ T cells activated with HDM-stimulated Fas-deficient BMDCs had higher IL-4 and IL-13 expression both in mRNA and in protein levels than those stimulated with wild-type BMDCs (**Figures 4A,B**). GATA3, the master transcription factor for Th2 cell differentiation, was also found increased in T cells activated by HDM-pulsed Fas-deficient BMDCs, while the expression of *Il9* and *Il10* was comparable (**Figure 4A**). The activation and proliferation of OT-II CD4$^+$ T cells activated by HDM-pulsed both wild-type and Fas-deficient BMDCs were comparable (**Figures 4C–E**). Collectively, these data indicate that Fas signaling mediates the direct crosstalk between BMDCs and Th2 cells upon HDM stimulation *in vitro*.

Fas-Deficient BMDCs Promote Th2 Differentiation by Inhibiting IL-12 Expression

Next we explored the molecular mechanism by which Fas signaling in BMDCs to shape Th2 differentiation upon HDM stimulation. We stimulated wild-type BMDCs with Fas agonistic antibody Jo2, the expression of *Cd86*, *Tslp*, *Il10*, *Il6*, and *Tnfsf4*, which had been reported to regulate Th2 polarization, had no difference compared to control group

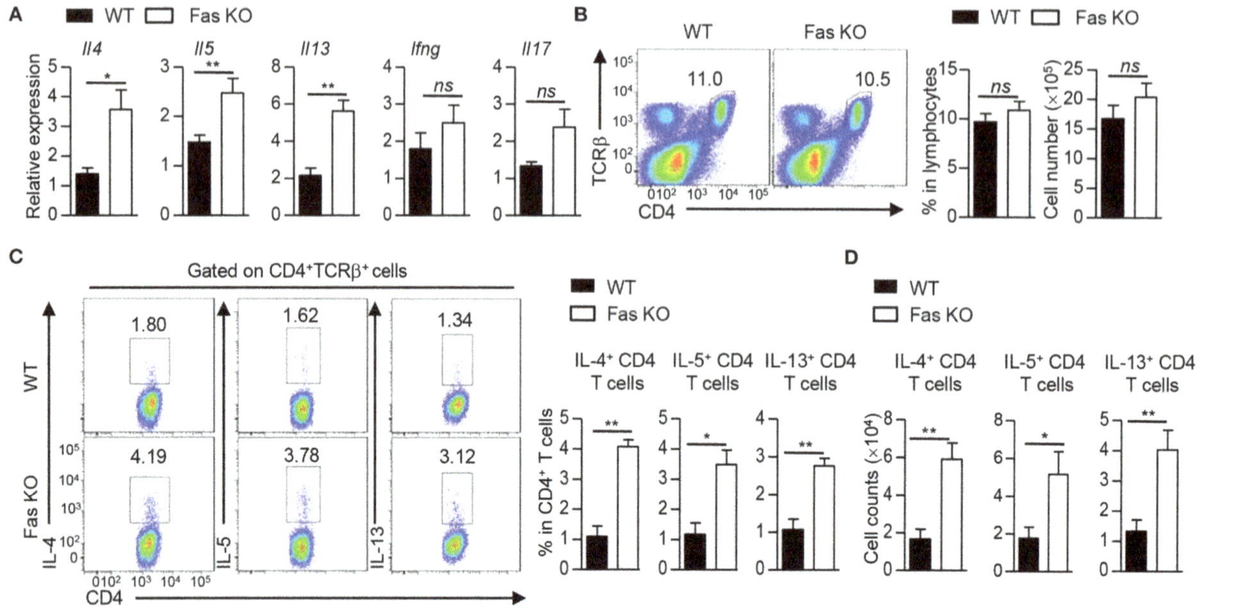

FIGURE 3 | Fas-deficient BMDCs promote Th2 responses upon HDM treatment. Mice were treated as **Figure 1A** described. **(A)** mRNA expression of *Il4*, *Il5*, *Il13*, *Ifng*, and *Il17* in lung tissues was detected by qPCR and normalized to *Hprt*. **(B)** Flow cytometry (left), percentage (middle), and cell number (right) of $CD4^+$ T cells in lung tissues. **(C)** Flow cytometry (left) and percentage of IL-4^+, IL-5^+, and IL-13^+ $CD4^+$ T cells in lung tissues. **(D)** Cell number of IL-4^+, IL-5^+, and IL-13^+CD4^+ T cells in lung tissues. $^*P < 0.05$, $^{**}P < 0.01$, *ns*, not significant. Data are representative of two independent experiments with 4–5 mice **(A–D)** per group. Student's *t*-tests **(A–D)** were performed and data were presented as mean ± SEM.

(**Figure 5A** and **Supplementary Figure 3A**). HDM stimulation could dramatically increase the expression of *Il6* and *Tnfsf4*, while Fas agonistic antibody Jo2 did not affect the expression of these two genes (**Figure 5A**), indicating that FAS signaling is not required for *Il6* and *Tnfsf4* expression in DCs upon HDM stimulation. IL-12 has been reported to affect Th2 differentiation (28). Fas agonistic antibody Jo2 stimulation could not affect the expression of *Il12p35* and *Il12p40* in wild-type BMDCs without HDM stimulation (**Figure 5A**). Upon HDM stimulation, the expression of *Il12p35* and *Il12p40* was significantly increased compared with non-HDM stimulation, and Fas agonistic antibody Jo2 could further enhance the expression of *Il12p35* and *Il12p40* in mRNA level and IL-12p70 in protein level (**Figures 5A,B**). Given that HDM-stimulated BMDCs had increased FasL, Fas antagonistic antibody kp7-6-treated HDM-pulsed wild-type BMDCs produced lower *Il12p40* in mRNA level and IL-12p70 in protein level than those of BMDCs stimulated with HDM alone, but the expression of *Il12p35* had no difference between HDM and HDM plus kp7-6 stimulated BMDCs (**Figures 5C,D** and **Supplementary Figure 3B**). Fas-deficient BMDCs had decreased expression of *Il12p35* and *Il12p40* compared to wild-type BMDCs upon HDM stimulation in the presence of Fas agonistic antibody Jo2 (**Figure 5E**). We next examined whether the lower expression of IL-12 in Fas-deficient BMDCs could contribute to the increased Th2 differentiation. We added exogenous IL-12 into the BMDC–T cell co-culture system and found that the IL-12 supplement could significantly decrease the expression of Th2-related cytokines, such as IL-4 and IL-13 in OT-II $CD4^+$ T cells activated by Fas-deficient BMDCs. The expression of IFNγ and IL-17 was comparable between wild-type and Fas-deficient BMDC activated T cells (**Figure 5F**). Altogether, these results indicate that Fas-deficient BMDCs promote Th2 differentiation through downregulation of IL-12 expression.

Fas Signaling Regulates IL-12 Expression by Modulation of ERK Activation in BMDCs

We next examined the downstream signaling of Fas involved in the regulation of IL-12 expression by analyzing the activation of p38, JNK, and ERK in BMDCs. We found that the phosphorylation of ERK was decreased in wild-type BMDCs treated with Fas agonistic antibody Jo2 and HDM compared to those treated with HDM alone (**Figure 6A**). Accordingly, the activation of ERK in Fas-deficient BMDCs was increased compared to that of wild-type BMDCs upon HDM and Fas agonistic antibody Jo2 stimulation (**Figure 6B**). To determine whether the increased ERK activation was contributed to the decreased IL-12 expression in Fas-deficient BMDCs, we treated Fas-deficient BMDCs with specific ERK inhibitor U0126, which resulted in a dramatically increased IL-12p70 expression in Fas-deficient BMDCs (**Figure 6C**). Consequently, U0126-treated Fas-deficient BMDCs completely restored the increased IL-4 and IL-13 expression in T cells to the level of T cells activated with wild-type BMDCs (**Figure 6D**). These results indicate that Fas signaling regulates IL-12 expression and Th2 differentiation through modulating the ERK activity in BMDCs.

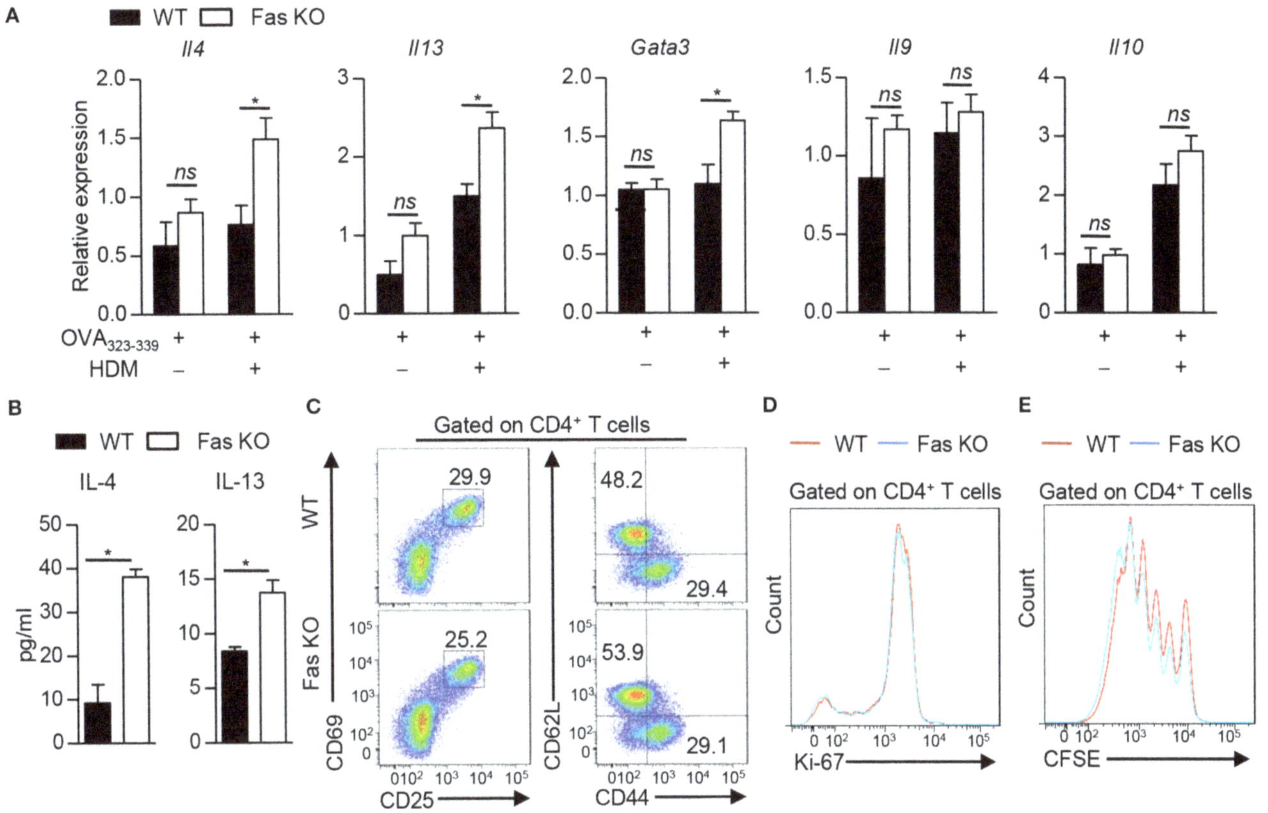

FIGURE 4 | Fas signaling in BMDCs instructs Th2 cell differentiation *in vitro*. **(A–D)** Co-culture of wild-type and Fas-deficient BMDCs with naïve OT-II $CD4^+$ T cells ($CD4^+CD25^-CD62L^+CD44^-$) in the presence of $OVA_{323-339}$ with or without HDM for 48 h **(A)**, 3 days **(B,D)**, 18 h **(C)**, and then $CD4^+$ T cells were harvested for analyses. **(A)** mRNA expression of *Il4*, *Il13*, *Gata3*, *Il9*, and *Il10* was detected by qPCR and normalized to *Hprt*. **(B)** Production of IL-4 and IL-13 was detected by ELISA. **(C)** Flow cytometry of the activation status of OT-II $CD4^+$ T cells. **(D)** Flow cytometry of Ki-67 expression in OT-II $CD4^+$ T cells. **(E)** Naïve OT-II $CD4^+$ T cells were labeled with CFSE and then co-cultured with wild-type or Fas-deficient BMDCs in the presence of $OVA_{323-339}$ and HDM for 4 days. Flow cytometry of $CD4^+$ T cell proliferation. $^*P < 0.05$, *ns*, not significant. Data are representative of two independent experiments with duplicate or triplicate wells per group **(A,B)**. Student's *t*-tests were performed and data were presented as mean ± SEM.

DISCUSSION

Numerous studies have reported that administration of allergen-pulsed DCs is sufficient to induce airway inflammation by polarizing Th2 responses (3, 29–31). However, the mechanism of DCs to regulate Th2 cell differentiation is still unclear (32). In this study, we used a BMDC-transfer protocol to investigate the important role of DC-specific Fas signaling in the pathogenesis of HDM-induced Th2-mediated allergic inflammation. We found that HDM-pulsed Fas-deficient BMDCs could promote Th2 responses and allergic eosinophilic inflammation, without affecting T cell apoptosis and proliferation in the recipients. Our study identified a crucial role of Fas signaling in regulating IL-12 expression by modulating ERK activity in DCs to direct Th2 differentiation upon HDM stimulation, which may provide an attractive treatment strategy for allergic diseases.

DCs constitutively express non-canonical costimulatory molecule Fas (13), which is activated by FasL or Fas agonistic antibody Jo2 to induce an apoptotic signaling. Numerous studies have shown that activated Fas signaling in DCs induces the secretion of cytokines such as IL-1β and CXC or CC chemokines (13, 33, 34), which may play important roles in the recruitment, activation and proliferation of naïve T cells (14, 35). Fas–FasL interaction on T cells has been proposed to promote the differentiation of naïve T cells into functional T cells (14), but little is known about how the Fas signaling in DCs regulating Th2 differentiation. DCs could promote Th2 differentiation through upregulation signal 2 (such as CD86, OX40L) (7, 36, 37) or signal 3 (such as IL-6, IL-10,TSLP) (38–40). In this study, we found that Fas agonistic antibody Jo2 stimulation did not affect the expression of OX40L and IL-6. However, Jo2 stimulation increased IL-12 expression in BMDCs stimulated with HDM. Accordingly, the ablation of Fas in DCs largely reduced the expression of IL-12, which contributed to the increased Th2 differentiation. Our results identify a new mechanism by which DC regulating Th2 responses through modulation of IL-12 production during inflammation development.

ERK signaling has been shown to play important roles in Fas-mediated non-apoptotic function. Ligation of Fas agonistic antibody Jo2 with Fas on DCs can promote the activation of

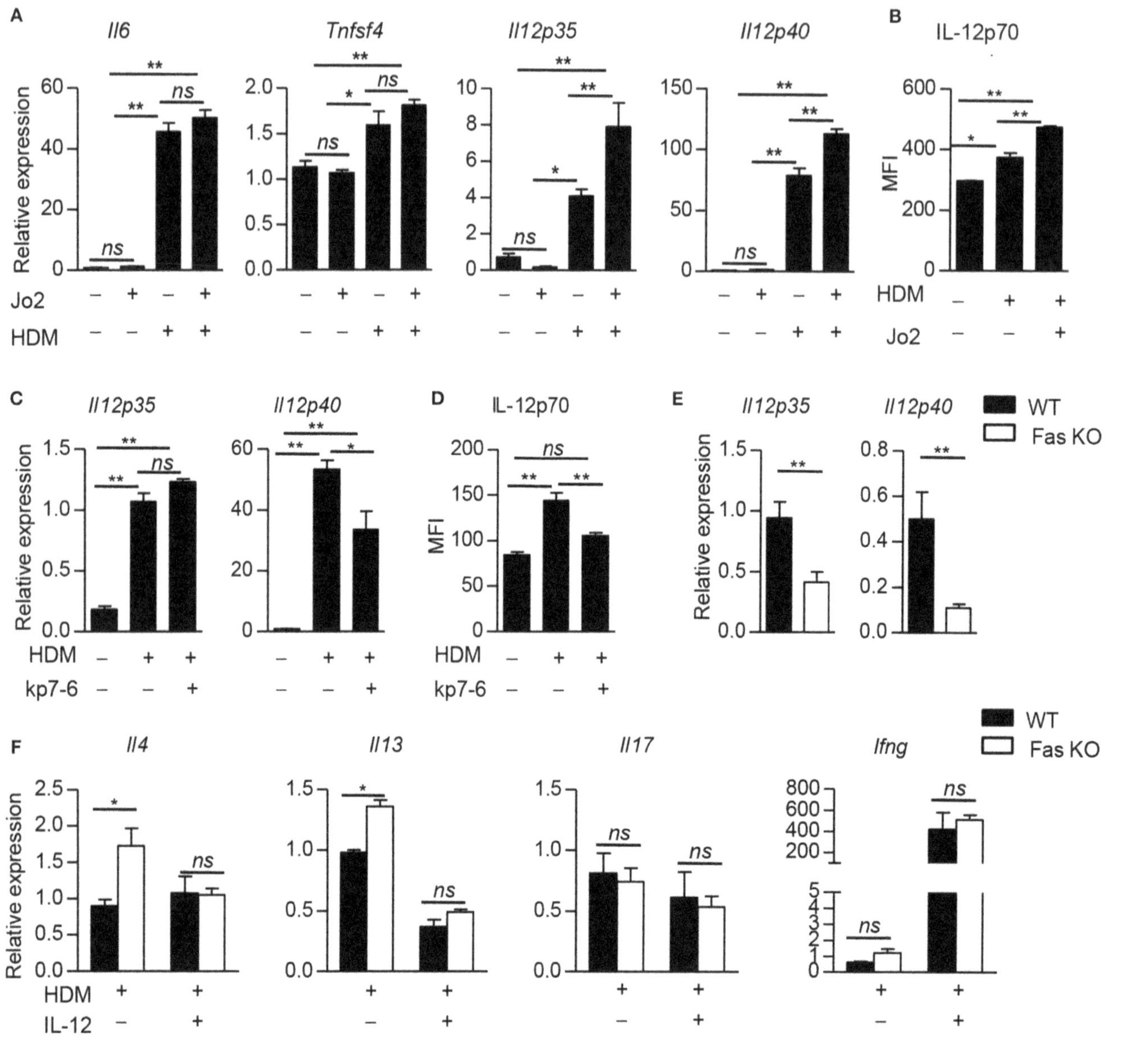

FIGURE 5 | Fas-deficient BMDCs promote Th2 differentiation by inhibiting IL-12 expression. **(A)** Wild-type BMDCs were stimulated with Fas agonistic antibody Jo2, HDM, and HDM with Jo2 for 5 h, un-stimulated BMDCs as control. Expression of *Il6*, *Tnfsf4*, *Il12p35,* and *Il12p40*, was detected by qPCR and normalized to *Hprt*. **(B)** Wild-type BMDCs were stimulated with HDM in the presence or absence of Fas agonistic antibody Jo2 for 8 h and Golgistop was added into the system in the last 4 h. The MFI of IL-12 was detected by intracellular staining. **(C)** Wild-type BMDCs were stimulated with HDM in the presence or absence of Fas antagonistic antibody kp7-6 for 5 h, un-stimulated BMDCs as control. Expression *Il12p35* and *Il12p40* was detected by qPCR normalized to *Hprt*. **(D)** Wild-type BMDCs were stimulated with HDM in the presence or absence of Fas antagonistic antibody kp7-6 for 10 h and Golgistop was added into the system in the last 4 h, un-stimulated BMDCs as control. The MFI of IL-12 was detected by intracellular staining. **(E)** Wild-type and Fas-deficient BMDCs were stimulated with HDM and Fas agonistic antibody Jo2 for 5 h. mRNA expression of *Il12p35* and *Il12p40* was detected by qPCR and normalized to *Hprt*. **(F)** IL-12 (1 ng/ml) was added into the BMDC–OT-II $CD4^+$ T cell co-culture system. mRNA expression of *Il4*, *Il13*, *Il17,* and *Ifng* in $CD4^+$ T cells was detected by qPCR and normalized to *Hprt*. $^*P < 0.05$, $^{**}P < 0.01$, *ns*, not significant. Data are representative of two independent experiments with duplicate or triplicate wells per group **(A–F)**. Student's *t*-tests **(E)**, one-way ANOVA **(A–D)** or two-way ANOVA **(F)** were performed and data were presented as mean ± SEM.

ERK and subsequent IL-1β secretion (34). In the current study, we found that Jo2 stimulation could dramatically decrease the activity of ERK in the presence of HDM. This different role might be caused by the type of stimuli and the status of the BMDCs, and further study need to be explored the potential mechanism for this different regulation by ERK. ERK signaling could profoundly influence the immune response of T cells. ERK activity in $CD4^+$ T cells has a key role in Th2 cell polarization (41). Blocking MEK-ERK signaling effectively suppresses IL-12p40 production from *Neospora caninum* infected peritoneal

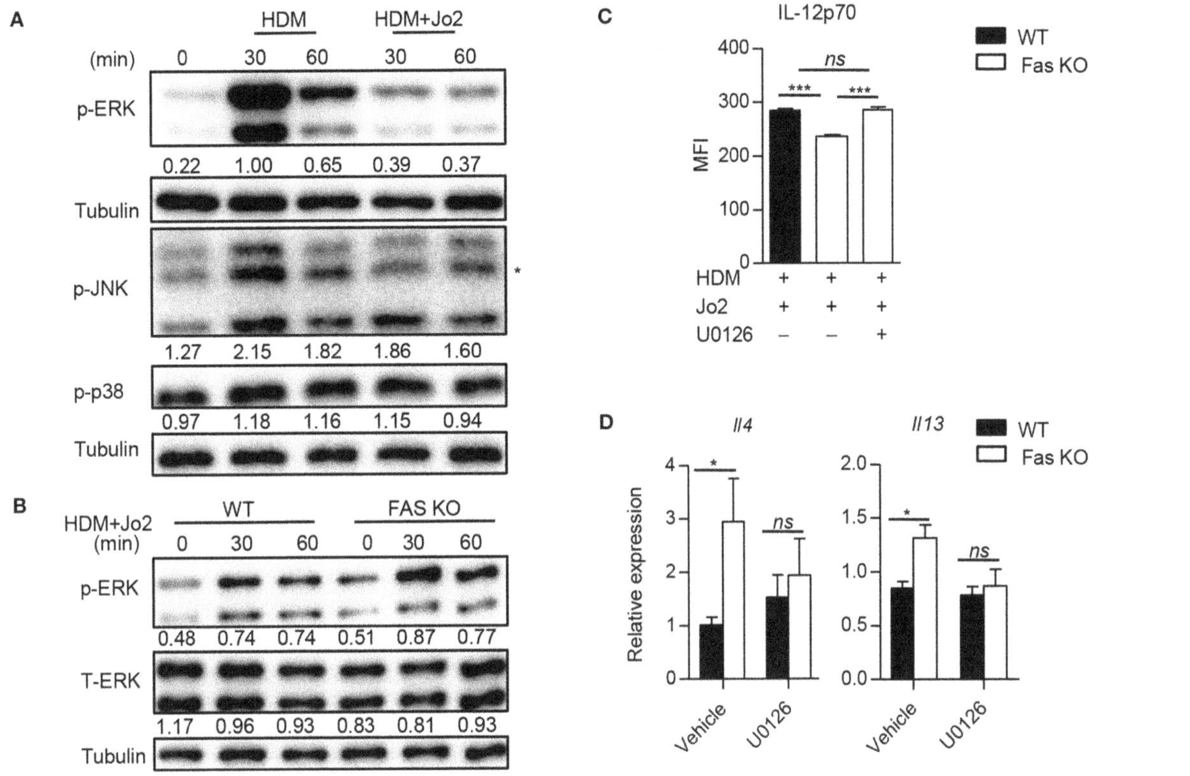

FIGURE 6 | Fas signaling regulates IL-12 expression by modulation of ERK activation in BMDCs. **(A)** Activity of ERK, JNK, and p38 in wild-type BMDCs stimulated with HDM in the presence or absence of Fas agonistic antibody Jo2 was detected by western blot. Asterisk indicates non-specific bands. Numbers under the lanes indicate band intensity related to that of alpha tubulin. **(B)** Activation of ERK in wild-type and Fas-deficient BMDCs stimulated with HDM plus Fas agonistic antibody Jo2. Numbers under the lanes indicate band intensity related to that of alpha tubulin. **(C)** Wild-type and Fas-deficient BMDCs were pre-treated with U0126 for 30 min and then stimulated with HDM and Fas agonistic antibody Jo2 for 8 h. Golgistop was added into the system in the last 4 h. The MFI of IL-12 was detected by intracellular staining. **(D)** Wild-type and Fas-deficient BMDCs were pre-treated with U0126 for 30 min and then stimulated with HDM for 5 h, washed and co-cultured with OT-II $CD4^+$ T cells for 48 h. Expression of *Il4* and *Il13* was detected by qPCR and normalized to *Hprt*. $^*P < 0.05$, $^{***}P < 0.001$, *ns*, not significant. Data are representative of two independent experiments with duplicate or triplicate wells per group **(C)** or combination of two experiments with consistent results **(D)**. One-way ANOVA **(C)** or two-way ANOVA **(D)** was performed and data were presented as mean ± SEM.

macrophages (42). In contrast, ERK signaling also has been reported to be an important negative regulator of IL-12 secretion in cigarette smoke extract (CSE) stimulated DCs (43). In this study, we found that a higher ERK activity could suppress IL-12 production in HDM-stimulated Fas-deficient BMDCs. Taken together, this study uncovers a specific role of Fas signaling in BMDCs in the regulation of Th2 differentiation and Th2-mediated allergic inflammation. Modulation of Fas signaling on DCs may provide a new strategy for treatment of allergic diseases.

AUTHOR CONTRIBUTIONS

MH designed and performed the *in vivo* and cellular experiments and contributed to manuscript writing. RH performed the *in vitro* and cellular experiments. JM contributed mouse models. CC contributed to animal colony management. BZ contributed to western blot analysis. HL and JY provided reagents. GH designed experiments, analyzed the data, wrote the manuscript, and provided overall directions.

ACKNOWLEDGMENTS

We thank Dr. Qibin Leng (Institut Pasteur of Shanghai, China) for kindly providing the J5 cell line.

REFERENCES

1. Lambrecht BN, Hammad H. The immunology of asthma. *Nat Immunol.* (2015) 16:45–56. doi: 10.1038/ni.3049
2. van Helden MJ, Lambrecht BN. Dendritic cells in asthma. *Curr Opin Immunol.* (2013) 25:745–54. doi: 10.1016/j.coi.2013.10.002
3. Chuang YH, Suen JL, Chiang BL. Fas-ligand-expressing adenovirus-transfected dendritic cells decrease allergen-specific T cells and airway inflammation in a murine model of asthma. *J Mol Med.* (2006) 84:595–603. doi: 10.1007/s00109-006-0047-3
4. Gregory LG, Lloyd CM. Orchestrating house dust mite-associated allergy in the lung. *Trends Immunol.* (2011) 32:402–11. doi: 10.1016/j.it.2011.06.006
5. Tjota MY, Hrusch CL, Blaine KM, Williams JW, Barrett NA, Sperling AI. Signaling through FcR gamma-associated receptors on dendritic cells drives IL-33-dependent T(H)2-type responses. *J Allergy Clin Immun.* (2014) 134:706–13.e8. doi: 10.1016/j.jaci.2014.06.013
6. Mayer A, Debuisson D, Denanglaire S, Eddahri F, Fievez L, Hercor M, et al. Antigen presenting cell-derived IL-6 restricts Th2-cell differentiation. *Eur J Immunol.* (2014) 44:3252–62. doi: 10.1002/eji.201444646
7. Krishnamoorthy N, Oriss TB, Paglia M, Fei M, Yarlagadda M, Vanhaesebroeck B, et al. Activation of c-Kit in dendritic cells regulates T helper cell differentiation and allergic asthma. *Nat Med.* (2008) 14:565–73. doi: 10.1038/nm1766
8. Ito T, Wang YH, Duramad O, Hori T, Delespesse GJ, Watanabe N, et al. TSLP-activated dendritic cells induce an inflammatory T helper type 2 cell response through OX40 ligand. *J Exp Med.* (2005) 202:1213–23. doi: 10.1084/Jem.20051135
9. Lambrecht BN, Hammad H. Biology of lung dendritic cells at the origin of asthma. *Immunity* (2009) 31:412–24. doi: 10.1016/j.immuni.2009.08.008
10. Shibaki A, Katz SI. Activation through CD40 ligation induces functional Fas ligand expression by Langerhans cells. *Eur J Immunol.* (2001) 31:3006–15. doi: 10.1002/1521-4141(2001010)31:10<3006::AID-IMMU3006>3.0.CO;2-L
11. Duez C, Tomkinson A, Shultz LD, Bratton DL, Gelfand EW. Fas deficiency delays the resolution of airway hyperresponsiveness after allergen sensitization and challenge. *J Allergy Clin Immunol.* (2001) 108:547–56. doi: 10.1067/mai.2001.118288
12. Tong J, Bandulwala HS, Clay BS, Anders RA, Shilling RA, Balachandran DD, et al. Fas-positive T cells regulate the resolution of airway inflammation in a murine model of asthma. *J Exp Med.* (2006) 203:1173–84. doi: 10.1084/jem.20051680
13. Rescigno M, Piguet V, Valzasina B, Lens S, Zubler R, French L, et al. Fas engagement induces the maturation of dendritic cells (DCs), the release of interleukin (IL)-1beta, and the production of interferon gamma in the absence of IL-12 during DC-T cell cognate interaction: a new role for Fas ligand in inflammatory responses. *J Exp Med.* (2000) 192:1661–8. doi: 10.1084/jem.192.11.1661
14. Meyer Zu Horste G, Przybylski D, Schramm MA, Wang C, Schnell A, Lee Y, et al. Fas promotes T Helper 17 cell differentiation and inhibits T Helper 1 cell development by binding and Sequestering Transcription Factor STAT1. *Immunity* (2018) 48:556–69 e7. doi: 10.1016/j.immuni.2018.03.008
15. Bien K, Zmigrodzka M, Orlowski P, Fruba A, Szymanski L, Stankiewicz W, et al. Involvement of Fas/FasL pathway in the murine model of atopic dermatitis. *Inflamm Res.* (2017) 66:679–90. doi: 10.1007/s00011-017-1049-z
16. Stewart SA, Dykxhoorn DM, Palliser D, Mizuno H, Yu EY, An DS, et al. Lentivirus-delivered stable gene silencing by RNAi in primary cells. *RNA* (2003) 9:493–501. doi: 10.1261/rna.2192803
17. Harris NL, Watt V, Ronchese F, Le Gros G. Differential T cell function and fate in lymph node and nonlymphoid tissues. *J Exp Med.* (2002) 195:317–26. doi: 10.1084/jem.20011558
18. Ji WJ, Ma YQ, Zhou X, Zhang YD, Lu RY, Sun HY, et al. Temporal and spatial characterization of mononuclear phagocytes in circulating, lung alveolar and interstitial compartments in a mouse model of bleomycin-induced pulmonary injury. *J Immunol Methods* (2014) 403:7–16. doi: 10.1016/j.jim.2013.11.012
19. Fulkerson PC, Fischetti CA, Hassman LM, Nikolaidis NM, Rothenberg ME. Persistent effects induced by IL-13 in the lung. *Am J Respir Cell Mol Biol.* (2006) 35:337–46. doi: 10.1165/rcmb.2005-0474OC
20. Kang Z, Swaidani S, Yin W, Wang C, Barlow JL, Gulen MF, et al. Epithelial cell-specific Act1 adaptor mediates interleukin-25-dependent helminth expulsion through expansion of Lin(-)c-Kit(+) innate cell population. *Immunity* (2012) 36:821–33. doi: 10.1016/j.immuni.2012.03.021
21. Zheng W, Flavell RA. The transcription factor GATA-3 is necessary and sufficient for Th2 cytokine gene expression in CD4 T cells. *Cell* (1997) 89:587–96.
22. Angkasekwinai P, Chang SH, Thapa M, Watarai H, Dong C. Regulation of IL-9 expression by IL-25 signaling. *Nat Immunol.* (2010) 11:250–6. doi: 10.1038/ni.1846
23. Slawek A, Maj T, Chelmonska-Soyta A. CD40, CD80, and CD86 costimulatory molecules are differentially expressed on murine splenic antigen-presenting cells during the pre-implantation period of pregnancy, and they modulate regulatory T-cell abundance, peripheral cytokine response, and pregnancy outcome. *Am J Reprod Immunol.* (2013) 70:116–26. doi: 10.1111/aji.12108
24. Bell BD, Kitajima M, Larson RP, Stoklasek TA, Dang K, Sakamoto K, et al. The transcription factor STAT5 is critical in dendritic cells for the development of TH2 but not TH1 responses. *Nat Immunol.* (2013) 14:364–71. doi: 10.1038/ni.2541
25. Huang G, Wang Y, Vogel P, Kanneganti TD, Otsu K, Chi H. Signaling via the kinase p38alpha programs dendritic cells to drive TH17 differentiation and autoimmune inflammation. *Nat Immunol.* (2012) 13:152–61. doi: 10.1038/ni.2207
26. Mesnil C, Raulier S, Paulissen G, Xiao X, Birrell MA, Pirottin D, et al. Lung-resident eosinophils represent a distinct regulatory eosinophil subset. *J Clin Invest.* (2016) 126:3279–95. doi: 10.1172/JCI85664
27. Holgate ST. Innate and adaptive immune responses in asthma. *Nat Med.* (2012) 18:673–83. doi: 10.1038/nm.2731
28. Lamhamedi-Cherradi SE, Martin RE, Ito T, Kheradmand F, Corry DB, Liu YJ, et al. Fungal proteases induce Th2 polarization through limited dendritic cell maturation and reduced production of IL-12. *J Immunol.* (2008) 180:6000–9. doi: 10.4049/jimmunol.180.9.6000
29. Lambrecht BN, De Veerman M, Coyle AJ, Gutierrez-Ramos JC, Thielemans K, Pauwels RA. Myeloid dendritic cells induce Th2 responses to inhaled antigen, leading to eosinophilic airway inflammation. *J Clin Invest.* (2000) 106:551–9. doi: 10.1172/JCI8107
30. Shao Z, Bharadwaj AS, McGee HS, Makinde TO, Agrawal DK. Fms-like tyrosine kinase 3 ligand increases a lung DC subset with regulatory properties in allergic airway inflammation. *J Allergy Clin Immunol.* (2009) 123:917–24.e2. doi: 10.1016/j.jaci.2009.01.052
31. Takagi T, Taguchi O, Toda M, Ruiz DB, Bernabe PG, D'Alessandro-Gabazza CN, et al. Inhibition of allergic bronchial asthma by Thrombomodulin is mediated by dendritic cells. *Am J Respir Critic Med.* (2011) 183:31–42. doi: 10.1164/rccm.201001-0107OC
32. Na H, Cho M, Chung Y. Regulation of Th2 cell immunity by dendritic cells. *Immune Network* (2016) 16:1–12. doi: 10.4110/in.2016.16.1.1
33. Guo Z, Zhang M, Tang H, Cao X. Fas signal links innate and adaptive immunity by promoting dendritic-cell secretion of CC and CXC chemokines. *Blood* (2005) 106:2033–41. doi: 10.1182/blood-2004-12-4831
34. Guo Z, Zhang M, An H, Chen W, Liu S, Guo J, et al. Fas ligation induces IL-1beta-dependent maturation and IL-1beta-independent survival of dendritic cells: different roles of ERK and NF-kappaB signaling pathways. *Blood* (2003) 102:4441–7. doi: 10.1182/blood-2002-11-3420
35. Kataoka T, Budd RC, Holler N, Thome M, Martinon F, Irmler M, et al. The caspase-8 inhibitor FLIP promotes activation of NF-kappaB and Erk signaling pathways. *Curr Biol.* (2000) 10:640–8. doi: 10.1016/S0960-9822(00)00512-1
36. van Rijt LS, Vos N, Willart M, Kleinjan A, Coyle AJ, Hoogsteden HC, et al. Essential role of dendritic cell CD80/CD86 costimulation in the induction, but not reactivation, of TH2 effector responses in a mouse model of asthma. *J Allergy Clin Immunol.* (2004) 114:166–73. doi: 10.1016/j.jaci.2004.03.044
37. Wu Q, Tang Y, Hu X, Wang Q, Lei W, Zhou L, et al. Regulation of Th1/Th2 balance through OX40/OX40L signalling by glycyrrhizic acid in a murine model of asthma. *Respirology* (2016) 21:102–11. doi: 10.1111/resp.12655
38. Lin YL, Chen SH, Wang JY. Critical role of IL-6 in dendritic cell-induced allergic inflammation of asthma. *J Mol Med.* (2015) 94:51–9. doi: 10.1007/s00109-015-1325-8

39. Laouini D, Alenius H, Bryce P, Oettgen H, Tsitsikov E, Geha RS. IL-10 is critical for Th2 responses in a murine model of allergic dermatitis. *J Clin Invest.* (2003) 112:1058–66. doi: 10.1172/Jci2003 18246
40. Zhang YL, Zhou XP, Zhou BH. DC-derived TSLP promotes Th2 polarization in LPS-primed allergic airway inflammation. *Eur J Immunol.* (2012) 42:1735–43. doi: 10.1002/eji.2011 42123
41. Tripathi P, Sahoo N, Ullah U, Kallionpaa H, Suneja A, Lahesmaa R, et al. A novel mechanism for ERK-dependent regulation of IL4 transcription during human Th2-cell differentiation. *Immunol Cell Biol.* (2012) 90:676–87. doi: 10.1038/icb.2011.87
42. Jin XX, Gong PT, Zhang XC, Li GJ, Zhu T, Zhang MG, et al. Activation of ERK signaling via TLR11 induces IL-12p40 production in peritoneal macrophages challenged by neospora caninum. *Front Microbiol.* (2017) 8:1393. doi: 10.3389/fmicb.2017.01393
43. Kroening PR, Barnes TW, Pease L, Limper A, Kita H, Vassall R. Cigarette smoke-induced oxidative stress suppresses generation of dendritic cell IL-12 and IL-23 through ERK-dependent pathways. *J Immunol.* (2008) 181:1536–47. doi: 10.4049/jimmunol.181.2.1536

13

ATP and its Metabolite Adenosine as Regulators of Dendritic Cell Activity

*Cinthia Silva-Vilches, Sabine Ring and Karsten Mahnke**

Department of Dermatology, Ruprecht-Karls-University Heidelberg, University Hospital, Heidelberg, Germany

Correspondence:
Karsten Mahnke
karsten.mahnke@med.uni-heidelberg.de

Adenosine (Ado) is a well-studied neurotransmitter, but it also exerts profound immune regulatory functions. Ado can (i) actively be released by various cells into the tissue environment and can (ii) be produced through the degradation of extracellular ATP by the concerted action of CD39 and CD73. In this sequence of events, the ectoenzyme CD39 degrades ATP into ADP and AMP, respectively, and CD73 catalyzes the last step leading to the production of Ado. Extracellular ATP acts as a "danger" signal and stimulates immune responses, i.e. by inflammasome activation. Its degradation product Ado on the other hand acts rather anti-inflammatory, as it down regulates functions of dendritic cells (DCs) and dampens T cell activation and cytokine secretion. Thus, the balance of proinflammatory ATP and anti-inflammatory Ado that is regulated by $CD39^+/CD73^+$ immune cells, is important for decision making on whether tolerance or immunity ensues. DCs express both ectoenzymes, enabling them to produce Ado from extracellular ATP by activity of CD73 and CD39 and thus allow dampening of the proinflammatory activity of adjacent leukocytes in the tissue. On the other hand, as most DCs express at least one out of four so far known Ado receptors (AdoR), DC derived Ado can also act back onto the DCs in an autocrine manner. This leads to suppression of DC functions that are normally involved in stimulating immune responses. Moreover, ATP and Ado production thereof acts as "find me" signal that guides cellular interactions of leukocytes during immune responses. In this review we will state the means by which Ado producing DCs are able to suppress immune responses and how extracellular Ado conditions DCs for their tolerizing properties.

Keywords: dendritic cells, adenosine, CD73, tolerance, ATP

ADENOSINE TRIPHOSPHATE (ATP) IN PERIPHERAL TISSUES

The chemical family of purines comprises of heterocyclic aromatic organic compounds, consisting of a pyrimidine ring fused to an imidazole ring. It comprehends biologically active molecules such as Adenosine-triphosphate (ATP) and its degradation product adenosine (Ado). ATP is widely known as an energy carrier within cells, but it can also be released from cells into the environment by cell membrane channels (gap junctions, pannexin channels) or specialized transporters (**Figure 1**) (1–4). Once located in the intercellular space, ATP transmits signals to other cells by engaging P2 receptors. P2 receptors can be divided into P2X and P2Y subtypes, which comprise different members as indicated by numbers, e.g., $P2X_1$ to $P2X_7$ and $P2Y_1$, $P2Y_2$, $P2Y_{11}$. While all P2X receptors bind ATP, only the $P2Y_1$, $P2Y_2$, and $P2Y_{11}$ receptors are engaged by ATP. The mode of action of P2X and P2Y receptors differs also and can be described as ionotropic for P2X receptors, or metabotropic G-protein coupled in case of P2Y types. The $P2X_7$ receptor is a well-studied example and serves as prototypic ATP receptor in many investigations. P2X receptors often form multimeric complexes that upon engagement open a pore for cations such as Na^+, Ca^{2+}, or K^+ (5). This ion flux will then induce further intracellular signaling events. The most important pathway triggered by P2X receptors involves activation of the NLRP3 inflammasome, leading to caspase-1 activation, which in turn activates interleukin (IL-) 1β and IL-18, two important pro inflammatory cytokines. But this is only one well studied example. In particular the transmembrane flux of Ca^{2+} ions can trigger multiple signaling events in cells involving mitogen activated kinases (MAPK), protein kinase C (PKC) and calmodulin. Therefore, many more effects of ATP induced signaling in leukocytes have been described These comprise the activation of T cells, (6–8), the release of IL-6, TNF (9, 10), prostaglandin (11), CXCL8, CCL2, CCL3 (12, 13) and metalloproteinase 9 (14), just to name a few [comprehensive list in Zimmermann. (15)]. The $P2Y_1$ receptor, which is binds ATP in rodents and the $P2Y_2$ receptor act via Gq coupled receptors and phospholipase C. Downstream, the second messengers inositol 1,4,5-triphosphate (IP3) that signals further via intracellular Ca^{2+} levels and diacylglycerol (DAC), which activates PKC, are produced. This rather general activation scheme illustrates the diverse groups of effects that can be induced by P2Y receptor engagement. Indeed, involvement of P2Y receptors in regulating hormone release and CNS activity has been documented in many instances. Beyond that, P2Y receptors are expressed by neutrophils, monocytes and T cells, indicating a role for immune regulation as well.

Due to the potent immune stimulatory actions of ATP, the extracellular concentrations are kept in check by enzymatic digestion of ATP. ATP is degraded fast within tissues, making it difficult to investigate its controlled release in defined organs *in vivo*. However, as skin is assessable for manipulation and measurement of ATP (16) and harbors several phenotypically distinct DC subtypes (17), it may be an organ of choice for investigating purine mediated signaling *in vivo*. At first, under non-inflammatory conditions the initial differentiation of skin keratinocytes (KCs) is guided by ATP. Upon binding of ATP the intracellular calcium levels rise gradually (as KCs express different subsets of ATP-specific P2X receptors depending on the layer), inducing the differentiation of the KCs (18, 19). Even the terminal differentiation and subsequent apoptosis of KC in the junction between stratum granulosum and stratum corneum seems to be dependent on ATP. Here, extensive colocalization of $P2X_7$ receptors with caspase-3 is evident (20), suggesting induction of cell death by ATP. This is corroborated by *in vitro* data, showing that prolonged engagement of $P2X_7$ receptors leads to extended pore-opening enabling even macromolecules of up to 900 Da to travel into cells, leading to induction of

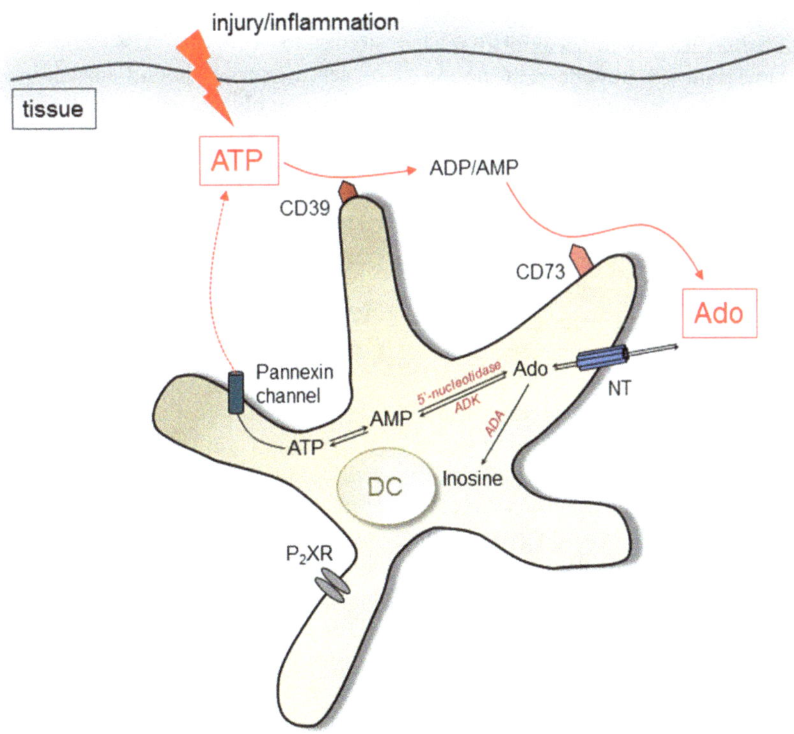

FIGURE 1 | Pathways of ATP/Ado generation in DCs. Intracellular Ado can be produced by degradation of AMP by 5′ectonucleotidases. Nucleoside transporters (NT) lead to extrusion of Ado. ATP can be released by cells via pannexin channels after injury and during inflammation, acting immune stimulatory by engagement of P2X receptors (P2XR). It can be degraded by the ectoenzymes CD39 and CD73, resulting in increased levels of Ado in the extracellular environment. Ado can be degraded by action of the enzyme Adenosine deaminase (ADA) intra- and extracellularly.

caspase-dependent cell death (21). Beyond serving as messenger involved in skin differentiation, ATP has also clear functions as a danger molecule. Due to its function as activator of the NLRP3 inflammasome, ATP is involved in triggering skin allograft rejection. Here it has been shown that ATP is released by host cells in response to transplantation leading to IL-18 production and Th1 responses. Moreover, the skin may "use" ATP even to alert the peripheral immune system, as monocytes during acute rejection of transplants exhibited higher expression of $P2X_7$ receptors (22). Skin, as opposed to most other organs, is exposed to UV irradiation. This causes DNA damage, which produces a special set of danger signals. In response to UV irradiation, ATP is released by KCs triggering activation and release of IL-17 by dendritic epidermal $\gamma\delta$ T cells (23). Once activated, $\gamma\delta$ T cells can release ATP by themselves, leading to an autocrine activation loop maintained by $P2X_4$ receptors (24). Functionally this sustained production of IL-17 is of importance for limiting adverse effects of UV, as it upregulates genes necessary for DNA-damage repair, such as TNF-related weak inducer of apoptosis (TWEAK) and the growth arrest gene GADD45 (23). Therefore, in case of UV induced cancers, therapeutic enhancement of extracellular ATP may offer a way for treatment.

Also in chronically diseased skin the distribution of ATP and its receptors change. For instance, in psoriatic plaques $P2X_7$ receptors were found to be upregulated in the basal cell layer, suggesting that activation of KCs is facilitated by ATP (25). ATP is indeed elevated under pathological conditions, as it can be released by IFNγ activated and/or dying leukocytes and KCs (26, 27). Moreover, early results demonstrated defective hydrolysis of ATP in the psoriatic epidermis, leading to accumulation of extracellular ATP in the diseased skin, which supports the notion that ATP is profoundly involved in development of psoriasis (28). These early studies were recently confirmed by Killeen et al. (29), showing in the dermis of psoriatic lesions in a skin explant model elevated expression of $P2X_7$ receptors as compared to healthy skin. This increased $P2X_7$ signaling lead also to a phenotype of skin-DCs that predominantly induced Th17 cells, which are the main drivers of psoriasis. Finally, the elevated ATP concentrations in skin can also activate neutrophils, which in conjunction with IL-23, form a local inflammatory circuit maintaining psoriasiform dermatitis in mice (30). Therefore, increased levels of ATP together with enhanced expression of ATP receptors seem to be involved in maintaining an inflammatory environment in psoriatic skin.

On the other hand counter regulatory mechanisms directly related to the degradation product of ATP, i.e., Ado, have been described too. For instance, chronically stimulated epidermal KCs have an altered expression pattern of different Ado receptor (AdoR) types, with the rather pro-proliferative acting A_2A receptor upregulated and reduced expression of the inhibitory A_2B receptor (31). These and other observations led to investigations that utilize topical application of AdoR agonists for the treatment of psoriasis. Indeed, engagement of the AdoR A_3 leads to reduced production of IL-17 and IL-23 in KCs of psoriatic patients, inducing amelioration of the disease (32, 33). Therefore, several drugs acting as agonist for different types of AdoR are currently used in clinical trials of skin- and other inflammatory diseases (34, 35). But not only in inflammatory diseases ATP plays a role, it is also important for induction of acute inflammation in skin. Weber et al. have shown that skin DCs without functioning $P2X_7$ receptors are unable to sensitize T cell responses, indicating a role for directed ATP release as mediator of innate immune reactions (16). At the same time it became clear that haptens only act as trigger for hypersensitivity reactions when they induce release of ATP. Therefore, even experimental attempts were made to predict the "allergic potential" of chemicals by their ability to induce ATP release in KC cultures (36).

ATP as Substrate for Adenosine Production

A major degradation product of ATP is Ado, which can be generated intracellularly as well as extracellularly. Ado derives from the dephosphorylation of ATP, catalyzed by different enzymes: the ectonucleoside triphosphate diphosphohydrolase 1 (CD39) and the ecto-5'-nucleotidase (CD73) (37, 38). Both enzymes act sequentially in degrading extracellular ATP to adenosine. In a first step CD39 converts ATP to adenosine-di-phosphate and adenosine-mono-phosphate. In a second step the action of CD73 clips off the last remaining phosphate group, producing Ado (39). Ado can be released by nucleoside transporters from the cytoplasm of cells (4), however, the extracellular degradation of ATP by CD39 and CD73 is thought to provide the major pathway for regulating extracellular Ado concentrations. Its degradation is accomplished by adenosine deaminase (ADA), which exists in intra- as well as extracellular forms (40, 41). Extracellular ADA can bind to CD26 (42). Thus, similar to ATP and ADP, Ado can be degraded to inosine by cell membrane bound enzymes. In summary, the regulated destruction of extracellular ATP to Ado by enzymatic digestions offers cells a possibility to shape the tissue environment from a pro-inflammatory (high concentrations of free ATP) to a rather immunosuppressive (elevated levels of Ado) ambiance (43). As DCs express CD39 and/or CD73 as well as AdoR, they actively participate in immune responses affected by Ado (**Figure 1**).

Regulation of Extracellular Ado and ATP Concentrations

In light of the opposing functions of the two mutually transformable signaling molecules ATP (activating) and Ado (suppressing) on immune reactions, their temporal/spatial distribution in tissues or along the plasma membranes of cells is of importance. Cells will presumably integrate activating (ATP) and suppressive (Ado) signaling pathways rendering a "final" outcome. Therefore, the half live as well as the diffusion speed through tissues is a critical factor determining the effects of ATP/Ado signaling. Real "in tissue" data of the distribution of extracellular ATP or Ado, respectively, are hardly available. However, contents in body fluids or organ cultures can be measured. For instance, in dog as well as human plasma Ado is only stable for a few seconds (44), making it a "short range" molecule. This rapid degradation may be useful to prevent a generalized immune suppression and it further prevents Ado from reaching the central nervous system, where it acts as neurotransmitter (45) and elevated levels may therefore disturb nerve functions. Moreover, a short half-life makes Ado a more defined tool for cellular communication. Because only cells that harbor CD73 on their surfaces are able to produce sufficient amounts of Ado that then acts locally by engaging AdoR of adjacent cells. This mechanism may in particular of importance for tolerance induction, as Ado production by CD73 expressing DCs is required during the intimate DC:T cell priming process in order to render T cells tolerant (own unpublished results). Finally, to regulate Ado concentrations in relation to ATP not only the half-life is important, also the regulation of expression of the Ado producing ectoenzyme CD73 provides a means to fine tune the extracellular Ado content. During ischemic preconditioning expression of CD73 is induced within 30 min (46), greatly enhancing the extracellular Ado concentration in tissues and thereby overcoming the degradation by ADA.

For ATP biosensors are available (47) making is more feasible to monitor extracellular ATP content in cell culture settings. The reported half live of ATP varies from up 2–20 min depending on the organ and the methods used (48–51). Of note, in the immune system ATP actions are rather fast, as neutrophils show a burst of ATP release for only 5 s after being stimulated with fMLP (52). However, these data are once more obtained in *in vitro* culture systems, which differ from the *in situ* situation, but after all these data give an impression on the speed and range of ATP or Ado signaling. It provides evidence that Ado may not act "cytokine-like" with distribution via the blood stream and exerting action(s) in tissues far from its origin.

EFFECTS OF Ado ON DCs

Expression of Ado Receptors by DCs

Four Ado Receptors (AdoR) are known so far (A_1, A_2A, A_2B, and A_3). Structurally they all belong to G-protein-coupled-receptors (GPCRs), but their intracellular signaling differs (**Figure 2**). In general the A_2 receptor types are $G_{\alpha s}$-protein coupled receptors, with the A_2B receptor additionally signaling via Gαq. In cells an activated G protein complex forms at the inner leaflet of the cell membrane after Ado engagement, which leads to activation of the adenylate cyclase (AC) and to rising cAMP levels (in case of $G_{\alpha s}$). As a consequence protein kinase A (PKA) is activated as secondary effector. On a molecular level this can directly be counteracted by engagement of A_1 or A_3 AdoR, which signal via $G_{\alpha i}/G_{\alpha q}$ complexes. Among them, the $G_{\alpha i/o}$ complex inhibits AC activity and thus dampens A_2 mediated signaling. The main signal transduction of A1 and A3 receptors downstream of G proteins is mediated by phospholipase C induced secondary messengers that ultimately leads to increased Ca^{2+} levels and PKC activation. Thus, a different secondary effector is induced by A_1 and A_3 AdoR, resulting in activation of different sets of genes. But nevertheless, even here a crosstalk with the A_2B receptors is possible, as A_2B AdoR via its coupling to $G_{\alpha q}$ can feed into the PLC mediated pathway and support A_1 and A_3 AdoR signaling (53, 54).

Many reports show expression of all four subtypes of AdoR by DCs in varying degrees (55, 56). However, the levels of expression and their distribution among defined subset of DC remain uncertain. When analysing the available data on AdoR expression by DCs at a glance it becomes clear that AdoR expression correlates with the maturation status of DC. Human immature DC express A_1 and A_3 AdoR, which after engagement activate and recruit DCs to inflammatory sites (57). Upon maturation A_2 AdoR emerge in DCs, now triggering rather inhibitory effects such as reduced secretion of IL-6, IL-12, and IFNγ (58). Here, differential expression of AdoR by DCs serves the purpose of regulating inflammatory processes. I.e., in the beginning of an insult, immature DCs are rendered active and are recruited to the inflammatory site whereas later A_2-type AdoR expression limits over boarding inflammatory reactions. However, with several ways of cross talk between AdoR (as described above), differential expression by different cell types as well as varying affinities for purines, it is nearly impossible to assign one defined effect on cell physiology to the sole action of one AdoR or to one ligand *in vivo*. But *in vitro* studies can at least give insight into general pathways modulated by Ado.

Effects of Ado on Functions of DCs

Despite the fact that four different AdoR can activate different pathways at the same time that may have opposite effects on immune cell activation, many reports unequivocally demonstrate immune suppressive actions of Ado on DCs. In particular cAMP elevating AdoR A_2A and A_2B mediate rather inhibitory functions in DCs (53). For instance, after stimulation of respective AdoR *in vitro*, human DCs downmodulate secretion of IL-12 and TNFα. The cells expressed low amounts of MHC class II and were functionally impaired in stimulating proliferation of allogenic T cells. Further parameters of DC activation such as CXCL10, CCL2 and CCL12 secretion were also downregulated by Ado (56, 59–62). All of these features are indicators for a less mature phenotype of DC, which can be regarded as a tolerogenic type of DC (63).

In an even broader context a $CD73^+$ cellular environment may be important to keep DC in "steady state" condition. *In vivo* genetic ablation of CD73 in mice leads to enhanced inflammatory reactions in a contact hypersensitivity model that is driven by increased migration of skin DCs to peripheral lymph nodes (64). Moreover, when analyzing the expression of T cell costimulatory molecules by different DC subsets after application of the hapten TNCB, we found increased expression of CD86 in subsets of skin DCs in CD73 deficient as compared to control mice. These data are further corroborated by findings using stimulation or blockade of Ado deaminase (ADA), an enzyme that is crucial for degradation of extracellular Ado. ADA is expressed by DCs during ongoing inflammation to degrade CD73 derived Ado and to maintain their hyper-reactive state (65). In contrast, in absence of ADA Ado levels in cellular environments are increased, as a consequence tolerogenic functions of DCs are enhanced (60). Moreover, addition of ADA to DC:T cell cultures, which leads to depletion of Ado from the cellular environment, enhanced priming of effector T cells and suppressed induction of Treg (66). In aggregate, adequate levels of extracellular Ado in peripheral tissues may be of importance to prevent overshooting DC activity

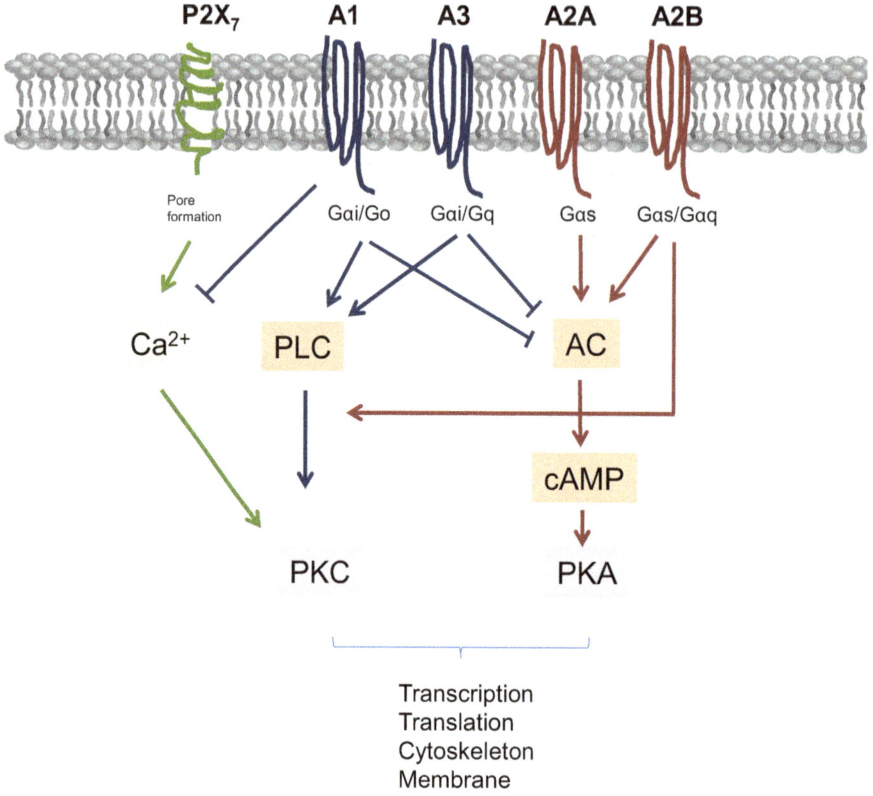

FIGURE 2 | Scheme of major pathways and interconnections of AdoR and $P2X_7$ ATP receptors. All receptors signal through G proteins. Different types of G proteins determine the further outcome. Briefly, A2A and A2B AdoR elevate adenylyl cyclase (AC) leading to activation of protein kinase A (PKA) through elevated cAMP levels. AC and thus cAMP is suppressed by A1 and A3 AdoR engagement, which themselves signal via phospholipase C (PLC) and proteinkinase C (PKC). However, raising Ca^{2+} levels, which transmit a $P2X_7$ derived signal are blocked by A1 AdoR. Finally, A2B AdoR can augment signals derived from A1 and A3 as it stimulates Ca^{2+} mediated PKC activation also.

and to maintain their "steady state," which has been shown to be crucial for the tolerogenic function of DCs (67).

But beyond the mere prevention of DC maturation by Ado, the DC phenotype may be impacted in more fundamental ways. For example engagement of A_2 AdoR in DCs enables them to actively suppress immune reactions. The mechanisms include the stimulation of IL-10 secretion or the upregulation of T cell inhibitory molecules such as B7H1, resulting in tolerant T cells as their proper activation by DCs is impaired (62, 68, 69).

Even "imprinting" tolerogenic functions in DCs has been attributed to AdoR engagement. Li et al. (70) were able to attenuate acute kidney injury by infusing DCs pretreated *ex vivo* with A_2A AdoR agonists. This phenotype of Ado tolerogenic DCs was stable for more than a week and its action *in vivo* relies on impeding NKT cell activation by a so far unknown mechanism. AdoR expression can also be intrinsically upregulated by already immunosuppressive DC subtypes to bolster their immunoregulatory functions. For instance, in a tolerogenic pediatric DC subtype, IL-10 is upregulated after Fc receptor mediated stimulation along with increased expression of the A_2A AdoR, which after Engagement further augments their IL-10 production (71). Thus, A_2A AdoR expression helps to reinforce the immunosuppressive capacity of the DCs.

SIGNALING OF AdoR IN DCs

The Molecular Mechanisms of cAMP in DCs

The main intracellular suppressive pathways triggered by A_2 AdoR types involve cAMP as a second messenger. Roughly, both A_2-type AdoR elevate cAMP levels by activating Adenylyl Cylase (AC). Further downstream cAMP signals via PKA that regulates gene transcription via NF-κB, HIF-1α and CREB. In addition, A_2B AdoR also acts on PLC, inducing raising intracellular Ca^{2+} levels.

In a recent transcriptomic approach performed in bone marrow derived DCs (72), elevated activity of AC was connected to both, inhibition of AKT signaling and to activation of PKA (**Figure 3**). PKA has relevance for host defense capacities, as inhibition of Salt induced kinases (SIK) by cAMP-activated and PKA-mediated phosphorylation was shown to suppress secretion of the pro-inflammatory cytokines IL-6, IL-12, and TNFα by DCs and macrophages (73–75). Moreover, one of the SIK targets is the CREB-regulated transcription co-activator 3 (CRTC3) that can be phosphorylated at several serine residues. Phosphorylation of CRTC3 is inhibited by the cAMP-activated PKA, leading to translocation of the

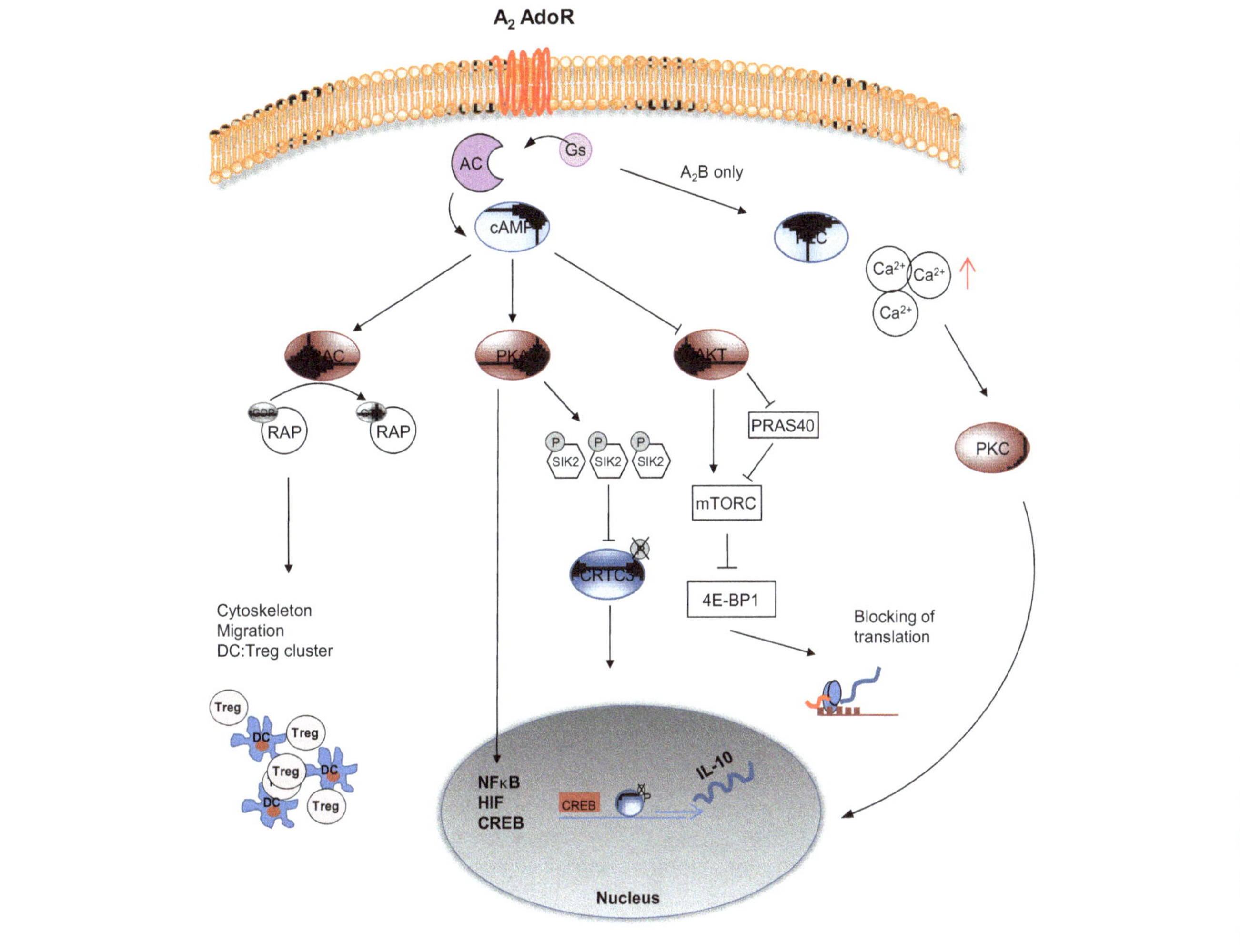

FIGURE 3 | cAMP mediated intracellular signaling of A2 AdoR. A2A and A2B AdoR activate adenylyl cyclase and elevate cAMP levels. The A2B AdoR can concomitantly activate Phospholipase C (PLC), thereby triggering elevated levels of free Calcium (Ca^{2+}). PKC mediated activation of NF-κB related gene expression follows. cAMP can suppress AKT activation leading to reduced mTORC activity either directly or via PRAS40. Without proper mTORC activity 4E-BP1 complex will terminate translation of proteins widely necessary for activation of cells. Additionally cAMP can signal via PKA, leading to hyper phosphorylation of Salt induced kinase (SIK) 2, allowing the phosphorylated transcription factor CRTC3 to cluster with CREB and to initiate translation of IL-10. Besides, further interaction of PKA with transcription factors such as NF-κB, HIF and CREB can induce "inhibitory" gene expression. A PKA independent pathway is mediated by EPAC, an enzyme that activates RAP via GTP binding, leading to profound changes in cytoskeleton and migration of DCs. As a result inhibitory DC:Treg clusters are formed and the immunological synapse may be changed in a tolerogenic fashion.

non-phosphorylated CRTC3 into the nucleus, where interaction with activated CREB upregulate IL-10 gene transcription (74).

In parallel to PKA activation, AKT activity is downregulated by elevated cAMP levels, promoting mTOR inhibition via PRAS40 (76). As a result, the downstream effectors of mTOR involved in the synthesis of cellular proteins, such as 4E-BP1 are hypophosphorylated. In this state, 4E-BP1 forms complexes with eukaryotic translation initiation factors and prevents translation (77). mTOR signaling regulation by AdoR driven cAMP content in DC may act as an important regulator of the antibacterial inflammatory response in monocytes, macrophages and primary dendritic cells (78, 79).

Effects of AdoR Triggered cAMP Levels on Phenotype and Function

Despite that AdoR triggered cAMP elevation has multiple molecular targets the overall effect is obvious, as several reports show clear induction of an immunocompromised and tolerogenic phenotype of DC by cAMP. This is indicated by reduced secretion of proinflammatory cytokines, reduced expression of MHC class-II but elevated secretion of IL-10. Also the capacity of DCs to prime $CD8^+$ T cells *in vitro* was impaired in DCs with elevated intracellular levels of cAMP after induction by Ado or defined AdoR agonists such as 5′-N-Ethylcarboxamidoadenosine (62, 68, 80–83). In turn, cAMP can feed back on AdoR expression. For example, high levels of cAMP induced by agents that trigger Gs-protein coupled receptors, upregulates expression of A_2 AdoR in PC12 tumor cells (84). This cycle may therefore vigorously enhance Ado mediated suppressive effects in cells, as cAMP triggered upregulation of AdoR provides a means that leads to an even more sustained cAMP production.

To further delineate the possible cAMP effects that are mediated by AdoR engagement, one can artificially raise the cAMP content in DCs with Cholera toxin to mimic A_2 AdoR triggering. This leads yet to another subtype of tolerogenic DCs, i.e., DCs that express both isoforms of the tolerogenic molecule cytotoxic T lymphocyte antigen 2 (CTLA-2α and CTLA-2β) (85). These DCs resembled a semi-mature state and were able to promote TGFβ-dependent Foxp3$^+$ "induced" Treg conversion. Of note expression of CTLA-2 was critical for this function as genetic downregulation by siRNA reduced Treg conversion, while addition of recombinant CTLA-2α increased Treg conversion *in vitro*. Finally, when Lee et al. (81) investigated the role of DCs in priming of Th2 cells, they showed that deletion of genes that encode the GTP binding protein Gαs, leads to decreased cAMP signaling in DCs and provokes Th2 T cells with a prominent allergic phenotype. In contrast, increases in cAMP levels inhibited these responses. These findings imply that G protein-coupled receptors in DCs, such as A_2 AdoR, which are natural regulators of cAMP formation, can prevent Th2-mediated immunopathologies by rendering DCs unable to induce potent Th2 answers.

Another major pathway induced by rising cAMP levels, but independent from PKA, depends on the exchange protein EPAC. Upon cAMP mediated activation, EPAC catalyzes the GTP binding of RAP1, a major regulator of the cytoskeleton. Via this axis cAMP seems to affect cell motility, cell adhesion, chemotaxis and phagocytosis (86). For DCs in particular it has been shown that Ado released by Treg is responsible for attracting them (mediated by an EPAC-RAP dependent pathway), leading to formation of DC:Treg aggregates (87). In these aggregates DC undergo "tolerogenic instruction," as they start to produce IL-10, upregulate T cell inhibitory molecules and simultaneously downregulate expression of MHC class II molecules. Moreover, even the directed induction of DC:Treg clusters themselves may serve immunosuppressive functions, as Onishi et al. (88) have shown that Treg insolate effector T cells from proper activation by DCs by simply outcompeting them and keeping DCs in clusters.

Priming of T Cells by DCs in Presence of Ado Is Altered

Despite the many well documented and long lasting effects of AdoR engagement on function of isolated DCs, the immediate presence of Ado during initial DC:T cell contact is crucially affecting the resulting immune response. For instance, *in vitro* engagement of A_2A AdoR during the cognate MHC:peptide (as presented by DCs) T cell interaction leads to induction of T cell anergy and not to activation of T cells that normally ensues after DC:T cell interaction (89). This effect seems to be dependent on altered signaling in T cells, as reduced activation of the MAPK pathway was observed under these conditions. Ado:DC induced anergic T cells are not only refractory to restimulation, they also develop a CD25$^-$ LAG3$^+$ "regulatory" phenotype that actively prevents autoimmunity. Thus, the initial tolerogenic effects of Ado during antigen presentation by DCs will further be disseminated into tissues by these induced "regulatory" T cells.

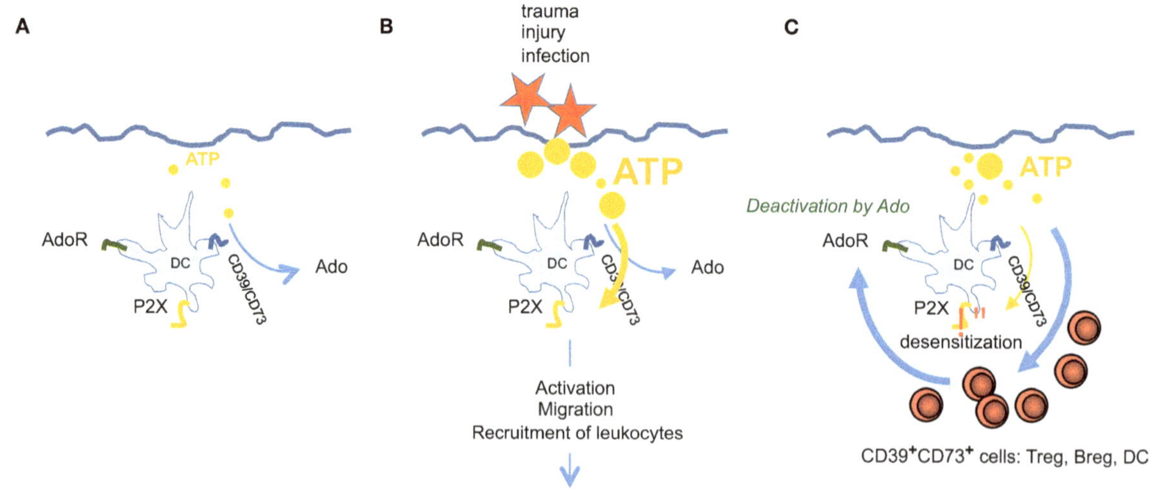

FIGURE 4 | ATP and Ado are involved in regulating tissue inflammation. Exemplary for skin it is shown that **(A)** during steady state only trace amounts of ATP, derived from cellular detritus, are present. ATP will be degraded immediately by CD39/CD73^{high} Langerhans cells. **(B)** After injury high amounts of ATP are set free, which cannot be degraded effectively and overrule Ado production. This stimulates DCs via $P2X_7$ receptors, leading to activation, to migration and to recruitment of different subsets of leukocytes. **(C)** When infection goes on, more CD39/CD73 expressing leukocytes are entering the tissue and $P2X_7$ signaling ceases due to receptor desensitization and by counteraction of Ado. ATP is degraded to Ado which now prevails and terminates effector functions of various immune cells. Thus, immune homeostasis is reestablished.

As DCs can express CD73 themselves, production of extracellular Ado by DCs is conceivable and regulated expression of CD73 by DC subsets may one way to tune DC function for either tolerance (high CD73) or immunity (low CD73). Indeed, in a skin model for contact hypersensitivity application of the tolerogen 2,4-dinitrothiocyanobenzene (DNTB) rendered mice tolerant toward sensitization with the hapten 2,4-dinitrofluorobenzene (DNFB) (90). We found that induction of tolerance with DNTB was accompanied by increased expression of CD73 by skin migrating DCs and of note, in CD73 deficient animals tolerance induction by DNTB ceased (unpublished data). This underlines the importance of tissue derived Ado in governing DC functions under inflammatory conditions.

The Complex Regulation of ATP–Ado Signaling During Inflammation

As DCs can express all four AdoR, the ectonucleotidases CD39/CD73 as well as $P2X_7$ receptors, disentangling the ATP and Ado effects is very complex (91). It becomes even more complicated, as the different receptors transmit either stimulatory or suppressive signals, differ in their affinity for the respective ligands and are expressed to different degrees. The well investigated example of ATP induced chemotaxis of neutrophils gives an example how important the actual physical distribution of the different receptor molecules within a cell membrane is for their function. In neutrophils the chemotactic signal induced by fMLP is translated into ATP release by panx1. It will autocrinely act back on $P2Y_2$ receptors. At the same time stimulatory A_3 AdoR as well as CD39/CD73 are recruited to this part of the membrane, creating a local excitation circuit by activating PIP3, MAPK pathways and forming a "leading edge" for migration. A_2A AdoR are excluded from this membrane site and are accumulating at the "trailing edge." At the same time Ado, produced at the "leading edge" by activity of CD39/CD73, diffuses to the "back" of the cell and engages A2A receptors. This signal is transmitted by means of cAMP-PKA activation and suppresses the activation of the cell locally. As a result neutrophils are polarized and find their way along chemotactic gradients (92–94). Altogether this was an elaborative effort of several research groups and similar investigation can be done for DCs too. Here we are just at the beginning, just investigating broad effects of ATP/Ado on DC migration and DC activation, without knowing how the individual pathways are interconnected at a molecular level.

Nevertheless, in a simplified scheme one can consider ATP as rather stimulatory and proinflammatory, and Ado (A_2A and A_2B receptors elevating cAMP) as being immune suppressive. In that sense CD39/CD73 expressing DCs are key cell for modulating homeostasis and inflammation and both receptor types (for ATP and Ado) are required to actually "measure" the degree of immune suppression or activation, respectively (**Figure 4**). Under non inflammatory conditions "steady state" DCs are patrolling through different tissues (95, 96) and sense only trace amounts of ATP, as tissues are intact and only limited amounts of extracellular ATP are produced, for instance by apoptotic cells. To maintain this homoeostatic status, high expression of CD39/CD73 ensures efficient degradation of ATP, preventing activation of the immune system. Examples are Langerhans cells in the epidermis that are highly positive for CD39 and degrade ATP effectively (37). Only when infection, tumor growth or trauma lead to elevated levels of extracellular ATP, the activating properties prevail, despite the fact that Ado receptors are expressed also. ATP simply outnumbers Ado effects. Subsets of immature peripheral DCs are recruited by ATP (58, 97) and an immune response is initiated. But counter regulatory mechanisms are initiated at the same time. For instance $P2X_7$ receptors become refractory to repeated stimulation by high ATP concentrations (37), making the DCs insensible to ATP mediated activation (58). Moreover, recruitment of regulatory T cells to inflammatory sites, which express high levels of CD39 and CD73, accelerates the degradation of ATP to Ado (98, 99). So the balance tips toward an Ado enriched ambiance that progressively exerts anti-inflammatory functions. More Ado means reduced proinflammatory functions of DCs (69, 70, 81, 100, 101), less migration of DCs from tissue to lymph nodes (64) and increased induction of regulatory T cells (60, 63, 87, 89). Thus, slowly immune homeostasis is reestablished.

CONCLUSION

The turnover of extracellular ATP to Ado by cell bound CD39 and CD73 offers a possibility to shape the tissue environment from an inflammatory (ATP high) to an immune suppressive habitat. DCs participate in this process as they (i) express ATP degrading enzymes CD39 and CD73 and (ii) harbor AdoR. Therefore, immunosuppressive effects of Ado can be mediated in two ways by DCs: First, DC derived Ado suppresses activation of T cells and fosters the induction of anergic and/or regulatory T cells during the cognate DC:T cell interactions. Secondly, Ado derived from adjacent cells act on DCs, preventing DC maturation and development of effector functions. These steady state DCs are considered tolerogenic. Thus, an Ado enriched tissue environment may be of importance to maintain the "steady state" of DCs to prevent autoimmunity.

AUTHOR CONTRIBUTIONS

CS-V and SR contributed equally. SR prepared figures and CS-V performed experiments. All authors wrote the paper.

REFERENCES

1. Seminario-Vidal L, Okada SF, Sesma JI, Kreda SM, Van Heusden CA, Zhu Y, et al. Rho signaling regulates pannexin 1-mediated ATP release from airway epithelia. *J Biol Chem.* (2011) 286:26277–86. doi: 10.1074/jbc.M111.260562
2. Onami K, Kimura Y, Ito Y, Yamauchi T, Yamasaki K, Aiba S. Nonmetal haptens induce ATP release from keratinocytes through opening of pannexin hemichannels by reactive oxygen species. *J Invest Dermatol.* (2014) 134:1951–60. doi: 10.1038/jid.2014.93
3. Dosch M, Gerber J, Jebbawi F, Beldi G. Mechanisms of ATP release by inflammatory cells. *Int J Mol Sci.* (2018) 19:E1222. doi: 10.3390/ijms19041222
4. Pastor-Anglada M, Perez-Torras S. Who is who in adenosine transport. *Front Pharmacol.* (2018) 9:627. doi: 10.3389/fphar.2018.00627
5. Browne LE, Compan V, Bragg L, North RA. P2X7 receptor channels allow direct permeation of nanometer-sized dyes. *J Neurosci.* (2013) 33:3557–66. doi: 10.1523/JNEUROSCI.2235-12.2013
6. Schenk U, Westendorf AM, Radaelli E, Casati A, Ferro M, Fumagalli M, et al. Purinergic control of T cell activation by ATP released through pannexin-1 hemichannels. *Sci Signal* (2008) 1:ra6. doi: 10.1126/scisignal.1160583
7. Yip L, Woehrle T, Corriden R, Hirsh M, Chen Y, Inoue Y, et al. Autocrine regulation of T-cell activation by ATP release and P2X7 receptors. *FASEB J.* (2009) 23:1685–93. doi: 10.1096/fj.08-126458
8. Woehrle T, Yip L, Elkhal A, Sumi Y, Chen Y, Yao Y, et al. Pannexin-1 hemichannel-mediated ATP release together with P2X1 and P2X4 receptors regulate T-cell activation at the immune synapse. *Blood* (2010) 116:3475–84. doi: 10.1182/blood-2010-04-277707
9. Yoshida H, Kobayashi D, Ohkubo S, Nakahata N. ATP stimulates interleukin-6 production via P2Y receptors in human HaCaT keratinocytes. *Eur J Pharmacol.* (2006) 540:1–9. doi: 10.1016/j.ejphar.2006.04.008
10. Inoue K, Hosoi J, Denda M. Extracellular ATP has stimulatory effects on the expression and release of IL-6 via purinergic receptors in normal human epidermal keratinocytes. *J Invest Dermatol.* (2007) 127:362–71. doi: 10.1038/sj.jid.5700526
11. Cheng SE, Lee IT, Lin CC, Wu WL, Hsiao LD, Yang CM. ATP mediates NADPH oxidase/ROS generation and COX-2/PGE2 expression in A549 cells: role of P2 receptor-dependent STAT3 activation. *PLoS ONE* (2013) 8:e54125. doi: 10.1371/journal.pone.0054125
12. Kataoka A, Tozaki-Saitoh H, Koga Y, Tsuda M, Inoue K. Activation of P2X7 receptors induces CCL3 production in microglial cells through transcription factor NFAT. *J Neurochem.* (2009) 108:115–25. doi: 10.1111/j.1471-4159.2008.05744.x
13. Shieh CH, Heinrich A, Serchov T, Van Calker D, Biber K. P2X7-dependent, but differentially regulated release of IL-6, CCL2, and TNF-alpha in cultured mouse microglia. *Glia* (2014) 62:592–607. doi: 10.1002/glia.22628
14. Gu BJ, Wiley JS. Rapid ATP-induced release of matrix metalloproteinase 9 is mediated by the P2X7 receptor. *Blood* (2006) 107:4946–53. doi: 10.1182/blood-2005-07-2994
15. Zimmermann H. Extracellular ATP and other nucleotides-ubiquitous triggers of intercellular messenger release. *Purinergic Signal* (2016) 12:25–57. doi: 10.1007/s11302-015-9483-2
16. Weber FC, Esser PR, Muller T, Ganesan J, Pellegatti P, Simon MM, et al. Lack of the purinergic receptor P2X(7) results in resistance to contact hypersensitivity. *J Exp Med.* (2010) 207:2609–19. doi: 10.1084/jem.20092489
17. Henri S, Guilliams M, Poulin LF, Tamoutounour S, Ardouin L, Dalod M, et al. Disentangling the complexity of the skin dendritic cell network. *Immunol Cell Biol.* (2010) 88:366–75. doi: 10.1038/icb.2010.34
18. Sharpe GR, Gillespie JI, Greenwell JR. An increase in intracellular free calcium is an early event during differentiation of cultured human keratinocytes. *FEBS Lett.* (1989) 254:25–8. doi: 10.1016/0014-5793(89)81002-6
19. Suter MM, Crameri FM, Slattery JP, Millard PJ, Gonzalez FA. Extracellular ATP and some of its analogs induce transient rises in cytosolic free calcium in individual canine keratinocytes. *J Invest Dermatol.* (1991) 97, 223–229. doi: 10.1111/1523-1747.ep12480162
20. Greig AV, Linge C, Terenghi G, Mcgrouther DA, Burnstock G. Purinergic receptors are part of a functional signaling system for proliferation and differentiation of human epidermal keratinocytes. *J Invest Dermatol.* (2003) 120:1007–15. doi: 10.1046/j.1523-1747.2003.12261.x
21. Di Virgilio F, Schmalzing G, Markwardt F. The Elusive P2X7 Macropore. *Trends Cell Biol.* (2018) 28:392–404 doi: 10.1016/j.tcb.2018.01.005
22. Amores-Iniesta J, Barbera-Cremades M, Martinez CM, Pons JA, Revilla-Nuin B, Martinez-Alarcon L, et al. Extracellular ATP activates the NLRP3 inflammasome and is an early danger signal of skin allograft rejection. *Cell Rep.* (2017) 21:3414–26. doi: 10.1016/j.celrep.2017.11.079
23. Macleod AS, Rudolph R, Corriden R, Ye I, Garijo O, Havran WL. Skin-resident T cells sense ultraviolet radiation-induced injury and contribute to DNA repair. *J Immunol.* (2014) 192:5695–702. doi: 10.4049/jimmunol.1303297
24. Manohar M, Hirsh MI, Chen Y, Woehrle T, Karande AA, Junger WG. ATP release and autocrine signaling through P2X4 receptors regulate gammadelta T cell activation. *J Leukoc Biol.* (2012) 92:787–94. doi: 10.1189/jlb.0312121
25. Tran JN, Pupovac A, Taylor RM, Wiley JS, Byrne SN, Sluyter R. Murine epidermal Langerhans cells and keratinocytes express functional P2X7 receptors. *Exp Dermatol.* (2010) 19:e151–7. doi: 10.1111/j.1600-0625.2009.01029.x
26. Pastore S, Mascia F, Gulinelli S, Forchap S, Dattilo C, Adinolfi E, et al. Stimulation of purinergic receptors modulates chemokine expression in human keratinocytes. *J Invest Dermatol.* (2007) 127:660–7. doi: 10.1038/sj.jid.5700591
27. Ishimaru M, Tsukimoto M, Harada H, Kojima S. Involvement of P2Y(1)(1) receptor in IFN-gamma-induced IL-6 production in human keratinocytes. *Eur J Pharmacol.* (2013) 703:67–73. doi: 10.1016/j.ejphar.2013.02.020
28. Mahrle G, Orfanos CE. Decreased membrane-bound ATP-hydrolytic activity in psoriatic epidermis. *Br J Dermatol.* (1974) 91:529–40. doi: 10.1111/j.1365-2133.1974.tb12941.x
29. Killeen ME, Ferris L, Kupetsky EA, Falo L Jr, Mathers AR. Signaling through purinergic receptors for ATP induces human cutaneous innate and adaptive Th17 responses: implications in the pathogenesis of psoriasis. *J Immunol.* (2013) 190:4324–36. doi: 10.4049/jimmunol.1202045
30. Diaz-Perez JA, Killeen ME, Yang Y, Carey CD, Falo LD Jr, Mathers AR. Extracellular ATP and IL-23 form a local inflammatory circuit leading to the development of a neutrophil-dependent psoriasiform dermatitis. *J Invest Dermatol.* (2018). doi: 10.1016/j.jid.2018.05.018. [Epub ahead of print].
31. Andres RM, Terencio MC, Arasa J, Paya M, Valcuende-Cavero F, Navalon P, et al. Adenosine A2A and A2B receptors differentially modulate keratinocyte proliferation: possible deregulation in psoriatic epidermis. *J Invest Dermatol.* (2017) 137:123–31. doi: 10.1016/j.jid.2016.07.028
32. Cohen S, Barer F, Itzhak I, Silverman MH, Fishman P. Inhibition of IL-17 and IL-23 in human keratinocytes by the A3 adenosine receptor agonist piclidenoson. *J Immunol Res.* (2018) 2018:2310970. doi: 10.1155/2018/2310970
33. Jacobson KA, Merighi S, Varani K, Borea PA, Baraldi S, Aghazadeh Tabrizi M, et al. A3 adenosine receptors as modulators of inflammation: from medicinal chemistry to therapy. *Med Res Rev.* (2018) 38:1031–72. doi: 10.1002/med.21456
34. Gessi S, Merighi S, Borea PA. Targeting adenosine receptors to prevent inflammatory skin diseases. *Exp Dermatol.* (2014) 23:553–4. doi: 10.1111/exd.12474
35. Merighi S, Borea PA, Varani K, Gessi S. Deregulation of adenosine receptors in psoriatic epidermis: an option for therapeutic treatment. *J Invest Dermatol.* (2017) 137:11–3. doi: 10.1016/j.jid.2016.08.001
36. Mizumoto N, Mummert ME, Shalhevet D, Takashima A. Keratinocyte ATP release assay for testing skin-irritating potentials of structurally diverse chemicals. *J Invest Dermatol.* (2003) 121:1066–72 doi: 10.1046/j.1523-1747.2003.12558.x
37. Mizumoto N, Kumamoto T, Robson SC, Sevigny J, Matsue H, Enjyoji K, et al. CD39 is the dominant Langerhans cell-associated ecto-NTPDase: modulatory roles in inflammation and immune responsiveness. *Nat Med.* (2002) 8:358–65. doi: 10.1038/nm0402-358
38. Romio M, Reinbeck B, Bongardt S, Huls S, Burghoff S, Schrader J. Extracellular purine metabolism and signaling of CD73-derived adenosine in murine Treg and Teff cells. *Am J Physiol Cell Physiol.* (2011) 301:C530–9. doi: 10.1152/ajpcell.00385.2010
39. Lazarowski ER, Boucher RC, Harden TK. Constitutive release of ATP and evidence for major contribution of ecto-nucleotide pyrophosphatase and

nucleoside diphosphokinase to extracellular nucleotide concentrations. *J Biol Chem.* (2000) 275:31061–8. doi: 10.1074/jbc.M003255200
40. Franco R, Valenzuela A, Lluis C, Blanco J. Enzymatic and extraenzymatic role of ecto-adenosine deaminase in lymphocytes. *Immunol Rev.* (1998) 161:27–42. doi: 10.1111/j.1600-065X.1998.tb01569.x
41. Hashikawa T, Hooker SW, Maj JG, Knott-Craig CJ, Takedachi M, Murakami S, et al. Regulation of adenosine receptor engagement by ecto-adenosine deaminase. *FASEB J.* (2004) 18:131–3. doi: 10.1096/fj.03-0011fje
42. Moreno E, Canet J, Gracia E, Lluis C, Mallol J, Canela EI, et al. Molecular evidence of adenosine deaminase linking adenosine A2A receptor and CD26 proteins. *Front Pharmacol.* (2018) 9:106. doi: 10.3389/fphar.2018.00106
43. Ohta A, Ohta A, Madasu M, Kini R, Subramanian M, Goel N, et al. A2A adenosine receptor may allow expansion of T cells lacking effector functions in extracellular adenosine-rich microenvironments. *J Immunol.* (2009) 183:5487–93. doi: 10.4049/jimmunol.0901247
44. Moser GH, Schrader J, Deussen A. Turnover of adenosine in plasma of human and dog blood. *Am J Physiol.* (1989) 256:C799–806. doi: 10.1152/ajpcell.1989.256.4.C799
45. Chiu GS, Freund GG. Modulation of neuroimmunity by adenosine and its receptors: metabolism to mental illness. *Metabolism* (2014) 63:1491–8. doi: 10.1016/j.metabol.2014.09.003
46. Eckle T, Krahn T, Grenz A, Kohler D, Mittelbronn M, Ledent C, et al. Cardioprotection by ecto-5'-nucleotidase (CD73) and A2B adenosine receptors. *Circulation* (2007) 115:1581–90. doi: 10.1161/CIRCULATIONAHA.106.669697
47. Wang C, Huang CY, Lin WC. Optical ATP biosensor for extracellular ATP measurement. *Biosens Bioelectron* (2013) 43:355–61. doi: 10.1016/j.bios.2012.12.027
48. Tennant JP, Hourani SM. Breakdown of extracellular ATP by the prostatic and epididymal ends of the guinea pig vas deferens. *Eur J Pharmacol.* (2000) 387:107–9. doi: 10.1016/S0014-2999(99)00789-X
49. Vekaria RM, Unwin RJ, Shirley DG. Intraluminal ATP concentrations in rat renal tubules. *J Am Soc Nephrol.* (2006) 17:1841–7. doi: 10.1681/ASN.2005111171
50. Frenguelli BG, Wigmore G, Llaudet E, Dale N. Temporal and mechanistic dissociation of ATP and adenosine release during ischaemia in the mammalian hippocampus. *J Neurochem.* (2007) 101:1400–13. doi: 10.1111/j.1471-4159.2006.04425.x
51. Sove RJ, Ghonaim N, Goldman D, Ellis CG. A computational model of a microfluidic device to measure the dynamics of oxygen-dependent ATP release from erythrocytes. *PLoS ONE* (2013) 8:e81537. doi: 10.1371/journal.pone.0081537
52. Ledderose C, Bao Y, Zhang J, Junger WG. Novel method for real-time monitoring of ATP release reveals multiple phases of autocrine purinergic signalling during immune cell activation. *Acta Physiol.* (2015) 213:334–45. doi: 10.1111/apha.12435
53. Borea PA, Gessi S, Merighi S, Varani K. Adenosine as a multi-signalling guardian angel in human diseases: when, where and how does it exert its protective effects? *Trends Pharmacol Sci.* (2016) 37:419–34. doi: 10.1016/j.tips.2016.02.006
54. Cekic C, Linden J. Purinergic regulation of the immune system. *Nat Rev Immunol.* (2016) 16:177–92. doi: 10.1038/nri.2016.4
55. Panther E, Idzko M, Herouy Y, Rheinen H, Gebicke-Haerter PJ, Mrowietz U, et al. Expression and function of adenosine receptors in human dendritic cells. *FASEB J.* (2001) 15:1963–70. doi: 10.1096/fj.01-0169com
56. Dickenson JM, Reeder S, Rees B, Alexander S, Kendall D. Functional expression of adenosine A2A and A3 receptors in the mouse dendritic cell line XS-106. *Eur J Pharmacol.* (2003) 474:43–51. doi: 10.1016/S0014-2999(03)02041-7
57. Hasko G, Cronstein BN. Adenosine: an endogenous regulator of innate immunity. *Trends Immunol.* (2004) 25:33–9. doi: 10.1016/j.it.2003.11.003
58. Schnurr M, Toy T, Shin A, Hartmann G, Rothenfusser S, Soellner J, et al. Role of adenosine receptors in regulating chemotaxis and cytokine production of plasmacytoid dendritic cells. *Blood* (2004) 103:1391–7. doi: 10.1182/blood-2003-06-1959
59. Ben Addi A, Lefort A, Hua X, Libert F, Communi D, Ledent C, et al. Modulation of murine dendritic cell function by adenine nucleotides and adenosine: involvement of the A(2B) receptor. *Eur J Immunol.* (2008) 38:1610–20. doi: 10.1002/eji.200737781
60. Novitskiy SV, Ryzhov S, Zaynagetdinov R, Goldstein AE, Huang Y, Tikhomirov OY, et al. Adenosine receptors in regulation of dendritic cell differentiation and function. *Blood* (2008) 112:1822–31. doi: 10.1182/blood-2008-02-136325
61. Wilson JM, Ross WG, Agbai ON, Frazier R, Figler RA, Rieger J, et al. The A2B adenosine receptor impairs the maturation and immunogenicity of dendritic cells. *J Immunol.* (2009) 182:4616–23. doi: 10.4049/jimmunol.0801279
62. Challier J, Bruniquel D, Sewell AK, Laugel B. Adenosine and cAMP signalling skew human dendritic cell differentiation towards a tolerogenic phenotype with defective CD8(+) T-cell priming capacity. *Immunology* (2013) 138:402–10. doi: 10.1111/imm.12053
63. Mahnke K, Johnson TS, Ring S, Enk AH. Tolerogenic dendritic cells and regulatory T cells: a two-way relationship. *J Dermatol Sci.* (2007) 46:159–67. doi: 10.1016/j.jdermsci.2007.03.002
64. Neuberger A, Ring S, Silva-Vilches C, Schrader J, Enk A, Mahnke K. Expression of CD73 slows down migration of skin dendritic cells, affecting the sensitization phase of contact hypersensitivity reactions in mice. *J Dermatol Sci.* (2017) 87:292–9. doi: 10.1016/j.jdermsci.2017.07.002
65. Desrosiers MD, Cembrola KM, Fakir MJ, Stephens LA, Jama FM, Shameli A, et al. Adenosine deamination sustains dendritic cell activation in inflammation. *J Immunol.* (2007) 179:1884–92. doi: 10.4049/jimmunol.179.3.1884
66. Naval-Macabuhay I, Casanova V, Navarro G, Garcia F, Leon A, Miralles L, et al. Adenosine deaminase regulates Treg expression in autologous T cell-dendritic cell cocultures from patients infected with HIV-1. *J Leukoc Biol.* (2016) 99:349–59. doi: 10.1189/jlb.3A1214-580RR
67. Pletinckx K, Dohler A, Pavlovic V, Lutz MB. Role of dendritic cell maturity/costimulation for generation, homeostasis, and suppressive activity of regulatory T cells. *Front Immunol.* (2011) 2:39. doi: 10.3389/fimmu.2011.00039
68. Kambayashi T, Wallin RP, Ljunggren HG. cAMP-elevating agents suppress dendritic cell function. *J Leukoc Biol.* (2001) 70:903–10. doi: 10.1189/jlb.70.6.903
69. Panther E, Corinti S, Idzko M, Herouy Y, Napp M, La Sala A, et al. Adenosine affects expression of membrane molecules, cytokine and chemokine release, and the T-cell stimulatory capacity of human dendritic cells. *Blood* (2003) 101:3985–90. doi: 10.1182/blood-2002-07-2113
70. Li L, Huang L, Ye H, Song SP, Bajwa A, Lee SJ, et al. Dendritic cells tolerized with adenosine A(2)AR agonist attenuate acute kidney injury. *J Clin Invest.* (2012) 122:3931–42. doi: 10.1172/JCI63170
71. Franco A, Kumar J, Lin G, Behnamfar N, Hsieh LE, Shimizu C, et al. Pediatric tolerogenic DCs expressing CD4 and immunoglobulin-like transcript receptor (ILT)-4 secrete IL-10 in response to Fc and adenosine. *Eur J Immunol.* (2018) 48:482–91. doi: 10.1002/eji.201747139
72. Novak J, Fabrik I, Linhartova I, Link M, Cerny O, Stulik J, et al. Phosphoproteomics of cAMP signaling of Bordetella adenylate cyclase toxin in mouse dendritic cells. *Sci Rep.* (2017) 7:16298. doi: 10.1038/s41598-017-14501-x
73. Clark K, Mackenzie KF, Petkevicius K, Kristariyanto Y, Zhang J, Choi HG, et al. Phosphorylation of CRTC3 by the salt-inducible kinases controls the interconversion of classically activated and regulatory macrophages. *Proc Natl Acad Sci USA.* (2012) 109:16986–91. doi: 10.1073/pnas.1215450109
74. Mackenzie KF, Clark K, Naqvi S, Mcguire VA, Noehren G, Kristariyanto Y, et al. PGE(2) induces macrophage IL-10 production and a regulatory-like phenotype via a protein kinase A-SIK-CRTC3 pathway. *J Immunol.* (2013) 190:565–77. doi: 10.4049/jimmunol.1202462
75. Sundberg TB, Choi HG, Song JH, Russell CN, Hussain MM, Graham DB, et al. Small-molecule screening identifies inhibition of salt-inducible kinases as a therapeutic strategy to enhance immunoregulatory functions of dendritic cells. *Proc Natl Acad Sci USA.* (2014) 111:12468–73. doi: 10.1073/pnas.1412308111
76. Sancak Y, Thoreen CC, Peterson TR, Lindquist RA, Kang SA, Spooner E, et al. PRAS40 is an insulin-regulated inhibitor of the mTORC1 protein kinase. *Mol Cell* (2007) 25:903–15. doi: 10.1016/j.molcel.2007.03.003

77. Gingras AC, Gygi SP, Raught B, Polakiewicz RD, Abraham RT, Hoekstra MF, et al. Regulation of 4E-BP1 phosphorylation: a novel two-step mechanism. *Genes Dev.* (1999) 13:1422–37. doi: 10.1101/gad.13.11.1422
78. Schmitz F, Heit A, Dreher S, Eisenacher K, Mages J, Haas T, et al. Mammalian target of rapamycin (mTOR) orchestrates the defense program of innate immune cells. *Eur J Immunol.* (2008) 38:2981–92. doi: 10.1002/eji.200838761
79. Weichhart T, Hengstschlager M, Linke M. Regulation of innate immune cell function by mTOR. *Nat Rev Immunol.* (2015) 15:599–614. doi: 10.1038/nri3901
80. Matsumoto T, Hasegawa H, Onishi S, Ishizaki J, Suemori K, Yasukawa M. Protein kinase C inhibitor generates stable human tolerogenic dendritic cells. *J Immunol.* (2013) 191:2247–57. doi: 10.4049/jimmunol.1203053
81. Lee J, Kim TH, Murray F, Li X, Choi SS, Broide DH, et al. Cyclic AMP concentrations in dendritic cells induce and regulate Th2 immunity and allergic asthma. *Proc Natl Acad Sci USA.* (2015) 112:1529–34. doi: 10.1073/pnas.1417972112
82. Rueda CM, Jackson CM, Chougnet CA. Regulatory T-cell-mediated suppression of conventional T-cells and dendritic cells by different cAMP intracellular pathways. *Front Immunol.* (2016) 7:216. doi: 10.3389/fimmu.2016.00216
83. Figueiredo AB, Souza-Testasicca MC, Mineo TWP, Afonso LCC. Leishmania amazonensis-Induced cAMP triggered by adenosine A2B receptor is important to inhibit dendritic cell activation and evade immune response in infected mice. *Front Immunol.* (2017) 8:849. doi: 10.3389/fimmu.2017.00849
84. Pleli T, Mondorf A, Ferreiros N, Thomas D, Dvorak K, Biondi RM, et al. Activation of adenylyl cyclase causes stimulation of adenosine receptors. *Cell Physiol Biochem.* (2018) 45:2516–28. doi: 10.1159/000488270
85. Silva-Vilches C, Pletinckx K, Lohnert M, Pavlovic V, Ashour D, John V, et al. Low doses of cholera toxin and its mediator cAMP induce CTLA-2 secretion by dendritic cells to enhance regulatory T cell conversion. *PLoS ONE* (2017) 12:e0178114. doi: 10.1371/journal.pone.0178114
86. Garay J, D'angelo JA, Park Y, Summa CM, Aiken ML, Morales E, et al. Crosstalk between PKA and Epac regulates the phenotypic maturation and function of human dendritic cells. *J Immunol.* (2010) 185:3227–38. doi: 10.4049/jimmunol.0903066
87. Ring S, Pushkarevskaya A, Schild H, Probst HC, Jendrossek V, Wirsdorfer F, et al. Regulatory T cell-derived adenosine induces dendritic cell migration through the Epac-Rap1 pathway. *J Immunol.* (2015) 194:3735–44. doi: 10.4049/jimmunol.1401434
88. Onishi Y, Fehervari Z, Yamaguchi T, Sakaguchi S. Foxp3+ natural regulatory T cells preferentially form aggregates on dendritic cells in vitro and actively inhibit their maturation. *Proc Natl Acad Sci USA.* (2008) 105:10113–8. doi: 10.1073/pnas.0711106105
89. Zarek PE, Huang CT, Lutz ER, Kowalski J, Horton MR, Linden J, et al. A2A receptor signaling promotes peripheral tolerance by inducing T-cell anergy and the generation of adaptive regulatory T cells. *Blood* (2008) 111:251–9. doi: 10.1182/blood-2007-03-081646
90. Iijima M, Katz SI. Specific immunologic tolerance to dinitrofluorobenzene following topical application of dinitrothiocyanobenzene: modulation by suppressor T cells. *J Invest Dermatol.* (1983) 81:325–30. doi: 10.1111/1523-1747.ep12519783
91. Ferrari D, Gorini S, Callegari G, La Sala A. Shaping immune responses through the activation of dendritic cells' P2 receptors. *Purinergic Signal* (2007) 3:99–107. doi: 10.1007/s11302-006-9024-0
92. Schrier DJ, Imre KM. The effects of adenosine agonists on human neutrophil function. *J Immunol.* (1986) 137:3284–9.
93. Thibault N, Burelout C, Harbour D, Borgeat P, Naccache PH, Bourgoin SG. Occupancy of adenosine A2a receptors promotes fMLP-induced cyclic AMP accumulation in human neutrophils: impact on phospholipase D activity and recruitment of small GTPases to membranes. *J Leukoc Biol.* (2002) 71:367–77. doi: 10.1189/jlb.71.2.367
94. Bao Y, Chen Y, Ledderose C, Li L, Junger WG. Pannexin 1 channels link chemoattractant receptor signaling to local excitation and global inhibition responses at the front and back of polarized neutrophils. *J Biol Chem.* (2013) 288:22650–7. doi: 10.1074/jbc.M113.476283
95. Mahnke K, Qian Y, Knop J, Enk AH. Induction of CD4+/CD25+ regulatory T cells by targeting of antigens to immature dendritic cells. *Blood* (2003) 101:4862–9. doi: 10.1182/blood-2002-10-3229
96. Mahnke K, Ring S, Enk AH. Antibody targeting of "Steady-State" dendritic cells induces tolerance mediated by regulatory T cells. *Front Immunol.* (2016) 7:63. doi: 10.3389/fimmu.2016.00063
97. Idzko M, Dichmann S, Ferrari D, Di Virgilio F, La Sala A, Girolomoni G, et al. Nucleotides induce chemotaxis and actin polymerization in immature but not mature human dendritic cells via activation of pertussis toxin-sensitive P2y receptors. *Blood* (2002) 100:925–32. doi: 10.1182/blood.V100.3.925
98. Deaglio S, Dwyer KM, Gao W, Friedman D, Usheva A, Erat A, et al. Adenosine generation catalyzed by CD39 and CD73 expressed on regulatory T cells mediates immune suppression. *J Exp Med.* (2007) 204:1257–65. doi: 10.1084/jem.20062512
99. Ring S, Oliver SJ, Cronstein BN, Enk AH, Mahnke K. CD4+CD25+ regulatory T cells suppress contact hypersensitivity reactions through a CD39, adenosine-dependent mechanism. *J Allergy Clin Immunol.* (2009)123:e1282. doi: 10.1016/j.jaci.2009.03.022
100. Huang S, Apasov S, Koshiba M, Sitkovsky M. Role of A2a extracellular adenosine receptor-mediated signaling in adenosine-mediated inhibition of T-cell activation and expansion. *Blood* (1997) 90:1600–10.
101. Lappas CM, Rieger JM, Linden J. A2A adenosine receptor induction inhibits IFN-gamma production in murine CD4+ T cells. *J Immunol.* (2005) 174:1073–80. doi: 10.4049/jimmunol.174.2.1073

14

Modulation of Immune Tolerance via Siglec-Sialic Acid Interactions

*Joyce Lübbers, Ernesto Rodríguez and Yvette van Kooyk**

Molecular Cell Biology and Immunology, Amsterdam UMC, Vrije Universiteit Amsterdam, Cancer Center Amsterdam, Amsterdam Infection and Immunity Institute, Amsterdam, Netherlands

Correspondence:
Yvette van Kooyk
Y.vanKooyk@vumc.nl

One of the key features of the immune system is its extraordinary capacity to discriminate between self and non-self and to respond accordingly. Several molecular interactions allow the induction of acquired immune responses when a foreign antigen is recognized, while others regulate the resolution of inflammation, or the induction of tolerance to self-antigens. Post-translational signatures, such as glycans that are part of proteins (glycoproteins) and lipids (glycolipids) of host cells or pathogens, are increasingly appreciated as key molecules in regulating immunity vs. tolerance. Glycans are sensed by glycan binding receptors expressed on immune cells, such as C-type lectin receptors (CLRs) and Sialic acid binding immunoglobulin type lectins (Siglecs), that respond to specific glycan signatures by triggering tolerogenic or immunogenic signaling pathways. Glycan signatures present on healthy tissue, inflamed and malignant tissue or pathogens provide signals for "self" or "*non-self*" recognition. In this review we will focus on sialic acids that serve as "self" molecular pattern ligands for Siglecs. We will emphasize on the function of Siglec-expressing mononuclear phagocytes as sensors for sialic acids in tissue homeostasis and describe how the sialic acid-Siglec axis is exploited by tumors and pathogens for the induction of immune tolerance. Furthermore, we highlight how the sialic acid-Siglec axis can be utilized for clinical applications to induce or inhibit immune tolerance.

Keywords: mononuclear phagocytes, dendritic cells, macrophages, Siglecs, tolerance, inflammation, sialic acid, cancer

HIGHLIGHTS

- Siglecs have an immune modulatory effect on TLR signaling.
- Sialic acids can be presented by pathogens through synthesis of "mimic" structures or the novo synthesis for survival advantage.
- Hyper sialic acid expression in the tumor microenvironments is linked to immune suppression.
- Targeting the sialic acid-Siglec axis could have beneficial effects in therapy in cancer, allergies and auto immune diseases.

INTRODUCTION

The human mononuclear phagocyte network consists of monocytes, different subsets of macrophages (MQ) and Dendritic cells (DCs) depending on their origin and tissue micro-environment. In each microenvironment, differentiation is dictated by various components such as stromal cell compartment, presence of immune cells and the diversity of chemokines and cytokines present (1). Moreover, mononuclear phagocytes are key instructors for inflammatory or tolerogenic programming of the immune system. The presence of MQ and DCs at multiple sites in the human body, like gut, lung, brain, oral mucosa, lymphnodes, spleen, skin and peripheral blood illustrates their importance in controlling immunity and tolerance (2–5). MQ are plastic cells that can polarize according to the signals they receive and this polarization is mainly described as classical activated M1, alternatively activated M2, or tumor-associated macrophages (TAM). The M1, depicted as pro-inflammatory cells, are induced by stimulating MQ with LPS and/or IFN-γ that produce IL-1, TNF-α and nitric oxide. On the other hand, M2 MQ are induced by stimulation with IL-4 and have anti-inflammatory and tissue repair properties, producing Il-10 and TGF-ß (6, 7). TAMs are found in the microenvironment of tumors, promoting tumor growth by among others release angiogenic factors like VEGF and EGF, attract regulatory T cells and inhibit effector T cells by the release of multiple cytokines and chemokines such as IL-10, TGF-ß, and CCL22 (8). DCs consists also of multiple subsets, were the conventional DCs (cDCs) and plasmacytoid DCs (pDCs) are the main populations in peripheral blood. The cDCs are the main antigen-presenting subset, able to present antigens to and activate antigen specific naïve $CD4^+$ and $CD8^+$ T cells and are able to secrete multiple proinflammatory and anti-inflammatory cytokines like IL12p70 and IL-10, respectively (9, 10). pDCs do not prime naïve T cells, however, there specialized function is the production of type I interferon (IFN-α/β) in response to viruses (11). Different cytokines like IFN-α, TNF-α and LPS can polarize cDCs into a more immunogenic state (12, 13), while other cytokines like IL-10 and TGF-ß induce tolerogenic cDCs that express checkpoint ligands like PD-L1 and produce the checkpoint molecule indoleamine 2,3-dioxygenase (IDO). *In-vitro* treatment of DCs with dexamethasone or vitamin D3 will also result in tolerogenic DCs (14). Functionally the main characteristics of MQ is their phagocytic capacity, while DCs are key in antigen presentation and stimulation of naïve T cells into antigen-specific effector T cells, however, some of these functions are not 100% restricted and are also shared between MQ and DCs.

In-vitro, human monocyte-derived DCs (moDCs) and monocyte-derived MQ (moMQ) can be generated from monocytes. Culturing monocytes with GM-CSF and IL-4 gives rise to moDCs, while culturing monocytes with M-CSF or GM-CSF alone creates moMQ (15, 16). moDCs and moMQ are often used as model systems for inflammatory DCs and MQ, respectively, as they are easily obtained in large numbers. moDCs are excellent antigen presenters, and able to induce antigen-specific $CD4^+$ and $CD8^+$ T cells, while culturing with IL-10 or TGF-β generates moDC prone to induce tolerance (4, 17–21). However, recent studies using mass cytometry as well as single cell RNA sequencing have revealed that moDCs are distinct from human peripheral blood and skin-derived DCs (2, 22).

Mononuclear phagocytes have an important function in maintenance of tissue homeostasis and the resolution of inflammation. They express multiple pattern recognition receptors (PRRs), like toll like receptors (TLR) and CLRs to recognize pathogen-associated molecular patterns (PAMPs), damaged self-antigens (DAMPs) or altered glycosylated self-antigens, such as tumor antigens (3, 23). The differentiation and maturation status of mononuclear phagocytes alters the expression levels of PRR (24, 25). CLRs is a large family of glycan-specific receptors that include, amongst others: DC-SIGN (CD209), Mannose receptor (MR, CD206), DEC-205 (CD205), Dectin-1, Macrophage galactose-type lectin (MGL, CD301) and Langerin (CD207) (26, 27). These CLRs are glycan-binding receptors, recognizing a wide variety of carbohydrate structures, like fucoses and mannoses found on host glycoproteins expressed by cells or pathogens or β-glucan structures that are only expressed on pathogens such as *Aspergillus fumigatus* and *Saccharomyces cerevisiae* (27–29). CLRs play an important role in the antigen uptake for processing and presentation of peptides on MHC class I and II, thereby stimulating antigen-specific T cell responses and T helper differentiation (27). Some CLRs, like Dectin-1, have the ability to directly modulate the DC or MQ phenotype and cytokine responses, while, other CLRs, like DC-SIGN and MGL are also highly expressed on tolerogenic DC/MQ and modulate TLR signaling through the acetylation of p65 and the induction of IL10 production (30–32).

Next to TLRs and CLRs, mononuclear phagocytes express Sialic acid binding immunoglobulin type lectins (Siglecs), that recognize sialic acids, a family of sugars with a nine-carbon sugar core structure derived from neuraminic acid, with the N-acetylneuraminic acid (Neu5Ac) being the main moiety present in humans (**Box 1** and **Figure 1**). Sialic acids are generally the last sugars added during the glycosylation process, thereby capping a diverse array of glycosylation structures (44, 45). Often, the presence of sialic acids functions as a self-associated molecular pattern (SAMP) and thus, Siglecs can serve as sensors for "self" (46). Most Siglecs possess an intracellular immunoreceptor tyrosine-based inhibition motif (ITIM) that induce strong inhibitory signaling when Siglecs bind sialic acids (47). Interestingly, both pathogens and tumor cells use enhanced expression of sialic acids as a mechanism to modify the immune system in their favor, illustrating that the sialic acid-Siglec axis is a key regulator in infection and cancer.

SIGLECS

The human genome contains 14 different Siglecs, which can be divided into two groups based on their genetic homology among mammalian species. The first group is present in all mammals and consists of Siglec-1 (Sialoadhesin), Siglec-2 (CD22), Siglec-4 (MAG), and Siglec-15 (48–50). The second group consists of the CD33-related Siglecs that have evolved rapidly and therefore their repertoire differs between species. The CD33 related Siglecs are Siglec-3 (CD33),–5,–6,–7,–8,–9,–10,–11,–14, and –16 (51). Monocytes, moMQ and moDCs have largely the same Siglec profile (**Figure 2**), namely high expression of Siglec-3,–7,–9, low Siglec-10 expression and upon stimulation with IFN-α, also Siglec-1 (52–60) is expressed. In contrast, MQ have primarily expression of Siglec-1,–3,–8,–9,–11,–15, and–16 depending on their differentiation status (49, 52, 61, 62). cDCs express Siglec-3,–7, and–9, similar to moDCs, but in addition also express low levels of Siglec-2 and Siglec-15 (49, 63–67). pDCs are

Box 1 | Sialic acid.

Sialic acids are a family of sugars with nine carbons derived from neuraminic acid that are negatively charged. Humans are able to synthetize Neu5Ac (**Figure 1A**), while other mammals can also synthetize the structure N-glycolylneuraminic acid (Neu5Gc). A deletion in the gene encoding the enzyme CMAH (Cytidine monophosphate-N-acetylneuraminic acid hydroxylase) is the reason why humans cannot produce Neu5Gc (33).

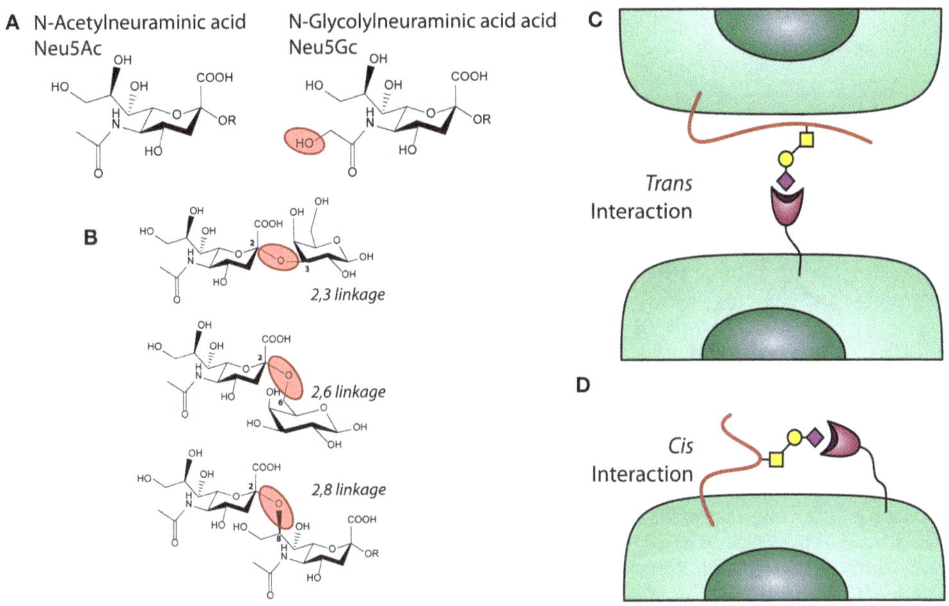

Figure 1 | Sialic acids, linkages, and interactions. **(A)** chemical structure of sialic acids Neu5Ac and Neu5Gc. **(B)** α2,3; α2,6, and α2,8 linked sialic acids. **(C)** Trans and **(D)** Cis interactions of Siglecs with sialic acids.

Synthesis

The expression of sialylated glycans is the result of glycosylation related enzymes able to catalyse the addition or removal of a glycan to growing carbohydrate structures. The transfer of sialic acid motifs from an activated donor (CMP-NeuAc, **C**ytidine 5′-**M**ono**P**hospho-N-**Ac**etyl**N**euraminic acid) to underlying glycans that serve as acceptors, is performed by a group of enzymes called sialyltransferases. Humans express more than 20 different sialyltransferases, each differing in their tissue expression, substrate specificity and linkages produced (34). The synthesis of sialylated structures depends also on the presence of the donor, which is synthetized in the nucleus by the enzyme CMAS (CMP-Neu5Ac synthetase) and subsequently transported into the Golgi via the transporter SLC35A1 (33, 35). Sialic acid blocking glycomimetic: $Ac_5 3F_{ax}$Neu5Ac is a metabolic inhibitor of sialyltransferases that blocks the addition of sialic acids to the glycan backbone (36).

Sialic Acid Linkages

Sialic acids can be linked to the underlying glycan via different types of linkages, which affects their recognition by glycan-binding receptors, such as Siglecs. These linkages mainly have an alpha configuration and are defined by which carbon in the acceptor glycan is connected to the anomeric carbon in the Neu5Ac (carbon 2). When sialic acid is transferred to a different glycan, the bond can involve the carbon 3 or 6 in the acceptor rising to α2,3 or a α2,6 linkages, respectively, (33, 35) (**Figure 2B**). In poly-sialic acid structures, one Neu5Ac is added to a strain of sialic acids in an α2,8 linkage. The different Sialic acid linkages are depicted in the complementary figure to this box.

Trans/Cis Interaction

Siglecs can interact with sialic acid on a different cell or protein/particulate (*trans* interaction) or with sialic acids present on the same cell that expresses the receptor (*cis* interaction), as depicted in the figure complementary with this box. An illustration of a *trans* interaction is α2,3 linked sialic acids expressed by lung epithelium under inflammatory conditions and Siglecs present on neutrophils (37, 38) (**Figure 1C**). An example of a *cis* interaction is α2,3 linked sialic acid present on the cell surface of moDCs, which bind to a Siglecs present on the same moDCs (39) (**Figure 1D**).

Degradation

Specific glycosidases, called neuraminidases or sialidases, can hydrolyse the sialic acid from oligosaccharides. Present mainly in intracellular vesicles, these enzymes can be secreted, thereby changing the profile of sialylated structures present on the cell membrane. Their expression is dysregulated in many different types of cancer.

Sialic Acid Immune Modulation

Sialic acids can modulate the immune system in diverse ways through Siglecs, influence on antibody mediated clearance of pathogens and through complement. Sialylation of the antibody immunoglobulin A (IgA) interferes with the cell surface attachment of influenza A and mediates anti-viral activity of IgA (40). Sialic acids can also bind to complement regulator factor H and by this negatively regulate the complement alternative pathway (41–43).

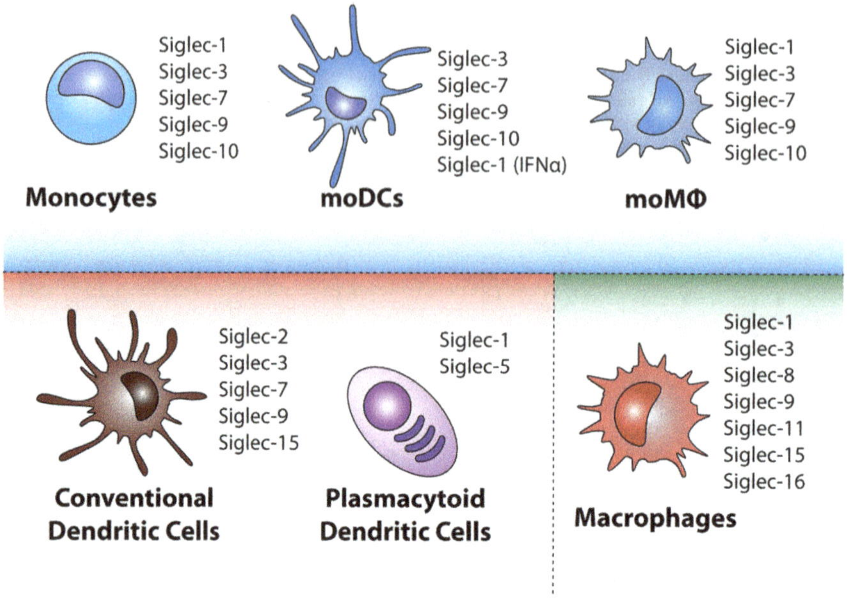

FIGURE 2 | Siglec expression by different mononuclear phagocytes in steady state. Depicted in the blue square are monocytes and *in-vitro* cultured monocyte-derived dendritic cells (moDC) and monocyte-derived macrophages (moMQ). In the red square the conventional dendritic cells and plasmacytoid dendritic cells that appear in peripheral blood are highlighted, whereas in the green square tissue resident macrophages (MQ) are depicted. Depending on microenvironmental triggers the immunogenic or tolerogenic status of the mononuclear phagocyte can change, leading to altered Siglec expression.

different in their expression of Siglecs, as they express Siglec-1 and Siglec-5 (54, 68). The presence of the Siglecs on mononuclear phagocytes is based on their steady state situation, however, microenvironmental triggers that change the maturation status of the cell, may influence the loss or gain of the expression of Siglecs. Downregulation of Siglecs-7 and Siglec-9 expression on moDCs is observed after stimulating moDCs for 48 h with LPS, however, on moMQ Siglec expression is not changed upon LPS triggering (54). Clearly, further research on the regulation of Siglec expression during cellular maturation is needed. Siglecs are also present on other immune cells [nicely reviewed by MacAuley et al. (69)], such as B cells, basophils, neutrophils, and NK cells, with different expression patterns for every cell subset.

Sialic acids, the ligands for Siglecs receptors, are widely expressed as they are exposed on the outermost end of glycosylated structures of glycoproteins expressed on immune and other cells in the body, secreted glycoproteins in tissues and blood and on extracellular matrix in tissues (70, 71). It is the glycosylation machinery of the cells that determines the type of sialic acids to be added on the carbohydrate backbone to be expressed by the glycoprotein (**Box 1**, **Figure 1**). A Siglec-expressing immune cell can bind to sialic acids present on another cell or secreted glycoprotein and this is called a *trans* interaction (72) (**Figure 1**). Siglec receptors can also bind sialic acids exposed on the same cell, called a *cis* interaction. Moreover, Siglec receptors have different binding affinities for different linkage and modifications of sialic acids (see **Box 1** for more information about sialic acid). Most Siglecs have a preference for a particular sialic acid linkage, being either α2,3, α2,6, or α2,8-linked sialic acid but Siglecs may also show redundant specificity toward more linkages (52, 58).

IMMUNE MODULATION THROUGH SIGLEC SIGNALING

The immune modulatory effect induced upon sialic acid binding to Siglec is regulated through downstream signaling pathways. Siglec-5 till Siglec-11, are the so-called inhibitory Siglecs, carrying ITIM and/or ITIM like motifs in their cytoplasmic domains, which can be phosphorylated by the Src family, thereby creating a binding site for the tyrosine phosphatases SHP-1 and SHP-2 (**Figure 3A**). Upon binding of SHP-1/2, de-phosphorylation of downstream targets can be achieved and ubiquitination, internalization, and phosphorylation of the receptor can be regulated (73, 74). The Src-mediated phosphorylation of ITIMs in Siglec-3 and possible also other ITIM-containing Siglecs can also lead to the binding of Cbl, a RING finger-containing E3 ligase, and suppressor of cytokine signaling 3 (SOCS3), resulting in the ubiquitination and protosomal degradation of Siglec-3. The same process also regulates the internalization and surface abundance of Siglec-3. SOCS proteins are upregulated by cytokines during inflammatory responses, leading to the loss of Siglec-3 and thereby higher proliferation of myeloid cells (75, 76) (**Figure 3A**). Signaling of different Siglecs through the binding of sialic acids or crosslinking via antibodies can lead to both an inflammatory or tolerogenic state in distinct mononuclear phagocytes. Antibodies against Siglec-3 and −7 inhibit the proliferation of myeloid cells (77) while monocytes

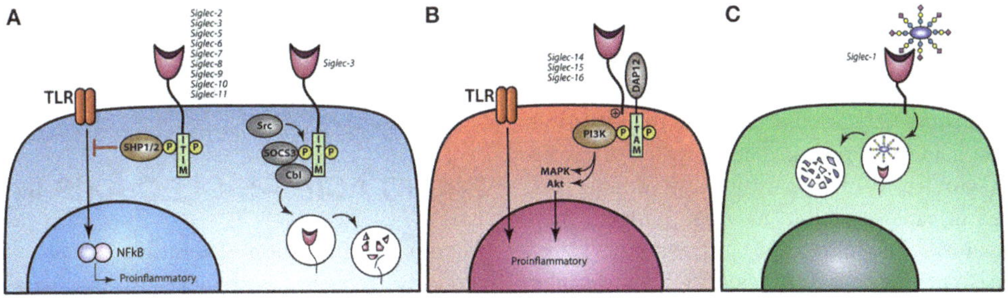

FIGURE 3 | Siglec signaling and the immune modulatory effect on TLR signaling. **(A)** Siglec-2,−3, and−5 till−11 modulate TLR signaling upon binding of sialic acids and thereby dampen proinflammatory responses. Ligand binding to Siglec-3 leads to phosphorylation of the ITIM motif and reveals a binding site for SOCS3 and Cbl, causing proteasomal degradation of Siglec-3 and SOCS3. **(B)** Activating Siglecs-14,−15, and−16 can associate with DAP12, resulting in the activation of the MAPK and AKT pathways, thereby stimulating a proinflammatory response. **(C)** Siglec-1 can internalize upon binding of its ligand and thereby present antigens to dendritic cells or B cell to initiate an immune response.

treated with Siglec-3 antibodies show increased production of the pro-inflammatory cytokines IL-1β, TNF-α, and IL-8 (78). These findings illustrate that crosslinking of Siglec-3 expressed on different myeloid cells induces opposite functional outcomes. Moreover, crosslinking Siglec-3 on monocytes via antibodies signals a pro-inflammatory effect, while *cis* binding of sialic acids to Siglec-3 represses IL-1β production by monocytes (78).

In contrast, Siglec-4 and Siglec-14 till Siglec-16 do not have an ITIM or ITIM like motif, but instead signal through the association of DNAX activation protein (DAP)12 and are therefore called activating Siglecs. DAP12 associates with these activating Siglecs through a positively charged lysine residue in the transmembrane domains and contain a cytosolic immunoreceptor tyrosine-based activation motifs (ITAM), which can recruit PI3K (**Figure 3B**) (49, 62). Furthermore, Siglec-14 can promote an inflammatory response by activating the MAPK pathway (46). The activating Siglecs most likely developed under evolutionary pressure, when pathogens adapted using the inhibitory Siglecs to circumvent the immune system, allowing sialic acids to also activate the immune system. There are a couple of paired Siglecs, consisting of an inhibitory and an activating Siglec, like Siglec-5 and Siglec-14 as well as Siglec-11 and Siglec-16. Polymorphisms in Siglec-5/14 have been described, whereby the Siglec-14 gene is deleted and the Siglec-5 gene is present under the Siglec-14 promotor. When monocytes from these individuals are challenged with LPS or with group B *streptococcus* (GBS) they produce less TNF-α than individuals that have normal Siglec-5 and Siglec-14 expression on their monocytes, indicating that Siglec-14 is tipping the balance toward the pro-inflammatory site when cells are confronted by pathogens (46, 61, 62).

Siglec-1 is a non-signaling Sigelc, that internalizes upon ligand binding (**Figure 3C**). Den Haan et al. showed in mice that antigen coupled to Siglec-1 antibodies targets Siglec-1 expressing marginal zone macrophages that transfer antigen to $CD8^+$ DC favoring effective antigen specific T cells to eradicate tumor growth (79, 80). Furthermore, it has been shown that Siglec-1^+ MQ promote germinal center B cell responses upon Siglec-1 antibody targeting (81).

Siglecs can also exert their immune modulatory effects by altering TLR signaling. LPS stimulation of TLR4 induces CCR7 upregulation of moMQ which is inhibited by anti-Siglec-9 antibodies or knock down of expression of Siglec-9 (53, 82). G. Chen and colleagues revealed that TLR4 forms a complex with Siglec E (mouse homologue for human Siglec-7 and Siglec-9) in murine DCs and macrophages (83). This *cis* interaction between Siglec-E and TLR4 is likely mediated by sialic acids present on the TLR (83). The TLR-Siglec-E interaction, is abrogated by NEU1 (a lysosomal sialidase that cleaves sialic acids from their glycoprotein backbone), which is translocated to the cell membrane upon LPS stimulation.

moDCs treated with the Ac_53F_{ax}Neu5Ac (**Box 1**), showed reduced sialic acid expression and a lower threshold of TLR activation, leading to increased sensitivity and response to poly I:C (TLR 3 agonist) and LPS, as reflected by the induction of moDC maturation and cytokine production by moDCs (55). Furthermore, it has been reported that sialic acid removal from moDCs uncovers Siglecs from their *cis* binding sialic acid ligands and increases expression of the maturation markers CD80 and CD86 and the secretion of IL-12 (84). Also, the cross presentation of melanoma antigens gp100 by DCs to antigen-specific $CD8^+$ T cells was increased upon removal of sialic acid on moDC, illustrating that the presence of sialic acid constraints, that occupy Siglecs in *cis*, inhibits the effectiveness of moDC to induce immunity (84). Alternatively, targeting Siglecs with sialic acids or sialic acid mimetics in *trans* can modulate TLR signaling leading to a more tolerogenic DC phenotype. This illustrates that interference in the sialic acid-Siglec axis is central in the balance between immunity and tolerance.

SIALIC ACIDS USED BY PATHOGENS TO MODULATE IMMUNITY

The co-evolution of the immune system and pathogens has led to the acquisition of several strategies for pathogens to evade the immune system, which also includes the expression of sialylated glycans to induce tolerance. One of the most notable examples is *Trypanosoma cruzi*, a protist parasite responsible for Chagas disease. During its infective stage in vertebrates, called trypomastigote, *T. cruzi* expresses a unique enzyme called *trans*-sialidase that catalyses the reversible transference of sialic acid from host glycoconjugates to glycan structures on the surface of the parasite. By doing this, *T. cruzi* uses host glycans to mask its own antigens and to modulate anti-parasitic responses (85). Parasitic sialylated glycans can interact with Siglec-E [homolog of human Siglec 7 and 9, Siglec comparison between Mammalians was recently reviewed by Bornhöfft et al. (86)] in murine dendritic cells to suppress the production of the pro-inflammatory cytokine IL-12 (87). Moreover, the addition of sialic acid to the surface of the parasite results in a negatively charged coat that inhibits complement-mediated killing. Furthermore, thanks to the *trans*-sialidase activity, *T. cruzi* is also able to alter the sialylation status of $CD8^+$ T cells, dampening their capacity to induce an effective anti-parasitic immune response (88).

Interestingly, several pathogenic bacteria also use the sialic acid-Siglec axis to dampen the immune system in favor of their survival. Despite the fact that sialic acids are mainly restricted to vertebrates, some bacteria have acquired the ability to take sialic acids or sialylated structures from the host, to synthetize "mimic" structures or even perform *de novo* synthesis of sialic acids, giving them a survival advantage. For example, Siglec-5 and−9 on neutrophils can be triggered by glycoconjugates present in *Pseudomonas aeruginosa* or *Group B streptococcus (GBS)* serotypes Ia and III, thereby inhibiting their ability to respond to the bacteria. Moreover, sialylated glycans present in *GBS* are able to inhibit the complement system, by reducing deposition of C3b on their surface and, therefore, the generation of C5a and the membrane attack complex (89–91).

The presence of sialic acids in envelope glycoproteins of viruses also contributes to enhanced infection of the host. This is the case for the *Human immunodeficiency virus* (HIV) and the *Porcine reproductive and respiratory syndrome virus* (PRRSV), which can bind to Siglec-1 to promote *trans* infection (92–94). Nevertheless, Siglec-1 ligands on *GBS* surface interact with Siglec-1 on marginal zone macrophages for the subsequent generation of anti-*GBS* immune responses (95).

Influenza A virus recognizes α2,3 and α2,6 linked sialic acids with its hemagglutinin (HA) glycoproteins to infect host cells. On the other hand, influenza A virus carries the neuraminidase (NA) glycoprotein that can cleave off sialic acids from cellular and viral glycoproteins that are expressed in infected cells and assembled in virions, to reduce HA causing aggregation of the virions to the cell surface. The HA and NA proteins are in perfect balance to warrant infection and to abolish detection by the immune system (96). Another example is the non-typeable *Haemophilus influenzae* (NTHi), which is also able to take up sialic acids through a tripartite ATP-independent periplasmic (TRAP) transporter. Incorporation of the sialic acids in the NTHi membrane protects it from serum-mediated killing (97).

Sialic acids are used by different pathogens to infect host cells and dampen the immune response. Knowledge on this mechanism can be exploited to design new therapeutic strategies in cancer or auto-immune diseases and asthma.

SIALIC ACID—SIGLEC AXIS IN CANCER

Aberrant glycosylation of multiple cancers and its influence on cancer progression and metastasis are well-known. Increased sialylation, α2,3; α2,6, and α2,8 linked sialic acids, has been demonstrated in multiple tumor tissues like renal cell carcinoma, prostate cancer, colon cancer, breast cancer, head and neck squamous cell carcinoma and oral cancer (98–101). This aberrant sialylation can also be detected in serum serving as potential biomarkers for cancer detection, progression and treatment responses (99, 101–103) (**Figure 4**).

In a mouse model for melanoma, hyper sialylation of B16 melanoma cells leads to increased tumor growth, associated with an enhanced T regulatory/T effector balance and reduced NK cell activity within the tumor and secondary lymphoid organs (110). DCs that interacted and sampled sialylated antigens via Siglec-E (murine homologue of human Siglec-7 and Siglec-9) induced regulatory T cells and inhibited effector T cell function *in-vivo*. These findings revealed that tumor sialylation impedes T cell-mediated anti-tumor immune responses, while promoting tumor-associated regulatory T cells (110). Blocking the inhibitory effects of sialic acids with a sialic acid blocking glycomimetic (**Box 1**) in a B16-OVA mouse model revealed reduced tumor growth, enhanced tumor killing by ovalbumin specific $CD8^+$ T cells and inhibition of metastasis (106, 107) (**Figure 4C**).

In breast cancer a specific glycoform of transmembrane mucin 1, MUC1-T is sialylated, creating MUC1-sT (111, 112). The MUC1-sT can interact with Siglec-9 on monocytes and thereby induce secretion of IL-6, M-CSF and chemokines associated with tumor progression. Binding of MUC1-sT to Siglec-9 on macrophages induces a tumor-associated macrophage (TAM) phenotype, that inhibits $CD8^+$ T cell proliferation and results in the upregulation of IDO, CD163 and PD-L1 *in-vivo* (113, 114). Another specific mucin glycoform, called MUC2-sT, has been shown to increase apoptosis of immature moDCs (115). Together, this points toward a broad immunological suppression by tumor-produced sialylated mucins.

Antibodies against Siglecs are explored for the treatment of different cancer types. For Acute Lymphoblastic Lymphoma (ALL) the FDA approved Inotuzumab Ozogamicin (Besponsa®), a monoclonal antibody against Siglec-2 coupled to the toxic agent calicheamicin is used. This antibody targets Siglec-2 positive B-lymphoblasts and causes cell death of these cells through the toxic agent (**Figure 4A**). Trials with this antibody revealed that an enhanced number of patients reached complete remission and had an increased overall progression free survival. However, serious adverse effects were seen like myeloid suppression (104), which could be due to the presence of Siglec-2 on DC subsets. Another Siglec that is targeted for the treatment

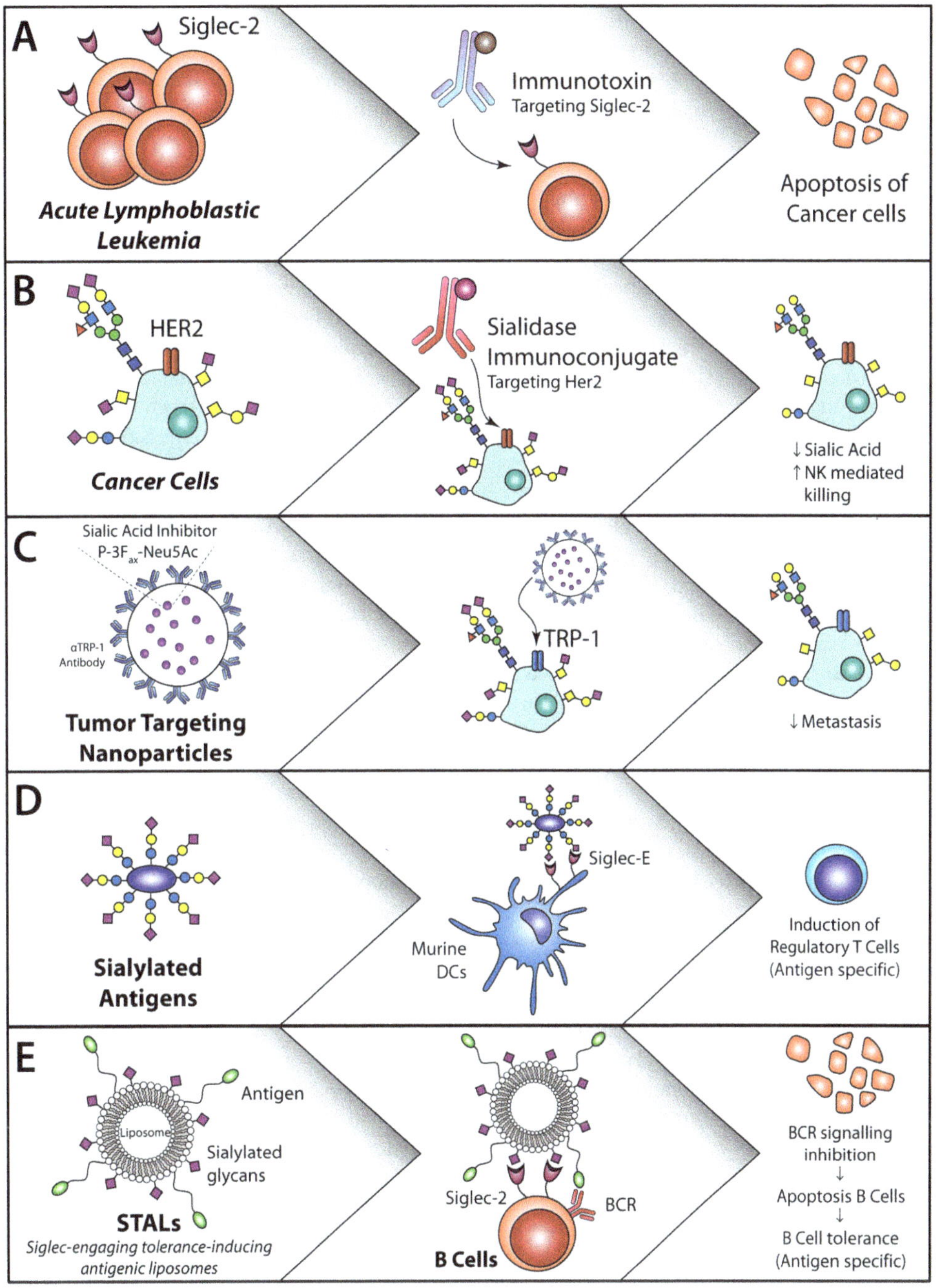

FIGURE 4 | Sialic acid–Siglec axis usage for the treatment of cancer or allergies and auto-immune diseases. **(A)** Siglec-2 antibodies coupled to an immunotoxin induce apoptosis of Siglec-2-expressing acute lymphoblastic leukemia cells (104). **(B)** HER2 targeting with a sialidase coupled to the HER2 antibody or locally applied non-targeted sialidases/synthesis inhibitors. This decreases sialic acid expression, reduce T reg induction and induced T cell activation and initiates NK cell killing (105). **(C)** Sialic acid inhibitor P-3F_{ax}-Neu5Ac inclusion in nanoparticles targeted to tumor cells inhibits the sialic acid expression on the tumor cells, thereby decreasing metastasis and increasing tumor cell killing (106, 107). **(D)** Sialylated antigens target DC to remove regulatory T cells (108). **(E)** Antigen-specific B cell apoptosis induction by STALs targeting Siglec-2 in combination with an antigen that inhibits B cell receptor signaling on B cells (109).

of acute myeloid leukemia (AML), is Siglec-3, using Siglec-3 antibody coupled to calicheamicin (116, 117). Hereby, the myeloid blasts that express Siglec-3 are targeted and this improved outcome in patients with relapsing disease as well as in elderly patients that were not eligible for extensive chemotherapy (116). Similar to the Siglec-2 antibody treatments, the Siglec-3 antibodies caused extensive adverse effects, probably due to the wide spread expression of Siglec-3 on (healthy) myeloid subsets. Therefore, it is of great imporatnce to have a complete and accurate overview of Siglec expression on immune cells. Other strategies to target Siglec-3 in AML include the use of CAR-T cells. Siglec-3 targeting CAR T-cells have shown to induce $CD8^+$ T cell degranulation against primary AML and AML cell lines *in-vitro* (118, 119). Although different CAR-T cells are already tested in the clinic for lymphoid leukemia (120), it is questionable whether Siglec3 targeting CAR-T cells have similar severe side effects as observed with Siglec-3 antibodies.

Instead of targeting the Siglecs using antibodies, modifying the phosphorylation status of Siglec-3 and Siglec-9, in particular dephosphorylation of the receptos, has shown to lead to increased immunity of moDCs, when treated with Dasatinib a SRC tyrosine kinase inhibitor that dephosphorylates Siglec-3 and Siglec-9 (121). Also, leukemia ($BCR\text{-}ABL^+$ AML) patients treated with Dasatinib, had a stronger $CD8^+$ T cell and NK cell response associated with long lasting remission (122). Another strategy to increase anti-tumor immunity through Siglecs has been developed by Xiao et al., where they target HER2 with a monoclonal antibody fused to a sialidase (105) (**Figure 4B**). This sialidase specifically cuts off the sialic acid ligands that are bound by Siglec-7 and Siglec-9 and thereby increase NK activity. *In vitro* these HER2 targeting antibodies fused to a sialidase, increased the NK cell mediated killing of HER2 positive tumor cells (105). As most breast cancer patients are HER2 positive, targeting of HER2 with this sialidase fused antibody could be an effective treatment strategy.

Most strategies that interfere with the sialic acids-Siglec Axis are developed for leukemic cells as they have high expression of Siglec-2 or Siglec-3 and are therefore easily targetable. Other cancer type treatments could also benefit from targeting Siglecs, blocking of Siglecs could abrogate the inhibitory effects on mononuclear phagocytes and lead to better migration and maturation of these cells, which subsequently stimulates tumor-specific T cell responses. Moreover, local removal of tumor-associated sialic acid may temporarily de-tolarize the tumor microenvironment and trigger immune activation at the tumor site. A combination with checkpoint inhibitors would than favor improved tumor eradication.

SIALIC ACID—SIGLEC AXIS TO INDUCE TOLERANCE FOR ALLERGIES AND AUTO-IMMUNE DISEASES

While in cancer it is important to induce immunity, in allergies and auto-immune diseases, an overactive immune system needs to be restored by inducing tolerance. Exploring the potential of the Sialic acid-Siglec Axis is an alternative to induce tolerance in an antigen specific manner. Because immune inhibitory Siglecs are found on mononuclear phagocytes, strategies can be designed aimed to actively induce tolerance via targeting inhibitory Siglecs on mononuclear phagocytes.

Modification of antigens such as OVA or MOG peptides with α2,3 or α2,6 sialyl-lactose has shown to increase targeting of these antigens to Siglec E, the human Siglec 7 and Siglec-9 homologue, and alter DC function in mice. Both *in-vitro* and *in-vivo* experiments demonstrated that sialic acid modified antigens induced antigen specific T reg induction and inhibition of inflammatory effector cells when activated with LPS (108) (**Figure 4D**).

Also, Siglec-engaging tolerance-inducing antigenic liposomes (STALs) are employed, in which sialic acid decorated nanoparticles, or sialo-glycoproteins or Siglec antibody targeting are used for Siglec targeting to induce tolerance. STALs with the peanut allergen Ara h2 (Ah2) and a high affinity Siglec-2 ligand (modified α2,6 linked sialic acid) incorporated in the outer membrane have shown high binding affinity to the B cell receptor and Siglec-2 simultaneously and to prevent peanut allergy against the Ah2 allergen in mice (109) (**Figure 4E**). This is acclaimed to the forced interaction between the B cell receptor and Siglec-2, thereby inducing apoptosis of autoreactive B cells. Pang et al. used the same STALs and incorporated rapamycin in the STALs and thereby enhanced the tolerogenic capacity in mice, which was the result of increased phagocytosis of these STALs by macrophages and DCs (123).

Sialic acid mimetics, such as the modified sialic acid coupled to liposomes discussed above, comprise of natural sialic acids as a backbone and are modified at certain positions in the sialic acid structures to develop high affinity ligands for Siglecs (124–126). Addition of hydrophobic groups at the C2 and C9 of α2,6 sialic acids results in a high affinity Siglec-2 ligands, which out-competing the *cis* interaction between the Siglec and its ligand. As a result better binding, endoyctosis, and eventually apoptosis of targeted B cells is acquired (126, 127).

Nanoparticles decorated with α2,8 linked sialic acids were developed to target murine Siglec-E (homologue of human Siglec-7 and Siglec-9) on macrophages. This approach limited the pro-inflammatory cytokines production by LPS-treated MQ *in-vitro*. Subsequently, these nanoparticles were able to limit the inflammation and increase levels of IL-10 in serum in a mouse model for LPS-induced systemic inflammation. Similar results were seen with human moMQ, resulting in an anti-inflammatory cytokine profile. In an *ex-vivo* human lung perfusion model the nanoparticles coated with α2,8 linked sialic acids reduced pulmonary oedema after LPS-induced injury (128).

Several studies have shown the importance of Siglec-sialic axes in auto-immune disease and allergy due to expression of Siglecs on other immune cells such as eosinophils and B-cells. Asthma is an eosinophil, expressing Siglec-8, mediated disease and it has been shown that polymorphisms in the SIGLEC8 gene are linked to the development of asthma (38, 129). Antibodies against Siglec-8 or the mouse homolog Siglec-F induce caspase and ROS dependent apoptosis of eosinophils (130, 131). Autoantibodies against Siglec-8 have been found in intravenous immunoglobulin preparations that are used in various chronic inflammatory disorders, although some cytotoxic effects are known (132). For asthma it would be beneficial to have specific Siglec-8 agonists to induce neutrophil apoptosis without the risk of side effects observed with intravenous immunoglobulin injections. Another example is the anti-Siglec-2 antibody (Epratuzumab) that has already been tested in seven clinical trials for the autoimmune disease systemic Lupus erythematosus (SLE). Although initial trials showed promising effects with reduced peripheral B cell numbers, the overall effect was not better than standard care for SLE (reviewed by D Geh) (133).

Most of these strategies are to date only tested in *in-vitro* or *ex-vivo* experiments and should be tested in *in-vivo* and clinical trials as they have great potential for future applications in the treatment of allergies and auto-immune diseases. It is also important to elucidate the Siglec expression on different human immune cell subsets in order to identify the potential risks on side-effects by targeting multiple Siglecs with one ligand.

CONCLUDING REMARKS

The last decade researchers identified the enormous potential of the sialic acid—Siglec axis to induce wanted or unwanted immune tolerance in cancer, allergies or auto-immune diseases. Both Siglec targeting antibodies, sialic acid mimetics, or glycan modifying agents can be used to interfere in this process and open new area's in the design of novel therapies for cancer, allergy and auto-immune diseases.

Still several questions need to be answered related to a better understanding of the biology of the Siglec-sialic acid axis. Those relate to the signaling capacity that sialic acid impose on immune cells to modify its function toward tolerance induction or activation of immunity. Interesting research topics to be addressed are: How do the various Siglecs expressed on one cell communicate with each other What is the exact specificity of these receptors for sialic-acids? Does multivalency of sialic acids or Siglec receptors matter? Other intriguing questions to be solved are: Do we need to inhibit only one Siglec receptor or more Siglec receptors simultaneously on one cell to alter function? What is the relation to *cis* and *trans* interaction on Siglec-sialic acid interactions? How important is the protein or lipid backbone on which the sialic acid is exposed? To answer these questions an urgent need for Siglec specific targeting molecules is needed, which can be sialic acid mimetics or Siglec specific antibodies.

As the Siglec—sialic axis plays a crucial role in tissue homeostasis and the resolution of inflammation, more studies are necessary to understand their involvement in these biomedical processes. A better understanding of its role in the resolution of inflammation is crucial for its application in the treatment of auto-immune diseases and allergies.

Moreover, both pathogens and tumors use the Siglec-sialic acid axis in their own benefit. It is therefore of vital importance to design new methods to modify glycosylation at site of infection or tumor location. Several studies already touch upon the investigation of targeting specific sialidases to the tumor micro-environment to remove the sialic acid content involved in the induction of tolerance in the tumor microenvironment. To unleash the sialic acid imposed tolerance in the local tumor microenvironment may be combined with other immune checkpoint inhibitors to stimulate tumor immunity in a multilevel manner. Alternatively, presence of sialic acid signatures in the tumor microenvironment may serve as new biomarkers to define immune tolerizing signatures in individual tumors and response therapy prediction (99).

Future studies are of great importance to unveil the complex Siglec-sialic acid axis and will warrant new discoveries in clinical application strategies in cancer, allergy and auto-immune diseases.

AUTHOR CONTRIBUTIONS

JL was involved in the writing, reading of literature, design and discussion of the figures. ER was involved in writing, critical reading of the manuscript and designing the figures. YvK was involved in the overall supervision of the review and editing of the manuscript.

ACKNOWLEDGMENTS

We gratefully thank Sandra J. van Vliet and Juan J. García-Vallejo, Amsterdam, UMC, Vrije University Amsterdam (Amsterdam, The Netherlands) for critical reading and fruitful discussions.

REFERENCES

1. Schlitzer A, McGovern N, Ginhoux F. Dendritic cells and monocyte-derived cells: two complementary and integrated functional systems. *Semin Cell Dev Biol.* (2015) 41:9–22. doi: 10.1016/j.semcdb.2015.03.011
2. Alcántara-Hernández M, Leylek R, Wagar LE, Engleman EG, Keler T, Marinkovich MP, et al. High-dimensional phenotypic mapping of human dendritic cells reveals interindividual variation and tissue specialization. *Immunity* (2017) 47:1037–50.e6. doi: 10.1016/j.immuni.2017.11.001
3. Ginhoux F, Jung S. Monocytes and macrophages: developmental pathways and tissue homeostasis. *Nat Rev Immunol.* (2014) 14:392–404. doi: 10.1038/nri3671
4. Haniffa M, Bigley V, Collin M. Human mononuclear phagocyte system reunited. *Semin Cell Dev Biol.* (2015) 41:59–69. doi: 10.1016/j.semcdb.2015.05.004
5. Kosten IJ, Van De Ven R, Thon M, Gibbs S, De Gruijl TD. Comparative phenotypic and functional analysis of migratory dendritic cell subsets from human oral mucosa and skin. *PLoS ONE* (2017) 12:1–15. doi: 10.1371/journal.pone.0180333
6. Nahrendorf M, Swirski FK. Abandoning M1/M2 for a network model of macrophage function. *Circ Res.* (2016) 119:414–7. doi: 10.1161/CIRCRESAHA.116.309194
7. Murray PJ, Allen JE, Biswas SK, Fisher EA, Gilroy DW, Goerdt S, et al. Macrophage activation and polarization: nomenclature and experimental guidelines. *Immunity* (2014) 41:14–20. doi: 10.1016/j.immuni.2014.06.008

8. Liu Y, Cao X. The origin and function of tumor-associated macrophages. *Cell Mol Immunol.* (2015) 12:1–4. doi: 10.1038/cmi.2014.83
9. Jongbloed SL, Kassianos AJ, McDonald KJ, Clark GJ, Ju X, Angel CE, et al. Human CD141+ (BDCA-3)+ dendritic cells (DCs) represent a unique myeloid DC subset that cross-presents necrotic cell antigens. *J Exp Med.* (2010) 207:1247–60. doi: 10.1084/jem.20092140
10. Collin M, McGovern N, Haniffa M. Human dendritic cell subsets. *Immunology* (2013) 140:22–30. doi: 10.1111/imm.12117
11. Liu Y-J. IPC: professional type 1 interferon-producing cells and plasmacytoid dendritic cell precursors. *Annu Rev Immunol.* (2005) 23:275–306. doi: 10.1146/annurev.immunol.23.021704.115633
12. Li MO, Flavell RA. Contextual regulation of inflammation: a duet by transforming growth factor-β and interleukin-10. *Immunity* (2008) 28:468–76. doi: 10.1016/j.immuni.2008.03.003
13. Schülke S. Induction of interleukin-10 producing dendritic cells as a tool to suppress allergen-specific T helper 2 responses. *Front Immunol.* (2018) 9:455. doi: 10.3389/fimmu.2018.00455
14. Yoo S, Ha SJ. Generation of tolerogenic dendritic cells and their therapeutic applications. *Immune Netw.* (2016) 16:52–60. doi: 10.4110/in.2016.16.1.52
15. Romani N. Proliferating dendritic cell progenitors in human blood. *J Exp Med.* (1994) 180:83–93. doi: 10.1084/jem.180.1.83
16. Ohradanova-Repic A, Machacek C, Fischer MB, Stockinger H. Differentiation of human monocytes and derived subsets of macrophages and dendritic cells by the HLDA10 monoclonal antibody panel. *Clin Transl Immunol.* (2016) 5:e55. doi: 10.1038/cti.2015.39
17. Cravens PD, Hayashida K, Davis LS, Nanki T, Lipsky PE. Human peripheral blood dendritic cells and monocyte subsets display similar chemokine receptor expression profiles with differential migratory responses. *Scand J Immunol.* (2007) 65:514–24. doi: 10.1111/j.1365-3083.2007.01933.x
18. Ruben JM, Bontkes HJ, Westers TM, Hooijberg E, Ossenkoppele GJ, de Gruijl TD, et al. Differential capacity of human interleukin-4 and interferon-α monocyte-derived dendritic cells for cross-presentation of free versus cell-associated antigen. *Cancer Immunol Immunother.* (2015) 64:1419–27. doi: 10.1007/s00262-015-1741-1
19. Tang-Huau TL, Gueguen P, Goudot C, Durand M, Bohec M, Baulande S, et al. Human *in vivo*-generated monocyte-derived dendritic cells and macrophages cross-present antigens through a vacuolar pathway. *Nat Commun.* (2018) 9:2570. doi: 10.1038/s41467-018-04985-0
20. Faure F, Jouve M, Lebhar-Peguillet I, Sadaka C, Sepulveda F, Lantz O, et al. Blood monocytes sample MelanA/MART1 antigen for long-lasting cross-presentation to CD8+T cells after differentiation into dendritic cells. *Int J Cancer* (2018) 142:133–44. doi: 10.1002/ijc.31037
21. Schultze JL, Aschenbrenner AC. Systems immunology allows a new view on human dendritic cells. *Semin Cell Dev Biol.* (2018). doi: 10.1016/j.semcdb.2018.02.017. [Epub ahead of print].
22. Balan S, Ollion V, Colletti N, Chelbi R, Montanana-Sanchis F, Liu H, et al. Human XCR1 + dendritic cells derived *in vitro* from CD34+ progenitors closely resemble blood dendritic cells, including their adjuvant responsiveness, contrary to monocyte-derived dendritic cells. *J Immunol.* (2014) 193:1622–35. doi: 10.4049/jimmunol.1401243
23. Akira S, Uematsu S, Takeuchi O. Pathogen recognition and innate immunity. *Cell* (2006) 124:783–801. doi: 10.1016/j.cell.2006.02.015
24. van Vliet SJ, van Liempt E, Geijtenbeek TBH, van Kooyk Y. Differential regulation of C-type lectin expression on tolerogenic dendritic cell subsets. *Immunobiology* (2006) 211:577–85. doi: 10.1016/j.imbio.2006.05.022
25. van Vliet SJ, Paessens LC, Broks-van den Berg VCM, Geijtenbeek TBH, van Kooyk Y. The C-type lectin macrophage galactose-type lectin impedes migration of immature APCs. *J Immunol.* (2008) 181:3148–55. doi: 10.4049/jimmunol.181.5.3148
26. Geijtenbeek TBH, Gringhuis SI. C-type lectin receptors in the control of T helper cell differentiation. *Nat Rev Immunol.* (2016) 16:433–48. doi: 10.1038/nri.2016.55
27. Geijtenbeek TBH, Gringhuis SI. Signalling through C-type lectin receptors: shaping immune responses. *Nat Rev Immunol.* (2009) 9:465–79. doi: 10.1038/nri2569
28. Monteiro J, Lepenies B. Myeloid C-type lectin receptors in viral recognition and antiviral immunity. *Viruses* (2017) 9:59. doi: 10.3390/v9030059
29. Akramien D, Kondrotas A, Did J, Egidijus K. Effects of b-glucans on the immune system. *Medicina* (2007) 43:597–606.
30. Feng D, Wang Y, Liu Y, Wu L, Li X, Chen Y, et al. DC-SIGN reacts with TLR-4 and regulates inflammatory cytokine expression via NF-κB activation in renal tubular epithelial cells during acute renal injury. *Clin Exp Immunol.* (2018) 191:107–15. doi: 10.1111/cei.13048
31. Gringhuis SI, den Dunnen J, Litjens M, van het Hof B, van Kooyk Y, Geijtenbeek TBH. C-type lectin DC-SIGN modulates toll-like receptor signaling via Raf-1 kinase-dependent acetylation of transcription factor NF-κB. *Immunity* (2007) 26:605–16. doi: 10.1016/j.immuni.2007.03.012
32. Gringhuis SI, Kaptein TM, Wevers BA, Mesman AW, Geijtenbeek TBH. Fucose-specific DC-SIGN signalling directs T helper cell type-2 responses via IKKε-and CYLD-dependent Bcl3 activation. *Nat Commun.* (2014) 5:1–13. doi: 10.1038/ncomms4898
33. Schnaar RL. Glycobiology simplified: diverse roles of glycan recognition in inflammation. *J Leukoc Biol.* (2016) 99:825–38. doi: 10.1189/jlb.3RI0116-021R
34. Harduin-Lepers A, Vallejo-Ruiz V, Krzewinski-Recchi MA, Samyn-Petit B, Julien S, Delannoy P. The human sialyltransferase family. *Biochimie* (2001) 83:727–37. doi: 10.1016/S0300-9084(01)01301-3
35. Varki A, Cummings RD, Esko JD, Stanley P, Hart GW, Aebi M, et al. *Essential of Glycobiology.* 3rd ed. Cold Spring Harbor, NY: Cold Spring Harbor Laboratory Press. Available online at: https://www.ncbi.nlm.nih.gov/books/NBK310274/
36. Rillahan CD, Antonopoulos A, Lefort CT, Sonon R, Ley K, Dell A, et al. Global metabolic inhibitors of sialyl- and fucosyltransferases cory. *Nat Chem Biol.* (2012) 8:661–8. doi: 10.1038/nchembio.999
37. Kiwamoto T, Katoh T, Tiemeyer M, Bochner BS. The role of lung epithelial ligands for Siglec-8 and Siglec-F in eosinophilic inflammation. *Curr Opin Allergy Clin Immunol.* (2013) 13:106–11. doi: 10.1097/ACI.0b013e32835b594a
38. Johansson M, Kelly E, Nguyen C, Jarjour N, Bochner BS. Characterization of Siglec-8 expression on lavage cells after segmental lung allergen challenge. *Int Arch Allergy Immunol.* (2018) 177:16–28. doi: 10.1159/000488951
39. Jenner J, Kerst G, Handgretinger R, Müller I. Increased α2,6-sialylation of surface proteins on tolerogenic, immature dendritic cells and regulatory T cells. *Exp Hematol.* (2006) 34:1211–7. doi: 10.1016/j.exphem.2006.04.016
40. Maurer MA, Meyer L, Bianchi M, Turner HL, Le NPL, Steck M, et al. Glycosylation of human IgA directly inhibits influenza A and other sialic-acid-binding viruses. *Cell Rep.* (2018) 23:90–9. doi: 10.1016/j.celrep.2018.03.027
41. Inzana TJ, Balyan R, Howard MD. Decoration of *Histophilus somni* lipooligosaccharide with N-acetyl-5-neuraminic acid enhances bacterial binding of complement factor H and resistance to killing by serum and polymorphonuclear leukocytes. *Vet Microbiol.* (2012) 161:113–21. doi: 10.1016/j.vetmic.2012.07.008
42. Schmidt CQ, Hipgrave Ederveen AL, Harder MJ, Wuhrer M, Stehle T, Blaum BS. Biophysical analysis of sialic acid recognition by the complement regulator Factor H. *Glycobiology* (2018) 28:765–73. doi: 10.1093/glycob/cwy061
43. Blaum BS. The lectin self of complement factor H. *Curr Opin Struct Biol.* (2017) 44:111–8. doi: 10.1016/j.sbi.2017.01.005
44. Angata T, Varki A. Chemical diversity in the sialic acids and related α-keto acids: an evolutionary perspective. *Chem Rev.* (2002) 102:439–70. doi: 10.1021/cr000407m
45. Varki A. Glycan-based interactions involving vertebrate sialic-acid-recognizing proteins. *Nature* (2007) 446:1023–9. doi: 10.1038/nature05816
46. Ali SR, Fong JJ, Carlin AF, Busch TD, Linden R, Angata T, et al. Siglec-5 and Siglec-14 are polymorphic paired receptors that modulate neutrophil and amnion signaling responses to group B *Streptococcus. J Exp Med.* (2014) 211:1231–42. doi: 10.1084/jem.20131853
47. Avril T, Attrill H, Zhang J, Raper A, Crocker PR. Negative regulation of leucocyte functions by CD33-related siglecs. *Biochem Soc Trans.* (2006) 34:1024–7. doi: 10.1042/BST0341024
48. Lehmann F, Gäthje H, Kelm S, Dietz F. Evolution of sialic acid-binding proteins: molecular cloning and expression of fish siglec-4. *Glycobiology* (2004) 14:959–68. doi: 10.1093/glycob/cwh120

49. Angata T, Tabuchi Y, Nakamura K, Nakamura M. Siglec-15: an immune system Siglec conserved throughout vertebrate evolution. *Glycobiology* (2007) 17:838–46. doi: 10.1093/glycob/cwm049
50. Crocker PR, Gordon S. Properties and distribution of a lectin-like hemagglutinin differentially expressed by murine stromal tissue macrophages. *J Exp Med.* (1986) 164:1862–75. doi: 10.1084/jem.164.6.1862
51. Angata T, Margulies EH, Green ED, Varki A. Large-scale sequencing of the CD33-related Siglec gene cluster in five mammalian species reveals rapid evolution by multiple mechanisms. *Proc Natl Acad Sci USA.* (2004) 101:13251–6. doi: 10.1073/pnas.0404833101
52. Barber EK, Crocker PR. Characterization of CD33 as a new member of the sialoadhesin family of cellular interaction molecules. *Blood* (1995) 85:2005–12.
53. Higuchi H, Shoji T, Iijima S, Nishijima KI. Constitutively expressed Siglec-9 inhibits LPS-induced CCR7, but enhances IL-4-induced CD200R expression in human macrophages. *Biosci Biotechnol Biochem.* (2016) 80:1141–8. doi: 10.1080/09168451.2016.1146070
54. Lock K, Zhang J, Lu J, Lee SH, Crocker PR. Expression of CD33-related siglecs on human mononuclear phagocytes, monocyte-derived dendritic cells and plasmacytoid dendritic cells. *Immunobiology* (2004) 209:199–207. doi: 10.1016/j.imbio.2004.04.007
55. Büll C, Collado-Camps E, Kers-Rebel ED, Heise T, Søndergaard JN, Den Brok MH, et al. Metabolic sialic acid blockade lowers the activation threshold of moDCs for TLR stimulation. *Immunol Cell Biol.* (2017) 95:408–15. doi: 10.1038/icb.2016.105
56. De Saint Jean A, Lucht F, Bourlet T, Delézay O. Transforming growth factor beta 1 up-regulates CD169 (sialoadhesin) expression on monocytederived dendritic cells: role in HIV sexual transmission. *AIDS* (2014) 28:2375–80. doi: 10.1097/QAD.0000000000000431
57. Nicoll G, Ni J, Liu D, Klenerman P, Munday J, Dubock S, et al. Identification and characterization of a novel Siglec, Siglec-7, expressed by human natural killer cells and monocytes. *J Biol Chem.* (1999) 274:34089–95. doi: 10.1074/jbc.274.48.34089
58. Angata T, Varki A. Cloning, characterization, and phylogenetic analysis of Siglec-9, a new member of the CD33-related group of Siglecs: evidence for co-evolution with sialic acid synthesis pathways. *J Biol Chem.* (2000) 275:22127–35. doi: 10.1074/jbc.M002775200
59. Zhang JQ, Nicoll G, Jones C, Crocker PR. Siglec-9, a novel sialic acid binding member of the immunoglobulin superfamily expressed broadly on human blood leukocytes. *J Biol Chem.* (2000) 275:22121–6. doi: 10.1074/jbc.M002788200
60. Li N, Zhang W, Wan T, Zhang J, Chen T, Yu Y, et al. Cloning and characterization of Siglec-10, a novel sialic acid binding member of the Ig superfamily, from human dendritic cells. *J Biol Chem.* (2001) 276:28106–12. doi: 10.1074/jbc.M100467200
61. Schwarz F, Landig CS, Siddiqui S, Secundino I, Olson J, Varki N, et al. Paired Siglec receptors generate opposite inflammatory responses to a human-specific pathogen. *EMBO J.* (2017) 36:751–60. doi: 10.15252/embj.2016 95581
62. Cao H, Lakner U, de Bono B, Traherne JA, Trowsdale J, Barrow AD. SIGLEC16 encodes a DAP12-associated receptor expressed in macrophages that evolved from its inhibitory counterpart SIGLEC11 and has functional and non-functional alleles in humans. *Eur J Immunol.* (2008) 38:2303–15. doi: 10.1002/eji.200738078
63. Reineks EZ, Osei ES, Rosenberg A, Auletta J, Meyerson HJ. CD22 expression on blastic plasmacytoid dendritic cell neoplasms and reactivity of anti-CD22 antibodies to peripheral blood dendritic cells. *Cytom Part B Clin Cytom.* (2009) 76B:237–48. doi: 10.1002/cyto.b.20469
64. Crespo I, Paiva A, Couceiro A, Pimentel P, Orfão A, Regateiro F. Immunophenotypic and functional characterization of cord blood dendritic cells. *Stem Cells Dev.* (2004) 13:63–70. doi: 10.1089/154732804773099263
65. Thomas R, Lipsky PE. Human peripheral blood dendritic cell subsets. Isolation and characterization of precursor and mature antigen-presenting cells. *J Immunol.* (1994) 153:4016–28. Available at: http://www.ncbi.nlm.nih.gov/pubmed/7523513
66. Varki A, Angata T. Siglecs - the major subfamily of I-type lectins. *Glycobiology* (2006) 16:1–27. doi: 10.1093/glycob/cwj008
67. Bochner BS, Zimmermann N. Role of siglecs and related glycan-binding proteins in immune responses and immunoregulation. *J Allergy Clin Immunol.* (2015) 135:598–608. doi: 10.1016/j.jaci.2014.11.031
68. Wilhelm TR, Taddeo A, Winter O, Schulz AR, Mälzer JN, Domingo C, et al. Siglec-1-positive plasmacytoid dendritic cells (pDCs) in human peripheral blood: a semi-mature and myeloid-like subset imbalanced during protective and autoimmune responses. *Clin Immunol.* (2016) 163:42–51. doi: 10.1016/j.clim.2015.12.001
69. MacAuley MS, Crocker PR, Paulson JC. Siglec regulation of immune cell function in disease. *Nat Rev Immunol.* (2014) 14:653–66. doi: 10.1038/nri3737
70. Cohen M, Varki A. The sialome—far more than the sum of its parts. *Omi A J Integr Biol.* (2010) 14:455–64. doi: 10.1089/omi.2009.0148
71. Varki A. Evolutionary forces shaping the Golgi glycosylation machinery: Why cell surface glycans are universal to living cells. *Cold Spring Harb Perspect Biol.* (2011) 3:1–14. doi: 10.1101/cshperspect.a005462
72. Crocker PR, Paulson JC, Varki A. Siglecs and their roles in the immune system. *Nat Rev Immunol.* (2007) 7:255–66. doi: 10.1038/nri2056
73. Avril T, Floyd H, Lopez F, Vivier E, Crocker PR. The membrane-proximal immunoreceptor tyrosine-based inhibitory motif is critical for the inhibitory signaling mediated by Siglecs-7 and−9, CD33-related Siglecs expressed on human monocytes and NK cells. *J Immunol.* (2004) 173:6841–9. doi: 10.4049/jimmunol.173.11.6841
74. Crocker PR, Redelinghuys P. Siglecs as positive and negative regulators of the immune system: figure 1. *Biochem Soc Trans.* (2008) 36:1467–71. doi: 10.1042/BST0361467
75. Walter RB, Häusermann P, Raden BW, Teckchandani AM, Kamikura DM, Bernstein ID, et al. Phosphorylated ITIMs enable ubiquitylation of an inhibitory cell surface receptor. *Traffic* (2008) 9:267–79. doi: 10.1111/j.1600-0854.2007.00682.x
76. Orr SJ, Morgan NM, Elliott J, Burrows JF, Scott CJ, McVicar DW, et al. CD33 responses are blocked by SOCS3 through accelerated proteasomal-mediated turnover. *Blood* (2007) 109:1061–8. doi: 10.1182/blood-2006-05-023556
77. Vitale C, Romagnani C, Falco M, Ponte M, Vitale M, Moretta A, et al. Engagement of p75/AIRM1 or CD33 inhibits the proliferation of normal or leukemic myeloid cells. *Proc Natl Acad Sci USA.* (1999) 96:15091–6. doi: 10.1073/pnas.96.26.15091
78. Lajaunias F, Dayer JM, Chizzolini C. Constitutive repressor activity of CD33 on human monocytes requires sialic acid recognition and phosphoinositide 3-kinase-mediated intracellular signaling. *Eur J Immunol.* (2005) 35:243–51. doi: 10.1002/eji.200425273
79. Backer R, Schwandt T, Greuter M, Oosting M, Jungerkes F, Tuting T, et al. Effective collaboration between marginal metallophilic macrophages and CD8+ dendritic cells in the generation of cytotoxic T cells. *Proc Natl Acad Sci USA.* (2010) 107:216–21. doi: 10.1073/pnas.0909541107
80. van Dinther D, Veninga H, Iborra S, Borg EGF, Hoogterp L, Olesek K, et al. Functional CD169 on macrophages mediates interaction with dendritic cells for CD8+T cell cross-priming. *Cell Rep.* (2018) 22:1484–95. doi: 10.1016/j.celrep.2018.01.021
81. Veninga H, Borg EGF, Vreeman K, Taylor PR, Kalay H, van Kooyk Y, et al. Antigen targeting reveals splenic CD169+macrophages as promoters of germinal center B-cell responses. *Eur J Immunol.* (2015) 45:747–57. doi: 10.1002/eji.201444983
82. Higuchi H, Shoji T, Murase Y, Iijima S, Nishijima KI. Siglec-9 modulated IL-4 responses in the macrophage cell line RAW264. *Biosci Biotechnol Biochem.* (2016) 80:501–9. doi: 10.1080/09168451.2015.1104238
83. Chen GY, Brown NK, Wu W, Khedri Z, Yu H, Chen X, et al. Broad and direct interaction between TLR and Siglec families of pattern recognition receptors and its regulation by Neu1. *Elife* (2014) 3:e04066. doi: 10.7554/eLife.04066
84. Silva M, Silva Z, Marques G, Ferro T, Gonçalves M, Monteiro M, et al. Sialic acid removal from dendritic cells improves antigen cross-presentation and boosts anti-tumor immune responses. *Oncotarget* (2016) 7:41053–66. doi: 10.18632/oncotarget.9419
85. Nardy AFFR, Freire-de-Lima CG, Pérez AR, Morrot A. Role of *Trypanosoma cruzi* Trans-sialidase on the escape from host immune surveillance. *Front Microbiol.* (2016) 7:348. doi: 10.3389/fmicb.2016.00348

86. Bornhöfft KF, Goldammer T, Rebl A, Galuska SP. Siglecs: a journey through the evolution of sialic acid-binding immunoglobulin-type lectins. *Dev Comp Immunol.* (2018) 86:219–31. doi: 10.1016/j.dci.2018.05.008
87. Erdmann H, Steeg C, Koch-Nolte F, Fleischer B, Jacobs T. Sialylated ligands on pathogenic *Trypanosoma cruzi* interact with Siglec-E (sialic acid-binding Ig-like lectin-E). *Cell Microbiol.* (2009) 11:1600–11. doi: 10.1111/j.1462-5822.2009.01350.x
88. Freire-de-Lima L, Alisson-Silva F, Carvalho ST, Takiya CM, Rodrigues MM, DosReis GA, et al. *Trypanosoma cruzi* subverts host cell sialylation and may compromise antigen-specific CD8+ T cell responses. *J Biol Chem.* (2010) 285:13388–96. doi: 10.1074/jbc.M109.096305
89. Carlin AF, Chang Y-C, Areschoug T, Lindahl G, Hurtado-Ziola N, King CC, et al. Group B *Streptococcus* suppression of phagocyte functions by protein-mediated engagement of human Siglec-5. *J Exp Med.* (2009) 206:1691–9. doi: 10.1084/jem.20090691
90. Carlin AF, Uchiyama S, Chang YC, Lewis AL, Nizet V, Varki A. Molecular mimicry of host sialylated glycans allows a bacterial pathogen to engage neutrophil Siglec-9 and dampen the innate immune response. *Blood* (2009) 113:3333–6. doi: 10.1182/blood-2008-11-187302
91. Khatua B, Bhattacharya K, Mandal C. Sialoglycoproteins adsorbed by *Pseudomonas aeruginosa* facilitate their survival by impeding neutrophil extracellular trap through siglec-9. *J Leukoc Biol.* (2012) 91:641–55. doi: 10.1189/jlb.0511260
92. Izquierdo-Useros N, Lorizate M, Puertas MC, Rodriguez-Plata MT, Zangger N, Erikson E, et al. Siglec-1 is a novel dendritic cell receptor that mediates HIV-1 trans-infection through recognition of viral membrane gangliosides. *PLoS Biol.* (2012) 10:e1001448. doi: 10.1371/journal.pbio.1001448
93. Vanderheijden N, Delputte PL, Favoreel HW, Vandekerckhove J, Damme J Van, Woensel P A Van, et al. Involvement of sialoadhesin in entry of porcine reproductive and respiratory syndrome virus into porcine alveolar macrophages involvement of sialoadhesin in entry of porcine reproductive and respiratory syndrome virus into porcine alveolar macrophages. *J Virol.* (2003) 77:8207–15. doi: 10.1128/JVI.77.15.8207-8215.2003
94. Delputte PL, Nauwynck HJ. Porcine arterivirus infection of alveolar macrophages is mediated by sialic acid on the virus. *J Virol.* (2004) 78:8094–101. doi: 10.1128/JVI.78.15.8094-8101.2004
95. Chang YC, Olson J, Louie A, Crocker PR, Varki A, Nizet V. Role of macrophage sialoadhesin in host defense against the sialylated pathogen group B *Streptococcus*. *J Mol Med.* (2014) 92:951–9. doi: 10.1007/s00109-014-1157-y
96. Byrd-Leotis L, Cummings RD, Steinhauer DA. The interplay between the host receptor and influenza virus hemagglutinin and neuraminidase. *Int J Mol Sci.* (2017) 18:1541. doi: 10.3390/ijms18071541
97. Heise T, Langereis JD, Rossing E, de Jonge MI, Adema GJ, Büll C, et al. Selective inhibition of sialic acid-based molecular mimicry in *Haemophilus influenzae* abrogates serum resistance. *Cell Chem Biol.* (2018) 25:1279–85.e8. doi: 10.1016/j.chembiol.2018.05.018
98. Bronikowska I, Swietochowska E, Oleksiak M, Czecior E. Sialic acids in head and neck squamous cell carcinoma. *Postep Hig Med Dosw.* (2016) 70:1300–8. doi: 10.5604/17322693.1227410
99. Rodríguez E, Schetters STT, van Kooyk Y. The tumour glyco-code as a novel immune checkpoint for immunotherapy. *Nat Rev Immunol.* (2018) 18:204–11. doi: 10.1038/nri.2018.3
100. Borzym-Kluczyk M, Radziejewska I, Cechowska-Pasko M, Darewicz B. Reduced expression of E-cadherin and increased sialylation level in clear cell renal cell carcinoma. *Acta Biochim Pol.* (2017) 64:465–70. doi: 10.18388/abp.2015_1215
101. Pihikova D, Kasak P, Kubanikova P, Sokol R, Tkac J. Aberrant sialylation of a prostate-specific antigen: electrochemical label-free glycoprofiling in prostate cancer serum samples. *Anal Chim Acta* (2016) 934:72–9. doi: 10.1016/j.aca.2016.06.043
102. Zhang Z, Wuhrer M, Holst S. Serum sialylation changes in cancer. *Glycoconj J.* (2018) 35:139–60. doi: 10.1007/s10719-018-9820-0
103. Adams OJ, Stanczak MA, von Gunten S, Läubli H. Targeting sialic acid–Siglec interactions to reverse immune suppression in cancer. *Glycobiology* (2017) 28:640–7. doi: 10.1093/glycob/cwx108
104. Kantarjian HM, DeAngelo DJ, Stelljes M, Martinelli G, Liedtke M, Stock W, et al. Inotuzumab ozogamicin versus standard therapy for acute lymphoblastic leukemia. *N Engl J Med.* (2016) 375:740–53. doi: 10.1056/NEJMoa1509277
105. Xiao H, Woods EC, Vukojicic P, Bertozzi CR. Precision glycocalyx editing as a strategy for cancer immunotherapy. *Proc Natl Acad Sci USA.* (2016) 113:10304–9. doi: 10.1073/pnas.1608069113
106. Büll C, Boltje TJ, Balneger N, Weischer SM, Wassink M, van Gemst JJ, et al. Sialic acid blockade suppresses tumor growth by enhancing T cell-mediated tumor immunity. *Cancer Res.* (2018) 78:3574–88. doi: 10.1158/0008-5472.CAN-17-3376
107. Büll C, Boltje TJ, Van Dinther EAW, Peters T, De Graaf AMA, Leusen JHW, et al. Targeted delivery of a sialic acid-blocking glycomimetic to cancer cells inhibits metastatic spread. *ACS Nano* (2015) 9:733–45. doi: 10.1021/nn5061964
108. Perdicchio M, Ilarregui JM, Verstege MI, Cornelissen LAM, Schetters STT, Engels S, et al. Sialic acid-modified antigens impose tolerance via inhibition of T-cell proliferation and *de novo* induction of regulatory T cells. *Proc Natl Acad Sci USA.* (2016) 113:3329–34. doi: 10.1073/pnas.1507706113
109. Orgel KA, Duan S, Wright BL, Maleki SJ, Wolf JC, Vichery BP, et al. Exploiting CD22 on antigen-specific B-cells to prevent allergy to the major peanut allergen ara h 2. *Allergy Eur J Allergy Clin Immunol.* (2017) 139:366–9.e2. doi: 10.1016/j.jaci.2016.06.053
110. Perdicchio M, Cornelissen LAM, Streng-Ouwehand I, Engels S, Verstege MI, Boon L, et al. Tumor sialylation impedes T cell mediated anti-tumor responses while promoting tumor associated-regulatory T cells. *Oncotarget* (2016) 7:8771–82. doi: 10.18632/oncotarget.6822
111. Burchell J, Poulsom R, Handby A, Whitehouse C, Cooper L, Clausen H, et al. An alpha2,3sialyltransferase (ST3Gal I) is elevated in primary breast carcinomas. *Glycobiology* (1999) 9:1307–11. doi: 10.1093/glycob/9.12.1307
112. Gendler SJ, Lancaster CA, Taylor-Papadimitriou J, Duhig T, Peat N, Burchell J, et al. Molecular cloning and expression of human tumor-associated polymorphic epithelial mucin. *J Biol Chem.* (1990) 265:15286–93.
113. Beatson R, Tajadura-ortega V, Achkova D, Picco G, Tsourouktsoglou T-D, Klausing S, et al. MUC1 modulates the tumor immune microenvironment through the engagement of Siglec-9. *Nat Immunol.* (2016) 17:1273–81. doi: 10.1038/ni.3552
114. Ohta M, Ishida A, Toda M, Akita K, Inoue M, Yamashita K, et al. Immunomodulation of monocyte-derived dendritic cells through ligation of tumor-produced mucins to Siglec-9. *Biochem Biophys Res Commun.* (2010) 402:663–9. doi: 10.1016/j.bbrc.2010.10.079
115. Ishida A, Ohta M, Toda M, Murata T, Usui T, Akita K, et al. Mucin-induced apoptosis of monocyte-derived dendritic cells during maturation. *Proteomics* (2008) 8:3342–9. doi: 10.1002/pmic.200800039
116. Amadori S, Suciu S, Selleslag D, Aversa F, Gaidano G, Musso M, et al. Gemtuzumab ozogamicin versus best supportive care in older patients with newly diagnosed acute myeloid leukemia unsuitable for intensive chemotherapy: results of the randomized phase III EORTC-GIMEMA AML-19 trial. *J Clin Oncol.* (2016) 34:972–9. doi: 10.1200/JCO.2015.64.0060
117. Castaigne S, Pautas C, Terré C, Raffoux E, Bordessoule D, Bastie JN, et al. Effect of gemtuzumab ozogamicin on survival of adult patients with de-novo acute myeloid leukaemia (ALFA-0701): a randomised, open-label, phase 3 study. *Lancet* (2012) 379:1508–16. doi: 10.1016/S0140-6736(12)60485-1
118. O'Hear C, Heiber JF, Schubert I, Fey G, Geiger TL. Anti-CD33 chimeric antigen receptor targeting of acute myeloid leukemia. *Haematologica* (2015) 100:336–44. doi: 10.3324/haematol.2014.112748
119. Minagawa K, Jamil MO, Al-Obaidi M, Pereboeva L, Salzman D, Erba HP, et al. *In vitro* pre-clinical validation of suicide gene modified anti-CD33 redirected chimeric antigen receptor T-cells for acute myeloid leukemia. *PLoS ONE* (2016) 11:e0166891. doi: 10.1371/journal.pone.0166891
120. Brentjens R, Davila ML, Riviere I, Park J, Cowell LG, Bartido S, et al. CD19-targeted T cells rapidly induce molecular remissions in adults with chemotherapy-refractory acute lymphoblastic leukemia. *Sci Transl Med.* (2013) 5:177ra38. doi: 10.1126/scitranslmed.3005930
121. Nerreter T, Köchel C, Jesper D, Eichelbrönner I, Putz E, Einsele H, et al. Dasatinib enhances migration of monocyte-derived dendritic cells by reducing phosphorylation of inhibitory immune receptors Siglec-9 and Siglec-3. *Exp Hematol.* (2014) 42:773–82.e1–3. doi: 10.1016/j.exphem.2014.05.010

122. Mustjoki S, Ekblom M, Arstila TP, Dybedal I, Epling-Burnette PK, Guilhot F, et al. Clonal expansion of T/NK-cells during tyrosine kinase inhibitor dasatinib therapy. *Leukemia* (2009) 23:1398–405. doi: 10.1038/leu.2009.46
123. Pang L, Macauley MS, Arlian BM, Nycholat CM, Paulson JC. Encapsulating an immunosuppressant enhances tolerance induction by Siglec-engaging tolerogenic liposomes. *ChemBioChem.* (2017) 18:1226–33. doi: 10.1002/cbic.201600702
124. Büll C, Heise T, Adema GJ, Boltje TJ. Sialic acid mimetics to target the sialic acid-siglec axis. *Trends Biochem Sci.* (2016) 41:519–31. doi: 10.1016/j.tibs.2016.03.007
125. Prescher H, Schweizer A, Kuhfeldt E, Nitschke L, Brossmer R. Discovery of multifold modified sialosides as Human CD22/Siglec-2 ligands with nanomolar activity on B-cells. *ACS Chem Biol.* (2014) 9:1444–50. doi: 10.1021/cb400952v
126. Abdu-Allah HHM, Watanabe K, Completo GC, Sadagopan M, Hayashizaki K, Takaku C, et al. CD22-antagonists with nanomolar potency: the synergistic effect of hydrophobic groups at C-2 and C-9 of sialic acid scaffold. *Bioorg Med Chem.* (2011) 19:1–16. doi: 10.1016/j.bmc.2011.01.060
127. Collins BE, Blixt O, Han S, Duong B, Li H, Nathan JK, et al. High-affinity ligand probes of CD22 overcome the threshold set by cis ligands to allow for binding, endocytosis, and killing of B cells. *J Immunol.* (2006) 177:2994–3003. doi: 10.4049/jimmunol.177.5.2994
128. Spence S, Greene MK, Fay F, Hams E, Saunders SP, Hamid U, et al. Targeting Siglecs with a sialic acid-decorated nanoparticle abrogates inflammation. *Sci Transl Med.* (2015) 7:303ra140. doi: 10.1126/scitranslmed.aab3459
129. Gao PS, Shimizu K, Grant A V., Rafaels N, Zhou LF, Hudson SA, et al. Polymorphisms in the sialic acid-binding immunoglobulin-like lectin-8 (Siglec-8) gene are associated with susceptibility to asthma. *Eur J Hum Genet.* (2010) 18:713–9. doi: 10.1038/ejhg.2009.239
130. Nutku E, Hudson SA, Bochner BS. Mechanism of Siglec-8-induced human eosinophil apoptosis: role of caspases and mitochondrial injury. *Biochem Biophys Res Commun.* (2005) 336:918–24. doi: 10.1016/j.bbrc.2005.08.202
131. Zimmermann N, McBride ML, Yamada Y, Hudson SA, Jones C, Cromie KD, et al. Siglec-F antibody administration to mice selectively reduces blood and tissue eosinophils. *Allergy Eur J Allergy Clin Immunol.* (2008) 63:1156–63. doi: 10.1111/j.1398-9995.2008.01709.x
132. von Gunten S, Vogel M, Schaub A, Stadler BM, Miescher S, Crocker PR, et al. Intravenous immunoglobulin preparations contain anti-Siglec-8 autoantibodies. *J Allergy Clin Immunol.* (2007) 119:1005–11. doi: 10.1016/j.jaci.2007.01.023
133. Geh D, Gordon C. Epratuzumab for the treatment of systemic lupus erythematosus. *Expert Rev Clin Immunol.* (2018) 14:245–58. doi: 10.1080/1744666X.2018.1450141

15

Dendritic Cells Actively Limit Interleukin-10 Production Under Inflammatory Conditions via DC-SCRIPT and Dual-Specificity Phosphatase 4

Jonas Nørskov Søndergaard[1†], Simon J. van Heeringen[2], Maaike W. G. Looman[1], Chunling Tang[1], Vassilis Triantis[1†], Pauline Louche[1], Eva M. Janssen-Megens[3], Anieta M. Sieuwerts[4], John W. M. Martens[4], Colin Logie[3], Hendrik G. Stunnenberg[3], Marleen Ansems[1] and Gosse J. Adema[1*]*

[1] Radiotherapy & OncoImmunology Laboratory, Department of Radiation Oncology, Radboud Institute for Molecular Life Sciences, Radboud University Medical Center, Nijmegen, Netherlands, [2] Department of Molecular Developmental Biology, Faculty of Science, Radboud Institute for Molecular Life Sciences, Radboud University, Nijmegen, Netherlands, [3] Department of Molecular Biology, Faculties of Science and Medicine, Radboud Institute for Molecular Life Sciences, Radboud University, Nijmegen, Netherlands, [4] Department of Medical Oncology and Cancer Genomics Netherlands, Erasmus MC Cancer Institute, Erasmus University Medical Center, Rotterdam, Netherlands

***Correspondence:**
Marleen Ansems
marleen.ansems@radboudumc.nl;
Gosse J. Adema
gosse.adema@radboudumc.nl

Dendritic cell (DC)-based immunotherapy makes use of the DC's ability to direct the adaptive immune response toward activation or inhibition. DCs perform this immune orchestration in part by secretion of selected cytokines. The most potent anti-inflammatory cytokine interleukin-10 (IL-10) is under tight regulation, as it needs to be predominantly expressed during the resolution phase of the immune response. Currently it is not clear whether there is active suppression of IL-10 by DCs at the initial pro-inflammatory stage of the immune response. Previously, knockdown of the DC-specific transcription factor DC-SCRIPT has been demonstrated to mediate an extensive increase in IL-10 production upon encounter with pro-inflammatory immune stimuli. Here, we explored how DC-SCRIPT contributes to IL-10 suppression under pro-inflammatory conditions by applying chromatin immunoprecipitation sequencing analysis of DC-SCRIPT and the epigenetic marks H3K4me3 and H3K27ac in human DCs. The data showed binding of DC-SCRIPT to a GA-rich motif at H3K27ac-marked genomic enhancers that associated with genes encoding MAPK dual-specificity phosphatases (DUSPs). Functional studies revealed that upon knockdown of DC-SCRIPT, human DCs express much less DUSP4 and exhibit increased phosphorylation of the three major MAPKs (ERK, JNK, and p38). Enhanced ERK signaling in DC-SCRIPT-knockdown-DCs led to higher production of IL-10, which was reverted by rescuing DUSP4 expression. Finally, DC-SCRIPT-knockdown-DCs induced less IFN-γ and increased IL-10 production in naïve T cells, indicative for a more anti-inflammatory phenotype. In conclusion, we have delineated a new mechanism by which DC-SCRIPT allows DCs to limit IL-10 production under inflammatory conditions and potentiate pro-inflammatory Th1 responses. These insights may be exploited to improve DC-based immunotherapies.

Keywords: ZNF366, ERK, chromatin immunoprecipitation sequencing, dual-specificity phosphatase 4, dendritic cells, MAPK, DC-SCRIPT, IL-10

INTRODUCTION

Immunotherapy has gained great success in recent years due to the success of checkpoint inhibitors targeting the PD-1/PD-L1 or CTLA-4 pathways (1–4). These checkpoint inhibitors act on T cells, and it is widely accepted that T cells are quintessential in the fight against cancer. However, T cells are not capable of eliciting an anti-tumor response by themselves, because without the right instructions, the T cells will remain naïve or become tolerogenic (5). The only cell type capable of efficiently educating naïve T cells is the dendritic cell (DC). We have come very far in our understanding of the role of cell surface receptors and secreted molecules involved in immune regulation by DCs, which has been exploited in therapies against cancer with promising results (6, 7). By contrast, information regarding intracellular regulatory circuits in DCs is far scarcer, and could possess potential for future therapeutic strategies as well.

DCs sample their environment, and sense foreign molecules using pattern-recognition receptors of which the toll-like receptors (TLRs) are the best known (8). Activation of DCs through TLR-triggering is needed for upregulation of antigen-presenting and co-stimulatory molecules, and production of cytokines that direct the T cell response toward activation (9). Thus, DCs hold the potential to induce either an immune-activating or immune-dampening response (10). Interleukin-10 (IL-10) has been demonstrated to play a crucial role in this process, by inhibiting development of pro-inflammatory Th1 cells and promoting development of anti-inflammatory Tr1 cells (11). Besides being involved in T cell education, several studies also reported on downregulation of MHC class II expression on antigen-presenting cells (APCs) and of MHC class I on tumor cells in cancer patients with elevated IL-10 levels in serum or tumors (12–18). Although high IL-10 production in cancer patients is associated with a poor prognosis, some recent reports have suggested that situations may exist in which elevated levels of IL-10 in cancer patients may also have beneficial effects *via* dampening the chronic inflammation in tumor microenvironments and by stimulation of cytotoxicity of already activated CD8+ T cells (19).

In the context of APCs, we have learned a great deal about how IL-10 is upregulated *via* activation of the MAP kinase ERK and the transcription factor NF-κB during the resolution phase of an immune response (20). Whether IL-10 expression is actively kept in check in DCs during the initial inflammatory phase of the immune response is currently unknown (20). Dendritic cell-specific transcript (DC-SCRIPT, *ZNF366*) is a transcription factor uniquely expressed by DCs in the immune system (21–23). DC-SCRIPT has been shown to have a complex collection of functions, including nuclear receptor co-regulatory activity (24–29), cell cycle regulation (30), NF-κB activity modulation (31), and mediating induction of T cell proliferation and IFN-γ production (23). Most strikingly, DC-SCRIPT knockdown leads to a massive increase in IL-10 production after pro-inflammatory TLR-triggering (23, 27, 31), suggesting that DC-SCRIPT may participate in active suppression of IL-10. In this study. we explored how DC-SCRIPT contributes to the active suppression of IL-10 production in human activated monocyte-derived DCs.

RESULTS

DC-SCRIPT Binds Genomic Enhancers Near MAPK Phosphatases

In order to delineate the molecular mechanism for how DC-SCRIPT regulates IL-10 expression in DCs under inflammatory conditions, we conducted a chromatin immunoprecipitation sequencing (ChIP-Seq) analysis using a DC-SCRIPT specific antibody on human monocyte-derived DCs. Antibodies specific for the epigenetic marks histone H3 lysine 4 tri-methylation [H3K4me3; associated with promoters of active genes (32)] and H3K27 acetylation (ac) [present at active enhancers and promoters (33)] were taken along in the same DC samples (**Figure 1**; GEO accession number: GSE78923). To account for donor variation and dynamics, three donors were assayed, using immature, 1 h, and 24 h TLR ligand R848 (Resiquimod)-stimulated DCs. Only DC-SCRIPT binding sites consistently present in all three donors in at least one of the assayed time points were used for subsequent analysis, yielding a total of 10,833 DC-SCRIPT binding sites in the human genome. Clustering of the DC-SCRIPT DNA binding sites with the genomic H3K27ac and H3K4me3 histone marks in DCs displayed a 37% overlap (**Figure 1A**, cluster 2–6). Out of these, 1,462 DC-SCRIPT binding sites overlapped with the promoter mark H3K4me3 (**Figure 1A**, clusters 2–4 and **Figure 1B**, *top*), and 2,550 DC-SCRIPT binding sites overlapped with histone marks characteristic for enhancers (high H3K27ac, low/no H3K4me3, clusters 5–6 **Figures 1A,B**, *middle*). Promoter-associated DC-SCRIPT binding sites are henceforth referred to as PA-SC binding sites and enhancer-associated DC-SCRIPT binding sites referred to as EA-SC binding sites. The DC-SCRIPT binding sites that did not co-localize with either of these marks (**Figures 1A,B**, *bottom*) were left out from the current analysis. To further characterize the sequence content of the genomic locations where DC-SCRIPT binds, a *de novo* motif analysis was performed on the DC-SCRIPT ChIP-Seq dataset using GimmeMotifs (34). This unguided comparison of the DNA sequence under all the DC-SCRIPT binding sites, yielded a GA-rich DC-SCRIPT binding motif (**Figure 1C**). To validate the motif in a different and independent assay, we also performed *in vitro* cyclic amplification and selection of targets (CAST) in a cell-free system (**Figure 1D**). The CAST motif successfully validated the *de novo* motif with the two independently generated motifs being 78% similar to each other [assayed by MAST in MEME (35), Figure S1 in Supplementary Material]. The *de novo* and the *in vitro* motif were found in up to 44% of the EA-SC binding sites and 38% of the PA-SC binding sites, respectively (Figure S1 in Supplementary Material).

Previously, we have shown that in the absence of DC-SCRIPT there is increased NF-κB binding to the *il10* enhancer (31), suggesting that DC-SCRIPT may also bind there. Surprisingly, there was no DC-SCRIPT binding site in the *il10* promoter or any *il10*-associated enhancer that could explain the effect of DC-SCRIPT expression on IL-10 production. Genomic Regions Enrichment of Annotations Tool [GREAT (36)] was then used to get more insight into the pathways that DC-SCRIPT may regulate to affect IL-10 expression. The gene ontology (GO)

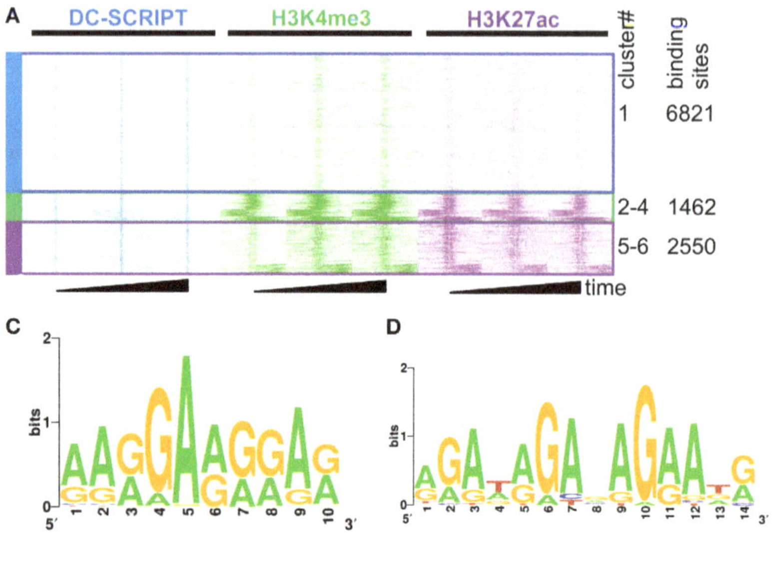

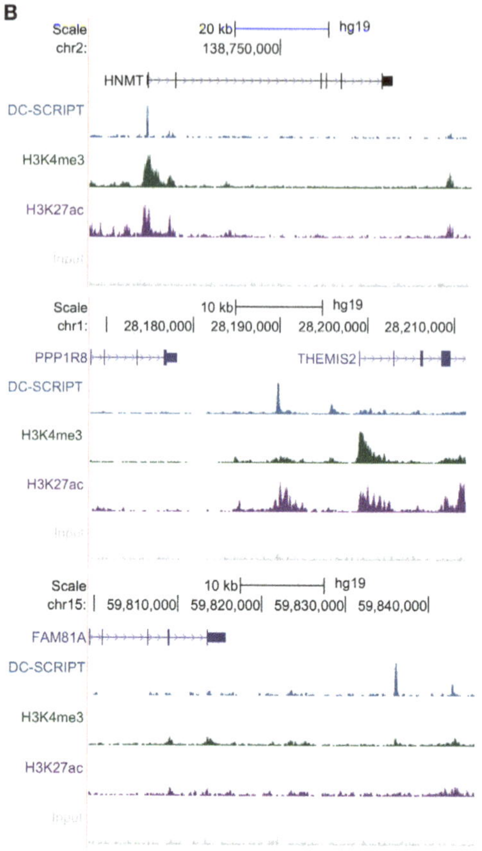

E

Term Name	FDR q-val	Enrich.	Regions	Genes
prenyltransferase activity	3.7E-03	8.3	8	4/16
protein transporter activity	3.3E-03	3.5	18	11/83
protease binding	4.3E-03	3.7	16	9/62
MHC class II receptor activity	4.0E-03	17.7	5	5/12
antigen binding	3.6E-03	5.3	11	10/56
complement binding	7.4E-03	14.3	5	4/9
MAP kinase tyrosine/serine/threonine phosphatase activity	9.1E-03	5.6	9	4/13
MAP kinase phosphatase activity	9.6E-03	5.5	9	4/14
non-membrane spanning protein tyrosine kinase activity	1.5E-02	3.4	14	10/46
purinergic receptor activity	1.7E-02	6.7	7	5/24

FIGURE 1 | Genome-wide mapping of DC-SCRIPT binding sites in human dendritic cells (DCs). Chromatin immunoprecipitation sequencing (ChIP-Seq) of human immature or R848 (toll-like receptors 7/8 ligand)-activated DCs using DC-SCRIPT, H3K4me3, or H3K27ac Abs ($n = 3$). **(A)** Heatmap of k-means clustering analysis ($k = 6$, Euclidean distance) of DC-SCRIPT (blue), H3K4me3 (green), and H3K27ac (purple) in 10-kb windows around DC-SCRIPT peak summits. Clusters 2–4 are merged into an enhancer-associated cluster; clusters 5–6 are merged into a promoter-associated cluster. The rows correspond to the peaks; the x-axis shows the position relative to the peak center. The intensity of the color represents the number of reads in 100-bp windows. **(B)** Representative UCSC Genome Browser tracks of a PA-SC binding site (top), an EA-SC binding site (middle), and a no mark binding site (bottom). The tracks from top to bottom show the gene annotation, the ChIP-Seq signal for DC-SCRIPT (blue), H3K4me3 (green), H3K27ac (purple), and input (gray). **(C)** *de novo* motif generated from DC-SCRIPT ChIP-Seq binding sites. **(D)** *In vitro* motif identified by cyclic amplification and selection of targets. **(E)** Genomic Regions Enrichment of Annotations Tool analysis of all DC-SCRIPT-binding sites containing the GA-rich motif. The table contains the top 10 most significant terms in the gene ontology category molecular function. See also Figure S1 and Tables S1 and S2 in Supplementary Material.

biological process term was dominated by immune regulatory processes (Table S1 in Supplementary Material), reinforcing the previously demonstrated role of DC-SCRIPT in immune regulation (23, 31). Interestingly, the molecular function GO showed that DC-SCRIPT binds in the vicinity of MAPK phosphatase genes (**Figure 1E**; Table S2 in Supplementary Material). MAPK phosphatases are a subgroup of the dual-specificity phosphatases (DUSPs) and are responsible for the dephosphorylation of MAPKs (37). Given that the MAPK ERK previously has been associated with IL-10 production (20), DC-SCRIPT may therefore potentially regulate DUSPs to modulate IL-10 production.

DC-SCRIPT Modulates the MAPK Pathway

The GREAT analysis showed that 4 out of 14 MAPK DUSPs were associated with a total of 9 EA-SC binding sites located on average 246 kb (range: 3–859 kb) from the transcription start site. In order to validate their expression in relation to DC-SCRIPT, we knocked down DC-SCRIPT using siRNA specific to DC-SCRIPT (SC-KD-DCs) or control non-targeting siRNA (Ctrl-DCs) (**Figure 2A**). The expression of the four DUSP genes that had DC-SCRIPT binding sites associated (DUSP1, DUSP4, DUSP5, and DUSP10) were assayed by RT-qPCR at different time points after R848 stimulation (**Figures 2B–E**). As a control, the well-known ERK phosphatase DUSP6 (38), that in this study did not have any DC-SCRIPT binding sites associated, was also assayed (**Figure 2F**). All five assayed DUSPs were upregulated after R848 stimulation, but only DUSP4 and DUSP6 displayed a significant difference in expression upon DC-SCRIPT knockdown. DUSP4 was consistently higher expressed in Ctrl-DCs, while DUSP6 was consistently higher expressed in SC-KD-DCs. Since the main role of DUSPs is to inhibit MAPK signaling, we next assayed if DC-SCRIPT silencing has an impact on the signaling of the MAPKs. The levels of phosphorylation of the three major MAPKs: ERK, JNK, and p38 were assayed by western blotting (WB)

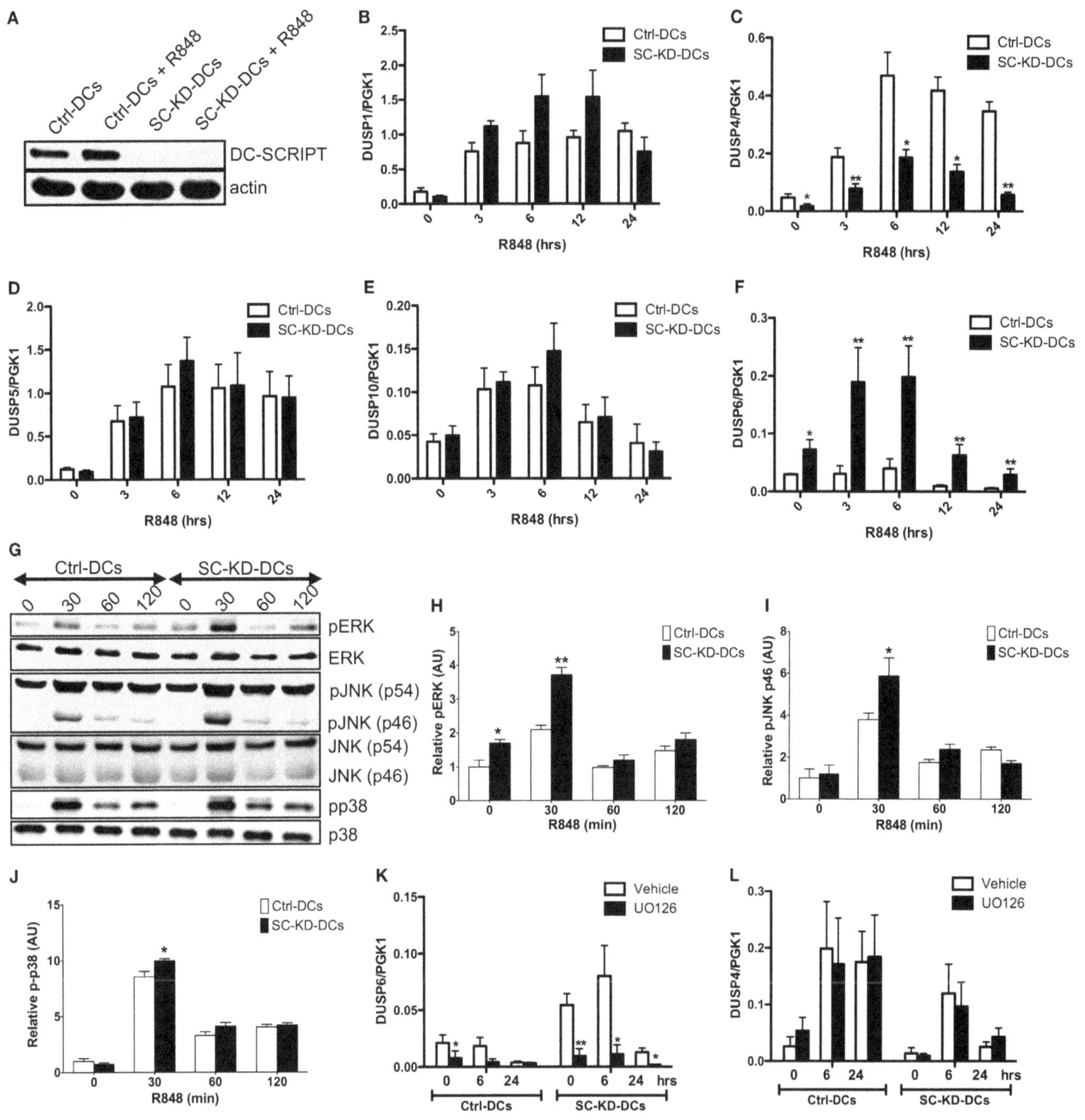

FIGURE 2 | DC-SCRIPT affects the MAPK pathway. **(A)** Representative western blot of siRNA-mediated DC-SCRIPT knockdown in immature and R848-stimulated dendritic cells (DCs). **(B–F)** R848-stimulated Ctrl-DC and SC-KD-DC time course for dual-specificity phosphatase (DUSP)1, 4, 5, 6, and 10 ($n = 4$, mean + SEM). **(G–J)** Phosphorylation and total protein expression of ERK, JNK, and p38 in Ctrl-DCs and SC-KD-DCs after stimulation with R848 ($n = 5$, mean + SEM). **(K,L)** DUSP6 and DUSP4 expression in Ctrl-DCs and SC-KD-DCs pretreated with UO126 (MEK inhibitor) or vehicle control for 1 h, followed by R848 stimulation ($n = 4$, mean + SEM). Statistics: Student's paired t test, Ctrl-DCs were compared to SC-KD-DCs at the same time point. $^*p < 0.05$, $^{**}p < 0.01$. See also Figure S2 in Supplementary Material.

(**Figures 2G–J**) and flow cytometry (Figure S2 in Supplementary Material). Stimulation with R848 led to a peak in phosphorylation of all three kinases after 30 min in both SC-KD-DCs and Ctrl-DCs. DC-SCRIPT knockdown significantly enhanced the phosphorylation of all three kinases, with the most potent increase in ERK, and only a minor change of phosphorylation on p38. As ERK signaling has previously been demonstrated to upregulate expression of DUSPs (39, 40), we pretreated the cells with a MEK inhibitor prior to stimulation, to investigate whether ERK signaling was responsible for the observed effect on

DUSP4 and DUSP6 expression (**Figures 2K,L**). Strikingly, pre treatment with the inhibitor diminished DUSP6 upregulation, while DUSP4 remained unaltered. This suggests that DUSP4 is regulated directly by DC-SCRIPT, whereas the effect on DUSP6 is rather part of an ERK signaling feedback loop.

DC-SCRIPT Enhances DUSP4 Expression

The DC-SCRIPT binding site associated with the DUSP4 gene was further validated by ChIP-qPCR in seven additional independent donors (Figure S3 in Supplementary Material). The binding site displayed enhancer characteristics (high H3K27ac and low H3K4me3 binding) and was located 285kB downstream of the DUSP4 transcription start site (**Figure 3A**). Both the *de novo* and the *in vitro* motif could be found toward the center of the binding site (**Figure 3B**). Intriguingly, this location falls within a local topological associated domain (TAD) previously found in all 19 different assayed cell lines and 13 different tissues, including immune cells (**Figure 3C**). Together this would suggest that this DC-SCRIPT binding position is an enhancer for DUSP4. To further evaluate this, a luciferase vector containing the DUSP4 promoter and the genomic DNA underlying the DUSP4 EA-SC-binding site was generated. For comparison, a control vector with a piece of genomic DNA of similar size, without the motif, and located between the DUSP4 TSS and

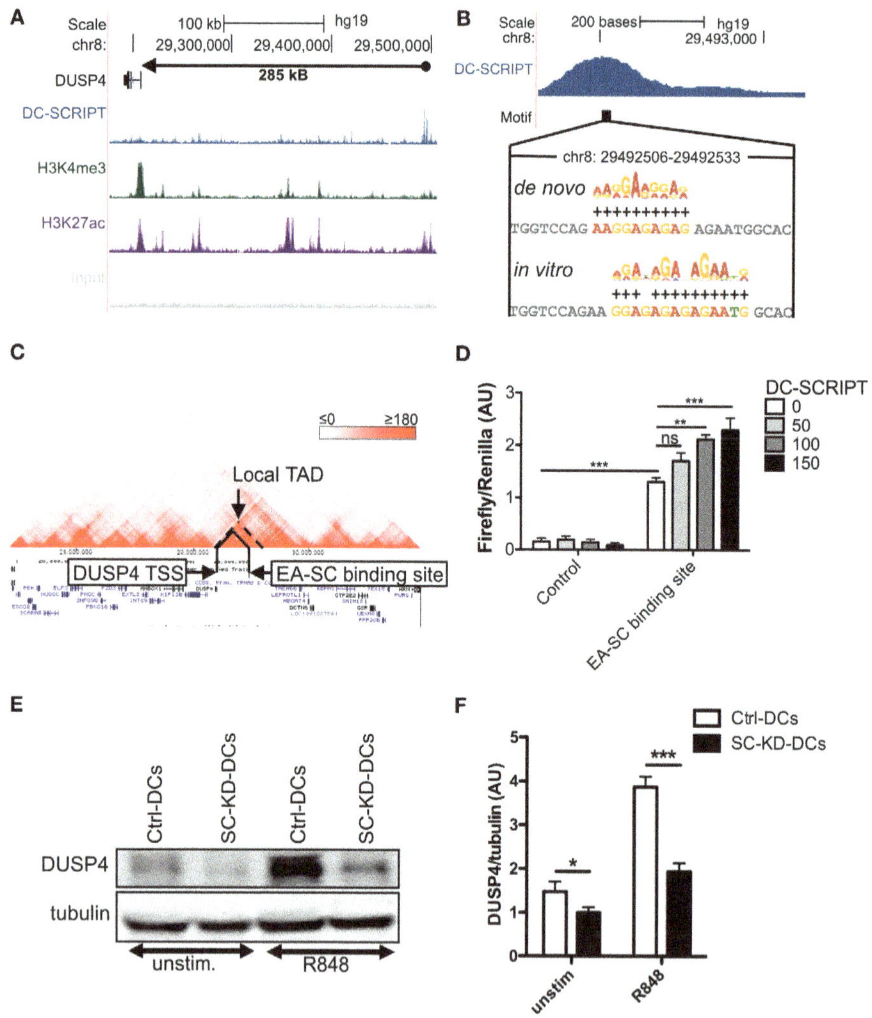

FIGURE 3 | DC-SCRIPT enhances dual-specificity phosphatase (DUSP)4 expression. **(A,B)** DUSP4 EA-SC binding site track from UCSC Genome Browser. **(A)** The tracks from top to bottom show the DUSP4 gene annotation, and the ChIP-Seq signal for DC-SCRIPT (blue), H3K4me3 (green), H3K27ac (purple), and input (gray). **(B)** Position of the GA-rich motifs identified *de novo* from this ChIP-Seq dataset or *in vitro* by cyclic amplification and selection of targets. **(C)** Topological associated domain (TAD) analysis was done using the Hi-C data browser from the Yue-lab at Penn State (http://promoter.bx.psu.edu/hi-c) containing data from Ref. (41–43). Highlighted in the figure is a local TAD that only contains the DUSP4 gene, and the EA-SC binding site. The example shown is from GM12878 (lymphoblastoid B cell line). **(D)** Luciferase assays with DUSP4 promoter-containing vector with either genomic DNA containing the DUSP4 gene-associated EA-SC binding site, or a control piece of DNA located in between the binding site and the DUSP4 TSS of similar length. Some conditions were cotransfected with increasing amounts of a DC-SCRIPT expression vector or corresponding amount of empty vector. Firefly luciferase is presented relative to TK renilla luciferase control (n = 3, mean + SEM). Statistics: ANOVA with Bonferroni post test. **(E,F)** Protein expression level of DUSP4 in unstimulated or 6 h R848-stimulated Ctrl-DCs and SC-KD-DCs (n = 7, mean + SEM). Statistics: Student's paired t test. $^{**}p < 0.01$, $^{***}p < 0.001$.

the DUSP4 EA-SC binding site was employed. Interestingly, the genomic DNA underlying the DUSP4 EA-SC genomic DNA lead to a 8.5-fold increase in luciferase activity (**Figure 3D**). Co-transfection with DC-SCRIPT further increased the luciferase signal in a dose-dependent manner (1.8-fold compared to no DC-SCRIPT). To confirm the impact of DC-SCRIPT expression on DUSP4 at the functional level, DUSP4 protein expression was determined in immature and R848-stimulated Ctrl-DCs and SC-KD-DCs (**Figures 3E,F**). In accordance with the mRNA expression, DUSP4 protein levels were significantly higher in Ctrl-DCs relative to DC-SCRIPT silenced DCs both at the immature state and after stimulation. Altogether, these data therefore indicate that the DUSP4 gene-associated EA-SC binding site works as an enhancer, and that DC-SCRIPT expression impacts the DUSP4 protein level.

The DC-SCRIPT-Induced Phenotype Is Mediated by DUSP4

The most dominant immunological phenotype reported for DC-SCRIPT in DCs so far is the major increase in IL-10 production following siRNA-mediated knockdown of DC-SCRIPT (23, 31). To assess whether the observed change in DUSP4 expression level could be responsible for this effect on IL-10 production, we evaluated Ctrl-DCs and SC-KD-DCs ability to produce IL-10 after MAPK inhibition and DUSP4 overexpression (**Figure 4**). While inhibition of JNK did not affect IL-10 secretion, both inhibition of the upstream kinase of ERK (MEK) and p38 lead to a major decrease in IL-10 (**Figure 4A**).

DUSP4 has previously been demonstrated to have a high affinity for dephosphorylating ERK (44), and could therefore explain the enhanced ERK phosphorylation after DC-SCRIPT knockdown. To confirm this in human DCs, we rescued DUSP4 expression by introducing DUSP4/GFP or GFP in SC-KD-DCs using Ctrl-DCs as controls and determined the level of phosphorylated ERK (**Figures 4B,C**; Figure S4 in Supplementary Material). Strikingly, rescuing DUSP4 expression changed phosphorylation of ERK in the SC-KD-DCs back to wild-type levels. As DC-SCRIPT knockdown also had an effect on phosphorylation of p38, the effect of DUSP4 on p38 phosphorylation was also assayed under the same settings (**Figures 4D,E**). Interestingly, like ERK, phosphorylation of p38 was also reduced to wild-type levels after rescuing DUSP4 in DC-SCRIPT knockdown DCs. Finally, rescuing DUSP4 expression in SC-KD-DCs also normalized levels of IL-10 production (similar level as Ctrl-DC) (**Figure 4F**).

DC-SCRIPT Expression in DCs Skews Naïve T Cells Toward Th1 Immune Activation

To determine the impact of DC-SCRIPT expression on the cytokine polarization of naïve CD4+ T cells, we co-cultured SC-KD-DCs or Ctrl-DCs with allogeneic naïve CD4+ T cells and assayed their cytokine production. Interestingly, the responding T cells produced less IFN-γ and more IL-10 upon incubation with SC-KD-DCs (**Figure 5A**). In line with these data, the expression of T cell subset restricted transcription factors revealed a significant decrease in T-bet (Th1 TF) expressing T cells, while the number of GATA3 (Th2 TF) and RORgT (Th17 TF) expressing T cells remained similar (**Figure 5B**).

Altogether, these data demonstrate that DC-SCRIPT-mediated enhancement of DUSP4 expression is responsible for restricting ERK and p38 signaling and subsequent IL-10 production by professional antigen-presenting DCs under inflammatory conditions (**Figure 6**), which in turn limits pro-inflammatory CD4+ T cell polarization.

DISCUSSION

Dendritic cells are the sentinels of the immune system, playing a decisive role in the balance between immunogenic and tolerogenic immune responses (10), however, the molecular mechanism of how DCs control production of the anti-inflammatory cytokine IL-10 in an inflammatory setting is still unclear. Here, we show that DC-SCRIPT, a DC-specific transcription factor in the immune system, binds to GA-rich sequences in enhancer- and promoter-associated DNA regions for many immune-related genes, including an enhancer for the MAPK phosphatase DUSP4. Moreover, we show that DC-SCRIPT knockdown limits DUSP4 expression resulting in an increase in the activity of the MAPK signaling pathway and subsequent IL-10 production by DCs. In addition, the knockdown of DC-SCRIPT also hindered differentiation of naïve CD4+ T cells into pro-inflammatory T cells. Altogether, these data show a novel mechanism by which professional antigen-presenting DCs limit IL-10 production, a pathway that needs to be tightly controlled to induce protective immune responses (20).

Many different immune cells can produce IL-10 and during cancer development, this has mainly been considered detrimental for successful eradication of the tumor cells due to IL-10's immunosuppressive capabilities on DCs (45) and T cells (46). Previously, we have demonstrated that DC-SCRIPT affects TLR-mediated IL-10 production in human DCs (23), and described that enhanced IL-10 production in SC-KD-DCs was partly caused by altered post-translational modifications of NF-κBp65 leading to increased binding of NF-κBp65 to an IL-10 enhancer element (31). In our current ChIP-Seq data, we did not find a DC-SCRIPT binding site at the same position as for NF-κBp65 in the enhancer of the IL-10 gene, i.e., it does not seem that DC-SCRIPT is part of the NF-κBp65 DNA binding complex. In line with these observations, knockdown of DC-SCRIPT affected the phosphorylation status of NF-κB (31), and with the current data linking DC-SCRIPT to phosphatases, it may suggest that DC-SCRIPT affects NF-κB activation indirectly. In support of this, a downstream kinase (MSK1) of the MAPKs ERK and p38 has been demonstrated to mediate phosphorylation of NF-κBp65 (47), and ERK has been shown to play a critical role for IL-10 production in DCs (20).

In the current work, we found that DC-SCRIPT knockdown leads to higher DUSP4 expression and that DC-SCRIPT binds a GA-rich DNA sequence with enhancer abilities within a local DUSP4-TAD. Using luciferase assays, we found that the largest enhancing effect was gained by cloning the enhancer close to the DUSP4 promoter, while co-transfecting DC-SCRIPT only

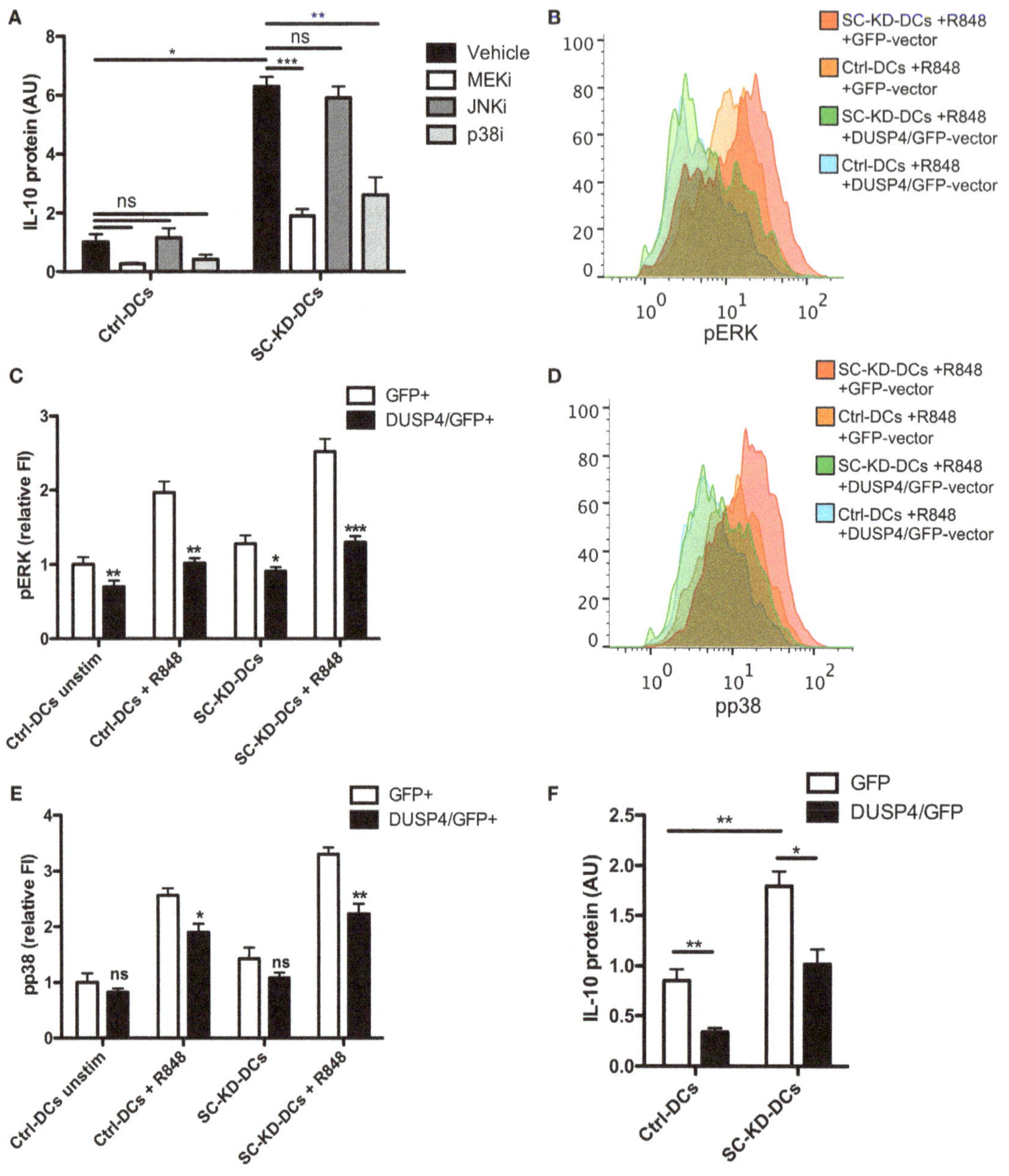

FIGURE 4 | DUSP4 expression prevents the DC-SCRIPT-knockdown-mediated change in ERK phosphorylation and IL-10 production. **(A)** IL-10 protein production by Ctrl-DCs and SC-KD-DCs pre-treated with inhibitors for MEK (upstream of ERK), JNK, p38 or with vehicle control and stimulated with R848 ($n = 6$, mean + SEM). **(B–E)** pERK and pp38 phosphorylation levels of Ctrl-DCs and SC-KD-DCs after overexpression of GFP or DUSP4/GFP by phosphoflow ($n = 8$, mean + SEM). **(F)** IL-10 protein production by Ctrl-DCs and SC-KD-DCs after overexpression of GFP or DUSP4/GFP ($n = 7$, mean + SEM). The IL-10 protein data have been normalized to account for donor variation and displayed as arbitrary units (SC-KD-DCs + vehicle range: 0.5–4.6 ng/mL) Statistics: Student's paired *t* test. Where no lines are shown, Ctrl-DCs were compared to SC-KD-DCs at the same time point. $^*p < 0.05$, $^{**}p < 0.01$, $^{***}p < 0.001$. FI, fluorescence intensity; AU, arbitrary unit. See also Figure S4 in Supplementary Material.

led to a subtle (but significant) further increase in the signal. These data could indicate that one of the roles of DC-SCRIPT in enhancing DUSP4 expression would be to bring the DUSP4 enhancer in close proximity to the promoter. Currently, only little is known about the functional role of DUSP4 in DCs. Gene expression analysis has revealed that immune cells express up to 17 different DUSPs to various extent, but only one or two DUSPs showed high expression in any single cell type (37). DUSP4 was predominantly expressed in DCs, and furthermore, high DUSP4 expression could distinguish DCs from the closely related monocyte-derived macrophages (37). Interestingly, accumulating evidence suggests that cell type-specific transcription factors often regulate cell type-specific genes *via* binding to enhancers (48).

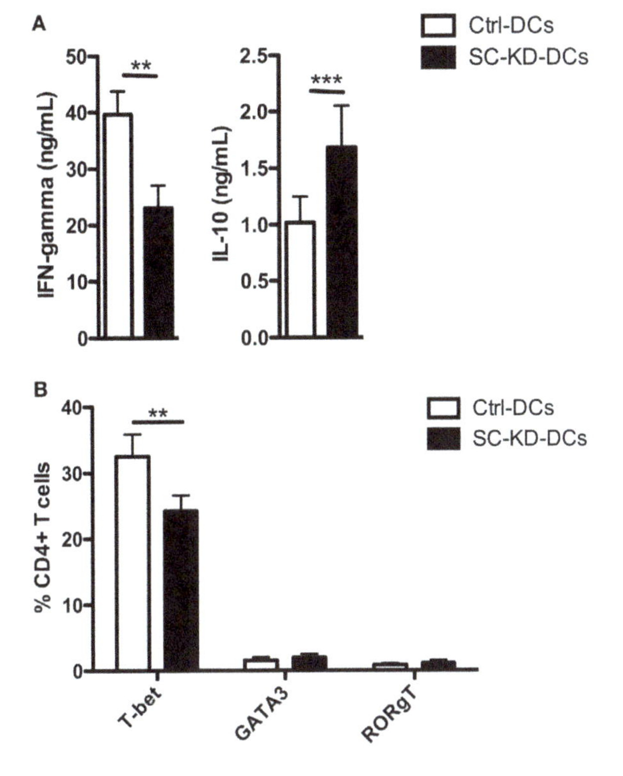

FIGURE 5 | Knockdown of DC-SCRIPT in DCs polarizes T cells toward immunosuppression. Naïve CD4+ T cells were co-cultured with SC-KD-DCs or Ctrl-DCs until in a resting state after 10–12 days. Upon re-stimulation, the phenotype of the T cells were assayed for **(A)** expression of T cell subset markers by FACS and **(B)** secreted cytokines by ELISA (n = 12 + SEM). Statistics: Student's paired t test. $^{**}p < 0.01$, $^{***}p < 0.001$.

One of DCs main function in the immune system is to educate T cells toward pro-inflammatory or anti-inflammatory responses. We observed that knockdown of DC-SCRIPT in DCs limited the DCs capability to induce pro-inflammatory CD4+ T cells when polarized from naïve cells. These T cells produced less IFN-γ and more IL-10, and in line with these data, the number of T-bet expressing T cells was also reduced. Surprisingly, even though DC-SCRIPT knockdown leads to increased production of IL-10, and IL-10 is a potent inducer of anti-inflammatory Tr1 cells (11), preliminary experiments did not show any skewing of naïve T cells into Tr1 cells (data not shown). As DC-SCRIPT levels affect a DC's capacity to induce inflammatory Th1 responses, one could consider monitoring DC-SCRIPT expression in DCs used in vaccination studies.

In summary, the transcription factor DC-SCRIPT binds regulatory DNA sequences linked to genes involved in the immune system and the MAPK pathway, including MAPK phosphatases. We identify regulation of expression of the MAPK phosphatase DUSP4 as the mode of action through which DC-SCRIPT restricts the expression of the crucial immune-inhibitory cytokine IL-10 in DCs. These data help to delineate the mechanisms that govern DCs unique molecular function, and its central role in controlling immune responses. As DC immunotherapy is a promising approach to treat cancer patients, specifically targeting tumor cells and having only few side effects (49, 50), much research has focused on which pattern-recognition receptor ligands or cytokine-cocktails would generate a DC-phenotype with a favorable cytokine profile, often focusing on high IL-12 and low IL-10 levels (51–53). The current data showing IL-10 being actively inhibited by DC-SCRIPT-induced phosphatases imply that maturing DCs with a combination of immune-activating adjuvants and either kinase inhibitors or

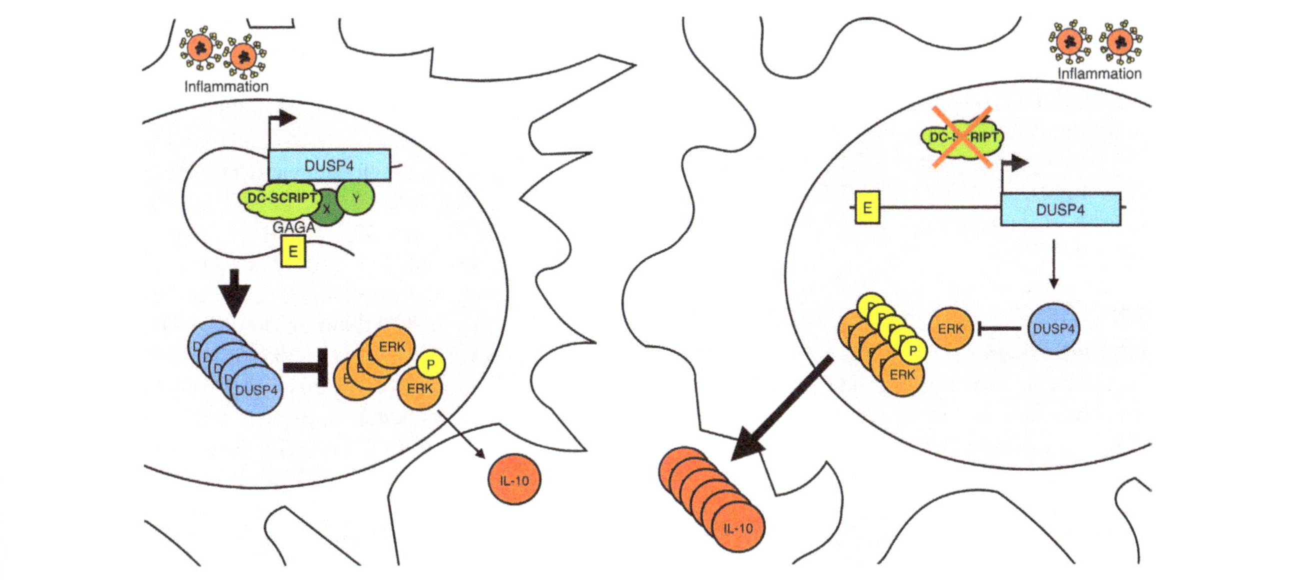

FIGURE 6 | Model of DC-SCRIPT mediated control of IL-10 production in DCs. In the presence of DC-SCRIPT (left figure), DC-SCRIPT binds an enhancer (E) for DUSP4 *via* a GA-rich motif. This leads to enhanced DUSP4 expression, which limits ERK signaling, and subsequent IL-10 production under inflammatory conditions. By contrast, in the absence of DC-SCRIPT (right figure), DUSP4 is only expressed at a low level, thereby enabling higher ERK signaling leading to an increase in IL-10 production. X and Y are potential protein partners in the enhancer complex.

phosphatase inducers may be beneficial to improve DC-based immunotherapy.

MATERIALS AND METHODS

Generation of Human Monocyte-Derived Dendritic Cells (moDCs)

Human moDCs were generated from PBMCs as described previously (54). Buffy coats were obtained from healthy volunteers (Sanquin, Nijmegen, The Netherlands) after informed consent and according to institutional guidelines. Plastic-adhered monocytes were cultured for a total of 6 days in RPMI 1640 medium (Life Technologies) supplemented with 1% ultra-glutamine (Cambrex), 0.5% antibiotic–antimycotic (Invitrogen), 10% (v/v) FCS (Greiner Bio-one), IL-4 (300 U/mL), and GM-CSF (450 U/mL) (both from Cellgenix). On day 3, moDCs were supplemented with new IL-4 (300 U/mL) and GM-CSF (450 U/mL).

Small Interfering RNA (siRNA)-Mediated Knockdown

On day 3–4 of DC differentiation, cells were harvested and subjected to electroporation. For DC-SCRIPT silencing, a 23-nt custom ZNF366 siRNA termed SC38 targeting the DC-SCRIPT gene at position 2,349–2,369 was used (Thermo Scientific). siRNA ON-TARGETplus Non-Targeting siRNA#1 (Thermo Scientific) was used as control. Cells were washed twice in PBS and once in OptiMEM without phenol red (Invitrogen). A total of 10 μg siRNA was transferred to a 4-mm cuvette (Bio-Rad), and 10×10^6 DCs were added in 200 μL OptiMEM and incubated for 3 min before being pulsed with an exponential decay pulse at 300 V, 150 μF, in a Genepulser Xcell (Bio-Rad), as previously described (55). Immediately after electroporation, the cells were transferred to pre-heated (37°C) phenol red-free RPMI 1640 culture medium supplemented with 1% ultra-glutamine, 10% (v/v) FCS, IL-4 (300 U/mL), and GM-CSF (450 U/mL).

Stimulations and Inhibitors

Immature DCs were stimulated with 4 μg/mL R848 (Axxora). In some experiments, DCs were pre-treated 1–2 h with one of the following inhibitors: 4 μM UO126 (MEK1/2, LC Laboratories), 2.5 μM SB203580 (p38, LC laboratories), 5 μM SP600125 (JNK, Tocris Bioscience).

RNA Isolation, Reverse Transcription, and Quantitative PCR

Total RNA was isolated from cells using Trizol (Ambion). RNA quantity and purity were determined on a NanoDrop spectrophotometer. RNA was treated with DNase I (amplification grade; Invitrogen) and reverse transcribed into cDNA by using random hexamers and Moloney murine leukemia virus reverse transcriptase (Invitrogen). mRNA levels for the genes of interest were determined with a CFX96 sequence detection system (Bio-Rad) with SYBR Green (Roche) as the fluorophore and gene-specific oligonucleotide primers. Primers used are as follows (forward, reverse): DC-SCRIPT (*ZNF366*): (5′-AAGCATGGAGTCATGGAG-3, 5′-TTCTGAGAGAGGTCAAAGG-3′), *PGK1*: (5′-CAAGAAGTATGCTGAGGCTGTCA-3, 5′-CAAATACCCCCACAGGACCAT-3′), *DUSP4*: (5′-AGTGGAAGATAACCACAAGG-3, 5′-GCTTAACGAACTCGAAGG-3′), *DUSP6*: (5′-GATCACTGGAGCCAAAAC-3, 5′-CAAGCAATGTACCAAGACAC-3′), *DUSP1*: (5′-AGTACCCCACTCTACGATCAGG-3, 5′-GAAGCGTGATACGCACTGC-3′), *DUSP5*: (5′-TGTCGTCCTCACCTCGCTA-3, 5′-GGGCTCTCTCACTCTCAATCTTC-3′), *DUSP10*: (5′-TTTGAAGAGGCTTTTGAGTT-3, 5′-GGGAGATAATTGGTCGTTT-3′). Reaction mixtures and program conditions were used as recommended by the manufacturer (Bio-Rad). Quantitative PCR data were analyzed with the CFX Manager software (Bio-Rad) and checked for correct amplification and dissociation of the products. mRNA levels of the genes of interest were normalized to mRNA levels of the housekeeping genes *GAPDH* or *PGK1* and were calculated according to the cycle threshold method (56).

ELISA

Secreted IL-10 was measured using the human IL-10 ready-set-go kit (eBioscience) in the supernatants of 16–24 h-stimulated DCs or T cells. Secreted IFN-γ was measured using IFN-γ monoclonal antibodies; coating clone 2G1, detection Ab-biotin, clone XMG1.2 (both Thermo Fisher).

Western Blotting

Monocyte-derived dendritic cells were lysed in a concentration of 10^6/100 μL 4°C cold lysis buffer consisting of 62.5 mM Tris (pH 6.8, Sigma-Aldrich), 1% SDS (Invitrogen), and freshly added complete protease inhibitor cocktail (Roche), 1 mM PMSF (Sigma-Aldrich), and for phosphorylation-specific western blot: phosphatase inhibitors 1 mM Na3VO4 (Sigma-Aldrich) and 10 mM NaF (Merck). Cell lysates were mixed 1:4 with sample buffer containing 5% glycerol (Invitrogen), 6% SDS, 125 mM Tris–HCl (pH 6.8), 0.1 mg/mL bromophenol blue (Gebr. Schmid), and 10% 2-ME (Sigma-Aldrich), heated at 95°C for 5 min, and then cooled on ice. The proteins were resolved by electrophoresis on a 10% polyacrylamide gel (ratio of acrylamide to bisacrylamide, 37.5:1) and transferred to Protran nitrocellulose transfer membranes (Amersham) at 4°C. The following Abs were used for staining in TBS with 0.1% tween 20 (TBST) and 5% BSA (all from Cell Signaling Technology): rabbit anti-DUSP4 (1:1,000 dilution, clone: D9A5), rabbit anti-ERK (1:1,000 dilution, cat: 9102), rabbit anti-pERK (Thr202/Tyr204) (1:2,000 dilution, clone: D13.14.4E), rabbit anti-JNK (1:1,000 dilution, cat: 9252), rabbit anti-p38 (1:2,000 dilution, clone: D13E1), and rabbit anti-p-p38 (Thr180/Tyr182) (1:1,000 dilution, clone: D3F9). Goat anti-DC-SCRIPT were used for staining in PBS with 0.1% tween 20 and 1% skimmed milk powder (Campina) and 3% BSA (1:600 dilution, cat: AF4707, R&D Systems). Mouse anti-p-JNK (Thr183/Tyr185) were used for staining in TBST with 2% skimmed milk powder and 2% BSA (1:250 dilution, clone: G9, Cell Signaling Technology). Membranes were blocked for 1 h at room temperature, stained overnight with primary Abs [including rabbit anti-actin (1:2,000 dilution, clone: 20–33, Sigma-Aldrich) or rat anti-tubulin (1:2,000 dilution, clone: YOL1/34, Novus Biologicals)], and stained for 1 h at room temperature with corresponding secondary Abs (diluted 1:5,000): goat anti-mouse IgG IRDye 800CW, goat anti-rabbit IgG IRDye 800CW, donkey anti-goat IgG IRDye 800CW, donkey anti-rabbit IgG IRDye 680 (all Li-cor Biosciences), and goat anti-rat Alexa Fluor 680 (Invitrogen). Membranes were scanned by using an Odyssey Infrared Imaging System (Li-cor Biosciences).

Flow Cytometry of DCs

For phosphorylation-specific flow cytometry, paraformaldehyde (Merck) was added directly to the culture medium at a final concentration of 1.6% at the end of the stimulation. Cells were fixed for 10 min at room temperature. Subsequently, culture medium was aspirated, resuspended in 100% ice-cold MeOH (Boom) and incubated at −20°C overnight, followed by extensive washing (4×) in PBS with 1% BSA, 0.05% NaN3 (Merck). Cells were blocked and stained in PBS with 1% BSA, 0.05% NaN3 (Merck), and 2% human serum (Sanquin), using 1:200 diluted pERK, 1:400 diluted p-p38 Abs, or isotype control (rabbit IgG, Jackson Immuno Research). Cells were stained with primary Ab/isotype control for 45 min on ice, followed by 30 min on ice with a secondary PE-Cy5.5 goat anti-rabbit IgG Ab (Invitrogen, cat# L42018). Data were acquired on an FACSCyan (Beckman Coulter). Isotype controls gave a staining intensity similar as unstimulated moDCs, indicating that blocking conditions were sufficient to avoid unspecific staining (data not shown). Viability was measured using a fixable viability dye eFluor780 (eBioscience), following the manufacturers instructions. Data were analyzed using FlowJo (Treestar).

Chromatin Immunoprecipitation Sequencing

Chromatin immunoprecipitation was performed as previously described (31), using 20 µg goat-α-DC-SCRIPT Ab (R&D Systems). 10 ng of input or ChIP-enriched DNA was end-paired using T4 DNA polymerase, *E. coli* DNA Pol I large fragment (Klenow polymerase, New England Biolabs), and T4 polynucleotide kinase (New England Biolabs), followed by purification using the QIAquick PCR purification kit (Qiagen). Subsequently, DNA was dA-tailed using the Klenow fragment (3′ to 5′ exo minus, New England Biolabs), followed by purification using the MinElute Reaction Cleanup kit (Qiagen). Next, DNA was ligated to multiplex NEXTflex adapters (Bioo Scientific). IP and input DNA were purified by the MinElute reaction Cleanup kit, and amplified by PCR using the KAPA HiFi HotStart ReadyMix PCR kit (KAPA Biosystems) with the following program: 45 s at 98°C for initial denaturation, 15 s at 98°C, 30 s at 65°C, 30 s at 72°C for four cycles, followed by 1 min at 72°C for final extension. Removal of excess adaptors and selection of 300 bp bands was done using 2% E-Gel SizeSelect Agarose Gels (Invitrogen). Adapter-modified DNA fragments were enriched by PCR using the KAPA HiFi HotStart ReadyMix PCR kit for 8–10 cycles with the aforementioned program. To get rid of the 120 bp adapter dimer, the PCR product was purified using Ampure beads (Beckman Coulter). Libraries were sequenced on the Illumina HiSeq 2000. H3K4me3 and H3K27ac antibodies were extensively characterized[1] and used for ChIP according to standard BLUEPRINT protocols.[1]

[1]www.blueprint-epigenome.eu (Accessed: April 18, 2018).

ChIP-Seq Data Processing

Peaks were called using the algorithm MACS2 version 2.0.10.20120913 (57) with default settings. In order to account for donor variation and dynamics, three donors were assayed, using immature, 1 h-, and 24 h-stimulated DCs. Peaks present in all three donors were determined using intersect with BEDTools version 2.20.1 (58), and only DC-SCRIPT peaks present in all three donors were used for subsequent analysis. All ChIP-Seq data have been submitted to the GEO database (accession number: GSE78923) k-Means clustering ($k = 6$, Euclidean distance) and heatmaps were generated using Fluff (59). *De novo* motif analysis was done using GimmeMotifs version 0.8.6 (34). The motif was trimmed to remove low information content containing bases.

Cyclic Amplification and Selection of Targets

Human DC-SCRIPT was cloned in the pCATCH vector (60), as BamHI-XbaI inserts. *In vitro* transcription/translation was performed with the TNT T7 Quick Coupled Transcription/Translation System (Promega) according to the manufacturer's recommendations, using 1 µg of DNA as input. Transcription/translation took place at 30°C for 90 min. 10% of the reaction was tested by western blot analysis to verify protein production, while 20% was used in each CAST round.

Oligo-nucleotides carrying defined ends and a 21-nt region of degeneracy (5′-GCCTCCATGGACGAATTCTGT-$(N)_{21}$-AGCG GATCCCGCATATGACCG-3′) and PCR primers (forward: 5′- G CCTCCATGGACGAATTCTGT-3′ and reverse: 5′-CGGTCAT ATGCGGGATCCGCT-3′) were used during CAST. As a first step, double-stranded oligo-nucleotides were prepared as follows. 8.5 µg of the degenerative nucleotides were mixed with 4.3 µg of the reverse primer in 50 µL of Tris–HCl (100 mM, pH 8) and heated at 80°C, then cooled down slowly to 4°C. 2 µL of the hybridized oligo-nucleotides were used together with 2 U of the Klenow fragment of DNA polymerase I (37°C for 1 h) to create dsDNA. dsDNA was precipitated and used in the first round of CAST. Each CAST round was performed in binding buffer containing 30 mM HEPES pH 7.4, 100 mM NaCl, 0.01% NP40, 0.01 mg/mL BSA, 0.05 mM $ZnSO_4$, 2 mM $MgCl_2$, 0.6 mM PMSF, and 10% glycerol. In brief, 500 µL of binding buffer were mixed with 20% *in vitro* transcribed/translated proteins and DNA and incubated for 30 min at 4°C. Then 10 µL of Protein G beads and 3 µg of mouse M2 anti-FLAG mAb (Sigma) were added and incubated overnight. Precipitated dsDNA was used for the first round of CAST, or 80% of the PCR reaction for the subsequent rounds. After the binding reaction, Protein G beads were washed twice with 600 µL of binding buffer and resuspended in 20 µL of 5 mM EDTA pH 8 for 10 min at 90°C. Beads were pelleted and supernatant was used for PCR. 20% of the PCR reaction was tested on gel to verify DNA precipitation and amplification by CAST.

PCR reactions for CAST were performed using 100 ng of forward and reverse primer, 0.5 mM of dNTPs, 5 mM of $MgCl_2$, and 2.5 U of Taq polymerase with 58°C as an annealing temperature. The number of PCR cycles was kept to a minimum, i.e., 15 cycles, in the first two rounds. Minimal PCR amplification helped to reduce the amplification of non-specific oligo-nucleotides and the formation of hetero-duplexes that resulted from the re-annealing of products that were mismatched in the 21-bp central-region. After the third round, however, 20 cycles of PCR ensured good amplification and abundance of specific oligo-nucleotides. Sequences from four rounds of CAST were used as input for MEME (35) to generate a consensus sequence for DC-SCRIPT.

Genomic Regions Enrichment of Annotations Tool

Genomic Regions Enrichment of Annotations Tool analysis was done in version 3.0.0 as previously described (36), with DC-SCRIPT binding sites with an H3K4me3 and/or H3K27ac histone mark, and containing the GA-rich motif. Default settings were employed, i.e., basal plus extension: proximal: 5.0 kb upstream, 1.0 kb downstream, plus distal: up to 1,000.0 kb. Statistical significance is based on false discovery rate (cutoff: 0.05). Displayed data contains minimum three genes in each GO.

Luciferase Assays

The DNA sequence underlying the ChIP-Seq-identified DUSP4 EA-SC-binding site was cloned into a pGL4.10 luciferase vector (Promega) behind a DUSP4 promoter. For comparison, a control pGL4.10 vector with the DUSP4 promoter and a piece of genomic DNA of similar size, and located between the DUSP4 TSS and the DUSP4 EA-SC binding site was also generated. These vectors were transfected into HEK293 [ATCC, tested to be mycoplasma free using mycoalert mycoplasma detection kit (Lonza), and used between passages 2–15 after thawing] together with a renilla control vector (pRL-TK, Promega) and increasing amounts of a pCATCH-DC-SCRIPT expression vector. HEK293s were plated 24 h before transfection using metafectene. Cells were harvested after 24 h, and cell lysates were analyzed for luminescence according to the manufacturer's protocol (Dual Luciferase Reporter assay, Promega) using a Victor3 luminometer (PerkinElmer). Relative light units were calculated after correction for transfection efficiency based on the activity of the cotransfected pRL-TK.

Overexpression of DUSP4

To generate a DUSP4/GFP expression vector, DUSP4 (NM_001394) was cloned into the expression vector pEGFP-N3 (Clontech, Mountain View, CA, USA), using the restriction enzyme sites BglII and BamHI. As a control, the empty pEGFP-N3 vector was used. Immature SC-KD-DCs and Ctrl-DCs were harvested on day 6 and electroporated using the Neon transfection system (Invitrogen) according to the manufacturer's instructions. Briefly, 10^6 DCs were mixed with 5 μg DNA, and electroporated with two pulses of 1,000 V for 40 ms. Subsequently, DCs were seeded in microtiter plates and rested for 5–6 h until GFP was visible. The cells were subsequently stimulated and used for functional assays.

Naïve T Cell Polarization

Naïve T cells were isolated from buffy coats using magnetic-associated cell sorting, and negative selection, by depleting cells expressing CD8a, CD14, CD15, CD16, CD19, CD36, CD56, CD132, TcRγ/δ, and CD235a (CD4+ T Cell isolation kit, human, Miltenyi), and CD45RO [anti-CD45RO-PE (DAKO) plus anti-PE microbeads (Miltenyi)]. Purity was checked using CD3-FITC (BD), CD4-PE-Cy7 (BioLegend), CD45RA-APC-Cy7 (BioLegend), and CD45RO-PE and determined to be >97% of CD3+ CD4+ CD45RO− CD45RA+ T cells.

SC-KD-DCs or Ctrl-DCs were stimulated for 16 h with R848, washed and counted, before co-culturing with naïve CD4+ T cells in a ratio of 5,000:20,000 DC:T. The super antigen SEB (Sigma-Aldrich) was added at 10 pg/mL. After 5, 7, and 9 days of co-culture, the T cells were split 1:2 and recombinant human IL-2 were added at a final concentration of 20 U/mL. On day 11, the T cells are in a resting state, which can be seen in a light microscope by the T cell clusters falling apart and cells are rounded. The resting T cells were assayed for intracellular transcription factor expression using the cytofix/cytoperm kit (BD). Prior to permeabilization cells were stained with fixable viability dye eFluor780 (eBioscience). Antibodies used for staining were: anti-human Gata-3-Alexa Fluor488, anti-human RORgamma(t)-APC, and anti-human T-bet-PE (all eBioscience).

For cytokine production, T cells were harvested, counted, and 100,000 cells re-plated in a 96-well round bottom plate, followed by addition of 100,000 anti CD3/CD28 beads (Gibco). Supernatant was harvested after 24 h and assayed by ELISA. Data presented in the figure consists of two T cell donors and six DC donors.

AUTHOR CONTRIBUTIONS

Conceptualization: JS, MA, and GA; methodology: JS, SH, MA, and GA; software: SH; formal analysis: JS and SH; investigation: JS, ML, CT, VT, PL, EJ-M, AS, and MA; writing—original draft: JS, SH, MA, and GA; writing—review and editing: JS, SH, ML, CT, VT, PL, EJ-M, AS, JM, CL, HS, MA, and GA; visualization: JS and SH; funding acquisition: JS, CT, JM, MA, and GA.

ACKNOWLEDGMENTS

MA is recipient of NWO-Veni 91615093 and a long-term fellowship (BUIT 2012-5347) from the Dutch Cancer Society. SH is supported by NWO, the Netherlands Organisation of Scientific Research (NWO-ALW grant 863.12.002). JM and AS received funding through Cancer Genomics Netherlands (CGC.nl) and a grant from the Netherlands Organization for Scientific Research (NWO).

REFERENCES

1. Wolchok JD, Kluger H, Callahan MK, Postow MA, Rizvi NA, Lesokhin AM, et al. Nivolumab plus ipilimumab in advanced melanoma. *N Engl J Med* (2013) 369:122–33. doi:10.1056/NEJMoa1302369
2. Weber JS, Kudchadkar RR, Yu B, Gallenstein D, Horak CE, Inzunza HD, et al. Safety, efficacy, and biomarkers of nivolumab with vaccine in ipilimumab-refractory or -naive melanoma. *J Clin Oncol* (2013) 31:4311–8. doi:10.1200/JCO.2013.51.4802
3. Yuan J, Adamow M, Ginsberg BA, Rasalan TS, Ritter E, Gallardo HF, et al. Integrated NY-ESO-1 antibody and CD8+ T-cell responses correlate with clinical benefit in advanced melanoma patients treated with ipilimumab. *Proc Natl Acad Sci U S A* (2011) 108:16723–8. doi:10.1073/pnas.1110814108
4. Brahmer JR, Drake CG, Wollner I, Powderly JD, Picus J, Sharfman WH, et al. Phase I study of single-agent anti-programmed death-1 (MDX-1106) in refractory solid tumors: safety, clinical activity, pharmacodynamics, and immunologic correlates. *J Clin Oncol* (2010) 28:3167–75. doi:10.1200/JCO.2009.26.7609
5. Grivennikov SI, Greten FR, Karin M. Immunity, inflammation, and cancer. *Cell* (2010) 140:883–99. doi:10.1016/j.cell.2010.01.025
6. Hamid O, Robert C, Daud A, Hodi FS, Hwu W-J, Kefford R, et al. Safety and tumor responses with lambrolizumab (anti-PD-1) in melanoma. *N Engl J Med* (2013) 369:134–44. doi:10.1056/NEJMoa1305133
7. Brahmer JR, Tykodi SS, Chow LQM, Hwu W-J, Topalian SL, Hwu P, et al. Safety and activity of anti-PD-L1 antibody in patients with advanced cancer. *N Engl J Med* (2012) 366:2455–65. doi:10.1056/NEJMoa1200694
8. Kawai T, Akira S. TLR signaling. *Cell Death Differ* (2006) 13:816–25. doi:10.1038/sj.cdd.4401850
9. Bakdash G, Sittig SP, van Dijk T, Figdor CG, de Vries IJM. The nature of activatory and tolerogenic dendritic cell-derived signal II. *Front Immunol* (2013) 4:53. doi:10.3389/fimmu.2013.00053
10. Steinman RM, Banchereau J. Taking dendritic cells into medicine. *Nature* (2007) 449:419–26. doi:10.1038/nature06175
11. Gregori S, Tomasoni D, Pacciani V, Scirpoli M, Battaglia M, Magnani CF, et al. Differentiation of type 1 T regulatory cells (Tr1) by tolerogenic DC-10 requires the IL-10-dependent ILT4/HLA-G pathway. *Blood* (2010) 116:935–44. doi:10.1182/blood-2009-07-234872
12. Boulland M-L, Meignin V, Leroy-Viard K, Copie-Bergman C, Brière J, Touitou R, et al. Human interleukin-10 expression in T/natural killer-cell lymphomas. *Am J Pathol* (1998) 153:1229–37. doi:10.1016/S0002-9440(10)65667-2
13. Sato T, McCue P, Masuoka K, Salwen S, Lattime EC, Mastrangelo MJ, et al. Interleukin 10 production by human melanoma. *Clin Cancer Res* (1996) 2:1383–90.
14. Nemunaitis J, Fong T, Shabe P, Martineau D, Ando D. Comparison of serum interleukin-10 (IL-10) levels between normal volunteers and patients with advanced melanoma. *Cancer Invest* (2001) 19:239–47. doi:10.1081/CNV-100102550
15. Chen Q, Daniel V, Maher DW, Hersey P. Production of IL-10 by melanoma cells: examination of its role in immunosuppression mediated by melanoma. *Int J Cancer* (1994) 56:755–60. doi:10.1002/ijc.2910560524
16. Boyano MD, Garcia-Vázquez MD, López-Michelena T, Gardeazabal J, Bilbao J, Cañavate ML, et al. Soluble interleukin-2 receptor, intercellular adhesion molecule-1 and interleukin-10 serum levels in patients with melanoma. *Br J Cancer* (2000) 83:847–52. doi:10.1054/bjoc.2000.1402
17. Adris SK, Klein S, Jasnis MA, Chuluyan E, Ledda MF, Bravo AI, et al. IL-10 expression by CT26 colon carcinoma cells inhibits their malignant phenotype and induces a T cell-mediated tumor rejection in the context of a systemic Th2 response. *Gene Ther* (1999) 6:1705–12. doi:10.1038/sj.gt.3301012
18. Steinbrink K, Graulich E, Kubsch S, Rgen Knop J, Enk AH. CD4+ and CD8+ anergic T cells induced by interleukin-10-treated human dendritic cells display antigen-specific suppressor activity. *Blood* (2002) 99:2468. doi:10.1182/blood.V99.7.2468
19. Mannino MH, Zhu Z, Xiao H, Bai Q, Wakefield MR, Fang Y. The paradoxical role of IL-10 in immunity and cancer. *Cancer Lett* (2015) 367:103–7. doi:10.1016/j.canlet.2015.07.009
20. Saraiva M, O'Garra A. The regulation of IL-10 production by immune cells. *Nat Rev Immunol* (2010) 10:170–81. doi:10.1038/nri2711
21. Triantis V, Trancikova DE, Maaike WG, Hartgers FC, Janssen RAJ, Adema GJ. Identification and characterization of DC-SCRIPT, a novel dendritic cell-expressed member of the zinc finger family of transcriptional regulators. *J Immunol* (2006) 176:1081–9. doi:10.4049/jimmunol.176.2.1081
22. Triantis V, Moulin V, Looman MWG, Hartgers FC, Janssen RAJ, Adema GJ. Molecular characterization of the murine homologue of the DC-derived protein DC-SCRIPT shown by real-time quantitative polymerase chain. *J Leukoc Biol* (2006) 79:1083–91. doi:10.1189/jlb.1005588
23. Hontelez S, Ansems M, Karthaus N, Looman MW, Triantis V, Adema GJ. Dendritic cell-specific transcript: dendritic cell marker and regulator of TLR-induced cytokine production. *J Immunol* (2012) 189:138–45. doi:10.4049/jimmunol.1103709
24. Ansems M, Hontelez S, Karthaus N, Span PN, Adema GJ. Crosstalk and DC-SCRIPT: expanding nuclear receptor modulation. *Biochim Biophys Acta* (2010) 1806:193–9. doi:10.1016/j.bbcan.2010.05.001
25. Ansems M, Hontelez S, Looman MWG, Karthaus N, Bult P, Bonenkamp JJ, et al. DC-SCRIPT: nuclear receptor modulation and prognostic significance in primary breast cancer. *J Natl Cancer Inst* (2010) 102:54–68. doi:10.1093/jnci/djp441
26. Ansems M, Karthaus N, Hontelez S, Aalders T, Looman MW, Verhaegh GW, et al. DC-SCRIPT: AR and VDR regulator lost upon transformation of prostate epithelial cells. *Prostate* (2012) 72:1708–17. doi:10.1002/pros.22522
27. Hontelez S, Karthaus N, Looman MW, Ansems M, Adema GJ. DC-SCRIPT regulates glucocorticoid receptor function and expression of its target GILZ in dendritic cells. *J Immunol* (2013) 190:3172–9. doi:10.4049/jimmunol.1201776
28. Lopez-Garcia J, Periyasamy M, Thomas RS, Christian M, Leao M, Jat P, et al. ZNF366 is an estrogen receptor corepressor that acts through CtBP and histone deacetylases. *Nucleic Acids Res* (2006) 34:6126–36. doi:10.1093/nar/gkl875
29. Sieuwerts AM, Ansems M, Look MP, Span PN, de Weerd V, van Galen A, et al. Clinical significance of the nuclear receptor co-regulator DC-SCRIPT in breast cancer: an independent retrospective validation study. *Breast Cancer Res* (2010) 12:R103. doi:10.1186/bcr2786
30. Ansems M, Søndergaard JN, Sieuwerts AM, Looman MWG, Smid M, de Graaf AMA, et al. DC-SCRIPT is a novel regulator of the tumor suppressor gene CDKN2B and induces cell cycle arrest in ERα-positive breast cancer cells. *Breast Cancer Res Treat* (2015) 149:693–703. doi:10.1007/s10549-015-3281-y
31. Søndergaard JN, Poghosyan S, Hontelez S, Louche P, Looman MWG, Ansems M, et al. DC-SCRIPT regulates IL-10 production in human dendritic cells by modulating NF-kBp65 activation. *J Immunol* (2015) 195:1498–505. doi:10.4049/jimmunol.1402924
32. Barski A, Cuddapah S, Cui K, Roh TY, Schones DE, Wang Z, et al. High-resolution profiling of histone methylations in the human genome. *Cell* (2007) 129:823–37. doi:10.1016/j.cell.2007.05.009
33. Welstead GG, Creyghton MP, Bilodeau S, Cheng AW, Markoulaki S, Young RA, et al. X-linked H3K27me3 demethylase Utx is required for embryonic development in a sex-specific manner. *Proc Natl Acad Sci U S A* (2012) 109:13004–9. doi:10.1073/pnas.1210787109
34. van Heeringen SJ, Veenstra GJC. GimmeMotifs: a de novo motif prediction pipeline for ChIP-sequencing experiments. *Bioinformatics* (2011) 27:270–1. doi:10.1093/bioinformatics/btq636
35. Bailey TL, Boden M, Buske FA, Frith M, Grant CE, Clementi L, et al. MEME Suite: tools for motif discovery and searching. *Nucleic Acids Res* (2009) 37:202–8. doi:10.1093/nar/gkp335
36. McLean CY, Bristor D, Hiller M, Clarke SL, Schaar BT, Lowe CB, et al. GREAT improves functional interpretation of cis-regulatory regions. *Nat Biotechnol* (2010) 28:495–501. doi:10.1038/nbt.1630
37. Jeffrey KL, Camps M, Rommel C, Mackay CR. Targeting dual-specificity phosphatases: manipulating MAP kinase signalling and immune responses. *Nat Rev Drug Discov* (2007) 6:391–403. doi:10.1038/nrd2289
38. Muda M, Boschert U, Dickinson R, Martinou J-C, Martinou I, Camps M, et al. MKP-3, a novel cytosolic protein-tyrosine phosphatase that examplifies a new class of mitogen-activated protein kinase phosphatase. *J Biol Chem* (1996) 271:4319–26. doi:10.1074/jbc.271.8.4319
39. Arthur JSC, Ley SC. Mitogen-activated protein kinases in innate immunity. *Nat Rev Immunol* (2013) 13:679–92. doi:10.1038/nri3495

40. Brondello JM, Brunet A, Pouysségur J, McKenzie FR. The dual specificity mitogen-activated protein kinase phosphatase-1 and -2 are induced by the p42/p44MAPK cascade. *J Biol Chem* (1997) 272:1368–76. doi:10.1074/jbc.272.2.1368
41. Dixon JR, Selvaraj S, Yue F, Kim A, Li Y, Shen Y, et al. Topological domains in mammalian genomes identified by analysis of chromatin interactions. *Nature* (2012) 485:376–80. doi:10.1038/nature11082
42. Rao SSP, Huntley MH, Durand NC, Stamenova EK, Bochkov ID, Robinson JT, et al. A 3D map of the human genome at kilobase resolution reveals principles of chromatin looping. *Cell* (2014) 159:1665–80. doi:10.1016/j.cell.2014.11.021
43. Dixon JR, Jung I, Selvaraj S, Shen Y, Antosiewicz-Bourget JE, Lee AY, et al. Chromatin architecture reorganization during stem cell differentiation. *Nature* (2015) 518:331–6. doi:10.1038/nature14222
44. Guan K-L, Butch E. Isolation and characterization of a novel dual specific phosphatase, HV2, which selectively dephosphorylates the mitogen-activated protein kinase. *J Biol Chem* (1995) 270:7197–203. doi:10.1074/jbc.270.13.7197
45. Banchereau J, Steinman RM. Dendritic cells and the control of immunity. *Nature* (1998) 392:245–52. doi:10.1038/32588
46. Brooks DG, Walsh KB, Elsaesser H, Oldstone MBA. IL-10 directly suppresses CD4 but not CD8 T cell effector and memory responses following acute viral infection. *Proc Natl Acad Sci U S A* (2010) 107:3018–23. doi:10.1073/pnas.0914500107
47. Reber L, Vermeulen L, Haegeman G, Frossard N. Ser276 phosphorylation of NF-kB p65 by MSK1 controls SCF expression in inflammation. *PLoS One* (2009) 4:e4393. doi:10.1371/journal.pone.0004393
48. Heinz S, Romanoski CE, Benner C, Glass CK. The selection and function of cell type-specific enhancers. *Nat Rev Mol Cell Biol* (2015) 16:144–54. doi:10.1038/nrm3949
49. Palucka K, Banchereau J. Dendritic-cell-based therapeutic cancer vaccines. *Immunity* (2013) 39:38–48. doi:10.1016/j.immuni.2013.07.004
50. Wayteck L, Breckpot K, Demeester J, De Smedt SC, Raemdonck K. A personalized view on cancer immunotherapy. *Cancer Lett* (2014) 352:113–25. doi:10.1016/j.canlet.2013.09.016
51. Jonuleit H, Kühn U, Müller G, Steinbrink K, Paragnik L, Schmitt E, et al. Pro-inflammatory cytokines and prostaglandins induce maturation of potent immunostimulatory dendritic cells under fetal calf serum-free conditions. *Eur J Immunol* (1997) 27:3135–42. doi:10.1002/eji.1830271209
52. Boullart ACI, Aarntzen EHJG, Verdijk P, Jacobs JFM, Schuurhuis DH, Benitez-Ribas D, et al. Maturation of monocyte-derived dendritic cells with toll-like receptor 3 and 7/8 ligands combined with prostaglandin E2 results in high interleukin-12 production and cell migration. *Cancer Immunol Immunother* (2008) 57:1589–97. doi:10.1007/s00262-008-0489-2
53. Schreibelt G, Benitez-Ribas D, Schuurhuis D, Lambeck AJA, Van Hout-Kuijer M, Schaft N, et al. Commonly used prophylactic vaccines as an alternative for synthetically produced TLR ligands to mature monocyte-derived dendritic cells. *Blood* (2010) 116:564–74. doi:10.1182/blood-2009-11-251884
54. de Vries IJM, Eggert AAO, Scharenborg NM, Vissers JLM, Lesterhuis WJ, Boerman OC, et al. Phenotypical and functional characterization of clinical grade dendritic cells. *J Immunother* (2002) 25:429–38. doi:10.1097/00002371-200209000-00007
55. Schuurhuis DH, Lesterhuis WJ, Kramer M, Looman MGM, van Hout-Kuijer M, Schreibelt G, et al. Polyinosinic polycytidylic acid prevents efficient antigen expression after mRNA electroporation of clinical grade dendritic cells. *Cancer Immunol Immunother* (2009) 58:1109–15. doi:10.1007/s00262-008-0626-y
56. Livak KJ, Schmittgen TD. Analysis of relative gene expression data using real-time quantitative PCR and the 2(-Delta Delta C(T)) Method. *Methods* (2001) 25:402–8. doi:10.1006/meth.2001.1262
57. Zhang Y, Liu T, Meyer CA, Eeckhoute J, Johnson DS, Bernstein BE, et al. Model-based analysis of ChIP-seq (MACS). *Genome Biol* (2008) 9:R137. doi:10.1186/gb-2008-9-9-r137
58. Quinlan AR, Hall IM. BEDTools: a flexible suite of utilities for comparing genomic features. *Bioinformatics* (2010) 26:841–2. doi:10.1093/bioinformatics/btq033
59. Georgiou G, van Heeringen SJ. fluff: exploratory analysis and visualization of high-throughput sequencing data. *PeerJ* (2016) 4:e2209. doi:10.7717/peerj.2209
60. Georgiev O, Bourquin JP, Gstaiger M, Knoepfel L, Schaffner W, Hovens C. Two versatile eukaryotic expression vectors permitting epitope tagging, radiolabelling and nuclear localisation of expressed proteins. *Gene* (1996) 168:165–7. doi:10.1016/0378-1119(95)00764-4

16

Current Concepts of Antigen Cross-Presentation

*Maria Embgenbroich and Sven Burgdorf**

Life and Medical Sciences (LIMES) Institute, University of Bonn, Bonn, Germany

***Correspondence:**
Sven Burgdorf
burgdorf@uni-bonn.de

Dendritic cells have the ability to efficiently present internalized antigens on major histocompatibility complex (MHC) I molecules. This process is termed cross-presentation and is important role in the generation of an immune response against viruses and tumors, after vaccinations or in the induction of immune tolerance. The molecular mechanisms enabling cross-presentation have been topic of intense debate since many years. However, a clear view on these mechanisms remains difficult, partially due to important remaining questions, controversial results and discussions. Here, we give an overview of the current concepts of antigen cross-presentation and focus on a description of the major cross-presentation pathways, the role of retarded antigen degradation for efficient cross-presentation, the dislocation of antigens from endosomal compartment into the cytosol, the reverse transport of proteasome-derived peptides for loading on MHC I and the translocation of the cross-presentation machinery from the ER to endosomes. We try to highlight recent advances, discuss some of the controversial data and point out some of the major open questions in the field.

Keywords: dendritic cells, cross-presentation, antigen processing, endosomes, antigen dislocation

INTRODUCTION

Dendritic cells (DCs) scan the peripheral tissue for antigens. Upon their recognition, antigens are internalized and the DCs activated and migrate toward the draining lymph node, where they can induce an adaptive immune response (1). In order to do so, they need to process the internalized antigens and load antigen-derived peptides on major histocompatibility complex (MHC) molecules. Peptides loaded onto MHC II molecules can be recognized by antigen-specific $CD4^+$ T helper cells. Similarly, peptides loaded on MHC I molecules can be recognized by antigen-specific $CD8^+$ T cells, leading to their proliferation and the activation of their cytotoxic capacities.

The presentation of internalized antigens on MHC I molecules is a process termed cross-presentation. Efficient cross-presentation has been shown to be crucial in, e.g., the induction of an adaptive immune response against tumors and viruses that do not infect DCs directly and in the induction of peripheral tolerance (2–5).

The molecular mechanisms that regulate classical antigen presentation on MHC II molecules and cross-presentation, however, have been shown to be quite divers. For MHC II-restricted presentation, internalized antigens are degraded in endo/lysosomal compartments by proteases such as cathepsins. Newly synthesized MHC II molecules, which are stabilized by binding to the invariant chain (Ii), are transported from the ER toward this compartment, where Ii is degraded by lysosomal proteases, resulting in the binding of only a small peptide fragment (CLIP) to MHC II. Subsequently, CLIP is replaced by antigen-derived peptides by the chaperon HLA-DM (6).

In contrast to MHC II-restricted presentation, the molecular mechanisms regulating cross-presentation are less understood and in part discussed controversially. There seems to be a whole variety of pathways leading to antigen cross-presentation and, despite intensive investigations, the molecular mechanisms and individual contribution of each pathway are rather unclear.

In this review, we try to describe some of the recent advances in cross-presentation, focusing on the major cross-presentation pathways and highlighting some of the controversial observations in the field.

CROSS-PRESENTING DC SUBSETS

Although many cells are able to present extracellular antigens on MHC I, DCs are considered to be the most prominent and most relevant cross-presenting cells.

In general, DCs are subdivided into conventional DCs (cDCs) and plasmacytoid DCs (pDCs). cDCs are further classified into cDC1 and cDC2 (7). In mice and human, cDC1 are characterized by the expression of the chemokine receptor XCR1 (7–9) and their development relies on the expression of the transcription factors IRF8 and Batf3 (10–12), whereas the development of cDC2 is mainly regulated by IRF4 (7, 13). Additionally, murine cDC1 express either CD8 (in lymphoid tissues) or CD103 (in non-lymphoid tissues), whereas human cDC1 are characterized by the expression of BDCA-3 (CD141) (8, 14–17).

The cDC1 are generally considered to be potent cross-presenting DCs *in vivo*. Accordingly, in murine lymphoid tissue, soluble and cell-associated OVA are cross-presented by resident $CD8^+$ DCs (18–20), whereas soluble and cell-associated antigens in lung (21, 22), intestine, and skin (23–25) are cross-presented by migratory $CD103^+$ DCs. Further functional properties of cDC1 are the uptake of apoptotic cells *via* Clec9A/DNGR1 (26–29) and the responsiveness to TLR3 stimulation (30).

cDC1 express high levels of MHC I pathway genes (31), show high intra-endosomal reactive oxygen species (ROS) production and low acidification in endosomes (32, 33), all features of efficient cross-presentation (see below). They express the small GTPase Rac2, which enables the assembly of the NAPDH oxidase complex NADPH oxidase 2 (NOX2), resulting in enhanced ROS production and active alkalization of endosomes (33). Additionally, cDC1 show only marginal expression levels of the C-type lectin Siglec-G, a potent inhibitor of NOX2 (34).

However, the cDC1 are not the only cross-presenting DC population. Many other DC subpopulations, including cDC2, have been shown to cross-present as well (35–39). For human DCs, it even has been demonstrated that $BDCA3^+$ (cDC1s), $BDCA1^+$ (cDC2s), and even pDCs all bear intrinsic capacities to cross-present extracellular antigens (40). The exact role of different cDC1 and cDC2 subpopulations in cross-presentation is, therefore, under debate and, especially since functional data on the physiological role of human DC subsets in cross-presentation is hard to obtain, future experiments will have to shed light on this question.

Although pDCs have been shown to be able to cross-present antigens (41), their role in cross-presentation *in vivo* is questionable, especially since their depletion did not affect cross-presentation and clearance of viral antigens (42).

MAJOR PATHWAYS OF ANTIGEN CROSS-PRESENTATION

Intensive research has clearly shown that there are a wide variety of mechanisms by which peptides derived from extracellular antigens can be presented on MHC I molecules. In general, there are two main cross-presentation pathways: the vacuolar pathway and the endosome-to-cytosol pathway (**Figure 1**). In the vacuolar pathway, antigen processing and loading onto MHC I molecules occurs within the endo/lysosomal compartment. After internalization, antigens are degraded by lysosomal proteases and antigen-derived peptides are loaded onto MHC class I molecules there. The lysosomal protease Cathepsin S has been demonstrated to play a crucial role in antigen degradation for the vacuolar pathway (43). In the endosome-to-cytosol pathway, internalized antigens need to be transported from the endosomal compartment into the cytosol, where they are degraded by the proteasome (44–46). Derived peptides are subsequently transported by the transporter associated with antigen processing (TAP) into the ER or back into the antigen-containing endosomes, where they can be loaded onto MHC class I (44, 45, 47–49). Although substantial evidence points out that some antigens indeed can be cross-presented independent of proteasomal degradation and TAP-mediated peptide transport by the vacuolar pathway (43, 50–53), most cross-presentation studies report of cross-presentation *via* the endosome-to-cytosol pathway. The dependency of cross-presentation on proteasomal degradation seems logical, since the functional outcome of cross-presentation is the activation of antigen-specific cytotoxic T cells. After migration toward to site of infection, these T cells are fully equipped to kill potential target cells, like virus-infected cells or tumor cells. In order to become functionally active, T cells must recognize the same epitope presented on MHC I by the target cells. Importantly, MHC I-loaded peptides on target cells do not emerge from cross-presentation but rather are the result of direct (classical) MHC I-restricted presentation of endogenous antigens, in which peptides are generated by the proteasome. Since it is hard to assume that for all antigens, the proteasome and lysosomal proteases generate exactly the same epitopes, the dependency of cross-presentation on proteasomal degradation for at least a substantial part of the antigens might circumvent this problem. Accordingly, DCs deficient in the LMP7 subunit of the immunoproteasome are impaired in cross-presentation *in vitro* and *in vivo* (46). However, it needs to be mentioned that very few information about the *in vivo* significance of the vacuolar vs. endosome-to-cytosol pathway is available, pointing out that future experiments are needed to further investigate the relative importance of both pathways *in vivo*.

DELAYED ANTIGEN DEGRADATION AND ITS ROLE IN CROSS-PRESENTATION

Over the last years, it has become clear that intra-endosomal antigen stability critically regulates cross-presentation, which efficiency is negatively affected by rapid lysosomal degradation of

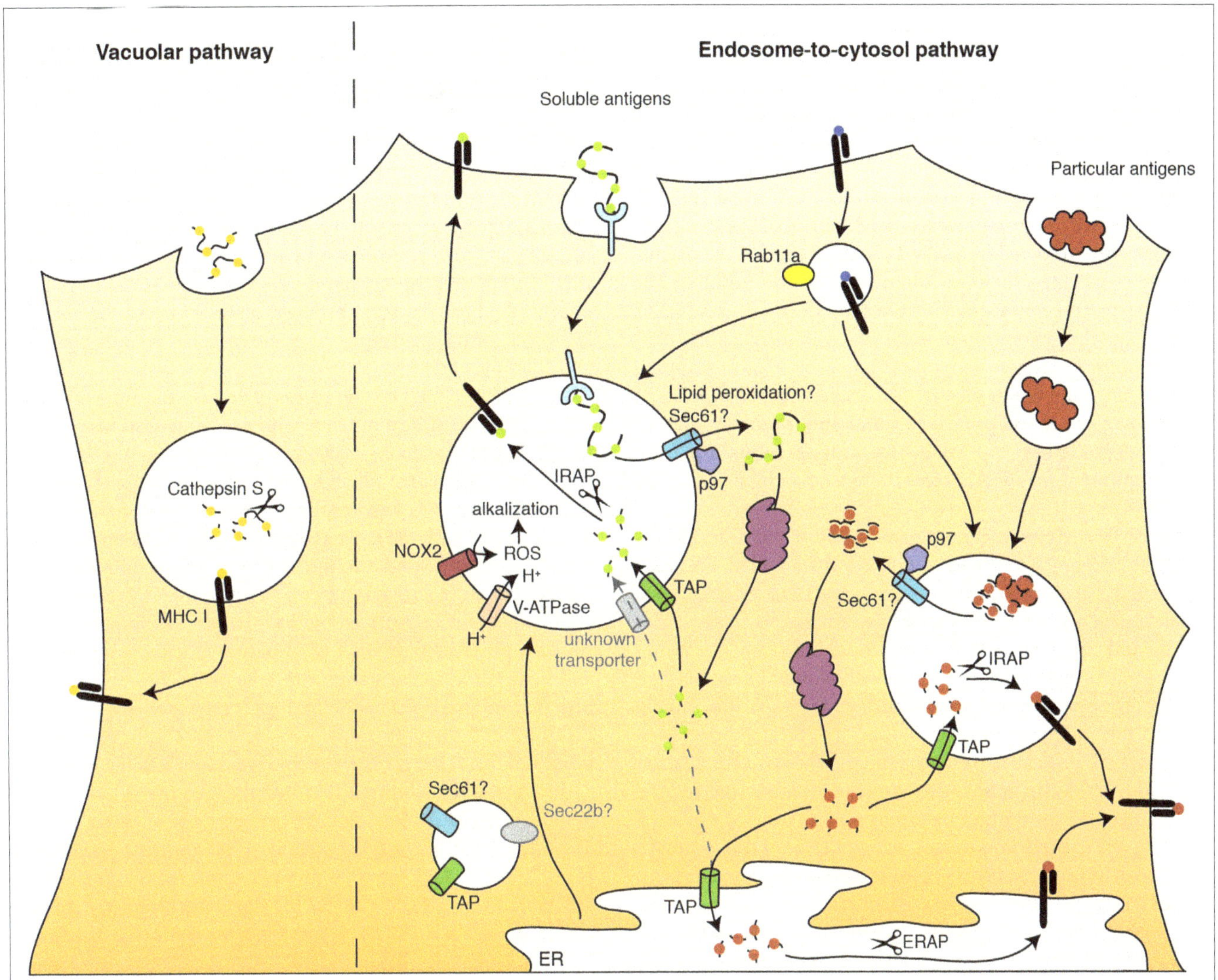

FIGURE 1 | Schematic overview of cross-presentation pathways. Internalized antigens can be presented *via* the vacuolar pathway or *via* the endosome-to-cytosol pathway. In the vacuolar pathway, antigens are degraded in endosomes by Cathepsin S and loaded onto major histocompatibility complex (MHC) I there. In the endosome-to-cytosol pathway, antigens are transported into the cytosol for proteasomal degradation. Afterward, antigen-derived peptides are transported back into the endosomes (soluble and particular antigens) or into the ER (particular antigens) *via* TAP. There, they are trimmed by IRAP (endosomes) or ERAP (ER) and loaded onto MHC I. They cross-presentation machinery might be translocated toward endosomes *via* Sec22b.

internalized antigens (54). Lysosomal maturation and activation of lysosomal proteases is fine-tuned by the transcription factor TFEB, an important regulator of cross-presentation (55).

It is generally assumed that rapid antigen degradation quickly destroys a large amount of epitopes before they can be processed properly and loaded onto MHC I molecules (56, 57). Additionally, peptide-loaded MHC I molecules have a limited life span at the cell membrane (58–60). In order to enable T cell activation after migration toward the draining lymph node, however, prolonged cross-presentation seems to be essential. Therefore, limited antigen degradation in antigen-presenting cells might be a mechanism to generate a kind of intracellular antigen depot, from where continuous antigen processing and presentation might ensure the presence of peptide-loaded MHC I molecules over a longer period of time (61). Such intracellular antigen storage depots have also been shown in human monocytes, which accumulate long-peptide antigens for over 5 days in non-lysosomal compartments, where day are protected from rapid degradation (62).

Since DCs are the most efficient cross-presenting cells, these cells possess several mechanisms by which they can actively prevent rapid lysosomal antigen degradation.

First, it was demonstrated that DCs express lower levels of lysosomal proteases (63) and display a reduced velocity of endosome maturation (64) compared to other immune cells. Expression of asparagine endopeptidase and Cathepsins L, S, D, and B in phagosomes of DCs was clearly reduced compared to macrophages, resulting in impaired phagolysosomal degradation and prolonged antigen stability after internalization by DCs (63). The delivery of lysosomal proteases toward phagosomes was even further reduced after stimulation of DCs with LPS (64).

Second, in DCs, an active alkalization of endosomes prevents pH-dependent activation of lysosomal proteases. During lysosome maturation, protons are transported into the luminal space by the V-ATPase, leading to the activation of pH-dependent lysosomal proteases. Reduced V-ATPase activity in DCs might contribute to prevent a rapid drop in pH after antigen internalization (65). Additionally, DCs seem to have the unique capacity to alkalize their endosomes by the recruitment the NOX2 toward the endosomal membrane (32, 66). There, NOX2 can mediate the generation of ROS, which in turn capture protons to build hydrogen peroxide (**Figure 1**). Proton trapping by ROS causes an active alkalization, impairing pH-dependent activation of lysosomal proteases, which in turn prevents rapid antigen degradation and stimulates cross-presentation (32). The recruitment of NOX2 toward endosomes is mediated by Rab27a (67).

Third, DCs express endocytosis receptors that specifically target non-degradative endosomal compartments. Previous studies have demonstrated that the endocytosis receptor used to internalize an antigen critically determines its intracellular routing and degradation (68). A previous study from our group demonstrated that antigens internalized by fluid phase pinocytosis or scavenger receptor-mediated endocytosis are rapidly targeted toward lysosomes, where they are efficiently degraded by lysosomal proteases, resulting in poor cross-presentation (68). However, if the same DCs simultaneously internalized the same antigen by the mannose receptor, it was targeted toward a distinct pool of early endosomes, which did not undergo rapid fusion with lysosomes and in which antigens were protected from lysosomal degradation, resulting in efficient cross-presentation of MR-internalized antigens (68). Although the role of the MR in *in vivo* cross-presentation has been discussed controversially (69, 70), it now is clear that CD103$^+$ DCs in liver and lung use this receptor for cross-presentation of, e.g., viral antigens (71). A correlation between antigen targeting into early endosomes clearly distinct from lysosomes and cross-presentation efficiency has also been confirmed in human DCs. Also in these cells, MR-mediated internalization resulted in its routing into early endosomes, retarded degradation and efficient cross-presentation, whereas uptake by DEC205 lead to antigen targeting into lysosomes, rapid lysosomal degradation, and hence poor cross-presentation (56). Interestingly, attenuating lysosomal degradation was sufficient to rescue the cross-presentation of DEC-205-internalized antigens (56), highlighting again the importance of intra-endosomal antigen stability for efficient cross-presentation. Additionally, the targeted region of the endocytosis receptor might also play a role in antigen degradation and presentation, adding even an additional degree of complexity. Figdor and colleagues demonstrated that antigen targeting toward the carbohydrate recognition domain of DC-SIGN delivers antigens to lysosomal compartments, resulting in rapid degradation and poor cross-presentation, whereas targeting the neck region of DC-SIGN causes antigen delivery in early endosomal compartments clearly distinct from lysosomes, causing prolonged stability and efficient cross-presentation (72, 73).

ANTIGEN TRANSLOCATION INTO THE CYTOSOL AS CRITICAL STEP IN ANTIGEN CROSS-PRESENTATION

After being internalized into a non-degradative endosomal compartment, antigens need to be processed before they can be loaded onto MHC I. In the endosome-to-cytosol pathway, internalized antigens, therefore, need to be transported across the endosomal membrane into the cytosol for proteasomal degradation. Although this is a key step in antigen cross-presentation and significant efforts have been made to shed light on this process, the underlying mechanisms mediating such intracellular antigen transport are still topic of debate.

In general, if DCs enable access of endosomal antigens to the cytosol, this must be a process, which is controlled very tightly. Uncontrolled lysosome leakage would lead to the cytosolic release of Cathepsins, which in turn would activate the NLRP3 inflammasome (74) and result in pyroptosis, an inflammatory form of cell death (75). To avoid this, total lysosomal content cannot just be released into the cytosol in an uncontrolled fashion. Accordingly, antigens need to be unfolded (76) and disulfide bridges need to be reduced by the γ-interferon-inducible lysosomal thiol reductase GILT (77) before efficient translocation and hence cross-presentation can take place. This supports the idea that antigen translocation is highly regulated, might involve dislocation through a transmembrane pore complex, and is presumably not the result of simple lysosome leakage.

It is generally assumed that members of the ER-associated degradation (ERAD) machinery contribute in enabling antigen dislocation for cross-presentation. First indirect indications for a role of ERAD in this process came from observations describing the presence of ERAD components in the phagosomal membrane (47, 48) and from experiments using the ERAD inhibitor Exotoxin A, which specifically represses cross-presentation (49, 78).

First direct evidence for the involvement of the ERAD machinery came from the Cresswell group, who demonstrated an important role of the AAA ATPase p97 in antigen dislocation (49). Whereas expression of a dominant-negative p97 mutant in DCs represses cross-presentation, the addition of purified wild-type p97 but not the dominant-negative mutant to purified phagosomes enhanced antigen translocation (49, 79–81), indicating that p97 indeed might provide the energy to pull endosomal antigens into the cytosol.

The identification of a dedicated translocon, which actually functions as a transmembrane pore complex to enable antigen dislocation across the endosomal membrane, has been (and still is) by far more difficult. One putative candidate, which has been proposed to mediate antigen dislocation into the cytosol over a decade ago, is the ERAD member Sec61 (49, 78), a trimeric protein whose downregulation has been shown to inhibit antigen translocation and cross-presentation (79, 82). However, since Sec61 plays an important role in the dislocation of proteins at the ER membrane, like, e.g., the dislocation of MHC I molecules themselves (83), it is very hard to distinguish endosome-specific effects of Sec61 from general effects at the ER. In an attempt to solve this problem, we generated

Sec61-specific intracellular antibody (intrabody), which we fused to an ER retention signal (84), leading to the trapping of Sec61 in the ER and preventing its transport toward endosomes (82). By this means, we could demonstrate that the transport of Sec61 toward endosomes indeed is essential for antigen dislocation and cross-presentation. Additionally, we could demonstrate that the expression of the intrabody did not alter overall Sec61 expression and did not affected the ERAD-mediated dislocation of MHC I, TCR, CD3δ and the split venus protein at the ER membrane. This points out that ERAD activity at the ER remained unaltered by the expression of the intrabody. These data suggest that Sec61 indeed might serve as a translocon for cross-presentation (**Figure 1**). However, it cannot be formally excluded that the translation of another pore complex at the ER membrane is changed by manipulating intracellular Sec61 transport or that another putative pore complex is translocated toward endosomes in a complex with Sec61, being influences by intrabody expression. Additionally, Grotzke et al. demonstrated that a chemical inhibitor of Sec61, mycolactone, does not seem to influence antigen dislocation from the cytosol (85). This inhibitor has been shown to directly bind Sec61 and targets proteins that are co-translationally imported in a Sec61-mediated fashion into the ER toward proteasomal degradation (86, 87). However, whether mycolactone could possibly affect Sec61-mediated protein dislocation from the ER into the cytosol is not clear, especially since such proteins are generally ubiquitinated and targeted for proteasomal degradation also in the absence of mycolactone (80). Indeed, mycolactone was shown to have no influence on ERAD (86) and also Grotzke et al. demonstrated that mycolactone does not affect protein retranslocation from the ER into the cytosol. Whether this is due to a missing role of Sec61 in this process or to specific properties of the inhibitor needs to be determined. Especially since addition of Exotoxin A, an inhibitor that blocks Sec61 channel openings (78, 88), clearly affects antigen translocation and cross-presentation (49, 82), there seems to be a need of information on the exact working mechanism of these inhibitors and on the role of Sec61 in dislocation from the ER to finally clear a potential role of Sec61 on cross-presentation.

In addition to antigen dislocation through a pore complex, a recent study postulated that lipid peroxidation in DCs might play a crucial role in antigen transport into the cytoplasm (89). Here, the authors proposed that the specific recruitment of NOX2 might cause lipid peroxidation in endosomes. As mentioned above, NOX2 captures protons to generate hydrogen peroxide, preventing rapid acidification of the endosome. Lipid peroxidation caused by such hydrogen peroxide was suggested to result in leakiness of the endosomal membrane and hence, antigen access into the cytosol and enhanced cross-presentation. However, it remains unclear how the antigen-presenting cell in this case would prevent inflammasome-induced cell death caused by unspecific release of cathepsins. Additionally, the necessity for endosomal antigens to be unfolded (76) and reduced by GILT (77) cannot be explained by simple leackage of the endosomal membrane. Therefore, the significance of such a pathway in cross-presentation *in vivo* remains to be elucidated.

TRANSPORT OF PROTEASOME-DERIVED PEPTIDES FOR LOADING ONTO MHC I

After being transported into the cytosol, internalized antigens are degraded by the proteasome. Subsequently, antigen-derived peptides can be transported through the TAP transporter into the ER or alternatively, by endosomal TAP, back into the endosomal compartments (44, 45, 47, 48, 90). There, peptides are trimmed into a suited size for loading onto MHC I molecules. Such trimming can occur *via* the peptidases ERAP (in the ER) or IRAP (in endosomes) (**Figure 1**) (91). Presentation of peptides derived from soluble antigens is mainly ERAP-independent *in vitro* and *in vivo* (92), but rather occurs in endosomes after transport by endosomal TAP and IRAP-mediated peptide trimming (90, 92). Proteasome-derived peptides derived from particulate antigens, however, can be transferred into both the ER and endosomes, where they are trimmed by ERAP or IRAP, respectively, and loaded onto MHC I (91). These underlying mechanisms for these differences are unknown.

Recently, it was demonstrated that, in addition to antigen translocation through endosomal TAP, some peptides might enter endosomes in an energy-consuming but TAP-independent fashion (93), pointing out the possibility of additional (unknown) transporters involved in peptide transport into endosomes for cross-presentation. Additionally, since TAP-independency was often used to demonstrate cross-presentation *via* the vacuolar pathway, there is the possibility that at least in part of these studies, antigens might have entered the endosome *via* the endosome-to-cytosol pathway, using alternative peptide transporters.

After peptide reimport into the endosomes, they can be loaded onto MHC I molecules. In general, there are two basic possibilities how MHC I molecules can enter the endosome. First, newly synthesized MHC I molecules could be transported from the ER to the endosomes and used for peptide loading in cross-presentation. Second, MHC I from the cell surface (that are already loaded with peptides) could be transported toward endosomes during endocytosis events. The Blander group demonstrated that for particulate antigens, MHC I molecules used for cross-presentation mainly originated from the cell membrane and were translocated into an endosomal recycling compartment in a Rab11a-dependent fashion (**Figure 1**) (94). From these organelles, MHC I molecules can be transported toward phagosomes, a process that is mediated by the SNARE protein SNAP23 and critically depends on MyD88 signaling (94). It remains unclear, however, whether peptide exchange on recycling MHC I molecules requires the help of additional chaperon proteins (similar to the function of HLA-DM in MHC II-restricted presentation) or can occur after simple weakening of the peptide–MHC I binding in endosomes. Additionally, it has been demonstrated that for cross-presentation of elongated peptides, a substantial part of the used MHC I molecules are newly synthesized molecules recruited from the ER (95). In this case, it needs to be determined whether such MHC I molecules are loaded with peptides in the ER and undergo peptide exchange in acidic endosomes, or whether the transport of the entire peptide loading complex, which stabilizes unbound MHC I molecules and assists in peptide binding, to the endosomes is required for cross presentation. Despite the presence of several members of the peptide loading machinery in endosomes (45, 47, 48), a functional relevance of these proteins in cross-presentation is missing.

TRANSPORT OF ER COMPONENTS TO ENDOSOMES

As described above, efficient cross-presentation requires the transport of ER proteins toward endosomes. The exact mechanisms, by which this transfer occurs, are not completely understood and in part contradictory data complicate a clear view on this process.

Since it is known that endosomes during their maturation directly interact with the ER to exchange a wide variety of molecules (96), such ER-endosome membrane contact sites would offer an easy explanation for the transfer of ER proteins toward endosomes. However, it has been proposed by Amigorena and Savina that the transport of cross-presentation components toward endosomes takes place from the ER-golgi intermediate compartment (ERGIC) (97). Membrane fusion between the ERGIC and the phagosomes has been postulated to be mediated by the SNARE proteins Sec22b (in the ERGIC) and syntaxin 4 (in the phagosome). Accordingly, shRNA-mediated downregulation of Sec22b resulted in impaired recruitment of ER proteins toward phagosomes, decreased antigen translocation into the cytosol, and hence reduced cross-presentation (94, 97). These observations support a critical role of the ERAD machinery in antigen dislocation into the cytosol for cross-presentation as described above. However, a recent study by Reddy and colleagues demonstrated that severe off target effects of the used shRNA might have caused the observed influence on cross-presentation (98), questioning the role of Sec22b in cross-presentation. Since such off target effects of shRNA molecules can be circumvented by the generation of Sec22b-deficient mice, one could expect that the use of conditional knockout mice would shed light on the situation and would clearly indicate whether Sec22b is indeed involved in cross-presentation. Mice bearing a conditional knockout of Sec22b in CD11c$^+$ DCs were generated by both the Reddy and the Amigorena group. Strikingly, whereas Reddy et al. reported complete independency of cross-presentation on Sec22b (98), Amigorena et al. showed a clear impairment of cross-presentation in Sec22b-knockout DCs, hence drawing completely opposite conclusions (99). Both groups used partially different *in vitro* and *in vivo* systems to substantiate their findings, but since also opposite effects of Sec22b on cross-presentation using the same cells (BM-DCs and splenic DCs) and the same antigens (soluble and bead-bound OVA) were observed, these contractionary results cannot be explained by different experimental setups only (100). Therefore, the exact role of Sec22b and ERGIC-mediated transport of ER proteins needs to be confirmed.

The recruitment of MHC I molecules toward antigen-containing phagosomes was shown to be induced by TLR ligands. TLR-induced and MyD88-dependent signaling resulted in the activation of IKK2, which phosphorylates SNAP23, mediating fusion events between phagosomes and MHC I-containing recycling endosomes (94). Also the transport of other ER proteins toward endosomes has been shown to be stimulated by TLR ligands (82, 90). Using flow cytometric analysis of individual endosomes (101), have demonstrated before that low amounts of Sec61 are present in endosomes also in the absence of TLR ligands, and that a clear recruitment of Sec61 toward antigen-containing endosomes was induced by LPS (82). Since it is very unlikely that Sec61 is also recruited *via* recycling endosomes, distinct mechanisms might come into play for the transport of these molecules.

One of these mechanisms might rely on the uncoordinated 93 homolog B1 (UNC93B1), which is activated by TLR triggering and mediates the transport of TLRs from the ER toward endosomes (102–104). Interestingly, UNC91B1 has been demonstrated to be critically involved in cross-presentation (105). Although a putative role of UNC93B has also been discussed controversially (106), it now becomes clear that an essential role of UNC93B1 in cross-presentation is based on its interaction with the store-operated-Ca^{2+}-entry regulator STIM1. UNC93B1 has been shown to be essential for oligomerization of hence activation of STIM1, which in turn alters local Calcium signaling regulating phago/endosome fusion events (107, 108). Ablation of UNC93B1 impairs antigen translocation into the cytosol and cross-presentation (107). Interestingly, antigen dislocation into the cytosol was impaired despite reduced endosomal antigen degradation, which is generally assumed to increase antigen export from the endosomes. Since UNC93B1 upon TLR stimulation mediates TLR transport from the ER toward endosomes, it, therefore, is thinkable that ER members of the cross-presentation machinery are transported from the ER toward endosomes in a similar UNC93B1-dependent fashion.

Additionally, DC activation by TLR ligands can have other effects on the cross-presentation machinery independent of ER to endosome transport, like the prevention of phagosome fusion with lysosomes and concomitant antigen stabilization (57) or increases in antigen internalization (109).

ALTERNATIVE CROSS-PRESENTATION PATHWAYS

In all cross-presentation pathways described above, cross-presented antigens entered the DC *via* endocytosis. However, there are some reports indicating that also distinct mechanisms can lead to cross-presentation.

One of these mechanisms is the transport of pre-processed antigens (peptides) from a donor cell to a DC. Such transport can occur *via* direct cell–cell contact, mediated by gap junctions (110, 111). After gap junction-mediated transport from one cell to another, antigen-derived peptides can enter the normal MHC I presentation pathway. Interestingly, the donor cell does not need to be an antigen-presenting cell, offering the possibility that DCs can obtain such peptides directly from infected cells. Infection of melanoma cells with *Salmonella* has been demonstrated to increase the expression of Connexin 43, an important gap junction protein, enabling efficient gap junction-mediated peptide transfer from the infected cell to the DC and hence efficient cross-presentation (112). However, given the limited stability of intracellular peptides (113), the physiological significance of such peptide transfer in cross-presentation remains unclear.

Another alternative cross-presentation pathway is termed cross-dressing, which generally implies that the cross-presenting DC becomes an MHC I molecule, which has already been loaded with an antigen-derived peptide, transferred from a donor cell (114, 115). Similar to gap junction-mediated peptide transfer, such donor cell does not necessarily need to be an antigen-presenting cell, suggesting that DCs can derive peptide-loaded MHC I molecules directly from infected cells or even apoptotic cells. The transfer of loaded MHC I molecules is thought to be mediated by cell–cell contact rather than secretory vesicles (114, 116) and overcomes the need of intracellular antigen processing within the DC. Cross-dressing has been shown to occur *in vivo* (114, 116) and cross-dressed DCs have been shown to activate memory T cells after viral infection (116). Remarkably, in this study, the activation of naive T cells did not depend on cross-dressing (116), offering the possibility that different cross-presentation pathways might be responsible for the activation of different T cell populations or for T cell activation under specific conditions. However, the exact physiological relevance of cross-dressing and especially its contribution compared to the other cross-presentation pathways in specific situations, however, remains to be elucidated.

CONCLUSION

Despite intensive research over the last decades, several questions regarding the molecular mechanisms of cross-presentation remain unsolved. How are antigens translocated into the cytosol? How are ER components recruited toward endosomes? What is the role of Sec22b and TLR ligands in this process? And probably most important: which of all these proposed mechanisms holds true *in vivo*? Are different cross-presentation pathways used *in vivo* by distinct cell types or antigens (e.g., particulate vs. soluble), or under different physiological conditions? Without any doubt, the elucidation of the molecular mechanisms underlying cross-presentation *in vivo* bears a high intrinsic potential to optimize various vaccination strategies. Therefore, future investigations will be required to shed more light into the exact pathways of cross-presentation and to solve remaining controversies. The publication of clearly contradicting data might suggest the need for common protocols to perform cross-presentation experiments, in particular in regard to cell culture procedures to generate the often used BM-DCs.

AUTHOR CONTRIBUTIONS

ME and SB designed the article and wrote the manuscript.

REFERENCES

1. Reis e Sousa C. Toll-like receptors and dendritic cells: for whom the bug tolls. *Semin Immunol* (2004) 16:27–34. doi:10.1016/j.smim.2003.10.004
2. Huang AY, Golumbek P, Ahmadzadeh M, Jaffee E, Pardoll D, Levitsky H. Role of bone marrow-derived cells in presenting MHC class I-restricted tumor antigens. *Science* (1994) 264:961–5. doi:10.1126/science.7513904
3. Sigal LJ, Crotty S, Andino R, Rock KL. Cytotoxic T-cell immunity to virus-infected non-haematopoietic cells requires presentation of exogenous antigen. *Nature* (1999) 398:77–80. doi:10.1038/18038
4. den Haan JM, Bevan MJ. Antigen presentation to CD8+ T cells: cross-priming in infectious diseases. *Curr Opin Immunol* (2001) 13:437–41. doi:10.1016/S0952-7915(00)00238-7
5. Heath WR, Carbone FR. Cross-presentation in viral immunity and self-tolerance. *Nat Rev Immunol* (2001) 1:126–34. doi:10.1038/35100512
6. Mellins ED, Stern LJ. HLA-DM and HLA-DO, key regulators of MHC-II processing and presentation. *Curr Opin Immunol* (2014) 26:115–22. doi:10.1016/j.coi.2013.11.005
7. Guilliams M, Ginhoux F, Jakubzick C, Naik SH, Onai N, Schraml BU, et al. Dendritic cells, monocytes and macrophages: a unified nomenclature based on ontogeny. *Nat Rev Immunol* (2014) 14:571–8. doi:10.1038/nri3712
8. Crozat K, Guiton R, Contreras V, Feuillet V, Dutertre C-A, Ventre E, et al. The XC chemokine receptor 1 is a conserved selective marker of mammalian cells homologous to mouse CD8alpha+ dendritic cells. *J Exp Med* (2010) 207:1283–92. doi:10.1084/jem.20100223
9. Dalod M, Chelbi R, Malissen B, Lawrence T. Dendritic cell maturation: functional specialization through signaling specificity and transcriptional programming. *EMBO J* (2014) 33:1104–16. doi:10.1002/embj.201488027
10. Aliberti J, Schulz O, Pennington DJ, Tsujimura H, Reis e Sousa C, Ozato K, et al. Essential role for ICSBP in the in vivo development of murine CD8alpha + dendritic cells. *Blood* (2003) 101:305–10. doi:10.1182/blood-2002-04-1088
11. Edelson BT, KC W, Juang R, Kohyama M, Benoit LA, Klekotka PA, et al. Peripheral CD103+ dendritic cells form a unified subset developmentally related to CD8alpha+ conventional dendritic cells. *J Exp Med* (2010) 207:823–36. doi:10.1084/jem.20091627
12. Merad M, Sathe P, Helft J, Miller J, Mortha A. The dendritic cell lineage: ontogeny and function of dendritic cells and their subsets in the steady state and the inflamed setting. *Annu Rev Immunol* (2013) 31:563–604. doi:10.1146/annurev-immunol-020711-074950
13. Schlitzer A, McGovern N, Teo P, Zelante T, Atarashi K, Low D, et al. IRF4 transcription factor-dependent CD11b+ dendritic cells in human and mouse control mucosal IL-17 cytokine responses. *Immunity* (2013) 38:970–83. doi:10.1016/j.immuni.2013.04.011
14. Bachem A, Güttler S, Hartung E, Ebstein F, Schaefer M, Tannert A, et al. Superior antigen cross-presentation and XCR1 expression define human CD11c+CD141+ cells as homologues of mouse CD8+ dendritic cells. *J Exp Med* (2010) 207:1273–81. doi:10.1084/jem.20100348
15. Jongbloed SL, Kassianos AJ, McDonald KJ, Clark GJ, Ju X, Angel CE, et al. Human CD141+ (BDCA-3)+ dendritic cells (DCs) represent a unique myeloid DC subset that cross-presents necrotic cell antigens. *J Exp Med* (2010) 207:1247–60. doi:10.1084/jem.20092140
16. Poulin LF, Salio M, Griessinger E, Anjos-Afonso F, Craciun L, Chen J-L, et al. Characterization of human DNGR-1+ BDCA3+ leukocytes as putative equivalents of mouse CD8alpha+ dendritic cells. *J Exp Med* (2010) 207:1261–71. doi:10.1084/jem.20092618
17. Haniffa M, Shin A, Bigley V, McGovern N, Teo P, See P, et al. Human tissues contain CD141hi cross-presenting dendritic cells with functional homology to mouse CD103+ nonlymphoid dendritic cells. *Immunity* (2012) 37:60–73. doi:10.1016/j.immuni.2012.04.012
18. den Haan JM, Lehar SM, Bevan MJ. CD8(+) but not CD8(-) dendritic cells cross-prime cytotoxic T cells in vivo. *J Exp Med* (2000) 192:1685–96. doi:10.1084/jem.192.12.1685

19. Pooley JL, Heath WR, Shortman K. Cutting edge: intravenous soluble antigen is presented to CD4 T cells by CD8- dendritic cells, but cross-presented to CD8 T cells by CD8+ dendritic cells. *J Immunol* (2001) 166:5327–30. doi:10.4049/jimmunol.166.9.5327
20. Busche A, Jirmo AC, Welten SPM, Zischke J, Noack J, Constabel H, et al. Priming of CD8+ T cells against cytomegalovirus-encoded antigens is dominated by cross-presentation. *J Immunol* (2013) 190:2767–77. doi:10.4049/jimmunol.1200966
21. Becker M, Güttler S, Bachem A, Hartung E, Mora A, Jäkel A, et al. Ontogenic, phenotypic, and functional characterization of XCR1(+) dendritic cells leads to a consistent classification of intestinal dendritic cells based on the expression of XCR1 and SIRPα. *Front Immunol* (2014) 5:326. doi:10.3389/fimmu.2014.00326
22. Cerovic V, Houston SA, Westlund J, Utriainen L, Davison ES, Scott CL, et al. Lymph-borne CD8α+ dendritic cells are uniquely able to cross-prime CD8+ T cells with antigen acquired from intestinal epithelial cells. *Mucosal Immunol* (2015) 8:38–48. doi:10.1038/mi.2014.40
23. Bedoui S, Whitney PG, Waithman J, Eidsmo L, Wakim L, Caminschi I, et al. Cross-presentation of viral and self antigens by skin-derived CD103+ dendritic cells. *Nat Immunol* (2009) 10:488–95. doi:10.1038/ni.1724
24. Henry CJ, Grayson JM, Brzoza-Lewis KL, Mitchell LM, Westcott MM, Cook AS, et al. The roles of IL-12 and IL-23 in CD8+ T cell-mediated immunity against *Listeria monocytogenes*: insights from a DC vaccination model. *Cell Immunol* (2010) 264:23–31. doi:10.1016/j.cellimm.2010.04.007
25. Kitano M, Yamazaki C, Takumi A, Ikeno T, Hemmi H, Takahashi N, et al. Imaging of the cross-presenting dendritic cell subsets in the skin-draining lymph node. *Proc Natl Acad Sci U S A* (2016) 113:1044–9. doi:10.1073/pnas.1513607113
26. Caminschi I, Proietto AI, Ahmet F, Kitsoulis S, Shin Teh J, Lo JCY, et al. The dendritic cell subtype-restricted C-type lectin Clec9A is a target for vaccine enhancement. *Blood* (2008) 112:3264–73. doi:10.1182/blood-2008-05-155176
27. Huysamen C, Willment JA, Dennehy KM, Brown GD. CLEC9A is a novel activation C-type lectin-like receptor expressed on BDCA3+ dendritic cells and a subset of monocytes. *J Biol Chem* (2008) 283:16693–701. doi:10.1074/jbc.M709923200
28. Sancho D, Joffre OP, Keller AM, Rogers NC, Martínez D, Hernanz-Falcón P, et al. Identification of a dendritic cell receptor that couples sensing of necrosis to immunity. *Nature* (2009) 458:899–903. doi:10.1038/nature07750
29. Hanč P, Fujii T, Iborra S, Yamada Y, Huotari J, Schulz O, et al. Structure of the complex of F-actin and DNGR-1, a C-Type lectin receptor involved in dendritic cell cross-presentation of dead cell-associated antigens. *Immunity* (2015) 42:839–49. doi:10.1016/j.immuni.2015.04.009
30. Jelinek I, Leonard JN, Price GE, Brown KN, Meyer-Manlapat A, Goldsmith PK, et al. TLR3-specific double-stranded RNA oligonucleotide adjuvants induce dendritic cell cross-presentation, CTL responses, and antiviral protection. *J Immunol* (2011) 186:2422–9. doi:10.4049/jimmunol.1002845
31. Dudziak D, Kamphorst AO, Heidkamp GF, Buchholz VR, Trumpfheller C, Yamazaki S, et al. Differential antigen processing by dendritic cell subsets in vivo. *Science* (2007) 315:107–11. doi:10.1126/science.1136080
32. Savina A, Jancic C, Hugues S, Guermonprez P, Vargas P, Moura IC, et al. NOX2 controls phagosomal pH to regulate antigen processing during crosspresentation by dendritic cells. *Cell* (2006) 126:205–18. doi:10.1016/j.cell.2006.05.035
33. Savina A, Peres A, Cebrian I, Carmo N, Moita C, Hacohen N, et al. The small GTPase Rac2 controls phagosomal alkalinization and antigen crosspresentation selectively in CD8(+) dendritic cells. *Immunity* (2009) 30:544–55. doi:10.1016/j.immuni.2009.01.013
34. Ding Y, Guo Z, Liu Y, Li X, Zhang Q, Xu X, et al. The lectin Siglec-G inhibits dendritic cell cross-presentation by impairing MHC class I-peptide complex formation. *Nat Immunol* (2016) 17:1167–75. doi:10.1038/ni.3535
35. Sheng J, Chen Q, Soncin I, Ng SL, Karjalainen K, Ruedl C. A discrete subset of monocyte-derived cells among typical conventional type 2 dendritic cells can efficiently cross-present. *Cell Rep* (2017) 21:1203–14. doi:10.1016/j.celrep.2017.10.024
36. Ji Q, Castelli L, Goverman JM. MHC class I-restricted myelin epitopes are cross-presented by Tip-DCs that promote determinant spreading to CD8? T cells. *Nat Immunol* (2013) 14:254–61. doi:10.1038/ni.2513
37. Ballesteros-Tato A, León B, Lund FE, Randall TD. Temporal changes in dendritic cell subsets, cross-priming and costimulation via CD70 control CD8(+) T cell responses to influenza. *Nat Immunol* (2010) 11:216–24. doi:10.1038/ni.1838
38. Backer R, van Leeuwen F, Kraal G, den Haan JM. CD8- dendritic cells preferentially cross-present *Saccharomyces cerevisiae* antigens. *Eur J Immunol* (2008) 38:370–80. doi:10.1002/eji.200737647
39. Mouriès J, Moron G, Schlecht G, Escriou N, Dadaglio G, Leclerc C. Plasmacytoid dendritic cells efficiently cross-prime naive T cells in vivo after TLR activation. *Blood* (2008) 112:3713–22. doi:10.1182/blood-2008-03-146290
40. Segura E, Durand M, Amigorena S. Similar antigen cross-presentation capacity and phagocytic functions in all freshly isolated human lymphoid organ-resident dendritic cells. *J Exp Med* (2013) 210:1035–47. doi:10.1084/jem.20121103
41. Di Pucchio T, Chatterjee B, Smed-Sörensen A, Clayton S, Palazzo A, Montes M, et al. Direct proteasome-independent cross-presentation of viral antigen by plasmacytoid dendritic cells on major histocompatibility complex class I. *Nat Immunol* (2008) 9:551–7. doi:10.1038/ni.1602
42. GeurtsvanKessel CH, Willart MAM, van Rijt LS, Muskens F, Kool M, Baas C, et al. Clearance of influenza virus from the lung depends on migratory langerin+CD11b- but not plasmacytoid dendritic cells. *J Exp Med* (2008) 205:1621–34. doi:10.1084/jem.20071365
43. Shen L, Sigal LJ, Boes M, Rock KL. Important role of cathepsin S in generating peptides for TAP-independent MHC class I crosspresentation in vivo. *Immunity* (2004) 21:155–65. doi:10.1016/j.immuni.2004.07.004
44. Kovacsovics-Bankowski M, Rock KL. A phagosome-to-cytosol pathway for exogenous antigens presented on MHC class I molecules. *Science* (1995) 267:243–6. doi:10.1126/science.7809629
45. Ackerman AL, Kyritsis C, Tampé R, Cresswell P. Early phagosomes in dendritic cells form a cellular compartment sufficient for cross presentation of exogenous antigens. *Proc Natl Acad Sci U S A* (2003) 100:12889–94. doi:10.1073/pnas.1735556100
46. Palmowski MJ, Gileadi U, Salio M, Gallimore A, Millrain M, James E, et al. Role of immunoproteasomes in cross-presentation. *J Immunol* (2006) 177:983–90. doi:10.4049/jimmunol.177.2.983
47. Guermonprez P, Saveanu L, Kleijmeer M, Davoust J, van Endert P, Amigorena S. ER-phagosome fusion defines an MHC class I cross-presentation compartment in dendritic cells. *Nature* (2003) 425:397–402. doi:10.1038/nature01911
48. Houde M, Bertholet S, Gagnon E, Brunet S, Goyette G, Laplante A, et al. Phagosomes are competent organelles for antigen cross-presentation. *Nature* (2003) 425:402–6. doi:10.1038/nature01912
49. Ackerman AL, Giodini A, Cresswell P. A role for the endoplasmic reticulum protein retrotranslocation machinery during crosspresentation by dendritic cells. *Immunity* (2006) 25:607–17. doi:10.1016/j.immuni.2006.08.017
50. Pfeifer JD, Wick MJ, Roberts RL, Findlay K, Normark SJ, Harding CV. Phagocytic processing of bacterial antigens for class I MHC presentation to T cells. *Nature* (1993) 361:359–62. doi:10.1038/361359a0
51. Liu T, Chambers B, Diehl AD, van Kaer L, Jondal M, Ljunggren HG. TAP peptide transporter-independent presentation of heat-killed Sendai virus antigen on MHC class I molecules by splenic antigen-presenting cells. *J Immunol* (1997) 159:5364–71.
52. Campbell DJ, Serwold T, Shastri N. Bacterial proteins can be processed by macrophages in a transporter associated with antigen processing-independent, cysteine protease-dependent manner for presentation by MHC class I molecules. *J Immunol* (2000) 164:168–75. doi:10.4049/jimmunol.164.1.168
53. Bertholet S, Goldszmid R, Morrot A, Debrabant A, Afrin F, Collazo-Custodio C, et al. *Leishmania* antigens are presented to CD8+ T cells by a transporter associated with antigen processing-independent pathway in vitro and in vivo. *J Immunol* (2006) 177:3525–33. doi:10.4049/jimmunol.177.6.3525
54. Accapezzato D, Visco V, Francavilla V, Molette C, Donato T, Paroli M, et al. Chloroquine enhances human CD8+ T cell responses against soluble antigens in vivo. *J Exp Med* (2005) 202:817–28. doi:10.1084/jem.20051106
55. Samie M, Cresswell P. The transcription factor TFEB acts as a molecular switch that regulates exogenous antigen-presentation pathways. *Nat Immunol* (2015) 16:729–36. doi:10.1038/ni.3196

56. Chatterjee B, Smed-Sörensen A, Cohn L, Chalouni C, Vandlen R, Lee B-C, et al. Internalization and endosomal degradation of receptor-bound antigens regulate the efficiency of cross presentation by human dendritic cells. *Blood* (2012) 120:2011–20. doi:10.1182/blood-2012-01-402370
57. Alloatti A, Kotsias F, Pauwels A-M, Carpier J-M, Jouve M, Timmerman E, et al. Toll-like receptor 4 engagement on dendritic cells restrains phagolysosome fusion and promotes cross-presentation of antigens. *Immunity* (2015) 43:1087–100. doi:10.1016/j.immuni.2015.11.006
58. Eberl G, Widmann C, Corradin G. The functional half-life of H-2Kd-restricted T cell epitopes on living cells. *Eur J Immunol* (1996) 26:1993–9. doi:10.1002/eji.1830260904
59. Cella M, Engering A, Pinet V, Pieters J, Lanzavecchia A. Inflammatory stimuli induce accumulation of MHC class II complexes on dendritic cells. *Nature* (1997) 388:782–7. doi:10.1038/42030
60. Rescigno M, Citterio S, Thèry C, Rittig M, Medaglini D, Pozzi G, et al. Bacteria-induced neo-biosynthesis, stabilization, and surface expression of functional class I molecules in mouse dendritic cells. *Proc Natl Acad Sci U S A* (1998) 95:5229–34. doi:10.1073/pnas.95.9.5229
61. van Montfoort N, Camps MG, Khan S, Filippov DV, Weterings JJ, Griffith JM, et al. Antigen storage compartments in mature dendritic cells facilitate prolonged cytotoxic T lymphocyte cross-priming capacity. *Proc Natl Acad Sci U S A* (2009) 106:6730–5. doi:10.1073/pnas.0900969106
62. Faure F, Jouve M, Lebhar-Pequillet I, Sadaka C, Sepulveda F, Lantz O, et al. Blood monocytes sample MelanA/MART1 antigen for long-lasting cross-presentation to CD8+ T cells after differentiation into dendritic cells. *Int J Cancer* (2018) 142:133–44. doi:10.1002/ijc.31037
63. Delamarre L, Pack M, Chang H, Mellman I, Trombetta ES. Differential lysosomal proteolysis in antigen-presenting cells determines antigen fate. *Science* (2005) 307:1630–4. doi:10.1126/science.1108003
64. Lennon-Duménil A-M, Bakker AH, Maehr R, Fiebiger E, Overkleeft HS, Rosemblatt M, et al. Analysis of protease activity in live antigen-presenting cells shows regulation of the phagosomal proteolytic contents during dendritic cell activation. *J Exp Med* (2002) 196:529–40. doi:10.1084/jem.20020327
65. Trombetta ES, Ebersold M, Garrett W, Pypaert M, Mellman I. Activation of lysosomal function during dendritic cell maturation. *Science* (2003) 299:1400–3. doi:10.1126/science.1080106
66. Mantegazza AR, Savina A, Vermeulen M, Pérez L, Geffner J, Hermine O, et al. NADPH oxidase controls phagosomal pH and antigen cross-presentation in human dendritic cells. *Blood* (2008) 112:4712–22. doi:10.1182/blood-2008-01-134791
67. Jancic C, Savina A, Wasmeier C, Tolmachova T, El-Benna J, Dang PM-C, et al. Rab27a regulates phagosomal pH and NADPH oxidase recruitment to dendritic cell phagosomes. *Nat Cell Biol* (2007) 9:367–78. doi:10.1038/ncb1552
68. Burgdorf S, Kautz A, Böhnert V, Knolle PA, Kurts C. Distinct pathways of antigen uptake and intracellular routing in CD4 and CD8 T cell activation. *Science* (2007) 316:612–6. doi:10.1126/science.1137971
69. Segura E, Albiston AL, Wicks IP, Chai SY, Villadangos JA. Different cross-presentation pathways in steady-state and inflammatory dendritic cells. *Proc Natl Acad Sci U S A* (2009) 106:20377–81. doi:10.1073/pnas.0910295106
70. Burgdorf S, Schuette V, Semmling V, Hochheiser K, Lukacs-Kornek V, Knolle PA, et al. Steady-state cross-presentation of OVA is mannose receptor-dependent but inhibitable by collagen fragments. *Proc Natl Acad Sci U S A* (2010) 107:E48–9. doi:10.1073/pnas.1000598107
71. Schuette V, Embgenbroich M, Ulas T, Welz M, Schulte-Schrepping J, Draffehn AM, et al. Mannose receptor induces T-cell tolerance via inhibition of CD45 and up-regulation of CTLA-4. *Proc Natl Acad Sci U S A* (2016) 113:10649–54. doi:10.1073/pnas.1605885113
72. Tacken PJ, de Vries I, Jolanda M, Gijzen K, Joosten B, Wu D, et al. Effective induction of naive and recall T-cell responses by targeting antigen to human dendritic cells via a humanized anti-DC-SIGN antibody. *Blood* (2005) 106:1278–85. doi:10.1182/blood-2005-01-0318
73. Tacken PJ, Ginter W, Berod L, Cruz LJ, Joosten B, Sparwasser T, et al. Targeting DC-SIGN via its neck region leads to prolonged antigen residence in early endosomes, delayed lysosomal degradation, and cross-presentation. *Blood* (2011) 118:4111–9. doi:10.1182/blood-2011-04-346957
74. Hornung V, Bauernfeind F, Halle A, Samstad EO, Kono H, Rock KL, et al. Silica crystals and aluminum salts activate the NALP3 inflammasome through phagosomal destabilization. *Nat Immunol* (2008) 9:847–56. doi:10.1038/ni.1631
75. Próchnicki T, Mangan MS, Latz E. Recent insights into the molecular mechanisms of the NLRP3 inflammasome activation. *F1000Res* (2016) 5:1–15. doi:10.12688/f1000research.8614.1
76. Giodini A, Cresswell P. Hsp90-mediated cytosolic refolding of exogenous proteins internalized by dendritic cells. *EMBO J* (2008) 27:201–11. doi:10.1038/sj.emboj.7601941
77. Singh R, Cresswell P. Defective cross-presentation of viral antigens in GILT-free mice. *Science* (2010) 328:1394–8. doi:10.1126/science.1189176
78. Koopmann JO, Albring J, Hüter E, Bulbuc N, Spee P, Neefjes J, et al. Export of antigenic peptides from the endoplasmic reticulum intersects with retrograde protein translocation through the Sec61p channel. *Immunity* (2000) 13:117–27. doi:10.1016/S1074-7613(00)00013-3
79. Imai J, Hasegawa H, Maruya M, Koyasu S, Yahara I. Exogenous antigens are processed through the endoplasmic reticulum-associated degradation (ERAD) in cross-presentation by dendritic cells. *Int Immunol* (2005) 17:45–53. doi:10.1093/intimm/dxh184
80. Zehner M, Chasan AI, Schuette V, Embgenbroich M, Quast T, Kolanus W, et al. Mannose receptor polyubiquitination regulates endosomal recruitment of p97 and cytosolic antigen translocation for cross-presentation. *Proc Natl Acad Sci U S A* (2011) 108:9933–8. doi:10.1073/pnas.1102397108
81. Ménager J, Ebstein F, Oger R, Hulin P, Nedellec S, Duverger E, et al. Cross-presentation of synthetic long peptides by human dendritic cells: a process dependent on ERAD component p97/VCP but Not sec61 and/or Derlin-1. *PLoS One* (2014) 9:e89897. doi:10.1371/journal.pone.0089897
82. Zehner M, Marschall AL, Bos E, Schloetel J-G, Kreer C, Fehrenschild D, et al. The translocon protein Sec61 mediates antigen transport from endosomes in the cytosol for cross-presentation to CD8(+) T cells. *Immunity* (2015) 42:850–63. doi:10.1016/j.immuni.2015.04.008
83. Wiertz EJ, Tortorella D, Bogyo M, Yu J, Mothes W, Jones TR, et al. Sec61-mediated transfer of a membrane protein from the endoplasmic reticulum to the proteasome for destruction. *Nature* (1996) 384:432–8. doi:10.1038/384432a0
84. Meli G, Lecci A, Manca A, Krako N, Albertini V, Benussi L, et al. Conformational targeting of intracellular Aβ oligomers demonstrates their pathological oligomerization inside the endoplasmic reticulum. *Nat Commun* (2014) 5:3867. doi:10.1038/ncomms4867
85. Grotzke JE, Kozik P, Morel J-D, Impens F, Pietrosemoli N, Cresswell P, et al. Sec61 blockade by mycolactone inhibits antigen cross-presentation independently of endosome-to-cytosol export. *Proc Natl Acad Sci U S A* (2017) 114:E5910–9. doi:10.1073/pnas.1705242114
86. Hall BS, Hill K, McKenna M, Ogbechi J, High S, Willis AE, et al. The pathogenic mechanism of the *Mycobacterium ulcerans* virulence factor, mycolactone, depends on blockade of protein translocation into the ER. *PLoS Pathog* (2014) 10:e1004061. doi:10.1371/journal.ppat.1004061
87. McKenna M, Simmonds RE, High S. Mechanistic insights into the inhibition of Sec61-dependent co- and post-translational translocation by mycolactone. *J Cell Sci* (2016) 129:1404–15. doi:10.1242/jcs.182352
88. Wirth A, Jung M, Bies C, Frien M, Tyedmers J, Zimmermann R, et al. The Sec61p complex is a dynamic precursor activated channel. *Mol Cell* (2003) 12:261–8. doi:10.1016/S1097-2765(03)00283-1
89. Dingjan I, Verboogen DR, Paardekooper LM, Revelo NH, Sittig SP, Visser LJ, et al. Lipid peroxidation causes endosomal antigen release for cross-presentation. *Sci Rep* (2016) 6:22064. doi:10.1038/srep22064
90. Burgdorf S, Schölz C, Kautz A, Tampé R, Kurts C. Spatial and mechanistic separation of cross-presentation and endogenous antigen presentation. *Nat Immunol* (2008) 9:558–66. doi:10.1038/ni.1601
91. Saveanu L, Carroll O, Weimershaus M, Guermonprez P, Firat E, Lindo V, et al. IRAP identifies an endosomal compartment required for MHC class I cross-presentation. *Science* (2009) 325:213–7. doi:10.1126/science.1172845
92. Firat E, Saveanu L, Aichele P, Staeheli P, Huai J, Gaedicke S, et al. The role of endoplasmic reticulum-associated aminopeptidase 1 in immunity to infection and in cross-presentation. *J Immunol* (2007) 178:2241–8. doi:10.4049/jimmunol.178.4.2241
93. Lawand M, Abramova A, Manceau V, Springer S, van Endert P. TAP-dependent and -independent peptide import into dendritic cell phagosomes. *J Immunol* (2016) 197:3454–63. doi:10.4049/jimmunol.1501925

94. Nair-Gupta P, Baccarini A, Tung N, Seyffer F, Florey O, Huang Y, et al. TLR signals induce phagosomal MHC-I delivery from the endosomal recycling compartment to allow cross-presentation. *Cell* (2014) 158:506–21. doi:10.1016/j.cell.2014.04.054
95. Ma W, Zhang Y, Vigneron N, Stroobant V, Thielemans K, van der Bruggen P, et al. Long-peptide cross-presentation by human dendritic cells occurs in vacuoles by peptide exchange on nascent MHC class I molecules. *J Immunol* (2016) 196:1711–20. doi:10.4049/jimmunol.1501574
96. Eden ER. The formation and function of ER-endosome membrane contact sites. *Biochim Biophys Acta* (2016) 1861:874–9. doi:10.1016/j.bbalip.2016.01.020
97. Cebrian I, Visentin G, Blanchard N, Jouve M, Bobard A, Moita C, et al. Sec22b regulates phagosomal maturation and antigen crosspresentation by dendritic cells. *Cell* (2011) 147:1355–68. doi:10.1016/j.cell.2011.11.021
98. Wu SJ, Niknafs YS, Kim SH, Oravecz-Wilson K, Zajac C, Toubai T, et al. A critical analysis of the role of SNARE protein SEC22B in antigen cross-presentation. *Cell Rep* (2017) 19:2645–56. doi:10.1016/j.celrep.2017.06.013
99. Alloatti A, Rookhuizen DC, Joannas L, Carpier J-M, Iborra S, Magalhaes JG, et al. Critical role for Sec22b-dependent antigen cross-presentation in antitumor immunity. *J Exp Med* (2017) 214:2231–41. doi:10.1084/jem.20170229
100. Montealegre S, van Endert P. MHC class I cross-presentation: stage lights on Sec22b. *Trends Immunol* (2017) 38:618–21. doi:10.1016/j.it.2017.07.002
101. Zehner M, Rauen J, Chasan AI, Embgenbroich M, Camps MG, Kaden S, et al. Intraendosomal flow cytometry: a novel approach to analyze the protein composition of antigen-loaded endosomes. *Eur J Immunol* (2012) 42:2187–90. doi:10.1002/eji.201142089
102. Latz E, Schoenemeyer A, Visintin A, Fitzgerald KA, Monks BG, Knetter CF, et al. TLR9 signals after translocating from the ER to CpG DNA in the lysosome. *Nat Immunol* (2004) 5:190–8. doi:10.1038/ni1028
103. Kagan JC, Su T, Horng T, Chow A, Akira S, Medzhitov R. TRAM couples endocytosis of toll-like receptor 4 to the induction of interferon-beta. *Nat Immunol* (2008) 9:361–8. doi:10.1038/ni1569
104. Kim Y-M, Brinkmann MM, Paquet M-E, Ploegh HL. UNC93B1 delivers nucleotide-sensing toll-like receptors to endolysosomes. *Nature* (2008) 452:234–8. doi:10.1038/nature06726
105. Tabeta K, Hoebe K, Janssen EM, Du X, Georgel P, Crozat K, et al. The Unc93b1 mutation 3d disrupts exogenous antigen presentation and signaling via toll-like receptors 3, 7 and 9. *Nat Immunol* (2006) 7:156–64. doi:10.1038/ni1297
106. Deguine J, Lee BL, Newman ZR, Barton GM. No antigen-presentation defect in Unc93b1(3d/3d) (3d) mice. *Nat Immunol* (2013) 14:1101–2. doi:10.1038/ni.2733
107. Maschalidi S, Nunes-Hasler P, Nascimento CR, Sallent I, Lannoy V, Garfa-Traore M, et al. UNC93B1 interacts with the calcium sensor STIM1 for efficient antigen cross-presentation in dendritic cells. *Nat Commun* (2017) 8:1640. doi:10.1038/s41467-017-01601-5
108. Nunes-Hasler P, Maschalidi S, Lippens C, Castelbou C, Bouvet S, Guido D, et al. STIM1 promotes migration, phagosomal maturation and antigen cross-presentation in dendritic cells. *Nat Commun* (2017) 8:1852. doi:10.1038/s41467-017-01600-6
109. Gil-Torregrosa BC, Lennon-Duménil AM, Kessler B, Guermonprez P, Ploegh HL, Fruci D, et al. Control of cross-presentation during dendritic cell maturation. *Eur J Immunol* (2004) 34:398–407. doi:10.1002/eji.200324508
110. Neijssen J, Herberts C, Drijfhout JW, Reits E, Janssen L, Neefjes J. Cross-presentation by intercellular peptide transfer through gap junctions. *Nature* (2005) 434:83–8. doi:10.1038/nature03290
111. Mendoza-Naranjo A, Saéz PJ, Johansson CC, Ramírez M, Mandakovic D, Pereda C, et al. Functional gap junctions facilitate melanoma antigen transfer and cross-presentation between human dendritic cells. *J Immunol* (2007) 178:6949–57. doi:10.4049/jimmunol.178.11.6949
112. Saccheri F, Pozzi C, Avogadri F, Barozzi S, Faretta M, Fusi P, et al. Bacteria-induced gap junctions in tumors favor antigen cross-presentation and antitumor immunity. *Sci Transl Med* (2010) 2:44ra57. doi:10.1126/scitranslmed.3000739
113. Reits E, Griekspoor A, Neijssen J, Groothuis T, Jalink K, van Veelen P, et al. Peptide diffusion, protection, and degradation in nuclear and cytoplas mic compartments before antigen presentation by MHC class I. *Immunity* (2003) 18:97–108. doi:10.1016/S1074-7613(02)00511-3
114. Dolan BP, Gibbs KD, Ostrand-Rosenberg S. Dendritic cells cross-dressed with peptide MHC class I complexes prime CD8+ T cells. *J Immunol* (2006) 177:6018–24. doi:10.4049/jimmunol.177.9.6018
115. Smyth LA, Harker N, Turnbull W, El-Doueik H, Klavinskis L, Kioussis D, et al. The relative efficiency of acquisition of MHC:peptide complexes and cross-presentation depends on dendritic cell type. *J Immunol* (2008) 181:3212–20. doi:10.4049/jimmunol.181.5.3212
116. Wakim LM, Bevan MJ. Cross-dressed dendritic cells drive memory CD8+ T-cell activation after viral infection. *Nature* (2011) 471:629–32. doi:10.1038/nature09863

17

The Nontoxic Cholera B Subunit is a Potent Adjuvant for Intradermal DC-Targeted Vaccination

Laura Antonio-Herrera[1,2]*, Oscar Badillo-Godinez*[3]*, Oscar Medina-Contreras*[4]*, Araceli Tepale-Segura*[1]*, Alberto García-Lozano*[1]*, Lourdes Gutierrez-Xicotencatl*[3]*, Gloria Soldevila*[5]*, Fernando R. Esquivel-Guadarrama*[6]*, Juliana Idoyaga*[7*] *and Laura C. Bonifaz*[1*]

[1] *Hospital de Especialidades, Centro Médico Nacional Siglo XXI, Instituto Mexicano del Seguro Social, Unidad de Investigación Médica en Inmunoquímica, Mexico City, Mexico,* [2] *Universidad Nacional Autónoma de México, Mexico City, Mexico,* [3] *Centro de Investigación Sobre Enfermedades Infecciosas, Instituto Nacional de Salud Pública, SS, Cuernavaca, Mexico,* [4] *Immunology and Proteomics Laboratory, Mexico Children's Hospital "Federico Gómez", Mexico City, Mexico,* [5] *Departamento de Inmunología, Instituto de Investigaciones Biomédicas, Universidad Nacional Autónoma de México, Mexico City, Mexico,* [6] *Laboratorio de Inmunología Viral, Facultad de Medicina, UAEM, Cuernavaca, Mexico,* [7] *Department of Microbiology and Immunology, Stanford University School of Medicine, Stanford, CA, United States*

***Correspondence:**
Juliana Idoyaga
jidoyaga@stanford.edu
Laura C. Bonifaz
labonifaz@yahoo.com

$CD4^+$ T cells are major players in the immune response against several diseases; including AIDS, leishmaniasis, tuberculosis, influenza and cancer. Their activation has been successfully achieved by administering antigen coupled with antibodies, against DC-specific receptors in combination with adjuvants. Unfortunately, most of the adjuvants used so far in experimental models are unsuitable for human use. Therefore, human DC-targeted vaccination awaits the description of potent, yet nontoxic adjuvants. The nontoxic cholera B subunit (CTB) can be safely used in humans and it has the potential to activate $CD4^+$ T cell responses. However, it remains unclear whether CTB can promote DC activation and can act as an adjuvant for DC-targeted antigens. Here, we evaluated the CTB's capacity to activate DCs and $CD4^+$ T cell responses, and to generate long-lasting protective immunity. Intradermal (i.d.) administration of CTB promoted late and prolonged activation and accumulation of skin and lymphoid-resident DCs. When CTB was co-administered with anti-DEC205-OVA, it promoted $CD4^+$ T cell expansion, differentiation, and infiltration to peripheral nonlymphoid tissues, i.e., the skin, lungs and intestine. Indeed, CTB promoted a polyfunctional $CD4^+$ T cell response, including the priming of Th1 and Th17 cells, as well as resident memory T (RM) cell differentiation in peripheral nonlymphoid tissues. It is worth noting that CTB together with a DC-targeted antigen promoted local and systemic protection against experimental melanoma and murine rotavirus. We conclude that CTB administered i.d. can be used as an adjuvant to DC-targeted antigens for the induction of broad $CD4^+$ T cell responses as well as for promoting long-lasting protective immunity.

Keywords: anti-DEC205, CTB, adjuvant, skin, memory, T cells, dendritic cells

INTRODUCTION

Formulation of successful subunit vaccines requires the optimal combination of antigen and adjuvant to ensure the development of long-lasting protective immunity. Expected responses should include the development of memory $CD4^+$ T cells, which play a major role in protecting against a myriad of pathogens (1–3) and against tumors (4, 5). To achieve this goal, delivering antigens via monoclonal antibodies (mAbs) targeting DCs, in combination with strong adjuvants, is one of the most promising strategies.

The administration of anti-DEC205-antigen mAbs can increase the efficiency of MHC-II antigen presentation relative to soluble antigen by 300-fold (4, 6). In combination with strong adjuvants, e.g., Poly IC, anti-CD40 mAbs, CpG, and flagellin (4, 7–9), it induces T helper (Th) cell differentiation and it mediates long-lasting immunity against experimental melanoma, malaria and influenza (4, 7, 10, 11). Moreover, DC-targeted vaccination can induce polyfunctional memory $CD4^+$ T cells that produce IFNγ, TNFα and IL-2 (7, 9). Therefore, DC-targeted vaccination serves as a powerful strategy to promote protective $CD4^+$ T cell responses.

Unfortunately, due to their toxicity, the adjuvants mentioned above are not approved for human use. Only synthetic derivatives, such as AS04 and phosphorothioate-backbone CpG adjuvants are undergoing trials with humans (12). However, these synthetic derivatives have shown adverse effects in murine models including splenomegaly, lymphoid follicle destruction and immunosuppression (12), which make them less promising for human use. Therefore, there is a need to identify adjuvants, which can be co-administered with DC-targeted antigens, for the induction of protective $CD4^+$ T cell responses in humans.

CTB has been proven to be safe for human use as an adjuvant (13–15). Its use has been approved for the killed whole-cell monovalent vaccine (WC-rBS) against cholera in humans, which has only induced mild adverse effects in a few individuals, and it has been safe for and well-tolerated by immunocompromized subjects (16). Unfortunately, the capacity of CTB to activate DCs is controversial. Some *in vitro* studies using bone marrow-derived DCs (BMDCs) and macrophages (BMDM) show that CTB can promote expression of TLRs, CD86 and production of IL-5, IL-12p70, IL-6, IL-10, IL-3, G-CSF, MIP-2 and eotaxin, as well as it can activate the NFkB pathway (17, 18). In contrast, other studies suggest that CTB does not induce the activation of *ex vivo* DCs (19–21). Therefore, it is necessary to evaluate the capacity of CTB to activate DCs *in vivo*.

Still, several reports have shown that CTB can be used as a strong adjuvant. When admixed or conjugated with pathogen derived antigens, it can promote the generation of long-lived $CD4^+$ T cells. Such responses mediate systemic immunity against several pathogens, including the influenza virus (22), *Helicobacter pylori* (23), *Streptococcus pneumoniae* (24), *Bordetella pertussis* (25), and *Francisella tularensis* (26). Furthermore, we have previously demonstrated that i.d. administration of soluble antigens in combination with CTB promotes $CD4^+$ T cell activation and differentiation of Th1 and Th17 cells (27). However, CTB adjuvant's capacity has never been tested with DC-targeted antigens administered i.d. Here, we asked whether CTB co-administration with anti-DEC205-antigen mAbs could induce DC activation and consequently promote long-lasting and protective $CD4^+$ T cell responses.

Abbreviations: CTB, cholera B subunit; i.d., intradermal; i.v., intravenous; s.c., subcutaneous; DC, dendritic cell; Ab, antibody; mAb, monoclonal antibody; SDLN, skin draining lymph node; T RM, resident memory T cell; T CM, central memory T cell; T EM, effector memory T cell.

MATERIALS AND METHODS

Mice

WT C57BL/6 mice and transgenic mice expressing green fluorescent protein (GFP) under the major histocompatibility complex class II molecule promoter were obtained from Unidad de Medicina Experimental, UNAM animal facility. BALB/c mice were obtained from INSP, SS animal facility. OT-II CD45.1 mice were obtained from Instituto de Investigaciones Biomédicas, UNAM animal facility. All animal experiments were performed following the Institutional Ethics Committee and the Mexican national regulations on animal care and experimentation. Experiments with DO11.10 $Thy1.1^+$ mice were performed at the Department of Microbiology and Immunology of the School of Medicine, at Stanford University, following institutional guidelines. Mice were sex (male or female)- and age (7–10 weeks)-matched.

$CD4^+$ T Cell Enrichment

Skin-draining lymph nodes (SDLN), spleen, and mesenteric lymph nodes were collected from OT-II $CD45.1^+$ or DO11 $Thy1.1^+$ mice, placed in RPMI medium (Gibco) supplemented with 5% fetal bovine serum (FBS) (HyClone), 300 μg/mL glutamine (Gibco) and 100 U/mL penicillin/100 μg/mL streptomycin (Biowest), and mashed separately to obtain cell suspensions. Red blood cells were lysed with RBC lysis buffer (Biolegend). Both LN and spleen suspensions were incubated for 30 min on ice with homemade rat hybridoma supernatants against CD8 (2.43), B cells (B220), MHCII-expressing cells (TIB120), and macrophages (F4/80). Next, cells were washed, suspended in supplemented RPMI and poured into petri dishes previously coated with rat anti-IgG (ThermoFisher) for 40 min at 4°C. Non-adherent cells were recovered, washed and suspended in PBS for injection through the retro orbital vein.

Cell Transfer and Immunization

Congenic mice received 4.5–5 × 10^6 $CD4^+$ T cells intravenously (i.v.). After 24 h, anesthetized mice were immunized i.d. in both ears (or in the right flank for melanoma and viral challenge experiments) with 1 μg of anti-DEC205-OVA (containing ~0.5 μg of OVA protein), 1 μg of a control mAb-OVA without receptor affinity or 3–30 μg of soluble unconjugated OVA in the presence or absence of 10 μg of CTB (Sigma-Aldrich). For proliferation experiments mice received 4.5–5 × 10^6 CFSE-labeled $CD4^+$ T cells 24 h before i.d. administration of 1 μg of anti-DEC205-OVA or 1, 3, or 10 μg of soluble unconjugated OVA. For prime/boost experiments, mice were immunized i.d. in both ears with 1 μg of anti-DEC205-OVA or 3 μg of soluble unconjugated OVA plus 10 μg of CTB. After 15 days, mice received i.p. 1 μg of anti-DEC205-OVA or 3 μg of soluble unconjugated OVA.

Tissue Processing

At 3 or 7 days post-immunization, mice were sacrificed to collect SDLN and skin. SDLN were enzymatically digested with 0.25 mg/mL Liberase TL (Roche) and 0.125 mg/mL DNAse (Roche) for 25 min at 37°C. Skin cell suspensions were also obtained by enzymatic digestion with 0.25 mg/mL Liberase TL and 0.125 mg/mL DNAse for 45 min at 37°C, then chopped with scissors and incubated under the same conditions with constant shaking. Next, enzymatic digestion was stopped by adding 0.5 μM EDTA, and cell suspensions were filtered through a 70 μm strainer (Corning), followed by the addition of 0.125 mg/mL DNAse. Finally, cells were washed, counted, stained and/or re-stimulated as needed.

To obtain cells from the lungs, mice were sacrificed 7 days post-immunization. Lungs were rinsed with water to remove excess blood, placed into polypropylene tubes and chopped into small pieces to digest with 0.25 mg/mL Liberase TL (Roche) and 0.125 mg/mL DNAse (Roche) for 1 h at 37°C with constant shaking. Next, enzymatic digestion was stopped by adding 0.5 μM EDTA, and cell suspensions were filtered through a 70 μm strainer (Corning), followed by the addition of 0.125 mg/mL DNAse. Next, cells were lysed with the RBC lysis buffer (Biolegend). Finally, cells were washed, counted and stained.

Isolation of intestinal cells was performed as previously described elsewhere (28). Briefly: intestines were removed and carefully cleaned off their mesentery lymph nodes and Peyer's patches were excised. Intestines were opened longitudinally, washed off fecal contents, cut into pieces 0.5 cm in length, and subjected to two sequential 20-min incubations in HBSS with 5% FCS and 2 mM EDTA at 37°C with agitation to remove epithelial cells. After each incubation step, media containing epithelial cells and debris were discarded. The remaining tissue was minced and incubated for 20 min in HBSS with 5% FCS, 1 mg/ml collagenase IV and 40 U/ml DNase I at 37°C in agitation. Cell suspensions were collected and passed through a 100-μm strainer and pelleted by centrifugation at 300 g. Cells were counted and divided for *in vitro* re-stimulation and cell surface staining.

In vitro Re-stimulation

Cells were resuspended in RPMI medium supplemented with 10% FBS, 300 μg/mL glutamine, 100 U/mL penicillin/100 μg/mL streptomycin, 110 μg/mL sodium pyruvate and 10 μM β-mercaptoethanol. SDLN cells were incubated for 48 h with OVA peptide 323–339 (in vivogen), followed by cell stimulation cocktail plus protein transport inhibitor, added according to the manufacturer's instructions (eBioscience), and cells were incubated for an additional 4 h at 37°C. Cells from the skin and intestine were only re-stimulated with cell cocktail stimulation plus protein transport inhibitor for 4 h without OVA.

Flow Cytometry

To allow for counting, cells were stained with anti-CD45-PECy7 (Biolegend) and DAPI (ThermoFisher), immediately mixed with CountBright absolute counting beads (ThermoFisher), acquired for flow cytometry. Cell surface staining was performed first by blocking Fc receptors (supernatant of 2.4G2 hybridoma against CD16/32) and then by staining using the following antibodies: anti-CD45-APC (Biolegend) or -PECy7 (Biolegend), anti-CD4-APC-Cy7 (Biolegend), anti-TCRVβ5.1, 5.2-PECy7 (Biolegend) or anti-Vα2-FITC (eBioscience), anti-CD45.2-Percp-Cy5.5 (Biolegend) or anti-CD45.1-Percp-Cy5.5 (Biolegend), anti-CD69-PE (ebioscience), and anti-CCR7-FITC (Biolegend). LIVE/DEAD Fixable Aqua (Thermofisher) staining was included. For DC analysis the following Abs were used: anti-CD45-APC (Biolegend), anti-Ter119-Percp-Cy5.5, anti-CD3-Percp-Cy5.5, anti-CD19-PercpCy5.5, anti-CD44b-Percp-Cy5.5, anti-MHCII-FITC (Biologend), and CD86-PE (eBioscience). To achieve intracellular staining, cell surface staining was first performed, followed by fixation and permeabilization using the intracellular fixation and permeabilization buffer set (Thermofisher), according to the manufacturer's instructions. To stain cytokine and transcription factors, the True-Nuclear transcription factor buffer set (Biolegend) was used according to the manufacturer's instructions. Intracellular staining included anti-IL-17-PE (BD Bioscience), anti-IFNγ-APC (Biolegend), anti-T-bet-BV421 (BD Biosciences), or anti-RORγT-APC (Thermofisher). Cells were acquired in a BD FACSCanto II or BD LSRFortessa cytometer (Becton, Dickinson and company). Data were analyzed with FlowJo software (Tree Star, Inc.).

Melanoma Challenge

Mice were transferred with OT-II CD45.1$^+$ cells 24 h before i.d. immunization with 1 μg of anti-DEC205-OVA or with 3 μg of soluble untargeted OVA ± 10 μg of CTB. After 30 days, mice received 2.5 × 10^5 MO4 cells subcutaneously (s.c.) in the right flank and then they were monitored for 21 days for survival. Alternatively, C57BL/6 naive mice were challenged i.v. in the tail vein 30 days after immunization to induce metastatic nodules in the lungs. For some experiments, anti-DEC205-OVA-vaccinated mice received i.p. 250 μg of anti-CD4 Ab (GK1.5, in house) or isotype control Ab (eBRG1, in house) as follows: 1 day before MO4 inoculation, on the day of MO4 inoculation and every 3 days after MO4 inoculation, up to day 12. Sixteen days after MO4 inoculation, mice were sacrificed and lungs were harvested for metastatic nodule count as described elsewhere (29). Briefly: lungs were rinsed with water to remove excess blood and bleached with Feket's solution, and metastatic nodules were counted under a stereoscope (Leica Microsystems). Uncountable nodules were reported as >250.

Viral Challenge

BALB/c mice were immunized i.d. in the right flank with 23 μg of anti-DEC205-VP6 (corresponding to 1.5 μg of VP6) or with 3 μg of *in vitro* synthetized soluble untargeted VP6 (produced from the murine rotavirus Ew *in vitro* with the Rapid Translation System, Roche), in the presence of 10 μg of CTB. After 20 days, mice were orally challenged with 1 × 10^4 focus forming units of murine RV EDIM$_{WT}$ as described elsewhere (30). For prime/boost experiments, mice were i.d. immunized with anti-DEC205-VP6 or 3 μg of VP6 plus 10 μg of CTB and, after 15 days, mice received i.p. anti-DEC205-VP6 or VP6 (same dose as before). For CD4$^+$ T cell depletion experiments, mice immunized with anti-DEC205-VP6 received either 250 μg of anti-CD4 Ab (GK1.5, in house) or isotype control Ab (eBRG1, in house) as follows: 3 days before the viral challenge, on the day of the challenge and 3 days after the challenge. Seven days after boost, mice were orally challenged with 1×10^4 focus forming units of murine RV $EDIM_{WT}$. Stool samples were collected daily for 8 days and kept at −20°C for further analysis of viral load by sandwich ELISA. Protection against infection was calculated as % protection = 100% − [area under the curve of the experimental group (Absorbance at 405 nm)/area under the curve of the control group (Absorbance at 405 nm)] × 100%. This represents a decrease in the quantity of rotavirus antigen shed after immunization, relative to control mice, during the 8 days after the challenge.

ELISA

Viral load in the stool was determined by sandwich ELISA, as described elsewhere (30). Briefly: diluted stool samples were poured into 96-well plates (Costar) previously coated with a goat polyclonal antibody (Ab) against different strains of RV (in house). After 2 h at 37°C, plates were washed, and a rabbit polyclonal Ab against RV RRV was added. After 1 h at 37°C, plates were washed and a PA-conjugated goat anti-rabbit IgG (Zymed) was added, which was incubated for 1 h at 37°C. Finally, after washing, the substrate (*p*-nitrophenyl phosphate, disodium; Sigma) was added, and plates were developed for 30–45 min at 37°C. The absorbance at 405 nm was read with a 96-well plate reader (BIO-TEK Instruments, Burlington, VT).

DC Activation

GFP-MHC-II mice received 10 μg of CTB or PBS i.d. in the ear. After 12, 24 or 72 h, epidermal sheets were obtained, stained with anti-CD86-PE (eBioscience), mounted with VectaShield (Vector Laboratories) and sealed. The images were obtained with a Leica TCS SP8x Confocal Microscope (Wetzlar, Germany) and analyzed with Leica Application Suite Advanced Fluorescent Lite software (Leica Microsystems, Mannheim, Germany). Alternatively, C57BL/6 mice received 10 μg of CTB or PBS i.d. in the ear. After 24, 72 h, or 7 days, mice were sacrificed to collect SDLN and skin. Tissues were processed and stained to be analyzed by flow cytometry.

Statistics

Statistical analysis was performed using Prism 6.0 (GraphPad Software Inc., La Jolla, CA, USA). Statistical significance was calculated when comparing two groups, using unpaired two-tailed Student's *t*-test. For comparison of more than two groups, one-way or two-way ANOVA with Tukey's multiple comparison test was used. A *P*-value <0.05 was considered significant.

RESULTS

CTB Induces Late and Prolonged Activation and Accumulation of SDLN and Skin DCs

We first aimed to determine whether CTB could induce *in vivo* activation of DCs. To this end, epidermal sheets of GFP-MHC-II mice were obtained at 12, 24, or 72 h after i.d. administration of CTB; followed by staining with fluorescent Ab specific for CD86. Using confocal microscopy, we observed co-expression of CD86 by epidermal MHC-II$^+$ cells, only after 72 h, and at no earlier time (**Supplementary Figure 1**). Next, we characterized skin DCs as viable CD45$^+$Lineage$^-$CD11c$^+$MHC-II$^+$ cells by multiparametric flow cytometry (**Supplementary Figure 2A**). We confirmed that CTB induces *in vivo* activation of DCs after 72 h by overexpression of CD86 (**Figure 1A**) and, interestingly, their accumulation in the inoculation site as well. It was striking that both the activation and accumulation were sustained 7 days after the i.d. administration of CTB (**Figure 1A**).

Next, we asked whether CTB could induce accumulation of activated DCs in the SDLN. To answer this question, we analyzed SDLN cells by multiparametric flow cytometry, which allowed us to discriminate between migrating (CD11c$^+$MHC-II^{hi}) and resident (CD11c$^+$MHC-II^{low}) DCs (**Supplementary Figure 2B**). Seventy-two hours after its administration, CTB induced the accumulation of migratory DCs in the SDLN, which displayed an increased expression of CD86 compared to the PBS control (**Figure 1B**). The accumulation of migrating DCs with an activated phenotype dropped after 72 h. However, it was still higher than the PBS control after 7 days. Interestingly, CTB also induced an increased expression of CD86 on resident DCs as well as their accumulation after 7 days (**Figure 1C**). It is worth noting that the accumulation and activation of DCs took place only at the inoculation site and the draining lymph node, as we did not find either effect on a distal organ, i.e., the mesenteric lymph nodes (**Supplementary Figure 2C**).

As a whole, our results demonstrate that skin administration of CTB acts as a potent stimulus to induce late and prolonged accumulation and activation of lymphoid-resident and skin DCs.

CTB Co-administration With a DC-Targeted or Soluble Antigen Promotes Expansion and Differential Activation of CD4$^+$ T Cells

To study the development of antigen specific CD4$^+$ T cell responses we used a DC-targeted OVA antigen and, for comparison, soluble OVA antigen. After 3 days, we observed a 20-fold increase in the proliferation of CD4$^+$ T cells after the i.d. inoculation of 1 μg of anti-DEC205-OVA, compared to 10 μg of soluble OVA (**Supplementary Figure 3B**). Furthermore, cells undergoing the last rounds of proliferation showed downregulation of CD69, which was more pronounced in cells from anti-DEC205-OVA-inoculated mice (**Figure 2A**). CD69 is rapidly activated after TCR engagement, but it decreases as T cells divide (31, 32). Even so, similar numbers of OVA-specific CD4$^+$ T cells were found in the SDLN of mice administered with 3 μg of soluble OVA or with 1 μg of anti-DEC205-OVA (**Figure 2B**).

Next, we evaluated the outcome of CTB co-administration in T cell activation. Three days post-immunization, cells from mice administered with CTB plus a DC-targeted antigen remained low for CD69 expression; while a soluble antigen admixed with CTB resulted in higher expression of CD69 (**Figure 2C**). The

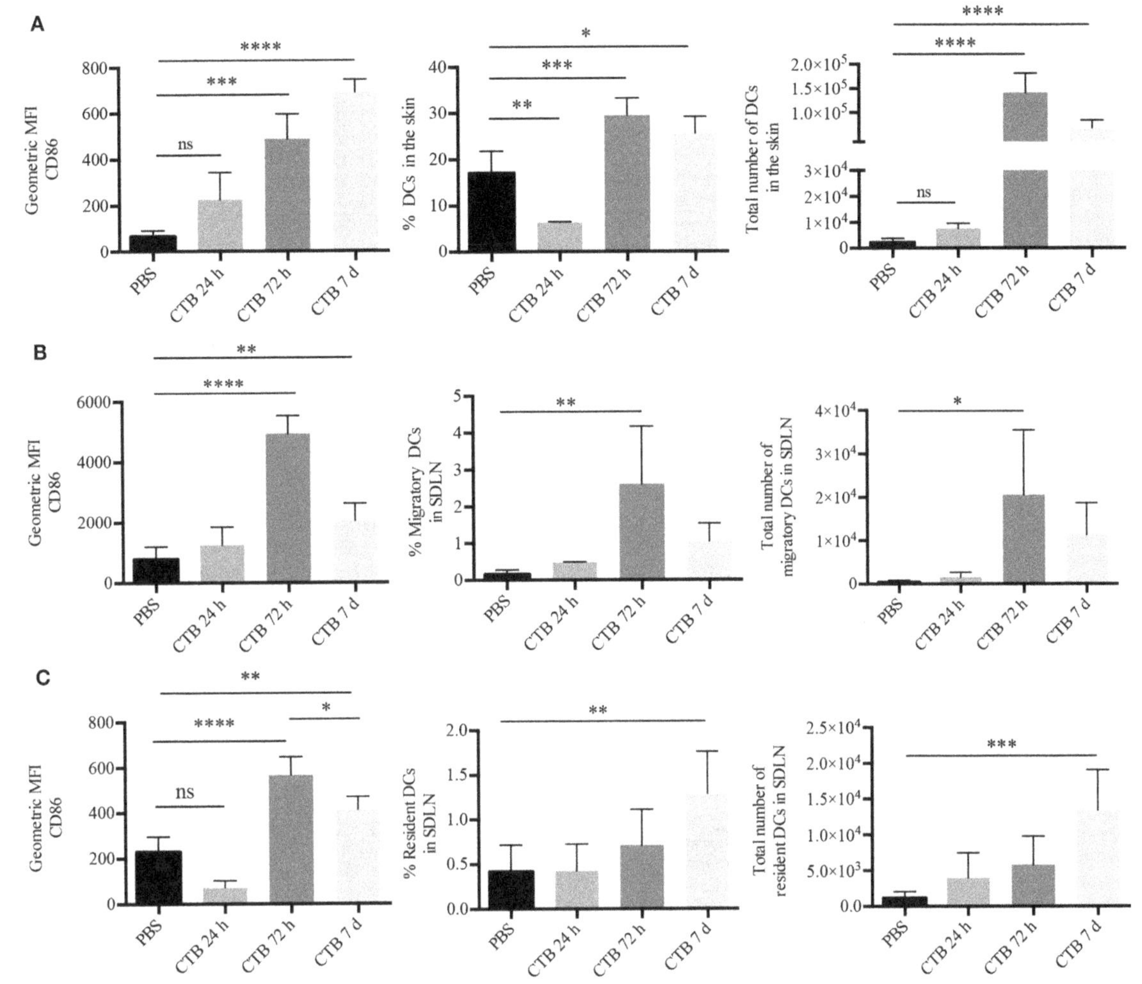

FIGURE 1 | Intradermal administration of CTB promotes recruitment and activation of DCs in the SDLN and the skin. C57BL6 mice received 10 μg of CTB or PBS i.d. in both ears, and they were sacrificed for skin and SDLN harvesting at the indicated times. **(A)** MHC-II$^+$CD11c$^+$ DCs were gated as in **Supplementary Figure 2A**. Graphs depicting the percentage, absolute cell numbers of DCs and geometric median fluorescence intensity (MFI) of CD86 on DCs in the skin. Mean ± SD, $N = 4$–6, data pooled from two independent experiments. One-way ANOVA with Tukey's multiple comparisons test (*$P < 0.05$, **$P < 0.005$, ***$P < 0.0005$, ****$P < 0.0001$). **(B)** Migratory and **(C)** resident DCs from the SDLN were gated as in **Supplementary Figure 2B**. Graphs of percentage, total numbers of DCs and geometric MFI of CD86 on DCs. Mean ± SD, $N = 4$–6, data pooled from two independent experiments. One-way ANOVA with Tukey's multiple comparisons test (*$P < 0.05$, **$P < 0.005$, ***$P < 0.0005$, ****$P < 0.0001$).

expression of CD69 promotes retention of T cells in the lymph node; while its deregulation allows cells to migrate to distal peripheral tissues (31, 32). Thus, similar to others (6, 33), our data suggest the possibility of systemic dissemination of CD4$^+$ T cells after DC-targeted antigen inoculation.

After 7 days, we observed a significant effect on T cell expansion, as CTB co-administered with a DC-targeted antigen promoted larger numbers of OVA-specific CD4$^+$ T cells (**Figure 2D**). This result was dependent on the antigen being targeted to DCs, since the administration of the isotype Ab conjugated with OVA, with or without CTB, did not promote expansion (**Figure 2D**; **Supplementary Figure 3B**). CTB co-administration with soluble OVA promoted larger accumulation of CD4$^+$ T cells in the SDLN as compared with the DC-targeted OVA group (**Figure 2D**), and it was consistent with a higher expression of CD69.

We next asked if CTB could promote the migration of antigen-specific CD4$^+$ T cells to the inoculation site. After 7 days of i.d. immunization, we observed a large infiltration of OT-II CD45.1$^+$ cells in the skin, which was promoted by the co-administration of CTB and not by the antigen alone (**Figure 2E**). Strikingly, higher numbers of OVA-specific T cells were observed in the skin of mice immunized with soluble OVA along with CTB compared to the DC-targeted vaccination group.

All together, these data demonstrate that CTB can be used as a strong adjuvant with a DC-targeted or soluble antigen to promote local expansion of antigen-specific CD4$^+$ T cells in the SDLN, and to induce their efficient migration to the inoculation site (i.e., skin). Remarkably, our data suggest that a DC-targeted

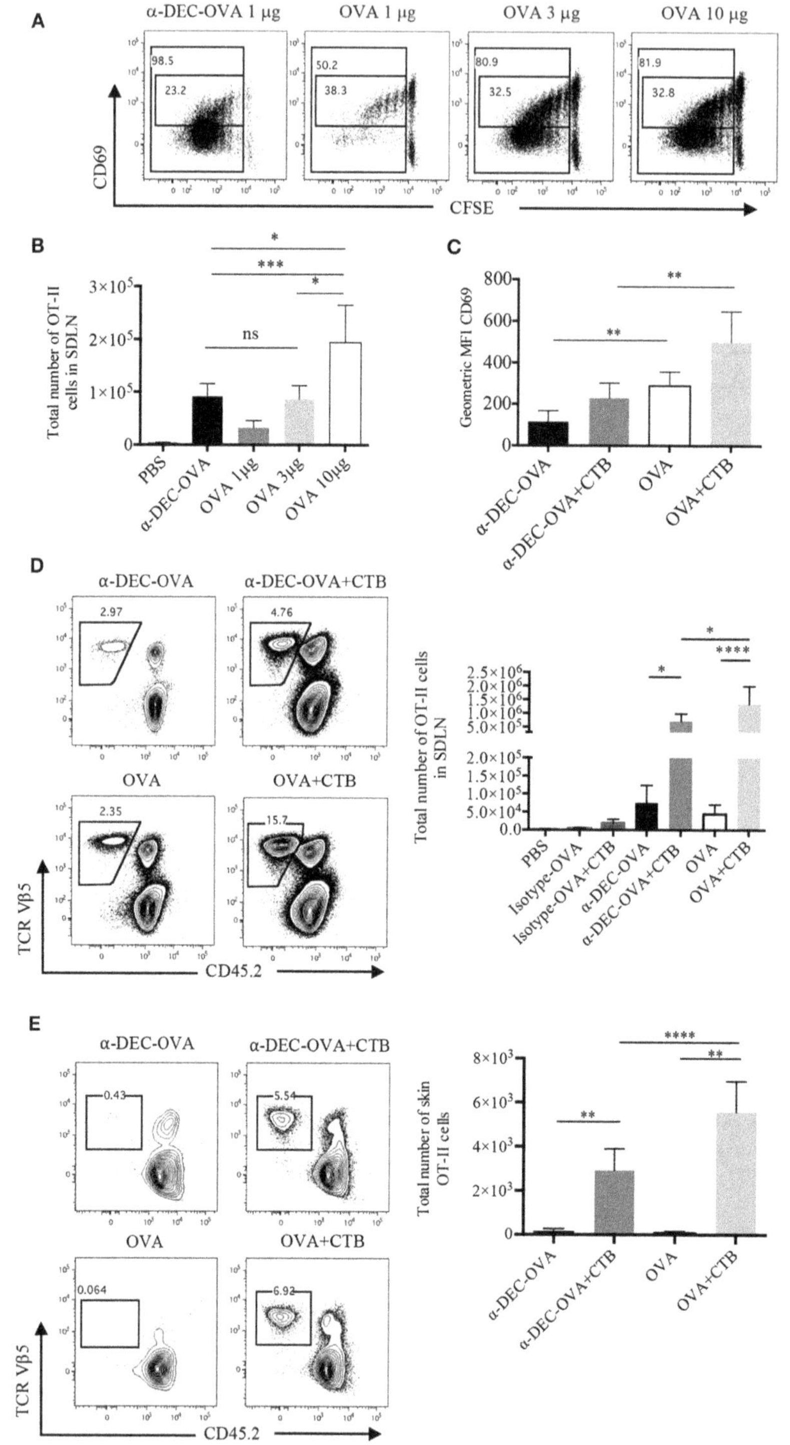

FIGURE 2 | CTB co-administration with a DC-targeted or soluble antigen promotes expansion and differential activation of CD4^{+} T cells. C57BL6 mice were adoptively transferred with OT-II CD45.1^{+} cells, 24 h later they were immunized i.d. in both ears, as indicated, and 3 or 7 days later, they were sacrificed for SDLN and skin harvesting. **(A)** Representative dot plot of CFSE dilution and CD69 expression by SDLN OT-II cells 3 days after inoculation of anti-DEC205-OVA or soluble OVA and **(B)** total numbers of OT-II cells. **(C)** Geometric median fluorescence intensity (MFI) of CD69 by OT-II cells 3 days after anti-DEC205-OVA or soluble OVA ± CTB's i.d. administration. Mean ± SD, $N = 4$–6, data pooled from four independent experiments. One-way ANOVA with Turkey's multiple comparisons test (ns, $P > 0.05$, $^{*}P < 0.05$, $^{**}P < 0.005$, $^{***}P < 0.0005$). **(D)** Representative dot plots and total number of SDLN OT-II cells 7 days after anti-DEC205-OVA or soluble OVA ± CTB's i.d. administration. Mean ± SD, $N = 5$–8 data pooled from four independent experiments. One-way ANOVA with Tukey's multiple comparisons test ($^{*}P < 0.05$, $^{****}P < 0.0001$). Transferred cells recovered from the SDLN were identified as viable CD4^{+}CD45.2^{-}TCRVβ 5.1, 5.2^{+} T cells (**Supplementary Figure 3A**). **(E)** Representative dot plot and total numbers of migrating OT-II cells identified as viable CD45^{+}CD4^{+}CD45.2^{-}TCRVβ 5.1, 5.2^{+} (**Supplementary Figure 3C**). Mean ± SD, $N = 4$–6, data pooled from four independent experiments. One-way ANOVA with Tukey's multiple comparisons test ($^{**}P < 0.005$, $^{****}P < 0.0001$).

antigen induces differential activation of CD4$^+$ T cells, which might impact their differentiation and, possibly, the differential anatomical localization of CD4$^+$ T cells after DC-targeted or soluble antigen immunization.

CTB Promotes a Combined Th1/Th17 Response When Co-administered With a DC-Targeted Antigen

We next asked whether CTB admixed with a DC-targeted antigen or a soluble antigen could promote the differentiation of CD4$^+$ T cells into Th1 or Th17 cells. At day 7 post-immunization, we observed antigen-specific IFNγ^+ cells in the SDLN, induced by the administration of CTB in combination with a DC-targeted antigen or a soluble antigen (**Supplementary Figure 4A; Figure 3A**). Remarkably, only DC-targeted vaccination promoted significant differentiation of IL-17$^+$ CD4$^+$ T cells (**Supplementary Figure 4A; Figure 3A**). These results were confirmed in the DO11.10 model (**Supplementary Figure 5A**), which is prone to Th2 and Treg responses. Moreover, IL-17$^+$ and IFNγ^+ cells expressed the transcription factors RORγt and T-bet, respectively (**Supplementary Figure 4A**). Thus, DC-targeted vaccination promoted a combined Th1/Th17 response in the SDLN, in contrast to soluble antigen, which induced mainly Th1 responses (**Figure 3B**).

We then analyzed skin-infiltrating T cells. Immunization with either DC-targeted OVA or soluble OVA together with CTB induced a similar percentage of Th1 CD4$^+$ T cells (**Figure 3C**). However, DC-targeted OVA + CTB induced a higher frequency of and absolute cell numbers of Th17, compared to soluble OVA + CTB (**Supplementary Figure 4B; Figure 3C**). Indeed, we confirmed that DC-targeted OVA + CTB promote a combined Th1/Th17 response in the skin, while immunization with the soluble OVA + CTB promotes a skewed Th1 response by calculating the Th1/Th17 ratio (**Figure 3D**). Similarly, we also observed great infiltration of Th17 cells and almost no Foxp3$^+$ regulatory T cell differentiation in the skin of BALB/c mice transferred with DO11.10 cells after DC-targeted OVA + CTB administration (**Supplementary Figures 5B,C**).

As a whole, our results demonstrate that CTB, in combination with a DC-targeted antigen, promotes a combined Th1 and Th17 response, while soluble antigen vaccination promotes a skewed Th1 response.

Antigen Targeting to DCs Along With CTB Promotes CD4$^+$ T RM Cell Differentiation in the Skin

We next aimed to dissect the memory response induced by a DC-targeted antigen or a soluble antigen in combination with CTB. We first characterized the circulating and re-circulating memory of the CD4$^+$ T cell pool in the SDLN of immunized mice. CD4$^+$ T cells were classified as central memory (T CM) T cells or effector memory (T EM) T cells, according to their expression of CD44 and CD62L. The CTB's co-administration promoted increased differentiation of both T CM and T EM antigen-specific CD4$^+$ T cells in the SDLN, in combination with a DC-targeted or soluble antigen (**Figure 4A**).

Next, we studied the differentiation of skin-resident memory CD4$^+$ T cells [T RM; CD69$^+$CCR7$^-$ (34)] after immunization. At the effector stage, a fraction of T cells that migrate to nonlymphoid organs acquire the expression of CD69 just upon their arrival to these sites (35), which can give rise to a smaller population of long-lived T RM cells (36). Accordingly, 7 days post i.d. immunization, we found that ~30% of OT-II cells were CD69$^+$CCR7$^-$ cells after DC-targeted OVA + CTB and, surprisingly, only ~15% after soluble OVA + CTB immunization (**Figure 4B**). Furthermore, 30 days post-immunization, most of the OVA-specific CD4$^+$ T cells from the skin of DC-targeted OVA + CTB mice were CD69$^+$ (**Figure 4C**). Interestingly, a DC-targeted antigen was more efficient at generating long-lived T RM cells, even in comparison with a high dose of soluble OVA (30 μg of OVA, which is ~60 times more than the amount of OVA contained in 1 μg of anti-DEC205-OVA; **Figure 4C**).

All together, our findings show that CTB can be used to enhance the differentiation of central and effector memory CD4$^+$ T cells, and that its combination with an antigen targeted to DCs efficiently promotes the differentiation of skin CD4$^+$ T RM cells.

Intradermal Immunization With CTB Along With a DC-Targeted Antigen Provides Local and Systemic Long-Lasting Immunity

The fact that the CTB's i.d. co-administration with a DC-targeted antigen promoted CD4$^+$ T cell activation, Th1/Th17 differentiation and migration to the skin, as well as CD4$^+$ TRM cell differentiation, prompted us to investigate whether this immunization strategy could translate into protective long-term immunity. Thus, we first made use of the subcutaneous OVA-expressing melanoma model (**Figure 5A**). We found that i.d. immunization with DC-targeted OVA or soluble OVA in combination with CTB promoted local protection against a subcutaneous challenge with an OVA-expressing melanoma (**Figure 5A**).

To evaluate if the CTB's co-administration with a DC-targeted antigen could elicit systemic activation of T cells, mice vaccinated i.d. were i.v. challenged with MO4 cells. Mice immunized with DC-targeted OVA developed ~5 times fewer metastatic nodules than control mice and superior systemic protection (~3 times less metastatic nodules) than mice immunized with soluble OVA + CTB (**Figure 5B**). Therefore, these data demonstrate that in comparison with the soluble antigen, CTB co-administered with a DC-targeted antigen can provide superior systemic immunity against melanoma. Interestingly, antigen specific CD4$^+$ T cells could be found in the lungs after i.d. priming, which were slightly increased after DC-targeted vaccination (**Supplementary Figure 4C**). However, the administration of an anti-CD4 Ab 30 days after priming, and prior to i.v. melanoma challenge, did not affect protection (**Figure 5B**). Nevertheless, our results show that the immune response induced by a single i.d. dose of CTB co-administered with a DC-targeted antigen provides long-term local and systemic immunity, and, as importantly, the infiltration of CD4$^+$ T cells in distal tissues.

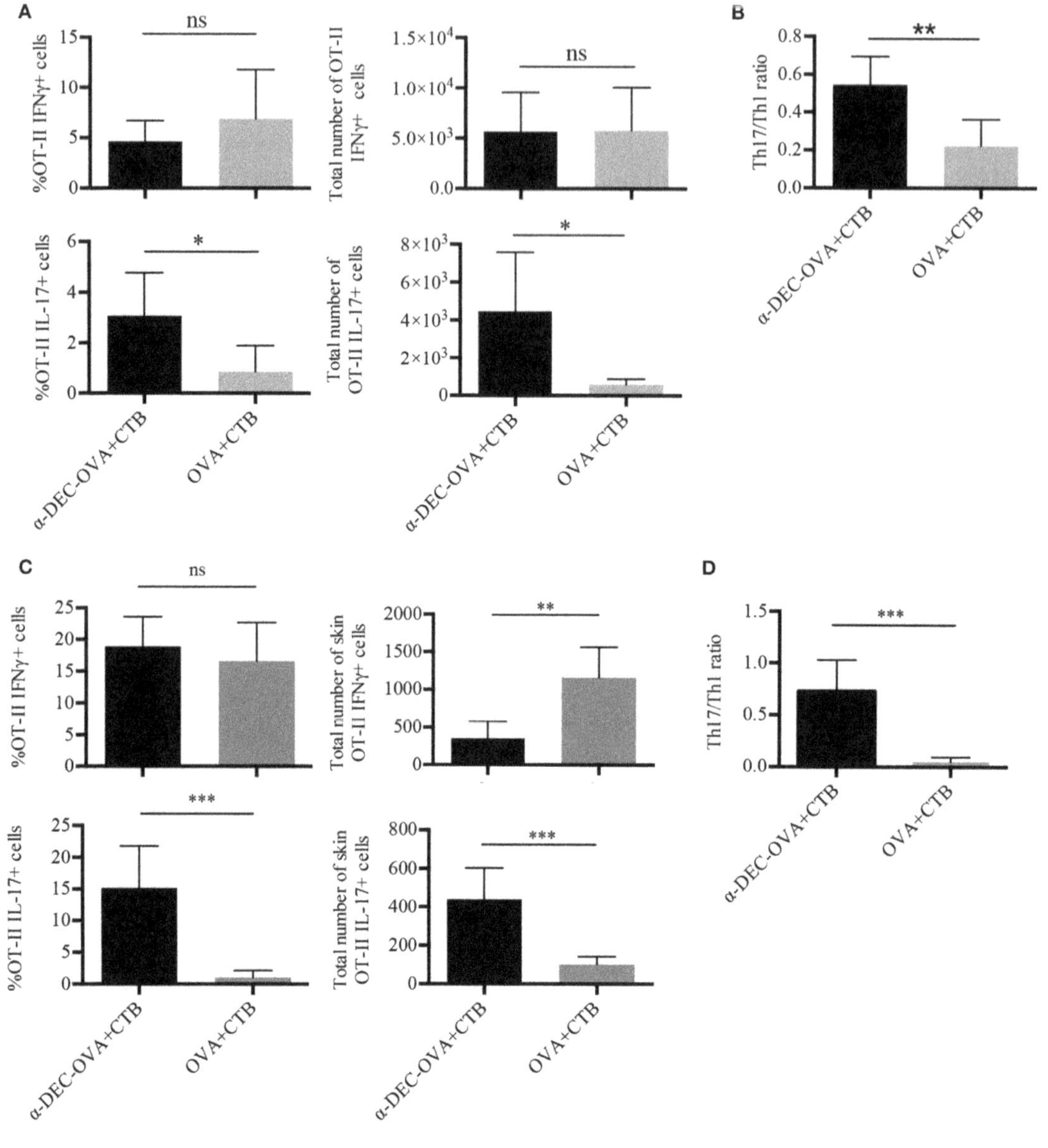

FIGURE 3 | CTB promotes Th1 and Th17 differentiation and recruitment to the skin after i.d. co-administration with a DC-targeted antigen. Mice were treated as in **Figure 2**, and 7 days after immunization, the SDLN and skin were collected to obtain cell suspensions for *in vitro* re-stimulation. **(A)** Cells from the SDLN were incubated for 48 h with OVA 323–339 peptide followed by 4 h with cell cocktail stimulation + protein transport inhibitor. Graphs of percentage and total numbers of IFNγ$^+$ and IL-17$^+$ OT-II cells (identified as in **Figure 2A**). **(B)** Ratio of SDLN Th17/Th1 cells. Mean ± SD, $N = 6$–8, data pooled from two independent experiments. Unpaired T-test (ns, $P > 0.05$, $^*P < 0.05$, $^{**}P < 0.005$). Skin cell suspensions were stimulated with cell cocktail stimulation + protein transport inhibitor for 4 h. **(C)** Graphs of percentage and total numbers of skin IFNγ$^+$ and IL-17$^+$ of OT-II cells (identified as in **Figure 2B**). **(D)** Ratio of skin Th17/Th1 cells. Mean ± SD, $N = 6$–8, data pooled from three independent experiments. Unpaired T-test (ns, $P > 0.05$, $^{**}P < 0.005$, $^{***}P = 0.0001$).

A DC Targeted Antigen Along With CTB Induces Infiltration of Polyfunctional CD4$^+$ T Cells in the Intestine and Provides CD4$^+$ T Cell Dependent Protection Against Rotavirus

Next, we asked whether the CTB's co-administration with a DC-targeted antigen could induce CD4$^+$ T cell responses in another distal tissue, i.e., the intestine. Indeed, very few cells were found in the intestine after i.d. immunization; however, DC-targeted vaccination promoted superior infiltration of OVA-specific CD4$^+$ T cells, as compared with the soluble antigen immunization (**Figures 6A,B**). Furthermore, a higher percentage and number of cells from the intestines of the DC-targeted vaccination group expressed the T RM marker CD69 (**Figure 6C; Supplementary Figure 4D**).

To evaluate whether i.d. DC-targeted vaccination could provide protection in the intestine we made use of a murine

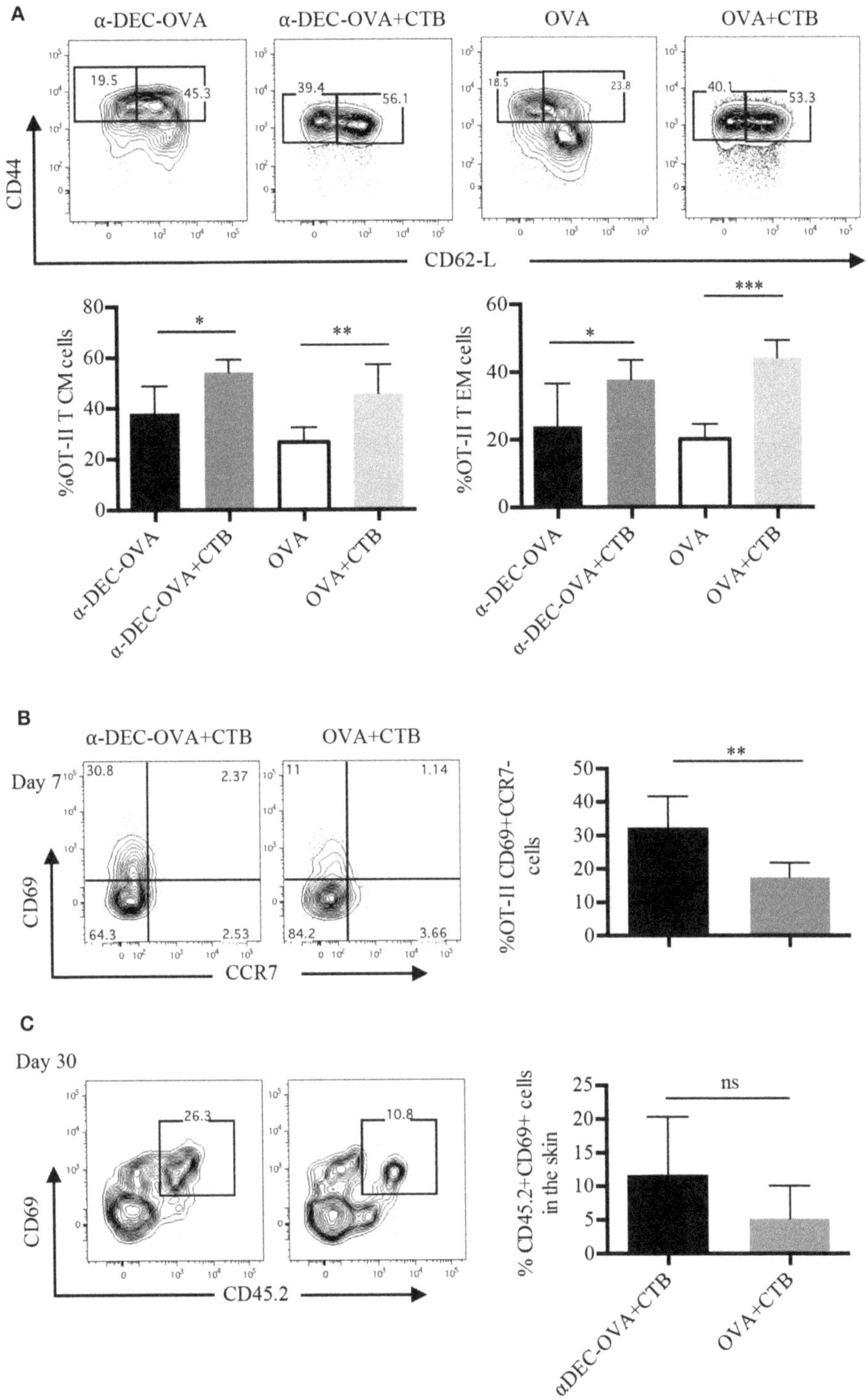

FIGURE 4 | Antigen targeting to DCs along with CTB promotes T EM, T CM and T RM cell differentiation. Mice were treated as in **Figure 2** and the SDLN along with the ears were collected at the indicated times. **(A)** Representative contour plots of T EM ($CD44^+CD62L^-$) and of T CM ($CD44^+CD62L^+$) cells from OT-II $CD45.1^+$ cells (identified as in **Figure 2A**), and graphs of the percentage of each population 7 days post-immunization. Mean ± SD, $N = 4$–6, data pooled from two independent experiments. One-way ANOVA with Tukey's multiple comparisons test (*$P < 0.05$, **$P < 0.005$, ***$P < 0.0005$). **(B)** Representative contour plots and a graph showing percentages of $CD69^+CCR7^-$ OT-II $CD45.1^+$ cells (identified as in **Figure 2B**) from the inoculation site 7 days post-immunization. Mean ± SD, $N =$ 5–6, data pooled from three independent experiments. **(C)** $CD45.1^+$ mice received i.v. OT-II $CD45.2^+$ cells and 1 μg of anti-DEC205-OVA or with 30 μg of OVA, both in combination with CTB. Representative contour plots and a graph showing percentages of $CD69^+$ OT-II $CD45.2^+$ cells 30 days post-immunization. Mean ± SD, $N = 3$–5 data pooled from two independent experiments. Unpaired T-test.

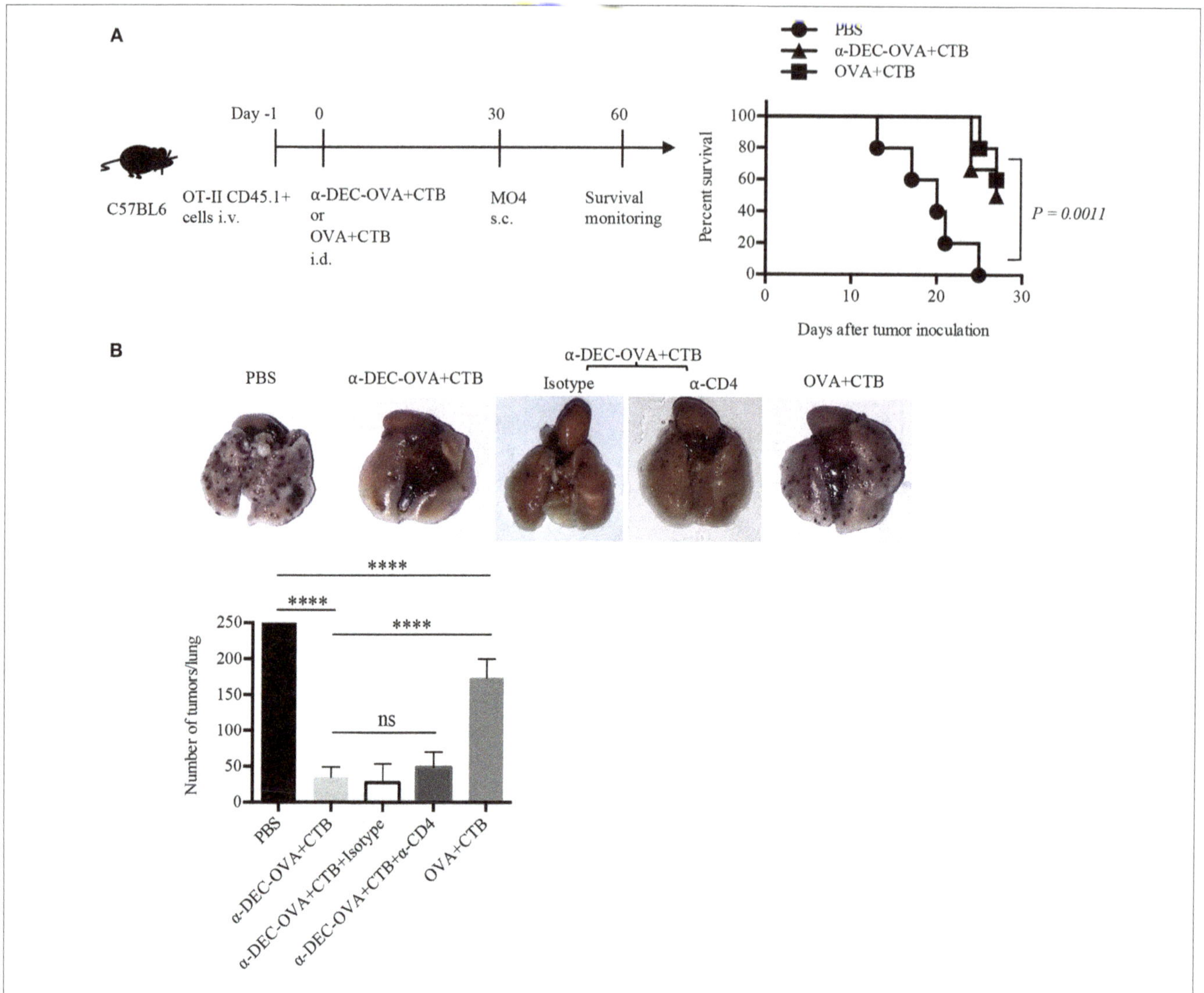

FIGURE 5 | Intradermal immunization with CTB, along with a DC-targeted antigen, provides local and systemic long-lasting immunity against melanoma. **(A)** Diagram showing the strategy followed for immunizations and a graph showing survival rate after MO4 s.c. challenge. $N = 5$ per group, data pooled from two independent experiments. Log-rank (Mantel-Cox) test. Naïve mice were i.d. immunized as indicated, and after 30 days i.v. challenged with MO4 cells. Mice immunized with anti-DEC-OVA+CTB received i.p. anti-CD4 or the control isotype Ab, before, during, and after the inoculation of MO4 cells. **(B)** Representative pictures of lungs and a graph of metastatic nodules per lung, 16 days after challenge. Mean ± SD, $N = 5$–10, data pooled from two independent experiments. One-way ANOVA with Tukey's multiple comparisons test (ns, $P > 0.05$, ****$P < 0.0001$).

rotavirus model. Rotavirus infection is mostly limited to the small intestine; therefore, the immune response is highly compartmentalized (37). Thus, we made use of a VP6-based vaccine model. VP6 is a highly conserved antigen among different strains of rotavirus (38), and it has been shown to promote protective immunity when targeted to DCs in the presence of Poly IC (30). Furthermore, protection against murine rotavirus, in models of soluble VP6 immunization, is dependent on $CD4^+$ T cells (39, 40). Thus, mice were i.d. administered with anti-DEC205−VP6+CTB or soluble VP6+CTB, 20 days before the challenge with oral rotavirus. Only antigen targeting immunization provided intestinal protection (~10%), while soluble immunization did not provide protection against the viral challenge (**Figure 6D**). Therefore, our results suggest that the immune response elicited by a single dose of i.d. DC-targeted antigen admixed with CTB provides partial long-term immunity in the intestine.

The development of partial protection after a single i.d. dose of a DC-targeted antigen could have been due to poor infiltration of functional T cells in the intestine. Therefore, we asked whether a prime/boost immunization scheme could expand the specific $CD4^+$ T cells. To answer this question, mice were i.d. immunized with a DC-targeted antigen or a soluble antigen admixed with CTB. Fifteen days later, mice received, i.p. the targeted or soluble antigen. After 5 days, we observed a greater expansion of antigen-specific $CD4^+$ T cells in the intestine after DC-targeted prime/boost, compared to the soluble antigen prime/boost group (**Figure 7A**). In addition, DC-targeted prime/boost promoted the

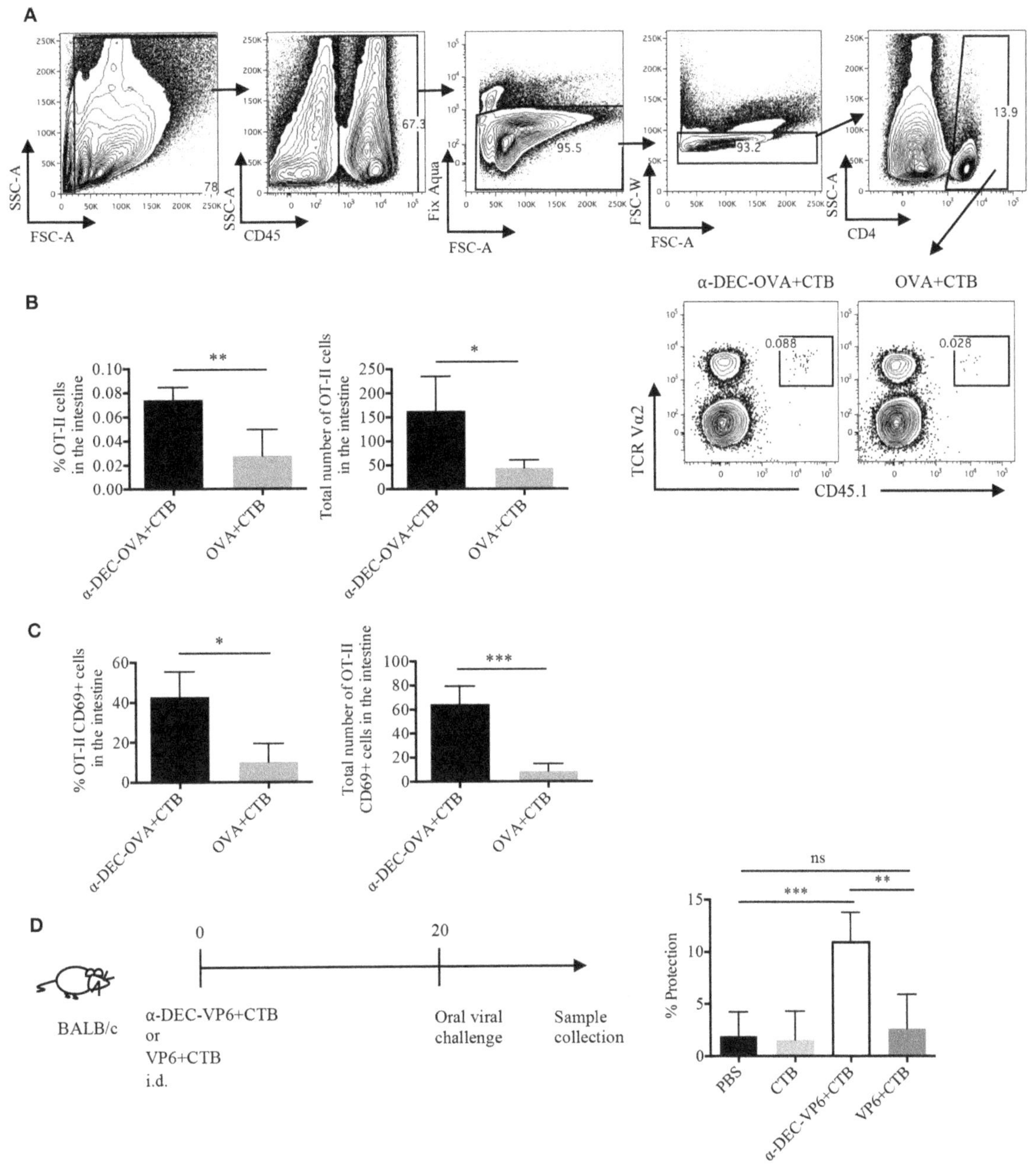

FIGURE 6 | A single dose of a DC-targeted antigen adjuvanted with CTB induces infiltration of antigen specific $CD4^+$ T cells in the intestine and partial protection against rotavirus. Mice were treated as in **Figure 2** and intestines were collected 7 days post-inoculation. **(A)** OT-II $CD45.1^+$ transferred cells were identified as viable $CD45^+CD4^+TCRV\alpha2^+CD45.1^+$ cells. **(B)** percentage and total numbers of OT-II $CD45.1^+$ cells in the intestines. Mean ± SD, $N = 5$ per group, data pooled from two independent experiments. Unpaired T-test ($^*P < 0.05$, $^{**}P < 0.005$). **(C)** Percentage and total numbers of OT-II $CD45.1^+$ cells expressing CD69. Mean ± SD, $N = 5$ per group, data pooled from two independent experiments. Unpaired T-test ($^*P < 0.05$, $^{**}P < 0.005$). **(D)** Diagram showing the immunization strategy followed for viral challenge with murine rotavirus. Stool samples were collected every day up to day 8 and viral load was determined by sandwich ELISA to calculate percentage of protection relative to control (vehicle) mice. Graph depicting percentage of protection after infection. Mean ± SD, $N = 5$ per group, data pooled from two independent experiments. One-way ANOVA with Tukey's multiple comparisons test (ns, $P > 0.05$, $^{**}P < 0.005$, $^{***}P < 0.0005$).

expansion of $IL\text{-}17^+$ $CD4^+$ T cells, that can also produce other cytokines like IFNγ and/or TNFα, in contrast to soluble antigen immunization (**Figure 7B**).

The above results prompted us to discern whether the prime/boost immunization strategy could improve protection in the murine rotavirus model. To this end, mice received anti-DEC205-VP6 or soluble VP6 admixed with CTB, via the i.d. route; 15 days later they received i.p. anti-DEC-VP6 or VP6 only. After 7 days, mice were orally challenged with rotavirus (**Figure 7C**). Four days after the challenge, the viral

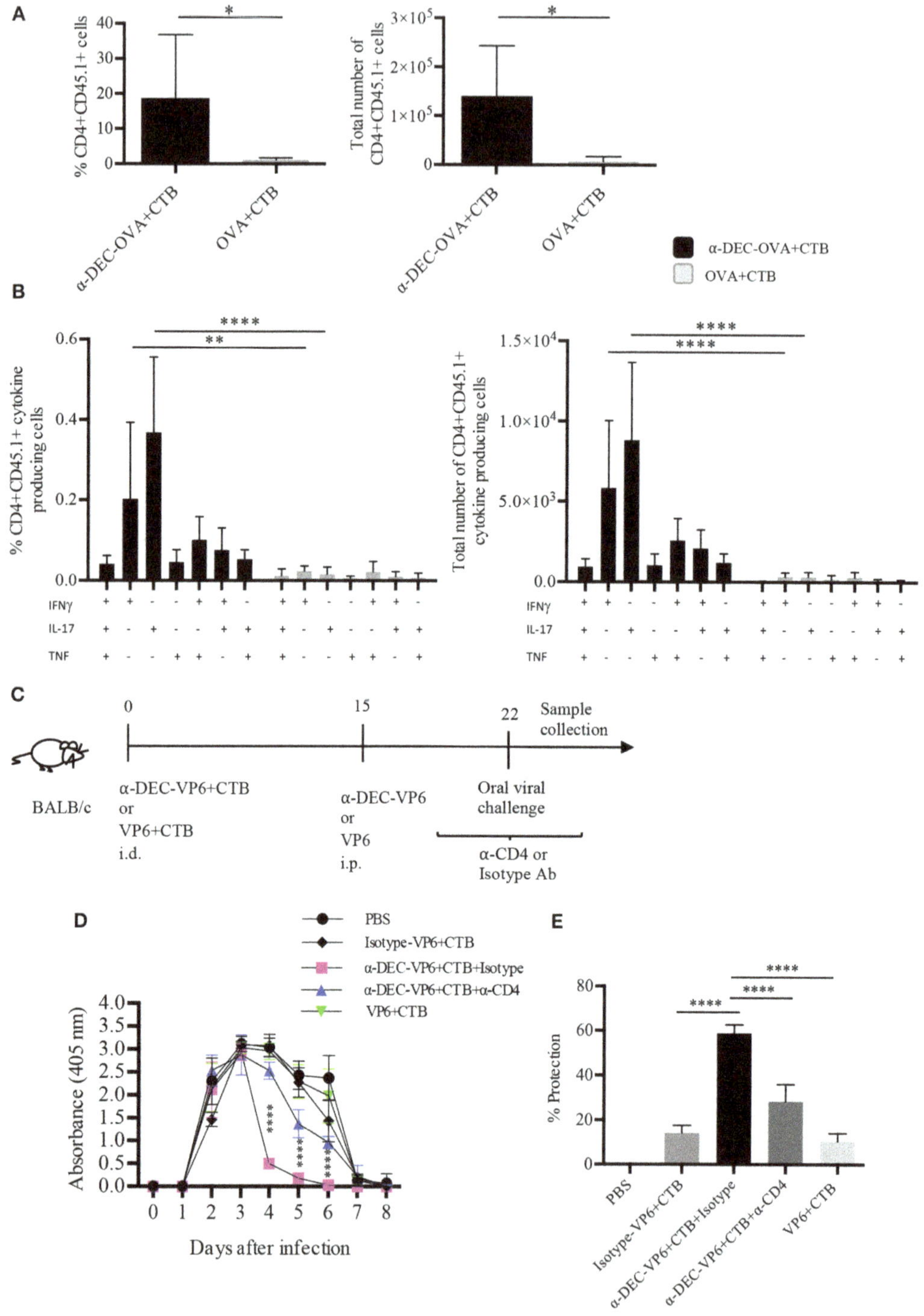

FIGURE 7 | Intradermal prime/i.p. boost immunization with a DC-targeted antigen + CTB induces functional CD4$^+$ T cells in the intestine and provides CD4$^+$ T cell dependent protection against rotavirus. C57BL6 mice were adoptively transferred with OT-II CD45.1$^+$ cells 24 h before i.d. anti-DEC205-OVA or soluble OVA with CTB. Fifteen days later, immune mice received i.p. anti-DEC205-OVA or soluble OVA and after 5 days, mice were sacrificed, and intestines were collected. **(A)** Cells were gated as viable CD45$^+$CD4$^+$CD45.1$^+$ cells to calculate percentage and total number of transferred cells present in the intestine. Mean ± SD, $N = 6$ per group, data pooled from two independent experiments. Unpaired T-test ($^*P < 0.05$). **(B)** Freshly isolated cells were stimulated 4 h with cell cocktail stimulation + protein transport inhibitor. Graphs of percentage and total numbers of CD4$^+$CD45.1$^+$ cytokine producing cells (gated as in **B**). Boolean combinations were calculated using FlowJo software. Mean ± SD, $N = 6$ per group, data pooled from two independent experiments. Two-way ANOVA with Bonferroni's multiple comparison test ($^{**}P = 0.0017$, $^{****}P < 0.0001$). **(C)** Strategy followed for oral viral challenge with murine rotavirus after i.d. immunizations and i.p. boost. Mice immunized with anti-DEC-VP6+CTB received i.p. anti-CD4 or the control isotype Ab, before, during and after the viral challenge. **(D)** Stool samples were collected every day up to day 8 and viral load was determined by sandwich ELISA. **(E)** Percentage of protection relative to control (vehicle) mice, calculated as area under the curve (From **D**). Mean ± SD, $N = 5$–8 per group, data pooled from two independent experiments. Two-way ANOVA with Tukey's multiple comparisons test.

load dramatically dropped in stool samples from the DC-targeted vaccination group (**Figure 7D**). This meant ~60% protection against infection relative to naïve mice (**Figure 7E**). Protection relied on the antigen being targeted to DCs, since the isotype Ab conjugated with VP6 and admixed with CTB only provided partial protection (~15%). Protection was significantly dampened when CD4$^+$ T cells were depleted by the administration of anti-CD4 antibody. On the other hand, soluble antigen vaccination provided only partial protection against infection (~15%; **Figures 7D,E**).

Collectively, our results show that i.d. administration of DC-targeted antigens admixed with CTB promotes the infiltration of polyfunctional CD4$^+$ T cells in the intestine. It is important to point out that our data suggest that this response provides long-term immunity against a pathogen whose clearance is partially dependent on CD4$^+$ T cells.

DISCUSSION

Immunization strategies that confer broad long-lasting immunity mediated by CD4$^+$ T cells are fundamental to eradicate modern pandemics. To achieve this goal, mAbs targeting antigen to DEC205$^+$ DCs, in combination with maturation stimuli, is one of the most promising strategies. Here we have demonstrated that DC-targeted antigens admixed with CTB promote the development of long-lasting systemic protective CD4$^+$ T cell responses.

Successful DC-targeted vaccination requires DC stimulation by strong adjuvants, which ultimately promotes T cell responses. Therefore, we studied the activation and accumulation of DCs following the CTB's i.d. administration. It took 72 h to observe both DC activation and accumulation in the skin; in contrast, other adjuvants (i.e., LPS, CpG, flagellin and the complete cholera toxin) can induce local activation as soon as 6 to 24 h (9, 41–45). Differences could be related to the receptors engaged by CTB on the DCs (17, 18). The late activation of skin DCs was also seen in the SDLN, where activated migratory DCs accumulated 72 h after CTB inoculation. These findings could explain why others have failed at demonstrating activation and accumulation of DCs in draining lymph nodes 2–24 h following CTB administration (44, 46). Therefore, while other adjuvants can promote rapid activation and accumulation of DCs, our results indicate that CTB induces late activation and accumulation of skin DCs.

Interestingly, the accumulation and the activated phenotype of DCs were still observed after 7 days, in both the skin and the SDLN. Similar observations have been reported after the administration of CpG, alum or the MF59 oil-in-water emulsion (47), which induced accumulation in the muscle of MHC-II$^+$ cells up to 4 days after inoculation. The same phenomenon was true for resident lymph node DCs following CTB administration. These findings suggest that CTB can stimulate various populations of DCs for a prolonged time, which could potentially lead to sustained and diverse DC-T cell interactions. Noticeably, the late accumulation of activated skin and lymph node-DCs correlated with the priming of CD4$^+$ T cell responses observed at day 7, following the CTB's co-administration with antigen. Together, our findings shed light on the CTB's controversial ability to activate DCs *in vivo*.

Antigen targeting to DEC205$^+$ DCs is a promising system to promote CD4$^+$ T cell responses (4, 6). Indeed, i.d administration of anti-DEC205-OVA increased the efficiency of antigen presentation relative to the soluble OVA. It was not, however, as large as reported by previous publications that used the s.c. or i.p. routes. Because the SDLN are very close to the inoculation site, i.d. administration of very small quantities of soluble antigen can efficiently promote CD4$^+$ T cell proliferation, in contrast with the s.c or i.p. routes (27). Furthermore, i.d. administration of anti-DEC205-OVA clearly induced a different activation of CD4$^+$ T cells as compared with soluble OVA. Not only did it induce cells to proliferate more, but it also induced a marked downregulation of CD69, which is necessary for T cells' egress to the periphery (31, 32). In this regard, the soluble antigen along with CTB promoted a localized CD4$^+$ T cell response, while a DC-targeted antigen admixed with CTB induced systemic CD4$^+$ T cell responses. Considering that we did not observe DC activation in distal sites, our results suggest that following i.d. DC-targeted vaccination; the priming occurs in the SDLN, and then, activated CD4$^+$ T cells migrate to infiltrate the site of inoculation and, remarkably, other peripheral tissues. Therefore, our results suggest that the priming induced by a DC-targeted antigen admixed with CTB promotes unique systemic CD4$^+$ T cell responses.

Indeed, a DC-targeted antigen along with CTB induced a combined and systemic Th1/Th17 response. In contrast, soluble antigen immunization promoted a skewed localized Th1 response, which is similar to that observed when using CTB as an adjuvant linked with antigens or admixed with pathogen derived antigens (22–24, 26). Furthermore, the CTB's combination with a DC-targeted antigen promoted the differentiation of polyfunctional Th cells. It has been documented that anti-DEC205-antigen Abs admixed with experimental adjuvants—i.e., CpG oligonucleotides, flagellin (9) and Poly IC (7)—induce differentiation of polyfunctional CD4$^+$ T cells that produce IFNγ, TNFα, and IL2. However, none of these adjuvants are able to induce Th17 differentiation (48–50). In our model, the superior induction of Th17 cells seemed to depend on both the adjuvant and the antigen being directly delivered to DEC205$^+$ DCs, since soluble antigen vaccination induced IL-17$^+$ antigen specific CD4$^+$ T cells only marginally. To our knowledge, this is the first report showing induction of systemic polyfunctional CD4$^+$ T cell responses that include IL-17$^+$ cells after antigen targeting to DEC205$^+$ DCs by genetically engineered mAbs admixed with CTB.

We also demonstrate that a DC-targeted antigen admixed with CTB efficiently promotes the generation of memory CD4$^+$ T cells, something that has not been extensively explored after performing DC-targeted vaccination. Here, using cell surface markers, we found in the SDLN the presence of circulating and re-circulating memory CD4$^+$ T cells after using a DC-targeted antigen or a soluble antigen admixed with CTB. Strikingly, the high infiltration of CD4$^+$ T cells after soluble antigen immunization did not translate into more T RM differentiation. In contrast, DC-targeted vaccination induced superior differentiation of CD4$^+$ T RM cells at the site of inoculation and, more importantly, at a distal nonlymphoid tissue, i.e., the intestine. This is similar to what has been observed

In studies inoculating recombinant vaccinia virus expressing OVA through skin scarification, which induces the differentiation of protective T RM cells in the skin and lungs (51–53). Thus far, there are only a couple of publications reporting CD8$^+$ T RM cell differentiation after immunization with anti-DEC205-antigen mAbs, using LPS (54) or Poly IC (55) as adjuvants. However, none of them have shown the presence of T RM cells in distal sites after local vaccination. Our observations suggest that antigen targeting to DEC205$^+$ DCs, in combination with CTB, is an effective strategy to promote systemic differentiation of CD4$^+$ T RM cells. This is of particular relevance in light of recent studies, pointing to T RM cells as essential players against several infections (34, 36, 56) and melanoma (53, 55) protection.

Following this line, DC-targeted and soluble antigen vaccination provided similar long-term protection against subcutaneous melanoma. This could be related to the protective capacity of both circulating and T RM cells against melanoma (53). However, we found that DC-targeted vaccination provided superior systemic protection against pulmonary tumor growth. Although we found antigen specific CD4$^+$ T cells in the lungs of immune mice, the administration of a neutralizing anti-CD4 Ab during the memory phase did not abrogate protection against i.v. melanoma. This is contrary to melanoma studies in CD4 knockout mice, where protection is partially dampened (4). Therefore, we cannot completely rule out the participation of CD4$^+$ T cells in the priming of protective CD8$^+$ T cell responses against i.v. melanoma. In this regard, our results suggest that protection in the lungs could be primarily mediated by memory CD8$^+$ T cells after DC targeted vaccination using CTB as adjuvant. This idea is supported by the fact that CD8$^+$ T cells are efficiently activated by anti-DEC205 Abs (4, 6) and by antigens linked to CTB (57, 58). Since priming occurred in the SDLN, our findings suggest that DC-targeted vaccination using CTB as adjuvant can be used as an efficient immunization strategy to provide systemic long-term immunity against melanoma.

Interestingly, DC-targeted vaccination-induced systemic CD4$^+$ T cell responses translated into protection in the intestine. This could have been mediated by the T RM and polyfunctional CD4$^+$ T cells found in the intestine after DC-targeted vaccination. However, a single immunization induced only small numbers of T cells in the intestine and partial protection. Since protective immunity correlates with high numbers of functional cells infiltrating the site of infection, we took advantage of the ability of anti-DEC205 Abs to disseminate systemically (6) to successfully expand the antigen specific CD4$^+$ T cells in the intestine through a DC-targeted antigen + CTB i.d. prime/DC-targeted antigen i.p. boost. Remarkably, this strategy promoted higher numbers of IL-17$^+$ CD4$^+$ T cells to be present in the intestine, as well as polyfunctional CD4$^+$ T cells. Furthermore, the prime/boost scheme dramatically improved protection against the oral viral challenge, but only when the antigen was targeted to DCs. Moreover, the protection observed was superior than the one reported by s.c. administration of the same antibody in the presence of Poly IC, which was related to the development of Th1 responses (30). Also, protection in our model was partially dependent on CD4$^+$ T cells, according with the CD4 blockade experiments. However, we cannot exclude the participation of CD8$^+$ T cells. These findings indicate that DC-targeted antigens admixed with CTB promote infiltration of the intestine with functional CD4$^+$ T cells capable of mediating protection against pathogens with intestine tropism.

Our results extend the advantages of immunization with antigens targeted to DEC205$^+$ DCs with mAbs in combination with strong adjuvants (CTB) to induce high quality systemic immune responses that translate into protection. We propose that a DC-targeted antigen can be co-administered with CTB i.d.; a suitable novel combination with potential human use, for the generation of protective, systemic and long-lasting Th17 CD4$^+$ and polyfunctional responses, which, importantly, are characterized by CD4$^+$ T RM cells. Furthermore, this immunization strategy could be used to fight infections and tumors.

AUTHOR CONTRIBUTIONS

LA-H performed the majority of the experiments, interpreted the data and drafted the manuscript. OB-G performed the murine rotavirus protection assay. OM-C processed intestine samples. AT-S helped with skin DCs analysis. AT-S and AG-L performed confocal microscopy experiments. FE-G and LG-X contributed to design the murine rotavirus experiments. GS provided transgenic OT-II CD45.1$^+$ mice and helped with the interpretation of data. JI helped to train the first author in experimental techniques, provided reagents necessary for the study (i.e., anti-DEC-OVA mAb), helped with the design of the study and the interpretation of results, and revised the manuscript. LB conceived and directed the project and revised the manuscript. All the authors reviewed the manuscript critically.

FUNDING

This study was funded by the Instituto Mexicano del Seguro Social (IMSS) R-2015-785-023 FIS/IMSS/PROT/G151435 and by Consejo Nacional de Ciencia y Tecnología (CONACyT) CB-2010-01157018 (to LB) 180441 (to FE-G) in Mexico, and by the National Institute of Arthritis, Musculoskeletal and Skin Diseases of the US National Institutes of Health (R00 AR062595 to JI) and the National Cancer Institute of the US National Institutes of Health (R01 CA219994 to JI). LA-H is a doctoral student from Programa de Doctorado en Ciencias Biomédicas at UNAM and she received a fellowship (275768) from Consejo Nacional de Ciencia y Tcenología (CONACYT) in Mexico, and a fellowship by the Coordinación de Investigación en Salud: Apoyo de movilidad internacional, programa de cooperación internacional. OB-G is a posdoctoral fellow from Programa Nacional para Estudios de Posdoctorado (CVU 348201) from CONACyT.

ACKNOWLEDGMENTS

We would like to thank the staff of the animal facility at the Experimental Medicine Unit, Faculty of Medicine, UNAM, and at the INSP, SS, for providing expert animal care. We also thank the members of Bonifaz' laboratory and of Idoyaga Lab for their advice and protocols. Finally, we extend our gratitude to the Flow Cytometry core facility, the Coordinación de Investigación en Salud, the CMN S XXI, and the IMSS, for their instrumental and technical support.

REFERENCES

1. Kannanganat S, Kapogiannis BG, Ibegbu C, Chennareddi L, Goepfert P, Robinson HL, et al. Human immunodeficiency virus type 1 controllers but not noncontrollers maintain CD4 T cells coexpressing three cytokines. *J Virol.* (2007) 81:12071–6. doi: 10.1128/JVI.01261-07
2. Darrah PA, Patel DT, De Luca PM, Lindsay RWB, Davey DF, Flynn BJ, et al. Multifunctional TH1 cells define a correlate of vaccine-mediated protection against Leishmania major. *Nat Med.* (2007) 13:843–50. doi: 10.1038/nm1592
3. Lindenstrom T, Agger EM, Korsholm KS, Darrah PA, Aagaard C, Seder RA, et al. Tuberculosis subunit vaccination provides long-term protective immunity characterized by multifunctional CD4 memory T cells. *J Immunol.* (2009) 182:8047–55. doi: 10.4049/jimmunol.0801592
4. Bonifaz LC, Bonnyay DP, Charalambous A, Darguste DI, Fujii S-I, Soares H, et al. *In vivo* targeting of antigens to maturing dendritic cells via the DEC-205 receptor improves T cell vaccination. *J Exp Med.* (2004) 199:815–24. doi: 10.1084/jem.20032220
5. He K, Liu P, Xu LX. The cryo-thermal therapy eradicated melanoma in mice by eliciting CD4$^+$ T-cell-mediated antitumor memory immune response. *Cell Death Dis.* (2017) 8:e2703. doi: 10.1038/cddis.2017.125
6. Bonifaz L, Bonnyay D, Mahnke K, Rivera M, Nussenzweig MC, Steinman RM. Efficient targeting of protein antigen to the dendritic cell receptor DEC-205 in the steady state leads to antigen presentation on major histocompatibility complex class I products and peripheral CD8$^+$ T cell tolerance. *J Exp Med.* (2002) 196:1627–38. doi: 10.1084/jem.20021598
7. Trumpfheller C, Caskey M, Nchinda G, Longhi MP, Mizenina O, Huang Y, et al. The microbial mimic poly IC induces durable and protective CD4$^+$ T cell immunity together with a dendritic cell targeted vaccine. *Proc Natl Acad Sci USA.* (2008) 105:2574–9. doi: 10.1073/pnas.0711976105
8. Idoyaga J, Lubkin A, Fiorese C, Lahoud MH, Caminschi I, Huang Y, et al. Comparable T helper 1 (Th1) and CD8 T-cell immunity by targeting HIV gag p24 to CD8 dendritic cells within antibodies to Langerin, DEC205, and Clec9A. *Proc Natl Acad Sci USA.* (2011) 108:2384–9. doi: 10.1073/pnas.1019547108
9. Antonialli R, Sulczewski FB, Amorim KN da S, Almeida B da S, Ferreira NS, Yamamoto MM, et al. CpG oligodeoxinucleotides and flagellin modulate the immune response to antigens targeted to CD8α^+ and CD8α^- conventional dendritic cell subsets. *Front Immunol.* (2017) 8:1727. doi: 10.3389/fimmu.2017.01727
10. Boscardin SB, Hafalla JCR, Masilamani RF, Kamphorst AO, Zebroski HA, Rai U, et al. Antigen targeting to dendritic cells elicits long-lived T cell help for antibody responses. *J Exp Med.* (2006) 203:599–606. doi: 10.1084/jem.20051639
11. Flacher V, Tripp CH, Mairhofer DG, Steinman RM, Stoitzner P, Idoyaga J, et al. Murine Langerin+ dermal dendritic cells prime CD8$^+$ T cells while Langerhans cells induce cross-tolerance. *EMBO Mol Med.* (2014) 6:1191–204. doi: 10.15252/emmm.201303283
12. Petrovsky N. Comparative safety of vaccine adjuvants: a summary of current evidence and future needs. *Drug Saf.* (2015) 38:1059–74. doi: 10.1007/s40264-015-0350-4
13. Kilander A, Jertborn M, Nordstro I, Czerkinsky C, Holmgren JAN. Local and systemic immune responses to rectal administration of recombinant cholera toxin B subunit in humans. *Infect Immun.* (2001) 69:4125–8. doi: 10.1128/IAI.69.6.4125-4128.2001
14. Concha A, Giraldo A, Castaneda E, Martinez M, de la HF, Rivas F, et al. Safety and immunogenicity of oral killed whole cell recombinant B subunit cholera vaccine in Barranquilla, Colombia. *Bull Pan Am Heal Organ.* (1995) 29:312–21.
15. Taylor DN, Cárdenas V, Sanchez JL, Bégué RE, Gilman R, Bautista C, et al. Two-year study of the protective efficacy of the oral whole cell plus recombinant B subunit cholera vaccine in Peru. *J Infect Dis.* (2000) 181:1667–73. doi: 10.1086/315462
16. World Health Organization. Cholera vaccines: WHO position paper–August 2017. *Wkly Epidemiol Rec.* (2017) 2017:477–500.
17. Hou J, Liu Y, Hsi J, Wang H, Tao R, Shao Y. Cholera toxin B subunit acts as a potent systemic adjuvant for HIV-1 DNA vaccination intramuscularly in mice. *Hum Vaccines Immunother.* (2014) 10:1274–83. doi: 10.4161/hv.28371
18. Phongsisay V, Iizasa E, Hara H, Yoshida H. Evidence for TLR4 and FcRγ-CARD9 activation by cholera toxin B subunit and its direct bindings to TREM2 and LMIR5 receptors. *Mol Immunol.* (2015) 66:463–71. doi: 10.1016/j.molimm.2015.05.008
19. Odumosu O, Payne K, Baez I, Jutzy J, Wall N, Langridge W. Suppression of dendritic cell activation by diabetes autoantigens linked to the cholera toxin B subunit. *Immunobiology* (2011) 216:447–56. doi: 10.1016/j.imbio.2010.09.008
20. D'Ambrosio A, Colucci M, Pugliese O, Quintieri F, Boirivant M. Cholera toxin B subunit promotes the induction of regulatory T cells by preventing human dendritic cell maturation. *J Leukoc Biol.* (2008) 84:661–8. doi: 10.1189/jlb.1207850
21. Eriksson K, Fredriksson M, Nordström I, Holmgren J. Cholera toxin and its B subunit promote dendritic cell vaccination with different influences on Th1 and Th2 development. *Infect Immun.* (2003) 71:1740–7. doi: 10.1128/IAI.71.4.1740-1747.2003
22. Li J, Arevalo MT, Chen Y, Posadas O, Smith JA, Zeng M. Intranasal immunization with influenza antigens conjugated with cholera toxin subunit B stimulates broad spectrum immunity against influenza viruses. *Hum Vaccines Immunother.* (2014) 10:1211–20. doi: 10.4161/hv.28407
23. Li Y, Chen Z, Ye J, Ning L, Luo J, Zhang L, et al. Antibody production and Th1-biased response induced by an epitope vaccine composed of cholera toxin B unit and *Helicobacter pylori* Lpp20 epitopes. *Helicobacter* (2016) 21:234–48. doi: 10.1111/hel.12268
24. Wiedinger K, Pinho D, Bitsaktsis C. Utilization of cholera toxin B as a mucosal adjuvant elicits antibody-mediated protection against *S. pneumoniae* infection in mice. *Ther Adv Vaccines* (2017) 5:15–24. doi: 10.1177/2051013617691041
25. Olivera N, Castuma CE, Hozbor D, Gaillard ME, Rumbo M, Gómez RM. Immunization with the recombinant cholera toxin B fused to fimbria 2 protein protects against bordetella pertussis infection. *Biomed Res Int.* (2014) 2014:421486. doi: 10.1155/2014/421486
26. Bitsaktsis C, Rawool DB, Li Y, Kurkure NV, Iglesias B, Gosselin EJ. Differential requirements for protection against mucosal challenge with *Francisella*

tularensis in the presence versus absence of cholera toxin B and inactivated *F. tularensis*. *J Immunol.* (2009) 182:4899–909. doi: 10.4049/jimmunol.0803242

27. Meza-Sánchez D, Pérez-Montesinos G, Sánchez-García J, Moreno J, Bonifaz LC. Intradermal immunization in the ear with cholera toxin and its non-toxic β subunit promotes efficient Th1 and Th17 differentiation dependent on migrating DCs. *Eur J Immunol.* (2011) 41:2894–904. doi: 10.1002/eji.201040997
28. Medina-Contreras O, Geem D, Laur O, Willianms IR, Lira SA, Nusrat A, et al. CX3CR1 regulates intestinal macrophage homeostasis, bacterial translocation, and colotogenic Th17 responses in mice. *J Clin Invest.* (2011) 121:4787–95. doi: 10.1172/JCI59150
29. Overwijk WW, Restifo NP. B16 as a mouse model for human melanoma. *Curr Protoc Immunol.* (2001) Chapter 20:Unit 20.1. doi: 10.1002/0471142735.im2001s39
30. Badillo-Godinez O, Gutierrez-Xicotencatl L, Plett-Torres T, Pedroza-Saavedra A, Gonzalez-Jaimes A, Chihu-Amparan L, et al. Targeting of rotavirus VP6 to DEC-205 induces protection against the infection in mice. *Vaccine* (2015) 33:4228–37. doi: 10.1016/j.vaccine.2015.03.080
31. Lambrecht BN, Pauwels RA, Fazekas de St. Groth B. Induction of rapid T cell activation, division, and recirculation by intratracheal injection of dendritic cells in a TCR transgenic model. *J Immunol.* (2000) 164:2937–46. doi: 10.4049/jimmunol.164.6.2937
32. Shiow LR, Rosen DB, Brdičková N, Xu Y, An J, Lanier LL, et al. CD69 acts downstream of interferon-α/β to inhibit S1P1and lymphocyte egress from lymphoid organs. *Nature* (2006) 440:540–4. doi: 10.1038/nature04606
33. Idoyaga J, Fiorese C, Zbytnuik L, Lubkin A, Miller J, Malissen B, et al. Specialized role of migratory dendritic cells in peripheral tolerance induction. *J Clin Invest.* (2014) 4:1–11. doi: 10.1172/JCI65260
34. Park CO, Kupper TS. The emerging role of resident memory T cells in protective immunity and inflammatory disease. *Nat Med.* (2015) 21:688–97. doi: 10.1038/nm.3883
35. Mackay LK, Braun A, Macleod BL, Collins N, Tebartz C, Bedoui S, et al. Cutting edge: CD69 interference with sphingosine-1-phosphate receptor function regulates peripheral T cell retention. *J Immunol.* (2015) 194:2059–63. doi: 10.4049/jimmunol.1402256
36. Stary G, Olive A, Radovic-Moreno AF, Gondek D, Alvarez D, Basto PA, et al. A mucosal vaccine against *Chlamydia trachomatis* generates two waves of protective memory T cells. *Science* (2015) 348:aaa8205. doi: 10.1126/science.aaa8205
37. Crawford SE, Ramani S, Tate JE, Parashar UD, Svensson L, Hagbom M, et al. Rotavirus infection. *Nat Rev Dis Prim.* (2017) 3:17083. doi: 10.1038/nrdp.2017.83
38. Ward RL, McNeal MM. VP6: a candidate rotavirus vaccine. *J Infect Dis.* (2010) 202:S101–7. doi: 10.1086/653556
39. Choi AH, Basu M, McNeal MM, Clements JD, Ward RL. Antibody-independent protection against rotavirus infection of mice stimulated by intranasal immunization with chimeric VP4 or VP6 protein. *J Virol.* (1999) 73:7574–81.
40. McNeal MM, VanCott JL, Choi AHC, Basu M, Flint JA, Stone SC, et al. CD4 T cells are the only lymphocytes needed to protect mice against rotavirus shedding after intranasal immunization with a chimeric VP6 protein and the adjuvant LT(R192G). *J Virol.* (2002) 76:560–8. doi: 10.1128/JVI.76.2.560-568.2002
41. Olguín-Alor R, De La Fuente-Granada M, Bonifaz LC, Antonio-Herrera L, García-Zepeda EA, Soldevila G. A key role for inhibins in dendritic cell maturation and function. *PLoS ONE* (2016) 11:e0167813. doi: 10.1371/journal.pone.0167813
42. De Smedt T, Pajak B, Muraille E, Lespagnard L, Heinen E, De Baetselier P, et al. Regulation of dendritic cell numbers and maturation by lipopolysaccharide *in vivo*. *J Exp Med.* (1996) 184:1413–24.
43. Behboudi S, Chao D, Klenerman P, Austyn J. The effects of DNA containing CpG motif on dendritic cells. *Immunology* (2000) 99:361–6. doi: 10.1046/j.1365-2567.2000.00979.x
44. Apte SH, Redmond AM, Groves PL, Schussek S, Pattinson DJ, Doolan DL. Subcutaneous cholera toxin exposure induces potent CD103$^+$ dermal dendritic cell activation and migration. *Eur J Immunol.* (2013) 43:2707–17. doi: 10.1002/eji.201343475
45. Anjuere F, Luci C, Lebens M, Rousseau D, Hervouet C, Milon G, et al. *In vivo* adjuvant-induced mobilization and maturation of gut dendritic cells after oral administration of cholera toxin. *J Immunol.* (2004) 173:5103–11. doi: 10.4049/jimmunol.173.8.5103
46. Anjuère F, George-Chandy A, Audant F, Rousseau D, Holmgren J, Czerkinsky C. Transcutaneous immunization with cholera toxin B subunit adjuvant suppresses IgE antibody responses via selective induction of Th1 immune responses. *J Immunol.* (2003) 170:1586–92. doi: 10.4049/jimmunol.170.3.1586
47. Mosca F, Tritto E, Muzzi A, Monaci E, Bagnoli F, Iavarone C, et al. Molecular and cellular signatures of human vaccine adjuvants. *Proc Natl Acad Sci USA.* (2008) 105:10501–6. doi: 10.1073/pnas.0804699105
48. Tigno-Aranjuez JT, Jaini R, Tuohy VK, Lehmann PV, Tary-Lehmann M. Encephalitogenicity of complete Freund's adjuvant relative to CpG is linked to induction of Th17 cells. *J Immunol.* (2009) 183:5654–61. doi: 10.4049/jimmunol.0900645
49. Joffre OP, Sancho D, Zelenay S, Keller AM, Reis E, Sousa C. Efficient and versatile manipulation of the peripheral CD4$^+$ T-cell compartment by antigen targeting to DNGR-1/CLEC9A. *Eur J Immunol.* (2010) 40:1255–65. doi: 10.1002/eji.201040419
50. Weber A, Zimmermann C, Meyer zu Hörste G, Kieseier BC, Hartung HP, Hofstetter HH. Bacterial flagellin and diphtheria toxin co-stimulate IL-17-producing thymocytes. *Cytokine* (2013) 64:221–6. doi: 10.1016/j.cyto.2013.06.318
51. Liu L, Fuhlbrigge RC, Karibian K, Tian T, Kupper TS. Dynamic programing of CD8$^+$ T cell trafficking after live viral immunization. *Immunity* (2006) 25:511–20. doi: 10.1016/j.immuni.2006.06.019
52. Liu L, Zhong Q, Tian T, Dubin K, Athale SK, Kupper TS. Epidermal injury and infection during poxvirus immunization is crucial for the generation of highly protective T cell-mediated immunity. *Nat Med.* (2010) 16:224–7. doi: 10.1038/nm.2078
53. Enamorado M, Iborra S, Priego E, Cueto FJ, Quintana JA, Martýnez-Cano S, et al. Enhanced anti-tumour immunity requires the interplay between resident and circulating memory CD8$^+$ T cells. *Nat Commun.* (2017) 8:1–11. doi: 10.1038/ncomms16073
54. Wakim LM, Smith J, Caminschi I, Lahoud MH, Villadangos JA. Antibody-targeted vaccination to lung dendritic cells generates tissue-resident memory CD8 T cells that are highly protective against influenza virus infection. *Mucosal Immunol.* (2015) 8:1060–71. doi: 10.1038/mi.2014.133
55. Gálvez-Cancino F, López E, Menares E, Díaz X, Flores C, Cáceres P, et al. Vaccination-induced skin-resident memory CD8$^+$ T cells mediate strong protection against cutaneous melanoma. *Oncoimmunology* (2018) 7:e1442163. doi: 10.1080/2162402X.2018.1442163
56. Teijaro JR, Turner D, Pham Q, Wherry EJ, Lefrancois L, Farber DL. Cutting edge: tissue-retentive lung memory CD4 T cells mediate optimal protection to respiratory virus infection. *J Immunol.* (2011) 187:5510–4. doi: 10.4049/jimmunol.1102243
57. Eriksson K, Sun JB, Nordström I, Fredriksson M, Lindblad M, Li BL, et al. Coupling of antigen to cholera toxin for dendritic cell vaccination promotes the induction of MHC class I-restricted cytotoxic T cells and the rejection of a cognate antigen-expressing model tumor. *Eur J Immunol.* (2004) 34:1272–81. doi: 10.1002/eji.200324368
58. Luci C, Hervouet C, Rousseau D, Holmgren J, Czerkinsky C, Anjuère F. Dendritic cell-mediated induction of mucosal cytotoxic responses following intravaginal immunization with the nontoxic B subunit of cholera toxin. *J Immunol.* (2006) 176:2749–57. doi: 10.4049/jimmunol.176.5.2749

Permissions

All chapters in this book were first published by Frontiers; hereby published with permission under the Creative Commons Attribution License or equivalent. Every chapter published in this book has been scrutinized by our experts. Their significance has been extensively debated. The topics covered herein carry significant findings which will fuel the growth of the discipline. They may even be implemented as practical applications or may be referred to as a beginning point for another development.

The contributors of this book come from diverse backgrounds, making this book a truly international effort. This book will bring forth new frontiers with its revolutionizing research information and detailed analysis of the nascent developments around the world.

We would like to thank all the contributing authors for lending their expertise to make the book truly unique. They have played a crucial role in the development of this book. Without their invaluable contributions this book wouldn't have been possible. They have made vital efforts to compile up to date information on the varied aspects of this subject to make this book a valuable addition to the collection of many professionals and students.

This book was conceptualized with the vision of imparting up-to-date information and advanced data in this field. To ensure the same, a matchless editorial board was set up. Every individual on the board went through rigorous rounds of assessment to prove their worth. After which they invested a large part of their time researching and compiling the most relevant data for our readers.

The editorial board has been involved in producing this book since its inception. They have spent rigorous hours researching and exploring the diverse topics which have resulted in the successful publishing of this book. They have passed on their knowledge of decades through this book. To expedite this challenging task, the publisher supported the team at every step. A small team of assistant editors was also appointed to further simplify the editing procedure and attain best results for the readers.

Apart from the editorial board, the designing team has also invested a significant amount of their time in understanding the subject and creating the most relevant covers. They scrutinized every image to scout for the most suitable representation of the subject and create an appropriate cover for the book.

The publishing team has been an ardent support to the editorial, designing and production team. Their endless efforts to recruit the best for this project, has resulted in the accomplishment of this book. They are a veteran in the field of academics and their pool of knowledge is as vast as their experience in printing. Their expertise and guidance has proved useful at every step. Their uncompromising quality standards have made this book an exceptional effort. Their encouragement from time to time has been an inspiration for everyone.

The publisher and the editorial board hope that this book will prove to be a valuable piece of knowledge for researchers, students, practitioners and scholars across the globe.

List of Contributors

Nikos E. Papaioannou and Maria Pasztoi
Biomedical Center, Institute for Cardiovascular Physiology and Pathophysiology, Ludwig-Maximilians University Munich, Munich, Germany

Barbara U. Schraml
Biomedical Center, Institute for Cardiovascular Physiology and Pathophysiology, Ludwig-Maximilians University Munich, Munich, Germany Walter-Brendel-Centre of Experimental Medicine, University Hospital, Ludwig-Maximilians-University Munich, Munich, Germany

Juliana de Souza Apostólico, Victória Alves Santos Lunardelli and Daniela Santoro Rosa
Laboratory of Experimental Vaccines, Department of Microbiology, Immunology and Parasitology, Federal University of São Paulo, São Paulo, Brazil Institute for Investigation in Immunology (iii)—INCT, São Paulo, Brazil

Marcio Massao Yamamoto
Department of Parasitology, Institute of Biomedical Sciences, University of São Paulo, São Paulo, Brazil

Edecio Cunha-Neto
Institute for Investigation in Immunology (iii)—INCT, São Paulo, Brazil Laboratory of Clinical Immunology and Allergy (LIM60), School of Medicine–University of São Paulo, São Paulo, Brazil

Silvia Beatriz Boscardin
Institute for Investigation in Immunology (iii)—INCT, São Paulo, Brazil Department of Parasitology, Institute of Biomedical Sciences, University of São Paulo, São Paulo, Brazil

Joanna Grabowska, Miguel A. Lopez-Venegas, Alsya J. Affandi and Joke M. M. den Haan
Department of Molecular Cell Biology and Immunology, Amsterdam University Medical Center, Cancer Center Amsterdam, Amsterdam Infection and Immunity Institute, Vrije Universiteit Amsterdam, Amsterdam, Netherlands

Arthur L. Kroczek
Molecular Immunology, Robert Koch-Institute, Berlin, Germany Protein Biochemistry, Institute for Biochemistry, Free University of Berlin, Berlin, Germany Institute of Biochemistry, Charité University Medicine Berlin, Berlin, Germany

Evelyn Hartung, Stephanie Gurka, Martina Becker, Nele Reeg, Hans W. Mages and Richard A. Kroczek
Molecular Immunology, Robert Koch-Institute, Berlin, Germany

Sebastian Voigt
Virology, Robert Koch-Institute, Berlin, Germany

Christian Freund
Protein Biochemistry, Institute for Biochemistry, Free University of Berlin, Berlin, Germany

Shuchi Smita and Abdul Ahad
Immuno-genomics and Systems Biology Laboratory, Institute of Life Sciences (ILS), Bhubaneswar, India Manipal Academy of Higher Education, Manipal, India

Arup Ghosh and Viplov K. Biswas
Immuno-genomics and Systems Biology Laboratory, Institute of Life Sciences (ILS), Bhubaneswar, India Department of Biotechnology, Kalinga Institute of Industrial Technology (KIIT), Bhubaneswar, India

Marianna M. Koga and Hans Acha-Orbea
Department of Biochemistry CIIL, University of Lausanne (UNIL), Epalinges, Switzerland

Bhawna Gupta
Department of Biotechnology, Kalinga Institute of Industrial Technology (KIIT), Bhubaneswar, India

Sunil K. Raghav
Immuno-genomics and Systems Biology Laboratory, Institute of Life Sciences (ILS), Bhubaneswar, India Manipal Academy of Higher Education, Manipal, India Department of Biotechnology, Kalinga Institute of Industrial Technology (KIIT), Bhubaneswar, India

Dirlei Nico
Departamento de Microbiologia Geral, Instituto de Microbiologia Paulo de Góes, Universidade Federaldo Rio de Janeiro, Rio de Janeiro, Brazil

Fernanda Martins Almeida
Programa de Pós Graduação em Anatomia Patológica, HUCFF, Universidade Federal do Rio de Janeiro, Rio de Janeiro, Brazil Programa de Graduação de Histologia, Instituto de Ciências Biomédicas, Universidade Federal do Rio de Janeiro, Rio de Janeiro, Brazil

Juliana Maria Motta
Programa de Glicobiologia, Instituto de Bioquímica Médica LeopoldoDe Meis, Universidade Federal do Rio de Janeiro, Rio de Janeiro, Brazil

Fellipe Soares dos Santos Cardoso and Ana Maria Blanco Martinez
Programa de Pós Graduação em Anatomia Patológica, HUCFF, Universidade Federal do Rio de Janeiro, Rio de Janeiro, Brazil

Celio Geraldo Freire-de-Lima
Programa de Imunobiologia, Instituto de BiofísicaCarlos Chagas Filho, Universidade Federal do Rio de Janeiro, Rio de Janeiro, Brazil

Leonardo Freire-de-Lima
Programa de Medicina Regenerativa, Instituto de Biofísica Carlos Chagas Filho, Universidade Federaldo Rio de Janeiro, Rio de Janeiro, Brazil

Paula Melo de Luca
Laboratório deImunoparasitologia, Instituto Oswaldo Cruz (IOC), Rio de Janeiro, Brazil

Alexandre Morrot
Laboratório deImunoparasitologia, Instituto Oswaldo Cruz (IOC), Rio de Janeiro, Brazil Centro de Pesquisas em Tuberculose, Faculdadede Medicina, Universidade Federal do Rio de Janeiro, Rio de Janeiro, Brazil

Clarisa Beatriz Palatnik-de-Sousa
Departamento de Microbiologia Geral, Instituto de Microbiologia Paulo de Góes, Universidade Federal do Rio de Janeiro, Rio de Janeiro, Brazil Instituto Nacional de Ciência e Tecnologia deInvestigação em Imunologia, São Paulo, Brazil

Nina Tel-Karthaus, Esther D. Kers-Rebel, Maaike W. Looman and Marleen Ansems
Department of Radiation Oncology, Radiotherapy & OncoImmunology Laboratory, Radboud Institute for Molecular Life Sciences, Radboud University Medical Center, Nijmegen, Netherlands

Hiroshi Ichinose
School of Life Science and Technology, Tokyo Institute of Technology, Yokohama, Japan

Carlie J. de Vries
Department of Medical Biochemistry, Academic Medical Center, Amsterdam Cardiovascular Sciences, Amsterdam, Netherlands

Kelly A. Prendergast
Malaghan Institute of Medical Research, Wellington, New Zealand School of Biological Sciences, Victoria University of Wellington, Wellington, New Zealand

Naomi J. Daniels
Department of Microbiology and Immunology, University of Otago, Dunedin, New Zealand

Troels R. Petersen
Malaghan Institute of Medical Research, Wellington, New Zealand

Ian F. Hermans
Malaghan Institute of Medical Research, Wellington, New Zealand, School of Biological Sciences, Victoria University of Wellington, Wellington, New Zealand, Maurice Wilkins Centre for Molecular Biodiscovery, Auckland, New Zealand

Joanna R. Kirman
Department of Microbiology and Immunology, University of Otago, Dunedin, New Zealand Maurice Wilkins Centre for Molecular Biodiscovery, Auckland, New Zealand

Raphaël Mattiuz, Christian Wohn, Sonia Ghilas, Marc Ambrosini, Yannick O. Alexandre, Cindy Sanchez, Anissa Fries, Thien-Phong Vu Manh, Marc Dalod and Karine Crozat
Centre d'Immunologie de Marseille-Luminy, Turing Center for Living Systems, CNRS, INSERM, Aix Marseille Univ, Marseille, France

Bernard Malissen
Centre d'Immunologie de Marseille-Luminy, Turing Center for Living Systems, CNRS, INSERM, Aix Marseille Univ, Marseille, France Centre d'Immunophénomique, Aix Marseille Univ, CNRS, INSERM, Marseille, France

Jennifer R. Richardson, Nicole S. Armbruster, Manina Günter, Jörg Henes and Stella E. Autenrieth
Department of Internal Medicine II, University of Tübingen, Tübingen, Germany

Adriana Flores-Langarica, Adam F. Cunningham, Nonantzin Beristain-Covarrubias and Juan Carlos Yam-Puc
Institute of Immunology and Immunotherapy, College of Medical and Dental Sciences, University of Birmingham, Birmingham, United Kingdom

Charlotte Cook and Ian R. Henderson
Institute of Microbiology and Infection, College of Medical and Dental Sciences, University of Birmingham, Birmingham, United Kingdom

Katarzyna Müller Luda, Madelene Dahlgren and Jenny J. Persson
Immunology Section, Department of Experimental Medical Science, Lund University, Lund, Sweden

Emma K. Persson
VIB-Ugent Center for Inflammation Research, Ghent, Belgium

Jennifer L. Marshall
Institute of Inflammation and Ageing, College of Medical and Dental Sciences, University of Birmingham, Birmingham, United Kingdom

Satoshi Uematsu
International Research and Development Centre for Mucosal Vaccine, Institute for Medical Science, The University of Tokyo, Tokyo, Japan, Department of Immunology and Genomics, Osaka City University Graduate School of Medicine, Osaka, Japan

Shizuo Akira
World Premier International Immunology Frontier Research Centre, Osaka University, Suita, Japan

Bengt Johansson Lindbom and William Agace
Immunology Section, Department of Experimental Medical Science, Lund University, Lund, Sweden Section of Biology and Chemistry, Department for Micro and Nanotechnology, Technical University of Denmark, Kongens Lyngby, Denmark

Miaomiao Han
Department of Otolaryngology-Head and Neck Surgery, Center for Allergic and Inflammatory Diseases, Affiliated Eye and ENT Hospital, Fudan University, Shanghai, China Shanghai Institute of Immunology, Shanghai Jiao Tong University School of Medicine, Shanghai, China Xin Hua Hospital Affiliated to Shanghai Jiao Tong University School of Medicine, Shanghai, China

Ran Hu, Jingyu Ma and Baohua Zhang
Shanghai Institute of Immunology, Shanghai Jiao Tong University School of Medicine, Shanghai, China

Ce Chen
Guangdong Provincial Key Laboratory of Medical Molecular Diagnostics, Guangdong Medical University, Dongguan, China

Huabin Li
Department of Otolaryngology-Head and Neck Surgery, Center for Allergic and Inflammatory Diseases, Affiliated Eye and ENT Hospital, Fudan University, Shanghai, China

Jun Yang
Xin Hua Hospital Affiliated to Shanghai Jiao Tong University School of Medicine, Shanghai, China

Gonghua Huang
Shanghai Institute of Immunology, Shanghai Jiao Tong University School of Medicine, Shanghai, China Guangdong Provincial Key Laboratory of Medical Molecular Diagnostics, Guangdong Medical University, Dongguan, China

Cinthia Silva-Vilches, Sabine Ring and Karsten Mahnke
Department of Dermatology, Ruprecht-Karls-University Heidelberg, University Hospital, Heidelberg, Germany

Joyce Lübbers, Ernesto Rodríguez and Yvette van Kooyk
Molecular Cell Biology and Immunology, Amsterdam UMC, Vrije Universiteit Amsterdam, Cancer CenterAmsterdam, Amsterdam Infection and Immunity Institute, Amsterdam, Netherlands

Jonas Nørskov Søndergaard, Maaike W. G. Looman, Chunling Tang, Vassilis Triantis, Pauline Louche, Marleen Ansems and Gosse J. Adema
Radiotherapy & OncoImmunology Laboratory, Department of Radiation Oncology, Radboud Institute for Molecular Life Sciences, Radboud University Medical Center, Nijmegen, Netherlands

Simon J. van Heeringen
Department of Molecular Developmental Biology, Faculty of Science, Radboud Institute for Molecular Life Sciences, Radboud University, Nijmegen, Netherlands

Eva M. Janssen-Megens, Colin Logie and Hendrik G. Stunnenberg
Department of Molecular Biology, Faculties of Science and Medicine, Radboud Institute for Molecular Life Sciences, Radboud University, Nijmegen, Netherlands

Anieta M. Sieuwerts and John W. M. Martens
Department of Medical Oncology and Cancer Genomics Netherlands, Erasmus MC Cancer Institute, Erasmus University Medical Center, Rotterdam, Netherlands

Maria Embgenbroich and Sven Burgdorf
Life and Medical Sciences (LIMES) Institute, University of Bonn, Bonn, Germany

Laura Antonio-Herrera
Hospital de Especialidades, Centro Médico Nacional Siglo XXI, Instituto Mexicano del Seguro Social, Unidad de Investigación Médica en Inmunoquímica, Mexico City, Mexico Universidad Nacional Autónoma de México, Mexico City, Mexico

Oscar Badillo-Godinez and Lourdes Gutierrez-Xicotencatl
Centro de Investigación Sobre Enfermedades Infecciosas, Instituto Nacional de Salud Pública, SS, Cuernavaca, Mexico

Oscar Medina-Contreras
Immunology and Proteomics Laboratory, Mexico Children's Hospital "Federico Gómez", Mexico City, Mexico

Araceli Tepale-Segura, Alberto García-Lozano and Laura C. Bonifaz
Hospital de Especialidades, Centro Médico Nacional Siglo XXI, Instituto Mexicano del Seguro Social, Unidad de Investigación Médica en Inmunoquímica, Mexico City, Mexico

Gloria Soldevila
Departamento de Inmunología, Instituto de Investigaciones Biomédicas, Universidad Nacional Autónoma de México, Mexico City, Mexico

Fernando R. Esquivel-Guadarrama
Laboratorio de Inmunología Viral, Facultad de Medicina, UAEM, Cuernavaca, Mexico

Juliana Idoyaga
Department of Microbiology and Immunology, Stanford University School of Medicine, Stanford, CA, United States

Index